How to Have Theory
in an Epidemic

How to Have Theory in an Epidemic

Cultural Chronicles of AIDS

Paula A. Treichler

DUKE UNIVERSITY PRESS   *Durham and London 1999*

© 1999 Duke University Press
All rights reserved
Printed in the United States of America on acid-free paper ∞
Typeset in Trump Mediaeval by Keystone Typesetting, Inc.
Library of Congress Cataloging-in-Publication Data appear
on the last printed page of this book.

For Cary,
the one and only—
my one and only

Contents

Acknowledgments

Acknowledgment must first be made to those whom AIDS/HIV has infected or killed; like those who continue to fight the epidemic every day, their courage is amazing and their examples inspiring.

Research for this project has been supported in part by grants from the National Council of Teachers of English and the University of Illinois at Urbana-Champaign Graduate College Research Board. Throughout its evolution, this work has also been supported in countless ways, both intellectual and material, by the academic units at the University of Illinois to which I have the good fortune to belong: the College of Medicine at Urbana-Champaign, the Institute of Communications Research, the Women's Studies Program, and the Unit for Criticism and Interpretive Theory. I am grateful to other institutions for furnishing me, at crucial points in this project, with a room of my own: the Ragdale Foundation in Lake Forest, Illinois; the Society for the Humanities at Cornell University; and the Women's Studies Program at the University of California, Santa Barbara.

Within the vast network of people committed to ending the AIDS/HIV epidemic, the following people have especially helped and inspired me: Dennis Altman, Allan M. Brandt, Douglas Crimp, Lisa Duggan, Paul Farmer, Elizabeth Fee, Jan Zita Grover, Nan Hunter, Stephanie Kane, Katie King, Emily Martin, Richard Parker, Cindy Patton, Steve Rabin, Eve Kosofsky Sedgwick, and Simon Watney. Intellectual debts to many others are reflected in the citations throughout this book.

I am indebted to many friends and colleagues for information, materials, and guidance in interpreting the cultural domains that this project spans: Kwame Anthony Appiah, Awour Ayudo, Shari Benstock, Edward Brunner, Lisa Cartwright, Wendy Dallas, Peter Ekstrom, Terry England, Faith Evans, Henry Finder, Daniel M. Fox, Francine W. Frank, Colin Garrett, Barrie Grenell, Evelynn Hammonds, Donna Haraway, Brad Hudson, Laurence H. Jacobs, Ibulaimu Kakoma, Stephen J. Kaufman, Alan Klusaček, Joan Lathrop, Allan Levy, Ana Lopez, Phil Mariani, Sally McConnell-Ginet, Richard Mohr, Timothy Murphy, Dorothy Nelkin, Rick Rambuss, Roddey Reid, Sheri Scott, Esther Sleator, Thomas Spech, Sarah Stein, John Stokes, Marita Sturken, John Tagg, Willard Visek, and Charles Whitney.

My profound thanks to the work of the Unit for Criticism and Interpretive Theory, a sustaining intellectual force for so many of us at Illinois since it was founded in 1977. A special debt is owed, collectively, to my colleagues in the Unit's Faculty Criticism Seminar, which has met regularly for more than twenty years. I especially thank Kal Alston, Amanda Anderson, Michael Bérubé, Edward Bruner, Cheryl Cole, Norman Denzin, Lisa Duggan, Peter Garrett, Larry Grossberg, Janet Lyon, Sonya Michel, Meaghan Morris, Carol Neely, Cary Nelson, Constance Penley, Andrew Ross, William Schroeder, Carole Stabile, Ellen Wartella, and Richard Wheeler.

To Howard Maclay, former director of the Institute of Communications Research, who makes being smart look easy, thanks for giving me a job and being an all-round champ. To Clifford Christians, the Institute's current director, thanks for leadership and generosity above and beyond the call of administrative duty. My gratitude also to Diane Tipps for expert help in many things, to the faculty of the Institute for being terrific colleagues, and to the Institute itself for the "rigorous intellectual pluralism," as our brochure puts it, that encourages interesting interdisciplinary work.

My colleagues in the Medical Humanities and Social Sciences Program, past and present, have contributed in innumerable ways to my knowledge, work, and spirits: Daniel K. Bloomfield, Clark Cunningham, Ann Barry Flood, Diane Gottheil, Evan Melhado, Leslie Reagan, and Harold M. Swartz. So have Suzanne Poirier and Barbara Sharf in the Medical Humanities Program, University of Illinois at Chicago.

To Daniel K. Bloomfield, founder, dean, and guiding light of the medical school—yes, there is a medical school at the University of Illinois in Urbana-Champaign—thanks for hiring me, having faith in me, and supporting my work.

Through its unusual collaborations with the Urbana campus over the last two decades, the medical school has contributed to the education of a stellar company of students, physicians, and physician-scholars for whom the biomedical sciences also encompass the humanities and the social sciences. They are part of a larger community of students and graduates of Illinois who are equally committed to progressive and interdisciplinary work. All have enriched my teaching and research in countless ways, often through their own outstanding scholarship. Thank you to Charles Acland, Martin Allor, Anne Balsamo, Lance Becker, Chloe Bird, Ernestine Briggs, Rachel Coel, Stacie Colwell, Matthew Doolittle, Anne Eckman, John Erni, Jamie Feldman, Gregory Flentje, Karen Foli, Allen Fremont, Paul Hattis, Christine Horak, Niranjan Karnik, Cris Mayo, Matthew McAllister, Daniel McGee, Robert McRuer, M. Kerry O'Banion, Karin Rhodes, Denise Roth, Marie V. Ruiz, Elisabeth Santos, Erik Stewart, Mary Vavrus, Catherine Warren, and Michael Witkovsky.

The list of graduate students and M.D.-Ph.D. students who have labored as research assistants on this project over the years is embarrassingly long, but it is certainly distinguished. Many thanks to Anne Balsamo, Theresa Conefrey, Jill Conway, Anne Eckman, Karen Ford, Matthew Hurt, Kirsten Lentz, Theresa Mangum, Robert McRuer, Shawn Miklaucic, William Murdoch, Carrie Rentschler, Maria T. Rodriguez, Denise Roth, Jay Stemmle, and Catherine Warren.

My thanks also to University of Illinois librarians John Littlewood (Documents) and Yvette Scheven (Africana) and to Phyllis Self and Victoria Pifalo (Medical Sciences Library).

Thanks to Denice Wells at the medical school for assistance in many ways over many years, including help preparing manuscripts and managing files for many drafts. For preparation of the final manuscript, I am grateful to the outstanding work of the Document Management Center at the College of Medicine and in particular to Candy Sullivan and Dianne Wickes.

To Ken Wissoker, for being everything an editor should be, my immense gratitude and thanks. Thanks also to Richard Morrison and the rest of the staff at Duke University Press.

To my dear friends Carol Neely, Sally McConnell-Ginet, and Constance Penley, with whom there will never be time enough to talk often or long enough, my deep thanks for inspiration, love, and immense help over many years for thinking through intellectual and professional challenges too numerous to count.

Finally, I come to that point where one acknowledges one's loving partner for support, sacrifice, and the patience of a saint. With wholehearted love and admiration, I give profound thanks to Cary Nelson, my longtime companion and best of friends, for unwavering support through good times and bad, professional wisdom both conceptual and practical, and true love. The less said about patience the better.

A Note on the Text

How to Have Theory in an Epidemic chronicles cultural, intellectual, and political engagements with AIDS/HIV over nearly two decades. Many chapters were originally written and published to address problems, events, or issues at particular points in the epidemic's evolution. In revising them to form a coherent intellectual narrative, I have nevertheless tried to preserve a strong sense of the occasions and imperatives that first shaped their composition. Even when material is largely new, I have tried to invoke and be true to the contemporary context of the events and issues described. Chapter 2, for example, examines evolving conceptions of gender in AIDS discourse from 1981 to 1988; although written in the mid-1990s, the chapter's critique is based less on hindsight than on the struggles surrounding knowledge and action that were taking shape throughout that first decade of crisis.

The term *AIDS* in this book refers to the AIDS epidemic as a broad social and cultural crisis; the terms *HIV disease* and *AIDS and HIV infection* are used interchangeably to mean the broad clinical spectrum of HIV-related conditions from asymptomatic infection to the specific diseases presently used to define AIDS (I use *AIDS* to mean the inclusive medical spectrum only if this sense is clear in context). I also use *AIDS/HIV* rather than *HIV/AIDS* to preserve continuity with earlier alphabetical listings.

Prologue

By the end of the 1980s, the AIDS epidemic had been invested with an abundance of meanings and metaphors. Scientists, physicians, and public health authorities argued repeatedly that AIDS represented "an epidemic of infectious disease and nothing more." This uncompromisingly medical argument, developed over the course of the twentieth century as medicine and public health wrenched themselves free of moral understandings of disease, has had value and power for the AIDS epidemic that must not be minimized. Continually eluding such containment efforts, however, the AIDS epidemic has produced a parallel epidemic of meanings, definitions, and attributions. This semantic epidemic, which I have come to call an *epidemic of signification*, has not diminished in the 1990s; it is the major subject of this book. In this prologue, I briefly sketch my argument and map for the reader the ground that I revisit in individual chapters.

The AIDS epidemic is cultural and linguistic as well as biological and biomedical. To understand the epidemic's history, address its future, and learn its lessons, we must take this assertion seriously. Moreover, it is the careful examination of language and culture that enables us, as members of intersecting social constellations, to think carefully about ideas in the midst of a crisis: to use our intelligence and critical faculties to consider theoretical problems, develop policy, and articulate long-term social needs even as we acknowledge the urgency of the AIDS crisis and try to satisfy its relentless demand for immediate action. This book documents cultural and linguistic dimensions of the AIDS epidemic and examines the tension between theory and practice as it recurs in diverse arenas. More broadly, *How to Have Theory in an Epidemic* is about the cultural evolution of the AIDS epidemic. Its subtitle, *Cultural Chronicles of AIDS*, signals its focus on the ways we have come to understand the AIDS epidemic, its interaction with culture and language, the intellectual debates and political initiatives that the epidemic has engendered, its function as a site for competing ideologies and sites of knowledge, and its possibilities for guiding us toward a more humane and enlightened future.

This enterprise focuses on a body of linguistic data and, through time, space, and multiple cultural venues, keeps this body in view. The evolution of the AIDS epidemic has coincided with a period of attention to language. Scientists commonly point out that AIDS arrived at the "right time"—that is, a time when basic scientific research in molecular biology, virology, and immunology could provide a foundation for an intensive research effort focused on AIDS. They point out that no other epidemic disease has been analyzed so quickly or had its cause so efficiently determined. At the same time, as the British critic and AIDS activist Simon Watney has often pointed out, investigation in the human sciences provides an equally crucial foundation for the understanding of AIDS. The apparatus of contemporary critical and cultural theory prepares us to analyze AIDS in relation to questions of language, representation, interpretation, narrative, ideology, social and intellectual difference, binary division, and contests for meaning. But the AIDS epidemic does not exist to demonstrate the value of contemporary theory. If anything, it puts theory stringently to the test, serving as a useful and often dramatic corrective for inadequate theoretical formulations. Of course, to my mind, *theory* is not the constellation of texts and thinkers demonized by William Bennett et al. Nor is it the creature disdained by other anti-intellectual traditions, including U.S. medicine, for whom *theory* is defined as that which is devoid of relevance for "practice" and real-life experience. At the end of the day, *theory* is another word for *intelligence*, that is, for a thoughtful and engaged dialectic between the brain, the body, and the world that the brain and the body inhabit.

My investigation of language in a medical and cultural crisis like AIDS is thus framed by a more profound question: What should be the role of theory in an epidemic? Of all the meanings and metaphors generated by the AIDS epidemic and identified throughout this book, AIDS as a war— a long, devastating, savage, costly, expensive, and continuing war—best helps us consider this question. When we try to account for the social and cultural impact, the economic toll, the multiplicity of understandings, and the unpredictable cultural upheavals and realignments that the AIDS crisis continues to generate, the major wars of our time offer a precedent as useful as plague, polio, and other more conventional comparisons. AIDS is a war whose participants have been in the trenches for years, surrounded daily by death and dying, yet only gradually has the rest of the population come to know that there is a war at all. To quote Simon Watney again, "for those of us living and working in the various constituencies most devastated by HIV it seems . . . as if the rest of the population were tourists, casually wandering through at the very height of a blitz of which they are totally unaware" (1994, 47).

The war metaphor also captures the dichotomy between theory and practice that marks the AIDS epidemic as well as U.S. cultural life more generally. The very mention of *theory, cultural construction,* or *discourse* may be exasperating or distressing to those face to face with the epidemic's enormity and overwhelming practical demands. Nowhere has this pressure for action been more poignant than in questions about treatment, an arena of the epidemic wholly informed by the sense of time passing and time lost. Martin Delaney, the AIDS treatment activist who founded Project Inform in San Francisco, participated in a forum on treatment options for people with HIV and AIDS at Columbia University in 1988; in a panel on AZT, Delaney argued that, however flawed or incomplete, results to date suggested AZT's benefits and that, in any case, it was at present the best hope. When other panelists urged caution and encouraged audience members to be skeptical of AZT's success, Delaney lost his patience with what he perceived as a quest for abstract truth: "This isn't an argument about how many angels can dance on the head of a pin. People's lives hang in the balance of this decision" (quoted in Douglas 1989, 33).

Yet theory is about "people's lives." As Stuart Hall (1992) has said, our inability to end this epidemic humbles us as intellectuals; at the same time, the epidemic demands our attention:

> AIDS is one of the questions which urgently brings before us our marginality as critical intellectuals in making real effects in the world. And yet it has often been represented for us in contradictory ways. Against the urgency of people dying in the streets, what in God's name is the point of cultural studies? What is the point of the study of representations, if there is no response to the question of what you say to someone who wants to know if they should take a drug and if that means they'll die two days later or a few months earlier? At that point, I think anybody who is into cultural studies seriously as an intellectual practice, must feel, on their pulse, its ephemerality, its insubstantiality, how little it registers, how little we've been able to change anything or get anybody to do anything. (pp. 284–85)

At the same time, Hall writes, AIDS

is indeed a more complex and displaced question than just people dying out there. The question of AIDS is an extremely important terrain of struggle and contestation. In addition to the people we know who are dying, or have died, or will, there are the many people dying who are never spoken of. How could we say that the question of AIDS is not also a question of who gets represented and who does not? AIDS is the site at which the advance of sexual politics is being rolled back. It's a site at which not only people will die, but desire and pleasure will also die if certain metaphors do not survive, or survive in the wrong way. Unless we operate in this tension, we don't know what cultural studies can do, can't, can never do; but also, what it has to do, what it alone has a privileged capacity to do. (p. 285)

This tension permeates the present book as it considers how the AIDS epidemic helps us understand the complex relation between language and reality, between meanings and definitions—and how those relations help us understand AIDS and develop interventions that are more culturally informed and socially responsible. Camus called the plague itself a kind of abstraction; "Still," he wrote, "when abstraction sets to killing you, you've got to get busy with it" ([1947] 1948, 81). But abstraction plays a central role in our ability to "get busy with it." To speak of AIDS as a linguistic construction that acquires meaning only in relation to networks of given signifying practices may seem politically and pragmatically dubious, like philosophizing in the middle of a war zone. But, as I argue throughout this book, making sense of AIDS compels us to address questions of signification and representation. When we deduce from the facts that AIDS is an infectious, sexually transmitted disease syndrome caused by a virus, what is it that we are making sense of? *Infection*, *sexually transmitted*, *disease*, and *virus* are also linguistic constructs that generate meaning and simultaneously facilitate and constrain our ability to think and talk about material phenomena. Language is not a substitute for reality; it is one of the most significant ways we know reality, experience it, and articulate it; indeed, language plays a powerful role in producing experience and in certifying that experience as "authentic."

This book, then, can be seen as a set of cultural chronicles that investigate these questions. In what follows, I sketch its basic structure and offer the reader a preliminary map of the themes, arguments, cultural domains, and evolving meanings that I revisit in individual chapters. But I want also, here, to say something about the nature of these chronicles. Written over the last decade, they can be read in several different ways. Their organization is roughly chronological, each chapter representing a particular era or phase in the AIDS epidemic and, in turn, a particular constellation of issues that seemed to me to be critically important. But, for someone working, as I have been for as long as I can remember, at the intersection of language, culture, medicine, gender, and institutional authority, neither *era* nor *phase* is very useful. No issue in the AIDS epidemic is ever fully settled, and no discursive term is ever free of its history. Rather, I see this book as a series of case studies, each centered around some unique conjunction in time and space of those questions that concern me, and each uniquely manifested through some particular set of texts. These case studies, then, serve to document the epidemic, to read its texts with some attention to contemporary theory, and to explore what theory does or does not do in this epidemic. I will not get ahead of myself in this prologue by summarizing the "findings" of this exploration—what theory tells us about AIDS, that is, and what AIDS tells us about theory. Rather, I will sketch the book's plan and get on with it, at the same time inviting the interested reader to join me for the epilogue, where I do offer several propositions about what I believe this study teaches us.

Chapter 1, "AIDS, Homophobia, and Biomedical Discourse," introduces a central question: How do people make sense of a novel cultural phenomenon that is complicated, frightening, and unpredictable? A preliminary approach involves framing the new phenomenon within familiar narratives, at once investing it with meaning and suggesting the potential for its control. One investment strategy is to link the new phenomenon with existing issues, social arrangements, or institutional sites, a linking that has been characterized as the process of "articulation" (as the bones of a human body are articulated to one another). I demonstrate in more detail what I have suggested above: that the AIDS epidemic has been articulated to a remarkable diversity of issues, perspectives, and agendas and that these different linkages may have differential material and ideological consequences. This inventory of narratives and meanings serves to illuminate alternative understandings of the epidemic as well as contradictory meanings and changing scientific accounts. An important point is that a complex cultural phenomenon produces diversity and contradiction but also that in a variety of ways "dominant" meanings emerge— default meanings, that is, that can be expressed with little fear of being challenged.

The early years of the epidemic functioned in part to link its fate with that of homosexuality, thereby constructing one such dominant meaning.

The widespread construction of AIDS as "a gay disease," I demonstrate, invested both AIDS and homosexuality with meanings neither had alone and produced specific material consequences across a broad social and scientific spectrum. The initial attribution of viral transmission to "gay lifestyle issues," for example, produced a burst of research in scientific journals that starkly revealed prevailing scientific conceptions and mythologies about the sexual practices of gay men—and, indeed, about sexuality and sexual behavior more generally. In turn, efforts to counter these mythologies by the gay community and others, beginning early in the epidemic, altered the course of AIDS's inscription in science by initiating the dialogue between physicians and patients, scientists and activists, so characteristic of this epidemic. This commitment to intervention and counterinscription led, too, to the development of safe sex recommendations, the drafting and dissemination of the Denver principles for the ethical representation of people with AIDS, and the establishment of crucial institutions for caretaking, fund-raising, and service. This articulation of AIDS to other cultural and theoretical questions reveals also, I argue here, the impossibility of identifying and isolating an element like *homophobia* within a given body of discourse, for any such characteristic enters into a system of binary divisions. If one pair of terms is repressed, others take on their function—hence, when the division between *homosexual* and *heterosexual* is called into question, it comes to be reenacted elsewhere, for example, by the division between the *vulnerable rectum* and the *rugged vagina*.

Chapter 2, on the role of gender in the AIDS epidemic from 1981 to 1988, examines how the semantic baggage attached to AIDS has had special consequences for women. Throughout the 1980s, deeply entrenched cultural stereotypes about sex, class, gender, and sexuality confused perceptions of who could get HIV disease, how it could be contracted, and the practices through which "a person with AIDS" was inevitably, if never totally, gendered. I document resistance to acknowledging HIV infection in nonhomosexual bodies, especially women and infants, and identify numerous points at which "the burdens of history" shaped policy, media treatment, and the choice of narratives through which the epidemic was understood. Taking the CDC's epidemiological account of AIDS as the bedrock data source for information about the epidemic in the 1980s, I trace the narrative threads about gender through the discourse of the *Morbidity and Mortality Weekly Report (MMWR)*. These close readings reveal the ambiguities and contradictions built into the official record and their suppression as this record was translated into myriad academic and popular discourses in the public arena. I then look at how the *MMWR*'s account was interpreted, translated, modified, negotiated, denounced, or explained in selected other publications. Representations in leading biomedical journals, mainstream media discourse including women's magazines, and alternative and feminist publications suggest that the insights of the women's health movement and of feminist theory did little to illuminate AIDS for women.

Chapter 3, "AIDS and HIV Infection in the Third World," explores representations of "Third World AIDS" as they occur in typical "First World" publications. With few exceptions, and in contrast to a sampling of images and stories that originate within the countries in question, Western representations reinforce familiar stereotypes about the less-developed world. In these predictable roundups of the usual suspects, most obvious are the limited set of words and images through which people themselves are portrayed: wasted, naive, and passive "natives" lie on mud floors, under trees, on bare mattresses in stark hospital wards. While to a degree these portrayals mimic Western photographic conventions for depicting the dying, nothing is provided to offset the portrait of hopeless, apocalyptic devastation: beyond officials from the World Health Organization or the country's health ministry, professionals and other experts are rarely shown, and even rarer are appearances of experienced and informed nonprofessionals. Underlying this discourse is another fundamental conviction: while the AIDS/HIV epidemic in industrial and postindustrial societies is believed to be complex, intellectually and politically contested, and theoretically interesting, Third World epidemics are seen to be simple material disasters. Examples drawn from AIDS commentary in a number of nations are used to discuss systematic differences between external and internal reporting; special problems of media and other resources in developing countries; the intersection of the local, the national, and the global; the role of ethnographies; and the function, value, and theoretical significance of conspiracy theories. I further explore the notion of articulation, identifying the ways that the global AIDS epidemic plays into preexisting social and cultural divisions.

How are media representations of the AIDS epidemic constituted, and why? Chapter 4 examines media treatments of AIDS and HIV, particularly on television network news programs. I discuss differences between mainstream, targeted, and specialized media outlets and note the widespread failure of liberal and left (straight) media, including feminist media, to cover AIDS adequately. In contrast, much of the gay media—including broadly based publications like the *Advocate*, regional and local newspapers, alternative and oppositional films, videos, and performance art—tells a different story and more often gets it right. AIDS coverage is sketched impressionistically through examples from newspapers and journals, independent videos, talk shows, news reports, documentaries, made-for-TV movies, and prime-time dramatic shows.

Chapter 5, "AIDS, HIV, and the Cultural Construction of Reality," forms the center of the book and the core of my argument, marking also a turning point in the intellectual construction of the AIDS epidemic. I try first to provide an intellectual and theoretical grounding for an analysis of science and medicine as "culturally constructed," drawing from work in sociology, history, and the philosophy of science as well as from anthropological writing on medicine and culture. I then examine shifting power relations, sites of knowledge, and regimes of credibility in terms of the right to define the reality of HIV and AIDS. The 1989 International Conference on AIDS in Montreal provides the specific context in which a series of contests for meaning are described and analyzed. While the vast majority of scientific papers at the 1989 conference further stabilized HIV as a reality in AIDS discourse, challenges to that reality also became more visible. ACT UP's debut at the conference introduced the media to the story it couldn't refuse. This chapter is the structural hinge from which the second half of the book unfolds, its last four chapters revisiting, in reverse order, the themes and preoccupations of the first four.

Chapter 6 takes up the media question again, this time to examine more extended AIDS narratives on television and to ask whose story they actually tell. Close readings of *An Early Frost* and *Our Sons* provide insights. On the one hand, a wholesome family movie like *An Early Frost* leaves out most of the problematic elements of sexual transmission; its blandness makes it hard to explain why this first AIDS drama about a gay man on prime-time television (1985) remained virtually the only one until *Our Sons* was broadcast in 1991. On the other hand, through its palatability, *An Early Frost* accomplished goals that other, more incisive and critical productions could not have. Its effectiveness as an educational vehicle requires us, I argue, to look closely at our common assumptions about identity and identification in narrative media and to recognize the value of the kinds of cultural work performed by different media genres and outlets. That said, I also argue, we can nevertheless hold some genres culpable for not doing the cultural work that they are uniquely suited to do. Network television could "do" condoms better than anyone and should be held responsible for colossal failure.

Chapter 7, "AIDS, Africa, and Cultural Theory," uses a *New York Times* series on AIDS in Africa to ask how we know what it is we think we know about AIDS "elsewhere." Returning to the conference scene via several conferences, including the San Francisco International AIDS Conference in 1990, I raise more questions about the production and politics of knowledge. Moving beyond the chronicles and accounts produced by First World narrators, I examine commentary on the epidemic originating in less-developed countries and argue for the importance of juxtaposing different accounts and representations.

Chapter 8, "Beyond *Cosmo*: AIDS, Identity, and Inscriptions of Gender," continues the story of women and AIDS and asks why, nearly twenty years into the epidemic, gender is still a conceptual muddle. Taking as my starting point a January 1988 article in *Cosmopolitan* claiming that "normal heterosexual women can't get AIDS," I review and update the evidence from chapter 2 that gender has been downplayed, ignored, stereotyped, alibied, and misrepresented. At the heart of these renditions are ongoing confusions surrounding identity, many introduced in chapter 2. Despite multiple impediments, however, by the end of the 1980s women had initiated many projects through which they could become active participants rather than passive receivers in the fight against the epidemic. Taking as exemplary the formation of the Women and AIDS Caucus within the activist group ACT UP New York, I document the relevance of women's AIDS activism and advocacy to other women's issues, including reproduction, birth control, benefits, access to health care, sex education, and poverty, and argue that collective activism is needed in order seriously to challenge the pervasive conservative agenda for women championed by the political and religious Right. The success of progressive projects worldwide now depends, in part, on their respect for such basic feminist tenets as the right to self-definition and self-representation as well as the recognition that *women* is not a monolithic category even while it is inscribed as unitary in discourse. What the role in the United States will be of the actual, historical feminist movement in the struggles ahead remains a question.

The final chapter, "How to Have Theory in an Epidemic: The Evolution of AIDS, Treatment, and Activism," returns to the title theme, the struggle for an intelligent vision to live by in the face of crisis, contradiction, and the urgent need to make life-or-death decisions. Using questions surrounding the pathophysiology of AIDS and the hypothesized effects of HIV on the body, I examine the strategies used by AIDS communities to develop educational materials and treatment regimens. The use of the human body as an experimental laboratory has long been a feature of clinical drug trials; in addition to the courage that such a decision demands, debates over AIDS drugs also address the terms of the debates themselves. They ask, for example, Am I eligible for experimental drugs? But they also ask, Who decides whether I am eligible? They ask, Is this drug safe and effective? But they also ask, What are the criteria that determine safety and efficacy? They ask, Should I take this drug? But they also ask, What theoretical vision of health and disease, of life and death, of science and medicine, guides me in deciding whether to take this drug? What, in the midst of this terrible epidemic disease—this "tidal wave of death" (Harrington 1997)—is acceptable as "good science"? What kind of "medicine" is required? As Steven Epstein has written, the engagement of AIDS activists with biomedical authorities is "no romantic tale of resistance that privileges the 'purity' of knowledge-seeking from below": "What makes the story . . . interesting and important are the ironies and tensions embedded in the process of forging novel scientific, political, and moral identities. This is a complicated history in which no party has had all the answers. All players have revised their claims and shifted their positions over time; all have had to wrestle with the unintended consequences of their actions" (1996, 4).

For readers who are comforted by closure, I use the epilogue to summarize the insights of this study about the operation of language in culture and the complicated circulation and status of meaning in a media-rich democracy. I try, in other words, to distill the linguistic lessons of the epidemic and the conclusions of my efforts to address the questions that I have identified in this prologue.

These "lessons" do not, of course, tell us how to determine the "truth" of the AIDS epidemic; yet, as continuing controversies surrounding AIDS and HIV make clear, they help us better understand how various kinds of knowledge are produced, the rules and universes of discourse through which truth is variously represented and understood, and the crucial role of theory in an epidemic. AIDS's lessons constitute a significant legacy and hold the key, I believe, to the kind of democracy and democratic technoculture that we will be able to build and inhabit in the years ahead.

I

AIDS, Homophobia,
and Biomedical Discourse:
An Epidemic of Signification

In multiple, fragmentary, and often contradictory ways, we struggle to achieve some sort of understanding of AIDS, a reality that is frightening, widely publicized, yet finally neither directly nor fully knowable. AIDS is no different in this respect from other linguistic constructions that, in the commonsense view of language, are thought to transmit preexisting ideas and represent real-world entities yet in fact do neither. The nature of the relation between language and reality is highly problematic; and *AIDS* is not merely an invented label, provided to us by science and scientific naming practices, for a clear-cut disease entity caused by a virus. Rather, the very nature of AIDS is constructed through language and in particular through the discourses of medicine and science; this construction is "true" or "real" only in certain specific ways—for example, insofar as it successfully guides research or facilitates clinical control over the illness.[1] The name *AIDS* in part *constructs* the disease and helps make it intelligible. We cannot therefore look "through" language to determine what AIDS "really" is. Rather, we must explore the site where such determinations *really* occur and intervene at the point where meaning is created: in language.

Of course, AIDS is a real disease syndrome, damaging and killing real human beings. Because of this, it is tempting—perhaps in some instances imperative—to view science and medicine as providing a discourse about AIDS closer to its "reality" than what we can provide ourselves. Yet, with its genuine potential for global devastation, the AIDS epidemic is simultaneously an epidemic of a transmissible lethal disease and an epidemic of meanings or signification. Both epidemics are equally crucial for us to understand, for, try as we may to treat AIDS as "an infectious disease" and nothing more, meanings continue to multiply wildly and at an extraordinary rate.[2] This epidemic of meanings is readily apparent in the chaotic assemblage of understandings of AIDS that by now exists. The mere enu-

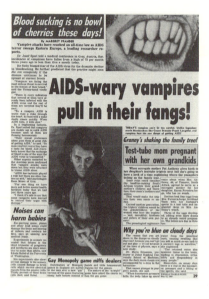

Readily grafting the AIDS epidemic onto their hardy narrative stock, the tabloids flooded the market with hybrid plague stories: of celebrities major and minor, innocent wives, predatory bisexuals, spread-of-aids sensations, cures and conspiracies, morality and mortality, and endless human oddities (1.1: Weekly World News, 12 May 1987, 29).

meration of some of the ways AIDS has been characterized suggests its enormous power to generate meanings:[3]

1. An irreversible, untreatable, and invariably fatal infectious disease that threatens to wipe out the whole world.
2. A creation of the media, which has sensationalized a minor health problem for its own profit and pleasure.
3. A creation of the state to legitimize widespread invasion of people's lives and sexual practices.
4. A creation of biomedical scientists and the Centers for Disease Control to generate funding for their activities.
5. A gay plague, probably emanating from San Francisco.
6. The crucible in which the field of immunology will be tested.
7. The most extraordinary medical chronicle of our times.
8. A condemnation to celibacy or death.
9. An Andromeda strain with the transmission efficiency of the common cold.
10. An imperialist plot to destroy the Third World.
11. A fascist plot to destroy homosexuals.
12. A CIA plot to destroy subversives.
13. A capitalist plot to create new markets for pharmaceutical products.
14. A Soviet plot to destroy capitalists.
15. The result of experiments on the immunological system of men not likely to reproduce.

16. The result of genetic mutations caused by "mixed marriages."
17. The result of moral decay and a major force destroying the Boy Scouts.
18. A plague stored in King Tut's tomb and unleashed when the Tut exhibit toured the United States in 1976.
19. The perfect emblem of twentieth-century decadence; of fin de siècle decadence; of postmodern decadence.
20. A disease that turns fruits into vegetables.
21. A disease introduced by aliens to weaken us before the takeover.
22. Nature's way of cleaning house.
23. America's Ideal Death Sentence.
24. An infectious agent that has suppressed our immunity from guilt.
25. A spiritual force that is creatively disrupting civilization.
26. A sign that the end of the world is at hand.
27. God's punishment of our weaknesses.
28. God's test of our strengths.
29. The price paid for the 1960s.
30. The price paid for anal intercourse.
31. The price paid for genetic inferiority and male aggression.
32. An absolutely unique disease for which there is no precedent.
33. Just another venereal disease.
34. The most urgent and complex public health problem facing the world today.
35. A golden opportunity for science and medicine.
36. Science fiction.
37. Stranger than science fiction.
38. A miserable and expensive way to die.

Such diverse conceptualizations of AIDS are coupled with fragmentary interpretations of its specific elements. Confusion about transmission now causes approximately half the U.S. population to refuse to *give* blood. Many believe that you can "catch" AIDS through casual contact, such as sitting beside an infected person on a bus. Many believe that lesbians—a population relatively free of sexually transmitted diseases in general—are as likely to be infected as gay men. Other stereotypes about homosexuals generate startling deductions about the illness: "I thought AIDS was a gay disease," said a man sitting near a friend of mine in an airport in October 1985, "but if Rock Hudson's dead it can kill anyone."

We cannot effectively analyze AIDS or develop intelligent social policy if we dismiss such conceptions as irrational myths and homophobic fantasies that deliberately ignore the "real scientific facts." Rather, they are part of the necessary work that people do in attempting to understand—

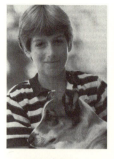
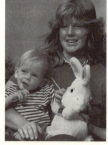
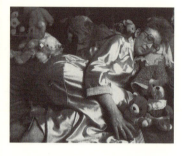

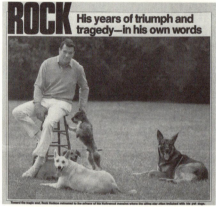

ROCK His years of triumph and tragedy—in his own words

Toward the tragic end, Rock Hudson retreated to the privacy of his Hollywood mansion where the ailing star often indulged with his pet dogs.

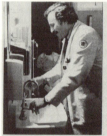
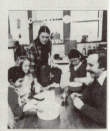

Preventive medicine: *He was constantly washing up*

Family doctor: *At home with Gail and their children*

He flew home weary from Paris. Gail was waiting at JFK airport to meet him. Maria died, she said. Last night.

He would not hesitate, he said, to send his own three youngsters to school with children who have AIDS.

Live or stuffed animals in photographs of persons with AIDS distinguish the "innocent" from the "guilty" or at least normalize their "otherness," as, for example, in these photos of Ryan White and of Matthew Kozup with his mother (1.2: both in Newsweek, 12 August 1985, 29). After Rock Hudson's death, many sympathetic stories showed him with his dogs (1.3: Star, 15 October 1985): he had AIDS, ran the subtext, but he was still a good person. Courageously going public in an interview with Macleans magazine (1.4: 31 August 1986, 34) Canadian PWA Candice Mossop offered herself as "living proof" that women, too, were vulnerable to AIDS; despite her desire to counter stereotypes about the epidemic, the magazine depicted her in a Camille-like deathbed pose, the bed heaped with stuffed animals (Walmsley 1986; photo by Mary Ann Donohue). Given widespread perceptions of AIDS as "a gay disease," the mainstream media also took pains to establish that at least some of the epidemic's featured heroes had wives and kids: they may study AIDS, but they're heterosexual (1.5: Dr. Gerald R. Friedland at work and at home, Newsweek 21 July 1986: 50, 48; story by Goldman and Beachy).

however imperfectly—the complex, puzzling, and quite terrifying phenomenon of AIDS. No matter how much we desire, with Susan Sontag, to resist treating illness as metaphor, illness *is* metaphor, and this semantic work—this effort to "make sense of" AIDS—must be done. Further, this work is as necessary and often as difficult and imperfect for physicians and scientists as it is for "the rest of us."[4]

I am arguing, then, not that we must take both the social and the biological dimensions of AIDS into account, but rather that the social dimension is far more pervasive and central than we are accustomed to believing. Science is not the true material base generating our merely symbolic superstructure. Our social constructions of AIDS (in terms of global devastation, the threat to civil rights, the emblem of sex and death, the "gay plague," the postmodern condition, whatever) are based not on objective, scientifically determined "reality" but on what we are told about this reality: that is, on *prior* social constructions routinely produced within the discourses of biomedical science.[5] (AIDS as infectious disease is one such construction.) There is a continuum, then, not a dichotomy, between popular and biomedical discourses (and, as Latour and Woolgar put it, "a continuum between controversies in daily life and those occurring in the laboratory" [(1979) 1986, 281]), and these play out in language. Consider, for example, the ambiguities embedded within this statement by an AIDS expert (an immunologist) on a television documentary in October 1985 designed to *dispel* misconceptions about AIDS:

> The biggest misconception that we have encountered and that most cities throughout the United States have seen is that many people feel that casual contact—being in the same room with an AIDS victim—will transmit the virus and may infect them. This has not been substantiated by any evidence whatsoever. . . . [This misconception lingers because] this is an extremely emotional issue. I think that when there are such strong emotions associated with a medical problem such as this it's very difficult for facts to sink in. I think also there's the problem that we cannot give any 100 percent assurances one way or the other about these factors. There may always be some exception to the rule. Anything we may say, someone could come up with an exception. But as far as most of the medical-scientific community is concerned, this is a virus that is actually very *difficult* to transmit and therefore the general public should really not worry about casual contact—not even using the same silverware and dishes would probably be a problem.[6]

The point is not merely that this particular scientist has not yet learned to "talk to the media" (see Fain 1985; and Check 1985) but that ambiguity and uncertainty are features of scientific inquiry to be socially and linguistically managed. Few scientists in the mid-1980s could produce more than common sense or contradiction—or both (as here: we can't be certain but the public should not worry). At issue here is a fatal infectious disease that is simply not fully understood; questions remain about the nature of the disease, its etiology, its transmission, and what individuals can do about it. It does not seem unreasonable that, in the face of these uncertainties, people's imaginations give birth to many different conceptions; to label them *mis-conceptions* implies what? Wrongful birth? Only "facts" can give birth to proper conceptions, and only science can give birth to facts? In that case, we may wish to avert our eyes from some of the "scientific" conceptions born in the course of the AIDS crisis:

> AIDS could be *anything*, considering what homosexual men do to each other in gay baths (cited in Leibowitch 1985).
> Heroin addicts won't use clean needles because they would rather get AIDS than give up the ritual of sharing them (cited in Barrett 1985).
> Prostitutes do not routinely keep themselves clean and are therefore "reservoirs" of disease (cited in Langone 1985).
> AIDS is homosexual; it can be transmitted only by males to males.
> AIDS in Africa is heterosexual but unidirectional: it can be transmitted only from males to females (cited in Langone 1985).
> AIDS in Africa is heterosexual because anal intercourse is a common form of birth control there (cited in L. Altman 1985b).

Such assertions blur the line between the facticity of scientific and nonscientific (mis)conceptions. Ambiguity, homophobia, stereotyping, confusion, doublethink, them versus us, blame the victim, wishful thinking: none of these popular forms of semantic legerdemain about AIDS is absent from biomedical communication. But scientific and medical discourses have traditions through which semantic epidemics as well as biological ones are controlled, and these may disguise contradiction and irrationality. In writing about AIDS, these traditions typically include characterizing ambiguity and contradiction as *nonscientific* (a no-nonsense let's-get-the-facts-on-the-table-and-clear-up-this-muddle approach), invoking faith in scientific inquiry, taking for granted the reality of quantitative and/or biomedical data, deducing social and behavioral reality from quantitative and/or biomedical data, setting forth fantasies and speculations as though they were logical deductions, using technical

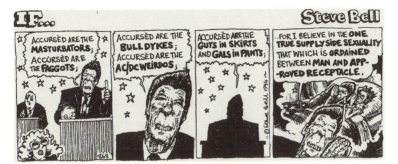

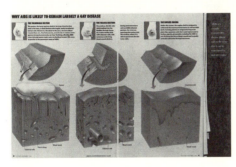

*What cartoonist Steve Bell
called "supply-side sexuality"
preoccupied conservative members of the U.S. Congress, the
Reagan-Bush administrations,
and the 1984–85 Meese Commission for the Study of Pornography (1.6: "If . . . ,"
Guardian, 16 October 1984, 29).
In the early years of the epi-
demic, even leading scientists equated "sex" with missionary-position orthodoxy: "How can AIDS be sexually transmitted?" they would ask. "It's a gay
disease: how can a virus carry a disease from one man's body to another man's?
Where would it get in?" Science writer John Langone explained it all but cautioned that nature never intended men to have sex with men and did not build
their bodies for it. The "rugged vagina," in contrast, "is designed to withstand the
trauma of intercourse as well as childbirth" (1.7: illus. by Lewis E. Calver, Discover, December 1985, 40–41). Plausible prose and decisive illustrations lent
credibility to the story's influential but flawed argument that "AIDS is, and will
continue to be, the fatal price paid for anal intercourse." Over the next decade,
women would be continuously bombarded by contradictory messages about
their biological vulnerability.*

euphemisms for sensitive sexual or political realities, and revising both
past and future to conform to present thinking.

Many of these traditions are illustrated in an article by John Langone in
the December 1985 general science journal *Discover*. In this lengthy review of research to date, entitled "AIDS: The Latest Scientific Facts,"
Langone suggests that the virus enters the bloodstream by way of the "vulnerable anus" and the "fragile urethra"; in contrast, the "rugged vagina"
(built to be abused by such blunt instruments as penises and small babies)
provides too tough a barrier for the AIDS virus to penetrate (pp. 40–41).

AIDS, Homophobia, Biomedical Discourse   17

"Contrary to what you've heard," Langone concludes—and his conclusion echoes a fair amount of medical and scientific writing at the time—"AIDS isn't a threat to the vast majority of heterosexuals. . . . It is now and is likely to remain—largely the fatal price one can pay for anal intercourse" (p. 52). (This excerpt from the article also ran as the cover blurb.) It sounded plausible, and detailed illustrations demonstrated the article's conclusion.[7]

But, by December 1986, the big news—what the major U.S. newsmagazines were running cover stories on—was the grave danger that AIDS posed to heterosexuals.[8] No dramatic discoveries during the intervening year had changed the fundamental scientific conception of AIDS.[9] What had changed was not "the facts" but the way in which they were now used to construct the AIDS text and the meanings that we were now allowed—indeed, at last encouraged—to read from that text.[10] The AIDS story, in other words, is not merely the familiar story of heroic scientific discovery. And until we understand AIDS's dual life as both a material and a linguistic reality—a duality inherent in all linguistic entities but extraordinarily exaggerated and potentially deadly in the case of AIDS—we cannot begin to read the story of this illness accurately or formulate intelligent interventions.

Sources outside biomedical science, however, have helped shape the discourse on AIDS. Almost from the beginning, through intense interest and informed political activism, members of the gay community have repeatedly contested the terminology, meanings, and interpretations produced by scientific inquiry. Such contestations had occurred a decade earlier in the struggle over whether homosexuality was to be officially classified as an illness by the American Psychiatric Association (see Bayer 1981). In the succeeding period, gay men and lesbians had achieved considerable success in political organizing. AIDS, then, first struck members of a relatively seasoned and politically sophisticated community. The importance of not relinquishing authority to medicine was articulated early in the AIDS crisis by Michael Lynch (1982): "Another crisis exists with the medical one. It has gone largely unexamined, even by the gay press. Like helpless mice we have peremptorily, almost inexplicably, relinquished the one power we so long fought for in constructing our modern gay community: the power to determine our own identity. And to whom have we relinquished it? The very authority we wrested it from in a struggle that occupied us for more than a hundred years: the medical profession."

Challenging biomedical authority—whose meanings are part of powerful and deeply entrenched social and historical codes—has required considerable tenacity and courage from people dependent in the AIDS crisis on science and medicine for protection, care, and the possibility of cure. These contestations provide the model for a broader social analysis, one that moves away from AIDS as a "lifestyle" issue and examines its significance for this country, at this time, with the cultural and material resources available to us. This, in turn, requires us to acknowledge and examine the multiple ways in which our social constructions guide our visions of material reality.

AIDS and Homophobia: Constructing the Text of the Gay Male Body

Whatever else it may be, AIDS is a story, or multiple stories, and read to a surprising extent from a text that does not exist: the body of the male homosexual. People so want—need—to read this text that they have gone so far as to write it themselves. AIDS is a nexus where multiple meanings, stories, and discourses intersect and overlap, reinforce and subvert each other. Yet clearly this mysterious male homosexual text has figured centrally in generating what I call here an *epidemic of signification*. Of course, "the virus," with mysteries of its own, has been a crucial influence. But we may recall Camus's ([1947] 1948) novel: "the word 'plague' . . . conjured up in the doctor's mind not only what science chose to put into it, but a whole series of fantastic possibilities utterly out of keeping" (p. 37) with the bourgeois town of Oran, where the plague struck. How could a disease so extraordinary as *plague* happen in a place so ordinary and dull? Initially striking people perceived as alien and exotic by scientists, physicians, journalists, and much of the U.S. population, AIDS did not pose such a paradox. The "promiscuous" gay male body—early reports noted that AIDS "victims" reported having had as many as a thousand sexual partners—made clear that, even if AIDS turned out to be a sexually transmitted disease, it would not be a commonplace one. The connections between sex, death, and homosexuality made the AIDS story inevitably, as David Black (1986) notes, able to be read as "the story of a metaphor."[11]

Ironically, a major turning point in the U.S. consciousness came when Rock Hudson acknowledged that he was being treated for AIDS. Through an extraordinary conflation of texts, the Rock Hudson case dramatized the possibility that the disease could spread to the "general population."[12] In fact, this possibility had been evident for some time to anyone who wished to find it: as Jean Marx summarized the evidence in *Science* in 1984, "Sexual intercourse both of the heterosexual and homosexual varieties is a major pathway of transmission" (p. 147). But only in late 1986 (and somewhat reluctantly at that) did the CDC (1986c) expand on its original "4-H list" of high-risk categories: *homosexuals, hemophiliacs, heroin addicts,* and *Haitians* and the sexual partners of people within these groups. The original list, developed during 1981 and 1982, has structured evidence collection in the intervening years and contributed to the view that the major risk factor in acquiring AIDS is being a particular kind of person rather than doing particular things.[13] Ann Giudici Fettner, AIDS reporter for the *New York Native*, pointed out in 1985 that "the CDC admits that at least ten percent of AIDS sufferers are gay *and* use IV drugs. Yet they are automatically counted in the homosexual and bisexual men category, regardless of what might be known—or not known—about how they became infected" ("AIDS: What Is to Be Done?" 1985, 43). So the "gay" nature of AIDS was in part an artifact of the way data were collected and reported. Although, almost from the beginning, scientific papers have cited AIDS cases that appeared to fall outside the high-risk groups, it has been generally hypothesized that these cases, assigned to the categories of *unknown, unclassified,* or *other,* would ultimately turn out to be one of the four Hs.[14] This commitment to categories based on monolithic identity filters out information. Shaw (1986) argues that when women are asked in CDC protocols "Are you heterosexual?" "this loses the diversity of behaviors that may have a bearing on infection." Even now, with established evidence that transmission can be heterosexual (which begins with the letter *h* after all), scientific discourse continues to construct women as "inefficient" and "incompetent" transmitters of HIV ("the AIDS virus"), passive receptacles without the projectile capacity of a penis or a syringe— stolid, uninteresting barriers that impede the unrestrained passage of the virus from brother to brother.[15] Exceptions include prostitutes, whose discursive legacy—despite their long-standing professional knowledge and continued activism about AIDS—is to be seen as so contaminated that their bodies are virtual laboratory cultures for viral replication.[16] Other exceptions are African women, whose exotic bodies, sexual practices, or who knows what are seen to be so radically different from those of women in the United States that anything can happen in them.[17] The term *exotic,* sometimes used to describe a virus that appears to have originated "elsewhere" (but *elsewhere,* like *other,* is not a fixed category), is an important theme running through AIDS literature (Leibowitch 1985, 73). The fact that one of the more extensive and visually elegant analyses of AIDS appeared in the *National Geographic* (Jaret 1986) is perhaps further evidence of its life on an idealized "exotic" terrain.

After the first cases appeared in New York, Los Angeles, and Paris, the early hypotheses about AIDS were sociological, relating it directly to the supposed "gay male lifestyle." In February 1982, for example, it was thought that a particular supply of amyl nitrate (poppers) might be contaminated. "The poppers fable," writes Jacques Leibowitch (1985), becomes

> a Grimm fairy tale when the first cases of AIDS-without-poppers are discovered among homosexuals absolutely repelled by the smell of the product and among heterosexuals unfamiliar with even the words *amyl nitrate* or *poppers*. But, as will be habitual in the history of AIDS, rumors last longer than either common sense or the facts would warrant. The odor of AIDS-poppers will hover in the air a long time—long enough for dozens of mice in the Atlanta epidemiology labs to be kept in restricted cages on an obligatory sniffed diet of poppers eight to twelve hours a day for several months, until, nauseated but still healthy, without a trace of AIDS, the wretched rodents were released—provisionally—upon the announcement of a new hypothesis: *promiscuity*. (p. 5)

This new perspective generated numerous possibilities. One was that sperm itself could destroy the immune system. "God's plan for man," after all, "was for Adam and Eve and not Adam and Steve."[18] Women, the "natural" receptacles for male sperm, have evolved over the millennia so that their bodies can deal with these foreign invaders; men, not thus blessed by nature, become vulnerable to the "killer sperm" of other men. In the lay press, AIDS became known as the "toxic cock syndrome." While scientists and physicians tended initially to define AIDS as a gay sociological problem, gay men, for other reasons, also tended to reject the possibility that AIDS was a new contagious disease. Not only would this make them sexual lepers, but it also did not make sense: "How could a disease pick out gays? That had to be medical homophobia" (Black 1986, 40).[19] Important to note here is a profound ambivalence about the origins of illness. Does one prefer an illness that is caused by who one is and that can therefore perhaps be prevented, cured, or contained through "self-control"—or an illness that is caused by some external "disease" that has a respectable medical name and can be addressed strictly as a medical problem, beyond individual control? The townspeople of Oran in *The Plague* experience relief when the plague bacillus is identified: the odd happenings—the dying rats, the mysterious human illnesses—are caused by something that has originated elsewhere, something external, something "objective," something that medicine can name, even if not cure. The tension between self and not-self becomes important as we try to understand the particular role of viruses and origin stories in AIDS.

But this anticipates the next chapter in the AIDS story. Another favored possibility in the early 1980s (still not universally discarded, for it is plausible so long as cases among monogamous homebodies are ignored) is that sex is a "cofactor": no *single* infectious agent causes the disease; rather, someone who is sexually active with multiple partners is exposed to a kind of bacterial/viral tidal wave that can crush the immune system.[20] Gay men on the sexual "fast track" would be particularly susceptible because of the prevalence of specific practices that would maximize exposure to pathogenic microbes. What were considered potentially relevant data came to be routinely included in scientific papers and presentations, with the result that the terminology of these reports was increasingly scrutinized by gay activists:[21] examples from *Science* from June 1981 through December 1985 (collected in Kulstad 1986) include "homosexual and bisexual men who are extremely active sexually" (Marx 1983, in Kulstad 1986, 22), "admitted homosexuals" (Gelmann et al. 1983, in ibid., 40), "homosexual males with multiple partners" (Barré-Sinoussi et al. 1983, in ibid., 49), "homosexual men with multiple partners" (Essex et al. 1983, in ibid., 65), "highly sexually active homosexual men" (Richards et al. 1984, in ibid., 142), and "promiscuous" versus "nonpromiscuous" homosexual males (Gallo et al. 1984, in ibid., 160). Also documented (examples are again from the *Science* collection) are exotic travels or practices: "a Caucasian who had visited Haiti" (Gallo et al. 1983, in ibid., 47), "persons born in Haiti" (Jaffe et al. 1983, in ibid., 130), "a favorite vacation spot for U.S. homosexuals" (Marx 1983, in ibid., 73), rectal insemination (Richards et al. 1984, in ibid., 142–46), "bisexual men" (Jaffe et al. 1983, in ibid., 130), "increased frequency of use of nitrite inhalants" (Curran et al. 1985, in ibid., 611), and "receptive anal intercourse" (Curran et al., 1985, in ibid., 611).

Out of this dense discursive jungle came the "fragile anus" hypothesis (tested by Richards et al. [1984, in Kulstad 1986], who rectally inseminated laboratory rabbits) as well as the vision of "multiple partners." Even after sociological explanations for AIDS gave way to biomedical ones involving a transmissible virus, these various images of AIDS as a "gay disease" proved too alluring to abandon. It is easy to see both the scientific and the popular appeal of the fragile anus hypothesis: scientifically, it confines the public health dimensions of AIDS to an infected population in the millions—merely mind-boggling, that is—enabling us to stop short of the impossible, the unthinkable billions that widespread heterosexual transmission might infect. Another appeal of thinking of AIDS as a gay disease is that it protects not only the sexual practices of heterosexuality but also heterosexuality's ideological superiority. In the service of this hypothesis, both homophobia and sexism are folded imperturbably into the language of the scientific text. As I noted above, women are characterized in the scholarly literature as "inefficient" transmitters of AIDS; Leibowitch refers to the "refractory impermeability of the vaginal mucous membrane" (1985, 36). In the *Journal of the American Medical Association* (Redfield et al. 1985) a study of German prostitutes who seemed to demonstrate female-to-male transmission of AIDS was interpreted by some as representing "quasi-homosexual" transmission with successive male clients infecting each other via deposits of contaminated semen (quoted in Langone 1985, 49).

But the conception and the conclusion are inaccurate. It is not monogamy or abstention per se that protects one from AIDS infection but practices that prevent the virus from entering one's bloodstream. Some evidence suggests that prostitutes are at greater risk not because they have multiple sex partners but because they are likely to use intravenous drugs; indeed, they may protect themselves better "than the typical woman who is 'just going to a bar' or a woman who thinks of herself as not sexually active but who 'just happens to have this relationship.' They may be more aware than women who are involved in serial monogamy or those whose self-image is 'I'm not at risk so I'm not going to learn more about it'" (Shaw and Paleo 1987, 144). At this point, COYOTE and other organizations of prostitutes had been addressing the issue of AIDS for several years.[22]

Donald Mager (1986) discusses the proliferation among heterosexuals of visions about homosexuality and their status as fantasy:

> Institutions of privilege and power disenfranchise lesbians and gay men because of stereotypic negative categorizations of them—stereotypes which engage a societal fantasy of the illicit, the subversive, and the taboo, particularly due to assumptions of radical sex role parodies and inversions. This fantasy in turn becomes both the object of fear and of obsessed fascination, while its status as fantasy is never acknowledged; instead, the reality it pretends to signify becomes the justification of suppression both of the fantasy itself and of those actual persons who would seem to embody it. Homophobia as a critique of societal sexual fantasy, in turn, enforces its primary location as a gay discourse, separate and outside the site of the fantasy which is normative male heterosexuality.

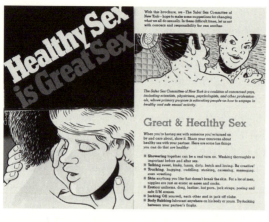

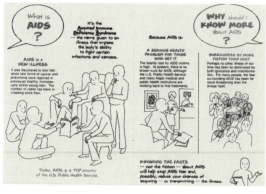

Beginning with How to Have Sex in an Epidemic, *gay communities pioneered "safe sex" initiatives in the 1980s. Departing from the long-standing anti-VD public health tradition, these campaigns demonized neither sex nor the contaminated Other, urging instead that safer sex practices be universally adopted by men who have sex with men (1.8: illus. by H. Cruze, panels from safe sex pamphlet, New York, 1984). The initial federal response to AIDS also broke historical precedent by farming out responsibility for public AIDS education to a private firm in Connecticut. Channing L. Bete's small "Scriptographic" booklets (1.9: Scriptographic AIDS booklet, 1984) were already recognized as a prolific fount of health education and public service messages. Whether the problem is AIDS, herpes, birth control, or proper food storage, generic Scriptographic citizens can be computer morphed as needed to represent the target audience (males, females, African Americans, grandmothers, whatever) and sent out into the world to help. Unlike the Public Health Service materials on AIDS/HIV eventually produced, the copyrighted Scriptographic booklets prohibited reproduction for wider distribution.*

Leibowitch (1985) comments as follows on AIDS, fantasy, and "the reality it pretends to signify": "When they come to write the history of AIDS, socio-ethnologists will have to decide whether the 'practitioners' of homosexuality or its heterosexual 'onlookers' have been the more spectacular in their extravagance. The homosexual 'life style' is so blatantly on display to the general public, so closely scrutinized, that it is likely we never will have been informed with such technicophantasmal complacency as to how 'other people' live their lives" (p. 3).

It was widely believed in the gay community that the connection of AIDS to homosexuality delayed and problematized virtually every aspect of the country's response to the crisis. That the response *was* delayed and problematic is the conclusion of various investigators (see, e.g., U.S. House 1984; Schwartz 1984; Office of Technology Assessment 1985; and Institute of Medicine and National Academy of Sciences 1986). Attempting to assess the degree to which prejudice, fear, or ignorance of homosexuality may have affected policy and research, Panem (1985, 24; 1988) concluded that homosexuality per se would not have deterred scientists from selecting interesting and rewarding research projects. But "the argument of ignorance appears to have more credibility." She quotes James Curran's 1984 judgment that policy, funding, and communication were all delayed because only people in New York and California had any real sense of crisis or comprehension of the gay male community. "Scientists avoid issues that relate to sex," he said, "and there is not much understanding of homosexuality." This was an understatement: according to Curran, many eminent scientists during this period rejected the possibility that AIDS was an infectious disease because they had no idea how a man could transmit an infectious agent to another man. Other instances of ignorance are reported by Patton (1985a, 1985b) and Black (1986). Physician and scientist Joseph Sonnabend (1985) attributes this ignorance to the sequestered ivory towers that many AIDS investigators (particularly those who do straight laboratory research as opposed to clinical work) inhabit and argues instead that AIDS needs to be studied in its cultural totality. Gay male sexual practices should not be dismissed out of hand because they seem "unnatural" to the straight (in both senses) scientist: "The rectum is a sexual organ, and it deserves the respect that a penis gets and a vagina gets. Anal intercourse is a central sexual activity, and it should be supported, it should be celebrated." An Institute of Medicine/National Academy of Sciences panel studying the AIDS crisis in 1986 cited an urgent need for accurate and *current* information about sex and sexual practices in the United States, noting that no comprehensive research had been carried out since Kinsey's studies in the 1940s; they recommended, as well, social science research on a range of social behaviors relevant to the transmission and control of AIDS.

It has been argued that the perceived *gayness* of AIDS was ultimately a crucial political factor in obtaining funding. Dennis Altman (1986) observes that the principle of providing adequate funding for AIDS research was institutionalized within the federal appropriations process as a result of the 1984 congressional hearings chaired by Representatives Henry Waxman and Theodore Weiss, members of Congress representing large and visible gay communities: "Here one sees the effect of the mobilization and organization of gays . . . ; it is salutary to imagine the tardiness of the response had IV users and Haitians been the only victims of AIDS, had Republicans controlled the House of Representatives as well as the Senate (and hence chaired the relevant oversight and appropriations committees) or, indeed, had AIDS struck ten years earlier, before the existence of an organized gay movement, openly gay professionals who could testify before the relevant committees and openly gay congressional staff" (pp. 116–17).

But these social and political issues were becoming, for many, essentially irrelevant. The hypothesis that AIDS was caused by an infectious agent, favored by some scientists, was strengthened when the syndrome began to be identified in a diversity of populations and found to cause apparently identical damage to the underlying immune system. By May 1984, a viral etiology for AIDS had been generally accepted. The real question became precisely what kind of viral agent this could be, and how the epidemic could now be re-read.

Rendezvous with 007

"Interpretations," write Bruno Latour and Steve Woolgar in *Laboratory Life* ([1979] 1986, 285), their analysis of the construction of facts in science, "do not so much *inform* as *perform*." And rarely do we see interpretation shaped toward performance so clearly as in the issues and controversies surrounding the identification and naming of "the AIDS virus."

As early as 1979, gay men in New York and California were coming down with and dying from illnesses unusual in young, healthy people. One of the actors who helped create the San Francisco *A.I.D.S. Show* (Adair and Epstein 1986) recalled that early period: "I had a friend who died way way back in New York in 1981. He was one of the first to go. We didn't know what AIDS was, there was no name for it. We didn't know it was contagious—we had no idea it was sexually transmitted—we didn't know it was anything. We just thought that he—alone—was ill. He was 26 years old and just had one thing after another wrong with him. . . . He was still coming to work—'cause he didn't *know* he had a terminal disease."

The oddness of these nameless isolated events gave way to an even more terrifying period in which gay men on both coasts gradually began to realize that too many friends and acquaintances were dying. As the numbers mounted, the deaths became "cases" of what was informally called in New York hospitals WOGS: the Wrath of God Syndrome. It all became official in 1981, when five deaths in Los Angeles from *pneumocystis* pneumonia were described in the 5 June issue of the CDC's bulletin *Morbidity and Mortality Weekly Report*, with an editorial note explaining, "The occurrence of pneumocystis in these 5 previously healthy individuals without a clinically underlying immunodeficiency is unusual. The fact that these patients were all homosexuals suggests an association between some aspect of a homosexual lifestyle or disease acquired through sexual contact and *Pneumocystis* in this population" (CDC 1981a, 250).

Gottlieb et al.'s (1981) paper in the *New England Journal of Medicine* described the deaths of young, previously healthy gay men from another rare but rarely fatal disease. The deaths were attributed to a breakdown of the immune system that left the body utterly unable to defend itself against infections not normally fatal. The syndrome was informally called GRID: Gay-Related Immunodeficiency. The published reports drew similar information from physicians in other cities (CDC 1981b), and, before too long, these rare diseases had been diagnosed in nongay people (e.g., hemophiliacs and people who had recently had blood transfusions). Epidemiological follow-up interviews over the next several months confirmed that the problem—whatever it was—was growing at epidemic rates, and a CDC task force was accordingly established to coordinate data collection, communication, and research. The name AIDS was selected at a 1982 conference in Washington (GRID was no longer applicable now that nongays were also getting sick): Acquired Immune Deficiency Syndrome ("reasonably descriptive," said Curran, "without being pejorative" [Black 1986, 60]).

Over the next two years, epidemiological and clinical evidence increasingly pointed toward the role of some infectious agent in AIDS. Researchers divided over this, with some searching for a single agent, others positing a "multifactorial cause." Most scientists affiliated with federal scientific agencies (primarily the National Institutes of Health, the Centers for Disease Control, the National Cancer Institute, and the National

Institute of Allergy and Infectious Disease) have tended toward the single-agent theory (as though "cofactors" were a kind of deuces-wild element that vulgarized serious investigation), and this view has tended to dominate scientific reporting. And, although some independent researchers, clinicians, and non-U.S. scientists protested the increasingly rigid party line of what has been called "the AIDS Mafia," multifactorial and environmental theories were subordinated to the quest for the single agent.[23] The National Cancer Institute (NCI), for example, developed a research strategy that focused on retroviruses, essentially to the exclusion of other lines of research (Panem 1985, 25), while other U.S. virology and immunology laboratories put forward their own favored possibilities. By 1983, the "leading candidate" for the AIDS virus seemed to be a member of the human T-cell leukemia family of viruses (HTLV), so called because they typically infect a particular kind of cell, the T-helper cells. But these were *retroviruses*, and there was doubt that a retrovirus could cause immunosuppression in humans.[24] Yet, by this time, it was widely agreed that AIDS was, indeed, a "new" disease—neither a statistical fluke nor a feature of the gay lifestyle. This generated excitement in the medical and scientific community not only because truly new diseases are rare but also because its *cause* might be new as well. In 1983, Luc Montagnier at the Pasteur Institute in Paris identified what he called LAV, a lymphoadenopathy-associated virus. In 1984, Robert Gallo at the NCI identified what *he* called HTLV-III, human T-cell lymphotropic virus type III (the third type identified by his laboratory). In accordance with Koch's postulates, both viruses were isolated in the blood and semen of AIDS patients; no trace was found in the healthy control population.[25]

These powerful findings—disputed and fractious though they were to be—narrowed almost at once the basic biomedical science agenda with regard to AIDS. In the construction of scientific facts, the existence of a name plays a crucial role in providing a coherent and unified signifier—a shorthand way of signifying what may be a complex, inchoate, or little-understood concept. Latour and Woolgar ([1979] 1986, 105–50) divide the research that they studied into the long and uncertain phase that led up to the identification, synthesis, and naming of TRF(H) (the thyrotropin-releasing factor [hormone], a substance involved in neuroendocrine hormone regulation) and the subsequent narrower and more routine phase in which the concept's status as "a fact" was taken for granted. So too with AIDS: before the isolation of the virus, there were considerably more universes of inquiry and open-ended speculation. Evidence for a virus as agent intensified scientific control over signification and enabled scientists to rule out less relevant hypotheses and lines of research. Of course, the existence of *two* names—LAV and HTLV-III—complicated the significa- tion process: did two signifiers entail two distinct signifieds? Despite the wrangling over this point between the involved parties, a consensus began to form that basic research should now relate directly to the hypothesis that a single virus was "the culprit" responsible for AIDS. Important issues included (1) etiology, (2) the identification of the virus's genetic struc- ture and precise shape, (3) clinical and other information about transmis- sion, (4) information about the clinical expression of the disease (the dis- covery that the virus infected brain cells encouraged its renaming since the names *LAV* and *HTLV* both presupposed an attack on lymph cells), (5) the scope and natural history of the disease, (6) differences among "risk groups," and (7) epidemiological information, including the long- term picture (circumstantial evidence but important nevertheless).

To most scientists, this process of narrowing inquiry and relinquishing peripheral lines of thought is simply the way science is done, the pro- cedural sine qua non for establishing anything that can be called a *fact*. But "a statement always has borders peopled by other statements" (Foucault 1972, 97), and it is important for us to keep in mind the provisional and consensual nature of this U.S. AIDS research agenda—each area of which exists within a heavily populated social, cultural, and ideological terri- tory. Consider the hypothesis that AIDS originated in Africa, for example (a view supported by the research of Gallo's colleague Myron Essex, whose African viruses are genetically similar to the virus Gallo's lab identified). Not surprisingly, some "geographic buck-passing" took place among the African countries themselves (Rwanda and Zambia say AIDS originated in Zaire, Uganda says it came from Tanzania, and so on). Beneath such public maneuvering, however, many Africans privately believe that AIDS may have originated somewhere else. And, despite Gallo's assertion that he cannot "conceive of AIDS coming from elsewhere into Africa," the view is by no means universal, especially among non-U.S. researchers (L. Altman 1985b, 8). Further, Americans refuse to acknowledge the possibility that exports of American blood products may have spread the disease to people elsewhere. In the Soviet Union, AIDS is considered a "foreign problem," attributable to the CIA or tribes in central Africa (Lee 1985). In the Carib- bean, and even within the United States (see Rechy 1983), AIDS is widely believed to come from U.S. biological testing. The French first believed that AIDS was introduced by way of an "American pollutant," probably contaminated amyl nitrate (they also believed that AIDS came from Mo- rocco). The Soviet Union, Israel, Africa, Haiti, and the U.S. armed forces deny the existence of indigenous homosexuality and thus claim that AIDS must always have originated "elsewhere."[26]

By 1986, five years after the initial article in *Morbidity and Mortality Weekly Report*, the Human Retrovirus Subcommittee of the International Committee on the Taxonomy of Viruses was at work "to propose an appropriate name for the retrovirus isolates recently implicated as the causative agents of the acquired immune deficiency syndrome (AIDS)"— to consider, that is, what "the AIDS virus" should officially be named. After more than a year of deliberation, the nomenclature subcommittee published its recommendations in the form of a letter to scientific journals (e.g., *Science*, 9 May 1986, 697). Its task has been made crucial, the subcommittee notes, by the widespread interest in AIDS and the multiplicity of names now in use:

> *LAV*: lymphadenopathy-associated virus (1983—Montagnier, Pasteur);
> *HTLV-III*: human T-cell lymphotropic virus type III (1984—Gallo, NCI);
> *IDAV*: immunodeficiency-associated virus;
> *ARV*: AIDS-associated retrovirus (1984—Levy, University of California, San Francisco);
> *HTLV-III/LAV* and *LAV/HTLV-III*: compound names used to keep peace (the CDC's use was perhaps a reprimand to the NCI for its perceived uncooperativeness in sharing data);
> *AIDS virus*: popular press

The subcommittee proposes *HIV*, Human Immunodeficiency Viruses. It reasons that this conforms to the nomenclature of other viruses, in which the first slot signals the host species (human), the second slot the major pathogenic property (immunodeficiency), and the last slot *V* for *virus*. (For some viruses, although not HIV, individual strains are distinguished by the initials of the thus "immortalized" patient from whom they originally came and in whose "daughter cells" they are perpetuated.) The multiple names of "the AIDS virus" point toward a succession of identities and offer a fragmented sense indeed of what this virus, or family of viruses, "really" is. The new name, in contrast, promises to unify the political fragmentations of the scientific establishment and certify the health of the single-agent hypothesis. The subcommittee argues in favor of its proposed name that it does not incorporate the term *AIDS*, on the advice of many clinicians; that it is distinct from all existing names and "has been chosen without regard to priority of discovery" (not insignificantly, Montagnier and Levy signed the subcommittee letter, but Gallo and Essex did not); and that it distinguishes the human immunodeficiency viruses from those with distinctly different biological properties, for example, the HTLV line (HTLV-I and HTLV-II), which this subcommittee calls *human T-cell leukemia viruses*, perhaps to chastise Gallo for changing the *L* in the nomenclature of the HTLVs from *leukemia* to *lymphotropic* so that HTLV-III (the AIDS virus) would appear to fit generically into the same series (and bear the stamp of his lab). In the same issue of *Science*, the editors chose to discuss this letter in their "News and Comment" column: "Disputes over viral nomenclature do not ordinarily command much attention beyond the individuals immediately involved in the fray"; but the current dissension, part of the continuing controversy over who should get credit for discovering the virus, "could provide 6 months' of scripts for the television series 'Dallas'" (Marx 1986a, 699–700).

Why such struggles over naming and interpretation? Because there are high stakes where this performance is concerned—not only patent rights to the lucrative test kits for the AIDS virus (Gallo fears that loss of the HTLV-III designation will weaken his claims) but the future and honor of immunology. As Donna Haraway (1979, 1985, 1989a, 1996) observes, modern immunology moved into the realm of high science when it reworked the military combat metaphors of World War II (battle, struggle, territory, enemy, truce) into the language of postmodern warfare: communication command control (coding, transmission, messages), interceptions, spies, lies. Scientific descriptions for general readers, like this one from the *National Geographic* article on the AIDS virus (Jaret 1986), accentuate this shift from combat to code: "Many of these enemies [of the body or the self] have evolved devious methods to escape detection. The viruses that cause influenza and the common cold, for example, constantly mutate, changing their fingerprints. The AIDS virus, most insidious of all, employs a range of strategies, including hiding out in healthy cells. What makes it fatal is its ability to invade and kill helper T-cells, thereby short-circuiting the entire immune response" (p. 709).

No ground troops here, no combat, not even generals: what we see instead is the evolution of a conception of the AIDS virus as a topflight secret agent—a James Bond of secret agents, armed with "a range of strategies" and licensed to kill. "Like Greeks hidden inside the Trojan horse," 007 enters the body concealed inside a helper T-cell from an infected host (Jaret 1986, 723; see also Anderson and Yunis 1983 and, for discussion, Sturken 1997, 296), but "the virus is not an innocent passenger in the body of its victims" (Krim 1985a):

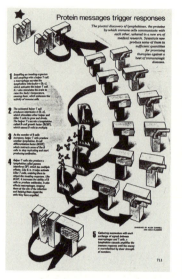

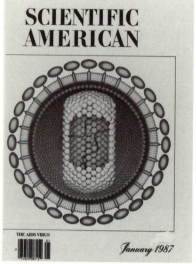

The military metaphors and images that pervade biomedical discourse are con-
tinuously upgraded and retooled. Illustrations for a National Geographic *story*
by Peter Jaret subtitled "The Wars Within" (1.10: "Protein messages trigger re-
sponses," illus. by Allen Carroll and Dale Glasgow, National Geographic, *June*
1986, p. 711) reflect a shift in the field of immunology, noted by Donna Haraway
(1989a), from conventional military metaphors to the communication and cod-
ing trope of postwar molecular biology. As represented on the cover of Scientific
American *in January 1987, the AIDS virus" is a smart grenade (1.11), genetically*
coded to detonate within the very DNA of its cellular target and hijack its com-
munication command center. Inside the journal, Robert C. Gallo told the story
of the virus he called HTLV-III (whose image, published earlier in Science *[4 May*
1984], had turned out to be that of LAV, isolated in Luc Montagnier's laboratory

In the invaded victim, helper T's immediately detect the foreign T-cell. But as the two T's meet, the virus slips through the cell membrane into the defending cell. Before the defending T-cell can mobilize the troops, the virus disables it. . . . Once inside an inactive T-cell, the virus may lie dormant for months, even years. Then, perhaps when another, unrelated infection triggers the invaded T-cells to divide, the AIDS virus also begins to multiply. One by one, its clones emerge to infect nearby T-cells. Slowly but inexorably the body loses the very sentinels that should be alerting the rest of the immune system. Phagocytes and killer cells receive no call to arms. B-cells are not alerted to produce antibodies. The enemy can run free. (Jaret 1986, 723–24) *at the Pasteur Institute). Indeed, these competing names (as well as ARV and others) had in 1986 led an international scientific commission to urge the adoption of an altogether new name: human immunodeficiency virus, or HIV. Wrote the commission chair Harold Varmus (1989, 4), "Since such names are in daily use by the working virologist, much ink and some blood have been spilled over them. The forces that influence decisions about them are as various as the forces that influence the naming of a baby, a book, a bridge, or a city. Scientific principles, political realities, convention, and justice must all be served" (1.12: still from video by Tom Kalin, They Are Lost to Vision Altogether [1988]). In April 1987, France and the United States announced the settlement of the dispute: henceforth, the two countries would share paternity for HIV and reapportion income from patents related to the virus formerly known as HTLV-III/LAV (1.13: French prime minister Jacques Chirac and U.S. president Ronald Reagan, photo by Jose R. Lopez, New York Times, 7 April 1987). A second Scientific American article (October 1988) represented a detailed coauthored account by Gallo and Montagnier.*

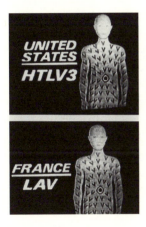 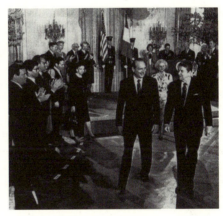

But on no mundane battlefield. The January 1987 *Scientific American* column "Science and the Citizen" warns of the mutability—the "protean nature of the AIDS virus"—that will make very difficult the development of a vaccine as well as the perfect screening of blood. "It is also possible," the column concludes, "that a more virulent strain could emerge"; indeed, even now, "the envelope of the virus seems to be changing." Clearly, 007 is a spy's spy, capable of any deception: evading the "fluid patrol officers" is child's play. Indeed, it is so shifting and uncertain that we might even acknowledge our own historical moment more specifically by giving the AIDS virus a postmodern metaphor and identity: a terrorist's terrorist, an Abu Nidal of viruses.[27]

So long as AIDS was seen as a battle for the body of the gay male—a battle linked to "sociological" factors at that—the biomedical establishment was not tremendously interested in it. The first professionals involved tended to be clinicians in the large urban hospitals where men with AIDS first turned up, epidemiologists (AIDS, writes Black [1986], is an "epidemiologist's dream," a mystery disease that is fatal), and scientists and clinicians who were gay themselves. Although from the beginning some saw the theoretical implications of AIDS, the possibility that AIDS was "merely" some unanticipated side effect of gay male sexual practices (about which, as I've noted above, there was considerable ignorance) limited its appeal to basic scientists. But with the discovery that the agent associated with AIDS appeared to be a virus—indeed, a *novel retrovirus*—what had seemed predominantly a public health phenomenon (clinical and service oriented) suddenly could be rewritten in terms of high theory and high science. The performance moved from off-off Broadway to the heart of the theater district, and the price of the tickets went way, way up. Among other things, identifying the viral agent made possible the development of a "definitive test" for its presence; not only did this open new scientific avenues (e.g., enabling researchers to map precise relations among diverse AIDS and AIDS-like clinical manifestations), but it also created opportunities for monetary rewards (e.g., revenue from patents on the testing kits). For these reasons, AIDS research became a highly competitive professional field.[28] Less-established assistant professors who had been working on the AIDS problem out of commitment suddenly found senior scientists peering at their data, while, in the public arena, the triumphs of pure basic science research were proclaimed. "The biomedical sciences is going brilliantly well" was how Dr. June Osborn summarized AIDS progress mid-decade (Eckholm 1986a, 19). "Indeed," wrote one science reporter, "had AIDS struck 20 years ago, we would have been utterly baffled by it" (Jaret 1986, 723). Ten years ago we had not even confirmed the *existence* of human retroviruses, noted *Scientific American*. Asked whether the NCI's strategy of focusing exclusively on retrovirus research was appropriate (considering that it might not have paid off), an official said that this would not have mattered: basic retroviral research was NCI's priority in any case (Panem 1985, 25). Because it *did* pay off, it could be said (as it could not have been said before 1984) that "AIDS may be a disease that has arrived at the right time" ("Science and the Citizen" 1987, 59). In the words of one biomedical scientist (quoted by Hunt 1986, 78), we face "an impending Armageddon of AIDS, and the salvation of the world through molecular genetics."[29]

Reconstructing the AIDS Text: Rewriting the Body

There is now broad consensus that AIDS—"plague of the millenium," "health disaster of pandemic proportions"—is the greatest public health problem of our era.[30] The epidemic of signification that surrounds AIDS is neither simple nor under control. AIDS exists at a point where many entrenched narratives intersect, each with its own momentum and context in which AIDS acquires meaning. It is extremely hard to resist the lure, familiarity, and ubiquity of these discourses. The AIDS virus enters the cell and integrates with its genetic code, establishing a disinformation campaign at the highest level and ensuring that replication and dissemination will be systemic. We inherit a series of discursive dichotomies; the discourse of AIDS attaches itself to these legacies of difference and reinvigorates them:

> self and not-self;
> the one and the other;
> homosexual and heterosexual;
> homosexual and "the general population";
> active and passive, guilty and innocent, perpetrator and victim;
> vice and virtue, us and them, anus and vagina;
> sins of the parent and innocence of the child;
> love and death, sex and death, sex and money, death and money;
> science and not-science, knowledge and ignorance;
> doctor and patient, expert and patient, doctor and expert;
> addiction and abstention, contamination and cleanliness;
> contagion and containment, life and death;
> injection and reception, instrument and receptacle;
> normal and abnormal, natural and alien;
> prostitute and paragon, whore and wife;
> safe sex and bad sex, safe sex and good sex;
> First World and Third World, free world and iron curtain;
> capitalists and Communists;
> certainty and uncertainty;
> virus and victim, guest and host.

As Brooke-Rose (1986) demonstrates, one must pay close attention to the way in which these apparently fundamental and natural semantic oppositions are put to work: What is self, and what is not-self? Who wears the white and who the black hat? (Or in Brooke-Rose's discussion, perhaps, who wears the pants and who the skirt?) As Turner observes with regard

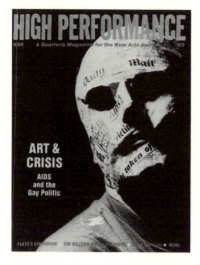

A special issue of High Performance *(no. 36, 1986) called* AIDS *"a crisis in our neighborhoods" and documented the explosion of* AIDS *art and activism. If art's only value in a crisis, wrote the editor, Steven Durland, "is as a fundraising commodity via benefit auctions and performances, then artists might just as well be manufacturing refrigerators"* (p. 6). The cover (1.14) showcased an image from London artist Tessa Boffin's Slings and Arrows of Outrageous Fortune: AIDS and the Body Politic, *a series of black-and-white photographs whose text transformed Hamlet's famous meditation on death into a call for life and safe sex.*

to sexually transmitted diseases in general, the diseased are seen not as "victims" but as "agents" of biological disaster (1984, 221). If Koch's postulates must be fulfilled to identify a given microbe with a given disease, perhaps, in rewriting the AIDS text, it would be helpful to take "Turner's postulates" into account: (1) disease is a language; (2) the body is a representation; and (3) medicine is a political practice (1984, 209).

There is little doubt that, for some people, the AIDS crisis lends force to their fear and hatred of gays; AIDS appears, for example, to be a significant factor in the increasing violence against them and other homophobic acts in the United States (Greer 1986). But to talk of *homophobia* as though it were a simple and rather easily recognized phenomenon is impossible. When we review the various conceptions of the gay male body produced within scientific research by the signifier *AIDS*, we find a discourse rich in signification as to what *AIDS* "means." At first, some scientists doubted that AIDS could be an infectious disease because they could not imagine wht gay men could do to each other to transmit infection. But intimate knowledge generated quite different conceptions:

> AIDS is caused by multiple and violent gay sexual encounters: exposure to countless infections and pathogenic agents overwhelms the immune system.

AIDS is caused by killer sperm, shooting from one man's penis to the anus of another.

Gay men are as sexually driven as alcoholics or drug addicts.

AIDS cannot infect females because the virus cannot penetrate the tough mucous membranes of the vagina.

Women cannot transmit AIDS because their bodies do not have the strong projectile capacity of a penis or a syringe.

Prostitutes can transmit the virus because their contaminated bodies harbor massive quantities of killer microbes.

Repeated hints that the male body is sexually potent and adventurous suggest that homophobia in biomedical discourse may play out as a literal "fear of the same." The text constructed around the gay male body—the epidemic of signification so evident in the conceptions cited above and elsewhere in this essay—is driven in part by the need for constant flight from sites of potential identity and thus the successive construction of new oppositions that will barricade self from not-self. The homophobic meanings associated with AIDS continue to be layered into existing discourse: analysis demonstrates ways in which the AIDS virus is linguistically identified with those it strikes: The penis is "fragile," the urethra is "fragile," the virus is "fragile." The African woman's body is "exotic," the virus is "exotic." The virus "penetrates" its victims; a carrier of death, it wears an "innocent" disguise. AIDS is "caused" by homosexuals; AIDS is "caused" by a virus. Homosexuality exists on a border between male and female, the virus between life and nonlife. This cross-cannibalization of language is not surprising. What greater relief than to find a final refuge from the specter of gay sexuality where the language that has obsessively accumulated around the body can attach to its substitute: the virus. This is a signifier that can be embraced forever.

The question is how to disrupt and renegotiate the powerful cultural narratives surrounding AIDS. Homophobia is inscribed within other discourses at a high level, and it is at a high level that these narratives must be interrupted and challenged. Why? The following scenario for Armageddon (believed by some, desired by many) makes clear why: AIDS will remain confined to the original high-risk groups (primarily gay males and IV drug users) because of their specific practices (like anal intercourse and sharing needles). At the Paris International AIDS Conference in June 1986, the ultimate spread of the disease was posed in terms of "containment" and "saturation." "Only" gay males and drug addicts will get infected—the virus will use them up and then have nowhere to go—the "general population" (which is also in epidemiological parlance a "virgin" population) will remain untouched. Even if this view is correct (which seems doubtful, given growing evidence of transmission through plain old everyday heterosexual intercourse) and the virus stops spreading once it has "saturated" the high-risk population, we would still be talking about a significant number of U.S. citizens: 2.5 million gay men, 7 million additional men who have at some time in the last ten years engaged in same-sex activity, 750,000 habitual intravenous drug users, 750,000 occasional drug users, 10,000 hemophiliacs already infected, the sex partners of these people, and the children of infected women—in other words, a total of more than 10 million people (the figures are from the June 1986 Paris conference). And "saturation" is currently considered a *best*-case scenario by the public health authorities.[31]

The fact is that any separation of not-self ("AIDS victims") from self (the "general population") is no longer possible. The U.S. surgeon general's and National Academy's reports make clear that "that security blanket has now been stripped away" ("Science and the Citizen" 1987, 58). Yet the familiar signifying practices that exercise control over meaning continue. The *Scientific American* column goes on to note fears that the one-to-one African ratio of females with AIDS to males may foreshadow U.S. statistics: "Experts point out, however, that such factors as the prevalence of other venereal diseases that cause genital sores, the use of unsterilized needles in clinics and the lack of blood-screening tests may explain the different epidemiology of AIDS in Africa" ("Science and the Citizen" 1987, 59). Thus, the African data are reinterpreted to reinstate the us/them dichotomy and project a rosier scenario for "us." (Well, maybe it improves on comic Richard Belzer's narrative: "A monkey in Africa bites some guy on the ass, and *he* balls a guy in Haiti, and now we're all gonna fuckin' die. THANKS A LOT!")[32]

Meanwhile, on the home front, monogamy is coming back into its own along with abstention, the safest sex of all. The virus itself—by whatever name—has come to represent the moment of truth for the sexual revolution: as though God has once again sent his only beloved son to save us from our high-risk behavior. Who would have thought that he would take the form of a virus: a viral Terminator ready to die for our sins.[33]

The contestations pioneered by the gay community over the last decade offer models for resistance. As old-fashioned morality increasingly infects the twentieth-century scenario, whether masquerading as "preventive health" or spiritual transformation, a new sampler can be stitched to hang on the bedroom wall: BETTER WED THAN DEAD. "It's just like the fifties," complains a gay man in San Francisco. "People are getting married again for all the wrong reasons" (quoted in FitzGerald 1986). One disruption of this narrative occurs in the San Francisco *A.I.D.S. Show* (Adair and Epstein 1986): "I *like* sex," a young man reminisces nostalgically; "I like to get drunk and smoke grass . . . and sleep with strangers: Call me old-fashioned, but that's what I like!" A gay pastor tells FitzGerald that the new morality threatens the gay community with pre-Stonewall repression: "If I had to go back to life in the closet again, I'm not sure I would not rather be dead." For Michel Foucault, the "tragedy" of AIDS was not intrinsically its lethal character but that a group that has risked so much—gays—is looking to standard authorities—doctors, the church—for guidance in a time of crisis. "How can I be scared of AIDS when I could die in a car?" Foucault asked a year or so before he died. "If sex with a boy gives me pleasure . . ." (Horvitz 1985, 80). And he adds: "Don't cry for me if I die."[34]

In AIDS, where meanings are overwhelming in their sheer volume and often explicitly linked to extreme political agendas, we do not know whose meanings will become "the official story." We need an epidemiology of signification—a comprehensive mapping and analysis of these multiple meanings—to form the basis for official definition that will in turn constitute the policies, regulations, rules, and practices that will govern our behavior for some time to come. As we have seen, these may rest on "facts," which in turn may rest on the deeply entrenched cultural narratives that I have been describing. For this reason, what AIDS signifies must be democratically determined: we cannot afford to let scientists or any other group of experts dismiss our meanings as "misconceptions" and our alternative views as noise that interferes with the pure processes of scientific inquiry. Rather, we must insist that many voices contribute to the construction of official definitions—and specifically certain voices that need urgently to be heard. Although the signification process for AIDS is by now very broad—just about everyone, seemingly, has offered a reading of what AIDS means—one excluded group continues to be users of illegal intravenous drugs. Caught between the "first wave" (gay white men) and the "second wave" (heterosexuals), drug users at high risk for AIDS remain silent and invisible (Barrett 1985; Joseph 1986). One public health official recently challenged the rush to educate heterosexuals about their risk when what is needed (and has been from the beginning) is "a massive effort directed at intravenous-drug abusers and their sex partners. This means treatment for a disease—chemical dependence on drugs. We have to prevent and treat one disease, drug addiction, to prevent another, AIDS" (Joseph 1986).[35]

If AIDS's dual life as both a material and a linguistic entity is important, the emphasis on *dual* is crucial. Symbolic and social reconceptualizations of AIDS are necessary but not sufficient to address the massive social questions that AIDS raises. The recognition that AIDS is heterosexually as well as homosexually transmitted certainly represents progress, but it does not interrupt fantasy. It is fantasy, for example, to believe that "safer sex" will protect us from AIDS; it may save us from becoming infected with the virus—New York City has instituted Singles Night at the Blood Bank, where people can meet and share their seropositivity status before they even exchange names. But AIDS is to be a fundamental force of twentieth-century life, and no barrier in the world can make us "safe" from its complex material realities. Malnutrition, poverty, and hunger are unacceptable, in our own country and in the rest of the world; the need for universal health care is urgent. Ultimately, we cannot distinguish self from not-self: "plague is life," and each of us has the plague within us; "no one, no one on earth is free from it" (Camus [1947] 1948, 229).

The discursive structures I have discussed in this essay are familiar to those of us in "the human sciences." We have learned that there is a disjunction between historical subjects and constructed scientific objects. There is still debate about whether, or to what extent, scientific discourse can be privileged—and relied on to transcend contradiction. My own view is unequivocal: it cannot be privileged in this way. Of course, where AIDS is concerned, science can usefully perform its interpretive part: we can learn to live—indeed *must* learn to live—as though there are such things as viruses. The virus—a constructed scientific object—is also a historical subject, a "human immunodeficiency virus," a real source of illness and death that can be passed from one person to another under certain conditions that we can apparently—individually and collectively—influence. The trick is to learn to live with this disjunction, and it is a lesson we must learn. Dr. Rieux, the physician-narrator of Camus's novel, acknowledges that, by dealing medically with the plague, he is allowing himself the luxury of "living in a world of abstractions." But not indefinitely, for, "when abstraction sets to killing you, you've got to get busy with it" (Camus [1947] 1948, 81).

But getting busy with it may require us to relinquish some luxuries of our own: the luxury of accepting without reflection the "findings" that science seems effortlessly able to provide us, the luxury of avoiding vigilance, the luxury of hoping that it will all go away. Rather, we need to use what science gives us in ways that are selective, self-conscious, and pragmatic ("as though" they were true). We need to understand that AIDS is and will remain a provisional and deeply problematic signifier. Above all, we need to resist, at all costs, the luxury of listening to the thousands of language tapes playing in our heads, laden with prior discourse, that tell us with compelling certainty and dizzying contradiction what AIDS "really" means.

2

The Burdens of History:

Gender and Representation in

AIDS Discourse, 1981–1988

It is a commonplace of feminist scholarship to claim that medical discourse represents women's bodies as pathological and contaminated.[1]
"What is woman?" asked Hippocrates: "Disease." Discussing the "longev-
ity of [the] male aversion to female bodies," Mary Poovey (1987, 166)
quotes a nineteenth-century Boston physician's approval of Hippocrates'
dictum: "The wise old physician was not far wrong in his judgment."
When AIDS arrived, the real and imagined links between women's bodies
and disease—especially infectious and sexually transmitted disease—were
many, complex, and long standing. This was a subject with heavy baggage:
indeed, with bags that in 1981 were already packed. Yet, as the decade
unfolded, women were repeatedly told that this time they would not be
traveling. If they were in the airport at all, it was for someone else's flight.
Despite documented cases of AIDS in women from almost the beginning
of the epidemic, AIDS was assumed by most of the medical and scientific
community to be a "gay disease" and a "male disease"—assumed, that is,
to be different from other sexually transmitted diseases. Moreover, despite intense concern with gendered human bodies in contemporary culture, the media of the 1980s were strikingly silent on the topic of women
and AIDS. And, despite the skepticism toward established science and
medicine fostered by two decades of feminist scholarship and activism,
few feminists challenged the biomedical account of AIDS or, with the
exception of some lesbian writers and activists, called for solidarity with
the gay male community. What a surprise, then, for many women to find
themselves at the end of the decade in midair over the Atlantic without
even a toothbrush, let alone a barrier contraceptive, on board.

It is against the background of medical and cultural beliefs that the
fractured story of women and AIDS must be read. Even as panic over the
possible "heterosexual transmission" of AIDS/HIV periodically erupted
and was quelled by biomedical experts, even as claims that female pros-

titutes were infecting their clients never materialized, the U.S. cultural archive was flush with stereotypes linking women to disease. Tracing the social history of venereal disease in the United States over the last century, the historian Allan M. Brandt (1987) provides memorable examples of this equation from the groundbreaking anti-VD campaigns of the two world wars. Regularly portraying venereal disease as a tireless enemy of the U.S. war effort and women as its deceitful handmaidens, the World War II campaign included a series of vivid posters aimed at servicemen. One shows the face of an attractive and wholesome young woman: "SHE MAY LOOK CLEAN," the text warns, "BUT PICK-UPS, GOOD TIME GIRLS, PROSTITUTES SPREAD SYPHILIS AND GONORRHEA. You can't beat the Axis if you get VD." In another, the disease itself is assigned a female identity. A painted prostitute walks down the street, arm in arm with Hitler and Hirohito; the caption reads: "VD: THE WORST OF THESE" (Brandt 1987, following p. 164). Except for the innocent wives and mothers back home, women in these texts are never quite what they seem.[2]

These phantoms were readily resurrected and revamped for the AIDS epidemic. For example, the following urban legend was circulating by at least the mid-1980s: a straight man meets an attractive young woman at a singles bar and takes her back to his apartment, where they have sex; she is gone the next morning, but written across the bathroom mirror in bright red lipstick he reads, "Welcome to the World of AIDS!" (Fine 1987, 192–97). And several anti-AIDS posters from the U.S. Public Health Service (circa 1989) would seem to have come straight from the archives. In one, a beautiful woman looks out at the viewer. The caption asks: "Does she or doesn't she?" The text answers: "People can carry the AIDS virus, but show no symptoms. Don't take chances. Get tested before you get sexually involved."[3]

It is not simply that medicine and public health have sometimes been "sexist," an accusation that in the end tells us little. The best research— Brandt's examination of representations of women in medical and public health discourses, historical studies of women's bodies by Poovey (1988, 1990), Lisa Cartwright (1995), Adele Clarke (e.g., Moore and Clarke 1995), and other contemporary scholars—aims to illuminate the social context in which specific representations are produced, disseminated, understood, and put to use. Hence, Brandt places the anti-VD campaigns and the posters that they generated within a universe of scientific debate, socioeconomic division, and ideological struggle at a particular historical moment. The World War I crusades, for example, relied on conventional distinctions between purity and prostitution, middle-class morality and lower-class decay, the nuclear family and the worldly temptations that jeopardized it; but they also sought to challenge the "conspiracy of silence" surrounding VD and educate the public, including women, about its dangers. One of the major strategies of VD fighters—perhaps their key strategy—was to capitalize on the realities and priorities of wartime. Depicting venereal disease as a significant threat to U.S. war efforts and to the country's social and economic health in general, progressive physicians and public health advocates formed important alliances with the military to advance a franker public health policy. Emphasizing modern medicine and technology to achieve measurable results, anti-VD activities came to be seen as patriotic rather than shameful or perverse. At the same time, conventional morality dictated the continued deployment of fire-and-brimstone exhortations to the troops, fearsomely graphic portrayals of end-stage syphilis, and the unrelenting targeting of prostitutes as the concrete embodiment of an evil empire.

The process by which specific initiatives and agendas are linked to pre-existing institutions and values is described in the field of cultural studies as *articulation* (see Hall 1992).[4] The concept in the case of anti-VD campaigns is further illuminated by Stacie Colwell (1998), who documents the production history of the 1919 film *The End of the Road*, a VD education film for women conceived as a companion piece to the World War I film for enlisted men, *Fit to Fight*. Developed by the U.S. Public Health Service in conjunction with the War Department and the American Social Hygiene Association (ASHA)—the latter itself formed from the contradictory agendas of its founding agencies—*The End of the Road* harnessed its didactic educational message to the vehicle of a narrative feature-length "women's film" complete with love story, patriotism, dramatic juxtapositions of wholesome heterosexual relationships with immorality and prostitution ("Two roads there are in life," begins the film ponderously), and graphic medical images of patients in advanced stages of syphilis. The film was well received in carefully organized screenings to women and girls over sixteen, but its subsequent release for viewing in commercial theaters provoked a storm of public debate. Charged with violating American femininity and standards of human decency, the ASHA felt compelled to withdraw the film from commercial circulation and ultimately discontinued it altogether. Indeed, no fully intact print of the film survives. The whole episode was a lost opportunity, Colwell argues, for, despite its euphemisms, moralistic story line, rigid good girl/ bad girl dichotomy, and narrative omissions, *The End of the Road* is rightly celebrated as a groundbreaking effort to provide education about sexuality and health to a wide female audience. The film ultimately failed to achieve its goals, in part because the return to the noncrisis conditions of peacetime enabled the film's warring constituencies to reach agreement on something at last: that sex education for women could now be safely abandoned.[5]

Again, it is too simple to call such chapters in history *sexist*. What they do make clear is that gendered representations bear complex historical burdens. And they make clear that, like other significant cultural crises, an epidemic intensifies existing social divisions and codifies cultural stereotypes because there seems to be no time to do otherwise. Ideas, metaphors, and images circulate efficiently. The long-standing use of the human body as a symbol of society—a body/society often conceptualized as female—takes on special force in an epidemic of sexually transmitted disease, where the images and terminology routinely associated with physical disease—sickness, contamination, infection, death, filth, malnutrition, breakdown, disorganization, and death, among others—seem to blend seamlessly with commentary on the society in which the epidemic is occurring.[6] Even as scientific and medical authorities work to discourage such populist semiosis, their own language, procedures, and stereotypes, which are equally permeated with metaphor, acquire elevated cultural authority—authority, that is, following Starr (1982), to define reality. Heirs of an ancient medical legacy of semantic and gendered imperialism, health experts acquire special license in an epidemic to define and categorize, codify and regulate, and contain and silence the diseased others whom they diagnose, treat, and study. For women, epidemics are rarely benign.

In the discourse of the AIDS epidemic, we see reenacted many of the semantic and regulatory battles that have marked relations between women and biomedical science for at least the last century—but with a difference. To sum this up crudely, when female prostitutes (and other "promiscuous" women) missed their cue to enter this latest venereal drama, biomedicine gave their role away to homosexual and bisexual men. Offered few other significant parts to play, women spent the first decade of the epidemic as little more than walk-ons whose real role in the epidemic was largely taking place offstage—unheralded, unbilled, and unpaid. To put this somewhat differently, once scientists decided that female-to-male sexual transmission of infection was less likely than male-to-male or male-to-female transmission, "heterosexual transmission" dropped out as a major plot element in stories of the epidemic.

This chapter examines how these plots were fashioned and how biomedical discourses came to enact and, by default, to reinforce deeply entrenched, pervasive, and stubbornly conservative cultural narratives about gender. I look first at the CDC's reports in the *Morbidity and Mortality Weekly Report* and their influence on interpretation in other biomedical discourse. I then explore how diverse media genres reworked these narratives into their own scripts about sex and sexuality to create the illusion that the "puzzle of women and AIDS" (as an Australian public health brochure was later to put it)[7] had already been solved—or was not a puzzle at all. Finally, it is about the failure of influential U.S. feminists and feminist institutions to challenge the messages of dominant discourses.

The MMWR's "AIDS Patient"

"Can women get this disease?"
"No."
"How do you know?"
"No one has looked."
—exchange in 1982 between women scientists and physician Joseph Sonnabend

Whose body stands as the model of social order, and whose social order is anatomized as a normal body?—Catherine Waldby, *AIDS and the Body Politic*

The existence of AIDS as an official, clinically defined entity is generally dated from the report of the deaths of five homosexual men in Los Angeles from *pneumocystis* pneumonia in the 5 June 1981 issue of the *Morbidity and Mortality Weekly Report (MMWR)*, published by the Centers for Disease Control in Atlanta, and follow-up reports published over subsequent months (CDC 1981a).[8] The men who died from these first official cases were reported to have histories of multiple sexual contacts and sexually transmitted diseases (STDS). The published report triggered the national surveillance apparatus as well as the suspicions of individual physicians in other cities where gay men were contracting and dying from strange diseases, including uncommon forms of pneumonia and cancer. What had unofficially been called *gay pneumonia, gay cancer, an epidemic of immunosuppression*, and *WOGS* (the Wrath of God Syndrome) came provisionally to be called *GRID* (Gay-Related Immune Deficiency), a term that sought to capture the syndrome's target organism and its disease process.[9]

Although *GRID* was never officially adopted, the name reinforced the presumption of the first *MMWR* article that the syndrome involved sexually active gay men and was likely related to "the homosexual lifestyle." As Oppenheimer (1988) has observed, this generalization about homosexuals—and with it the "lifestyle hypothesis"—was surprisingly broad given that it was based on only five cases (see also Oppenheimer 1992). But it proved remarkably tenacious, creating a persistent tension between the *in*cluded and the *ex*cluded even as the clinical conditions outlined in the *MMWR* report began to be seen in a larger and more heterogeneous population, both gay and nongay, male and female. By mid-1982, the syndrome had been identified in intravenous drug users who shared needles, men and women from Haiti living in the United States, adult males with hemophilia who had received Factor VIII blood concentrate, and people who had received blood transfusions, including infants and elderly men and women. Although scientists continued to investigate the potential role of lifestyle factors, notably multiple sexual encounters and the heavy use of recreational drugs, these new cases lent support to the "viral hypothesis," the view that an infectious agent, transmitted sexually and/or through blood or blood products, was probably responsible. Moreover, the transfusion cases (where exposure could usually be dated precisely) suggested that a substantial period of time—even years—could elapse between exposure to the agent and the development of symptoms.

By mid-1982, women with AIDS had been identified who reported no other potential source of infection than sexual contact with a male partner; likewise, a small number of men with AIDS claimed no other source of exposure than female sexual partners, suggesting that this condition was sexually transmissible and transmissible to and from women. When babies with no history of transfusion also began developing AIDS-like symptoms, it seemed likely that the virus could be transmitted "vertically" (to the next generation), from an infected woman to her baby during gestation or childbirth (or perhaps after birth through breast-feeding). By late 1982, enough nonhomosexual cases had been documented to render GRID an unsuitable diagnosis, and, at a conference in Washington, D.C., the CDC accepted the recommendation to change the name of the syndrome to *AIDS*, Acquired Immune Deficiency Syndrome (Shilts 1987, 191). In 1983, while widespread media attention raised the specter of transmission through "routine household contact," increasing evidence attributed the reported cases to vertical transmission. By 1984, reports from other countries established that AIDS was taking hold regardless of national borders—further, that in many areas the virus appeared to be transmitted primarily through male-female sexual intercourse, with almost as many women infected in some locations as men. By 1985, when Rock Hudson confirmed that he had been diagnosed with AIDS, the epidemic was increasingly perceived as a national and international public health crisis. By 1987, when President Ronald Reagan first spoke the word

AIDS in public, media polls showed the public acutely aware of the epidemic and supportive of increased research and treatment spending. By 1988, when postal service workers delivered copies of the U.S. surgeon general's booklet *Understanding AIDS* to every household in the United States, the public—whatever its beliefs, attitudes, and practices—was adept at reciting the AIDS 101 catechism (see Kaiser Family Foundation 1996).

This summary of the early evolution of AIDS and the virus that we now call HIV sounds conventional enough in retrospect; largely undisputed, it is standard boilerplate for stories about the epidemic's history. Yet today's scientific consensus obscures interpretive ambiguities at each stage of AIDS's evolution, ambiguities that history inevitably appears to resolve but often simply overwrites. Nor does today's understanding explain why this seemingly straightforward account could be so disputed, so resisted, that almost twenty years into the epidemic women diagnosed with HIV or AIDS—and sometimes their physicians as well—still express astonishment at finding themselves with a "gay man's disease." At the same time, in the United States in the late 1990s, the quantitative burden of this epidemic continues to be borne by gay men, and, today, with recognition of the profound irony of the move, the very communities who labored throughout the 1980s to disarticulate "AIDS" from "gay male sexuality" are striving to "re-gay" AIDS so that resources will not be withdrawn when they are as needed as ever. The management of the AIDS crisis thus continues to be highly public, and, more than most epidemic diseases, its epidemiology is extraordinarily layered, marked by the periodic resurrection of old data, sudden shifts in interpretation, the appearance of revised chronologies, an ongoing dialectic between official and less official definitions and accounts, and intense negotiations among a substantial number of interested constituencies. It is therefore instructive to look more closely at AIDS as it unfolded in the pages of the *Morbidity and Mortality Weekly Report*, the narrative that formed the bedrock for accounts in many other scientific journals and the general media.

The 5 June 1981 *MMWR* report, we will recall, had been submitted by the clinical researchers Michael Gottlieb and Wayne Shandera of the University of California, Los Angeles. The paper had been routed in May by Dr. Mary Guinan to Dr. James W. Curran, head of the CDC's venereal disease division; according to Randy Shilts, he returned it to her with a note: "Hot stuff. Hot stuff." Although at first Gottlieb had reportedly thought nothing of the fact that his first *pneumocystis* patient was gay (he considered it, says Shilts [1987, 43], equivalent to "the fact that the guy might drive a Ford"), by the time the paper was written he had decided that the outbreak represented a new illness specific to gay men. The *MMWR* bulletin put it this way: "The occurrence of pneumocystosis in these 5 previously healthy individuals without a clinically apparent underlying immunodeficiency is unusual. The fact that these patients were all homosexuals suggests an association between some aspect of homosexual lifestyle or disease acquired through sexual contact and *Pneumocystis* pneumonia in this population" (CDC 1981a, 251). By mid-1982, a small number of women had been diagnosed with Kaposi's sarcoma and other opportunistic infections (which CDC shorthand was now reducing to KSOI). This was the lead paragraph in the CDC's first-year update on the epidemic: "Between June 1, 1981, and May 28, 1982, CDC received reports of 355 cases of Kaposi's sarcoma (KS) and/or serious opportunistic infections (OI), especially *Pneumocystis carinii* pneumonia (PCP), occurring in previously healthy persons between 15 and 60 years of age. Of the 355, 281 (79%) were homosexual (or bisexual) men, 41 (12%) were heterosexual men, 20 (6%) were men of unknown sexual orientation, and 13 (4%) were heterosexual women. This proportion of heterosexuals (16%) is higher than previously described" (CDC 1982a, 294; see also CDC 1981b). Unlike prior *MMWR* reports on the epidemic, this sixth report designated the patient population as "previously healthy persons" rather than "previously healthy homosexual males." Dates of the onset of symptoms in the women were distributed across 1980, 1981, and 1982. The report commented as follows about race and drug use: "Both male and female heterosexual PCP patients were more likely than homosexual patients to be black or Hispanic. Of patients with PCP for whom drug-use information was known, 14% of homosexual men had used intravenous drugs at some time compared with 63% of heterosexual men and 57% of heterosexual women" (CDC 1982a, 294).

In other words, some—but not all—of the infected women had reportedly used drugs. The report's choice of language is interesting here. Although use of the term *person* is technically "gender inclusive," it may have represented not the CDC's wish to emphasize reports of KSOI in women as well as men but rather its view that the data were still ambiguous. *Persons*, like *patients*, provided plausible deniability, making possible either a retrospective reading in which gender (and race, for that matter) had consistently been included as a factor (should gender turn out to be significant) or one that denied the relevance of gender, subsuming it under the category "intravenous drug users" if this turned out to be the overarching factor in etiology. Yet, in July 1982, when KSOI cases were reported in twenty Haitian patients living in the United States, the report's title designated the population as "Haitians," although three of the twenty were women (CDC 1982b, 353): here, the puzzling choice was made to collapse a small number of cases that were in other respects heterogeneous (age, gender, marital status, sexual history, etc.) into a single ethnic/national "risk group." (On the "Haitian connection," see Schwartz [1984], Feldman and Johnson [1986], Fettner and Check [1985], Connor and Kingman [1989], Johnson and Pape [1989], Farmer et al. [1996], and Bond et al. [1997].)

PCP was next reported among "persons with hemophilia A." After describing the cases—"all three were heterosexual males"—the report noted that the "clinical and immunologic features these three patients share are strikingly similar to those recently observed among certain individuals from the following groups: homosexual males, heterosexuals who abuse IV drugs, and Haitians who recently entered the United States. Although the cause of the severe immune dysfunction is unknown, the occurrence among the three hemophiliac cases suggests the possible transmission of an agent through blood products" (CDC 1982c, 366). No mention was made of "heterosexuals" who do *not* abuse intravenous drugs, although such a "group" had been explicitly identified in an earlier report, which concluded that "similarities between homosexual and heterosexual cases in diagnoses and geographic and temporal distribution suggest that all are part of the same epidemic" (CDC 1982a, 294).

In September 1982, the *MMWR* ruled out hepatitis B virus vaccine as the source of the new epidemic, characterized immune deficiency as its central clinical feature, and introduced the official designation *AIDS*: "Beginning in 1978, a disease or group of diseases was recognized, manifested by Kaposi's sarcoma and opportunistic infections, associated with a specific defect in cell-mediated immunity. This group of clinical entities, along with its specific immune deficiency, is now called acquired immune deficiency syndrome (AIDS)" (CDC 1982d, 465).

In a September 1982 update on AIDS in the United States, the CDC offered the following overview:

> Approximately 75% of AIDS cases occurred among homosexual or bisexual males, among whom the reported prevalence of intravenous drug abuse was 12%. Among the 20% of known heterosexual cases (males and females), the prevalence of intravenous drug abuse was about 60%. Haitians residing in the United States constituted 6.1% of all cases, and 50% of the cases in which both homosexual activity and intravenous drug abuse were denied. Among the 14 AIDS cases involving males under 60 years old who were not homosexuals, intravenous drug abusers, or Haitians, two (14%) had hemophilia A.

Reported AIDS cases may be separated into groups based on these risk factors: homosexual or bisexual males—75%, intravenous drug abusers with no history of male homosexual activity—13%, Haitians with neither a history of homosexuality nor a history of intravenous drug abuse—0.3%, and persons in none of the other groups—5%. (CDC 1982e, 508)

Having established this rather complicated scheme of categories and percentages, some of which intersected or overlapped with each other and some of which, apparently, did not, the *MMWR* editors emphasized that, in this rapidly escalating epidemic, members of the "4-H Club" were still the folks to watch: the "reported incidence of AIDS has continued to increase rapidly. Only a small percentage of cases have none of the identified risk factors (male homosexuality, intravenous drug abuse, Haitian origin, and perhaps hemophilia A)." Nonetheless, the CDC cautioned, "To avoid a reporting bias, physicians should report cases regardless of the absence of these factors" (CDC 1982e, 508).

But the "risk groups" were fraying at the edges. Following reports of the syndrome in men with hemophilia, the CDC began confirming other cases in recipients of blood transfusions. The nation's blood-banking industry denied the possibility that the blood supply could be contaminated even while advising blood-bank centers to follow the CDC blood donor deferral guidelines and asking homosexuals (lesbians as well as gay men) to refrain voluntarily from donating blood. (A January 1983 CDC workshop would explore the possible transmission of AIDS via the blood supply and debate the proper steps, if any, to screen the nation's blood donors and blood supply. Reported *Science* on January 21, "The CDC is also investigating the cases of two adults who developed AIDS after receiving blood transfusions during surgery. The two did not belong to any of the known high-risk groups, which include, in addition to hemophiliacs, homosexual and bisexual men who are extremely active sexually, users of intravenous drugs, and Haitians" [Jean L. Marx, quoted in Kulstad 1986, 22]). The *MMWR* recommendations of 4 March 1983 listed "sexually active homosexual or bisexual men with multiple partners" as the only homosexual population at increased risk for AIDS (1983b), but, as numerous sources testified, the gender distinction was largely lost in translation (see Patton 1985a; Ostrow 1987c, 19–26). In December the CDC reported cases of immune deficiency and opportunistic infections in infants in New York, New Jersey, and California that could not be attributed to transfusions (CDC 1982f). On the basis of the "sociodemographic profiles of the mothers," the CDC suggested that "transmission of an 'AIDS agent' from mother to child, either in utero or shortly after birth, could account for the early onset of immunodeficiency in these infants." In other words, the mothers were presumed to be carrying the "AIDS agent," having themselves acquired it through sexual contact with an infected man or through intravenous drug use (sharing contaminated needles with an infected person), and to have then transmitted it vertically to their infants. By the end of December 1982, fifty-seven adult women, or 6 percent of total cases, had been diagnosed with AIDS. The CDC also reported two cases of AIDS in women who were longtime partners of men with AIDS, noting also forty-three reports of PCP and other AIDS-related conditions in previously healthy women, apparently contracted primarily through sexual contact with intravenous drug users who were not yet themselves overtly ill (CDC 1983a; Shilts [1987, 225] identifies this report as a turning point in U.S. media coverage). The finding of AIDS and AIDS-like conditions in women, concluded the CDC, supported "the infectious-agent hypothesis" as well as "the possibility that transmission of the putative 'AIDS agent' may occur among both heterosexual and male homosexual couples" (CDC 1983a, 698). Moreover, while evidence mounted that an infectious agent was responsible for AIDS and was probably transmitted through penetrative sexual contact and infected blood products, other modes of transmission were not emerging. As of spring 1983, nearly two years into the epidemic, the CDC had found *no* evidence that "casual contact" contributed to the transmission of the infectious agent believed to cause AIDS (CDC 1983c, 311).

The 30 November 1984 *MMWR* (CDC 1984) reported a total of 6,993 cases in the United States—72 patients under thirteen, 6,921 adult patients. Of these, 59 percent were white, 25 percent were black, 14 percent were Hispanic, and 2 percent were "other/unknown." The report noted that, among "the 54 AIDS patients who were heterosexual sex partners of persons with AIDS or with an increased risk for acquiring AIDS, 49 (91%) were women." The report introduced the category "noncharacteristic patients": "Of the adult AIDS patients, 263 (4%) have not been placed in any of the identified risk groups and are classified as noncharacteristic patients. One hundred eighty-six (71%) of the noncharacteristic patients were male; 34%, white; 43%, black; and 19%, of Hispanic origin. Investigations of 65 of the male noncharacteristic patients have identified 17 (26%) who reported a history of sexual contact with female prostitutes. Five of the seventeen gave a history of over 100 heterosexual partners in the past five years. . . . One of the nine noncharacteristic women interviewed claimed to be a former prostitute" (CDC 1984, 661).

The appearance in 1984 of "prostitutes" and "heterosexual partners" (meaning, in this context, women) on the AIDS scene in the United States coincided with growing reports of heterosexual transmission of AIDS in both the United States and Africa, reports confirmed in 1985 by the World Health Organization, the U.S. Public Health Service, and other scientific organizations. At the same time, problems with the "risk-group" model and its hierarchical modes of exposure led the CDC to develop several "multiple" and "overlapping" categories. In the *MMWR*'s January 1985 update for Europe, for example, "homosexual/bisexual + IV drug exposure" appears for the first time as a "risk group" (CDC 1985). But, still, no interest was expressed in "women."

Very early in the epidemic, some versions of the CDC's "4-H Club" did include women: "homos, heroin addicts, Haitians, and hookers" was how David Black reported it in 1986. A number of researchers had pursued the exploration of risk for HIV in prostitutes. Joyce Wallace (1984), for example, a New York City physician, tested T-cell ratios of working prostitutes in the early 1980s; although finding normal ratios, she concluded that other symptoms of immune system impairment suggested that this population could be at risk for developing AIDS. Even so, given the high incidence of intravenous drug use among women prostitutes, the potential source of their risk from *sexual* contact was ambiguous. In the absence of evidence that prostitutes were transmitting the virus to their male clients, "hookers" were summarily bounced off the risk-group list (just in time to open a slot for hemophiliacs), and women as a whole lost their only presence on the AIDS research agenda.

Sporadic reports of male exposure to AIDS through "prostitutes" did keep alive, however, the historical axiom that prostitutes constitute a major "reservoir" or "harbor" for venereal disease as well as a major "vector" along which it is spread (e.g., see Corea [1992, 22–23, 34] on the cases of Elizabeth Prophet and Helen Cover). Following historical tradition, investigators were interested in female prostitutes as potential transmitters of "the AIDS virus" to males—as infec*tors*, in other words, not as infec*tees*. The development of serologic testing for the "putative AIDS agent"—widely misunderstood as "a test for AIDS"—opened new possibilities for identifying infection in particular individuals and groups. This suggested a practical way to investigate AIDS in "prostitutes"—a group, moreover, whose rights to privacy and civil liberties had played little part in the history of epidemics. No move was made, however, to determine whether the clinical symptoms and precursors of AIDS might look different in women than in men: not until 1992 would selected gynecological conditions be added to the suspected clinical profile of HIV infection and AIDS.

Under pressure to study women, the CDC initiated a multicenter study of female prostitutes known as "Project 72" to determine the prevalence of antibodies to AIDS in this population. Existing CDC data on "women" as of 10 March 1987—at that point totaling 2,159 U.S. cases of AIDS—were used for comparison. *Prostitution* was defined for the study as "the exchange of physical-sexual services for money or drugs" in at least one instance since 1 January 1978. The findings, published in March 1987 (CDC 1987a), revealed roughly the same overall rate of seroprevalence—4 percent—in both populations as well as parallel variation across seven geographic research sites (i.e., both HIV seroprevalence and AIDS cases among both groups were highest in New Jersey and Miami and lowest in southern Nevada). In all seven areas, rates were higher in both groups for black and Hispanic than for white and other women. Unprotected vaginal intercourse and a history of intravenous drug use were associated with seroprevalence and AIDS regardless of race. Consistent and correct use of latex condoms reduced the risk of HIV infection; prostitutes were considerably more likely to use condoms regularly with clients than with their husbands and boyfriends. Despite problems with the study (for a general critique of "prostitute studies," see Shaw and Paleo [1987]), its findings allayed fears that AIDS/HIV was "exploding" among female prostitutes, thus placing their clients—the "general population"—at greater risk. No further studies of "women" or "prostitutes" were undertaken until the mid-1990s. Although the Board of Health in Nevada (where prostitution is regulated) began requiring that prostitutes be tested for HIV antibody as a condition of employment in county-licensed brothels and, once employed, be tested monthly thereafter (Campbell 1991), and although media reports and urban legends circulating about "prostitutes with AIDS" regularly triggered calls for mandatory testing and quarantine, the CDC remained opposed to both measures as drastic, expensive, and futile. Adding in its characteristic flat prose that, traditionally, "medical care, therapy for drug addiction, welfare benefits, and vocational rehabilitation have not been routinely offered to women apprehended for prostitution," the CDC took note of several "innovative approaches to male, as well as female, prostitutes" (CDC 1987a, 160; see also Shaw and Paleo 1987; Ostrow 1987c; Schneider 1988a, 1988b; Stephens 1988; Cohen and Wofsy 1989; Campbell 1990a; Corea 1992; and Saunders 1997).

This did not mean that the CDC ruled out the spread of HIV to heterosexual women and men. Although "the prostitute study" and other targeted studies, such as they were, failed to turn up unequivocal evidence of increasing incidence through heterosexual sex, HIV infection was reported by some other sources to be increasing in this population even while the large cohort studies of new infection rates among gay men appeared to show a leveling off (but new AIDS cases and deaths remained high). In late 1986, CDC interviews with female members of two heterosexual singles clubs in Minneapolis documented that some were infected with HIV yet had made virtually no modifications in their sexual practices (CDC 1986b). Another study found that adolescents in San Francisco, a city where public health information about AIDS had been extensive, were not well informed about its seriousness, causes, or prevention (DiClemente et al. 1986). A 1987 "Review of Current Knowledge" (CDC 1987b and 1987c) reinforced the view that AIDS/HIV was probably not uniquely distinct from other sexually transmitted infections and, without intervention, could and probably would spread to large numbers of sexually active women and men—gradually, perhaps, but steadily.

These worrisome possibilities were not communicated clearly to the public. Although, as early as 1983, nine of ten Americans had heard of AIDS, most people did not yet think of AIDS/HIV as an epidemic that could gain purchase in a population slowly and undramatically; nor did most really believe that they could become infected through heterosexual intercourse, despite the theoretical possibility. Certainly, most women didn't have a clue. As public health officials debated how—and whether—to call attention to this unfamiliar conception of the AIDS epidemic, the question was taken out of their hands. AIDS/HIV may not have been "exploding" in the "heterosexual population," but the idea of "heterosexual AIDS" now exploded in the general media. "Suddenly," proclaimed the cover story of *U.S. News and World Report* on 12 January 1987, "the disease of *them* is the disease of *us*." The magazine's cover graphic represented "us" as a young white urban professional man and woman, a graph of rising AIDS deaths cutting across their faces. "The Big Chill" was the title of *Time*'s 16 February 1987 cover story; in an accompanying illustration (55), a tiny heterosexual couple is being swamped by a dark wave of AIDS. Leishman's (1987) cover story for the *Atlantic*, subtitled "The Second Stage of the Epidemic," showed a man and woman blankly huddled in bed. Other publications followed suit.

As I noted in the last chapter, this media explosion was the product of several factors. In December 1986, having reviewed a number of cases that "could not be classified by recognized risk factors for AIDS," the CDC reassigned a significant number of cases to the category of heterosexual transmission (CDC 1986a). Analyzing the CDC review data and related research for *Mobilizing against AIDS*, a collection of papers from a high-powered scientific conference in 1985, Eve K. Nichols concluded that "these facts suggest a possible association between a small number of

AIDS cases and heterosexual promiscuity in this country" (Nichols 1986, 28; Nichols 1989, 46). Despite the hedging and the use of the loaded term *promiscuity*, the conclusion represented a new biomedical construction of AIDS within the official scientific establishment and was interpreted as such by the media (e.g., Associated Press 1986b). But Nichols also acknowledged that "researchers disagree about the extent to which the virus will spread in the heterosexual population in the United States. Numerous studies indicate that men can transmit the virus to women, although vaginal intercourse may be a less efficient mode of transmission than anal intercourse. The focus of the disagreement is the likelihood of female-to-male transmission" (p. 39). Yet, as *Science* editor Jean L. Marx summarized the evidence in 1984, "sexual intercourse both of the heterosexual and homosexual varieties is a major pathway of transmission" (Marx 1984, 147).

Confronting AIDS, a 1986 report from the National Institute of Medicine and the National Academy of Sciences, predicted the future course of the epidemic as follows:

> New AIDS cases in men and women acquired through heterosexual contact will increase from 1,100 in 1986 to almost 7,000 in 1991. . . . Although there is a broad spectrum of opinion on the likelihood of further spread of HIV infection in the heterosexual population, there is a strong consensus that the surveillance systems and studies presently in place have very limited ability to detect such spread. Better approaches to tracking this spread can be instituted, but general population surveys are probably neither practical nor ethical. The committee believes that over the next five to ten years there will be substantially more cases of HIV infection in the heterosexual population and that these cases will occur predominantly among the population subgroups at risk for other sexually transmitted diseases. . . .
>
> Because in the United States the majority of AIDS patients are men, the implications of HIV infection in women have often been overlooked. Women need to know that if they are infected with HIV they may transmit the virus to their sexual partners and possibly to their future offspring. The message is particularly important for IV drug users and their sexual partners. (Institute of Medicine and National Academy of Sciences 1986, 3, 9, 10)

U.S. Surgeon General C. Everett Koop held a press conference to release the *U.S. Surgeon General's Report on Acquired Immune Deficiency Syndrome* and announced that he, too, now viewed AIDS as a potential threat to every sexually active person and would advocate immediate explicit sex education for everyone over eight years of age (U.S. Surgeon General 1986; see also Koop 1991). And the World Health Organization confirmed what many had suspected: AIDS had become a serious health problem in a number of central African countries, and nearly half of those with AIDS were women; moreover, AIDS had now been reported in at least seventy-five countries around the world and constituted a crisis of potentially catastrophic proportions (see Netter 1986; and "Official Warns" 1987).

This wave of "spread of AIDS" coverage had several consequences. At the very point that aggressive, intelligent public health outreach was called for, the panicked representations of "heterosexual AIDS" forced the CDC instead to downplay its potential threat. On 1 April 1987, President Ronald Reagan finally made a public address about the AIDS epidemic, speaking with approval of mandatory antibody testing. (One political cartoon had the president asking his staff, "The AIDS speech ready yet?" as he pulled on latex gloves.) Although Koop's hard-hitting Surgeon General's Report had in 1986 unequivocally declared the need for widespread AIDS and sex education in all populations in the United States, no real federal AIDS initiative was launched until the 1987–88 America Responds to AIDS (ARTA) education and prevention campaign. Although the heterosexual scare certainly gave impetus to ARTA, it did nothing to simplify the process of producing the centerpiece of the initiative, a Public Health Service mailing slated to be delivered to "every household in America." Koop's 1986 report had been prepared and released with virtually no clearance from the conservative Reagan administration; his subsequent efforts were more highly policed. In addition, the far-reaching Helms amendment had drastically constrained the language and message that could lawfully be employed in federally funded AIDS efforts. By the time the surgeon general's mailer Understanding AIDS arrived on U.S. doorsteps in early 1988, it successfully sent the important message that "America" considered AIDS important. But it also looked like what it was: a document developed amid conflicting data, warring agendas, and multiple drafts. Gay men looked for themselves in vain among the apparent target groups pictured in the mailer's photos and had to settle for the construction worker whose hard hat might—in a stretch—be seen as an effort at gay iconography. Except in their maternal capacity, women got little attention in the mailer. In the heat of concern over heterosexual transmission, a new category had been proposed to catch women's attention: "women at risk." But, at the last minute, this category was collapsed with another new category called "multiple partners of sexually active adults." A category called "women at risk" might be useful, but "multiple partners" sounds like a duplicate bridge tournament, and a politically correct gender-neutral one at that. The AIDS epidemic has generated many useful acronyms, but Women at Risk and Multiple Partners of Sexually Active Adults is not one of them. Not only did WARMPSAA collapse gender, risk behaviors, sex, and the inscrutable identity "multiple partner," it couldn't even be pronounced.[10]

I have not quoted so heavily from the *MMWR* because it is great poetry. On the contrary, as a formative AIDS discourse, its utilitarian prose and clunky categories are a poor fit with the world most of us inhabit. In part because of that, the *MMWR* indexes the challenges of translating specialized academic concepts—specifically, epidemiological statistics and surveillance categories—into meaningful everyday knowledge. Reading the *MMWR* closely also points to the problems of constructing a chronology of women and AIDS. While chronologies—whether drawn from scientific journals, media coverage, or any other set of texts—appear to chronicle history, they also create it through selection, emphasis, language, and omission: this may be as true of my chronology as of the *MMWR's*. And what is to count as the "*MMWR's* discourse"?[11] Indeed, surely one of the most persistently vexing questions in AIDS's epidemiological history is, Who are to count as "women"? Acknowledging these difficulties, I want nevertheless to try to extract several lessons from this chronological "narrative of women and AIDS."

In September 1982, when the CDC published its first update on the U.S. epidemic and officially adopted the term *AIDS*, 593 cases of AIDS had been reported. Of this total, 34 cases, or 5.7 percent, occurred in women; sexual orientation for all 34 was listed as "heterosexual," while 20 were identified as having some history of intravenous drug use (CDC 1982d). Taking the CDC categories at face value for the moment, what is the inescapable logic of this communication?

1. Some people with AIDS are women.
2. All women with AIDS are "heterosexual."
3. Some women with AIDS have a history of intravenous drug use.
4. Some women with AIDS have *no* history of intravenous drug use.
5. Therefore, some women with AIDS have acquired AIDS through heterosexual sexual contact.

The significance of this conclusion is threefold. First, if some women acquired AIDS through heterosexual sex, the listing of transmission categories for women should have been modified *immediately*—either by expanding "sexual contact" explicitly to include both homosexual and heterosexual or by adding "heterosexual contact" as a new category. Second, if some women with AIDS reported a history of both intravenous drug use and heterosexual sexual contact (with an infected or "high-risk" partner), surveillance reporting should have reflected these dual sources of potential exposure—either by including both categories for women or by creating a category comparable to that established for men called "dual (or multiple) sources of exposure: heterosexual contact and intravenous drug use." Third, if some women have AIDS, no matter what the mode of exposure, the listing of risk groups should have been modified to reflect gender explicitly, paralleling the listing of existing groups: "male and female homosexuals," "male and female heterosexuals," "men and women who use intravenous drugs," "men and women of Haitian origin," and so on.

Yet, interestingly, as the next paragraph in this *MMWR* account indicates, the CDC elected instead to finesse this point, deemphasizing the conclusion inherent in its own data: "The incidence of AIDS has continued to increase rapidly. Only a small percentage of cases have none of the identified risk factors (male homosexuality, intravenous drug abuse, Haitian origin, and perhaps hemophilia A). To avoid a reporting bias, physicians should report cases regardless of the absence of these factors." This cautionary emphasis puts the burden for identifying exceptions on the reporting physician. By December 1982, fifty-seven adult women, or 6 percent of total cases, had been diagnosed with AIDS. This time we were not told how many had a history of intravenous drug use or how many labeled themselves "heterosexual." Instead, women were on their way into the categorical limbo only hinted at in the September update: "none of the above" and "other."[12]

Biomedicine's "AIDS Patient"

Women are often discussed as a single group defined chiefly by biological sex, members of an abstract, universal (and implicitly white) category. In reality, we are a mixed lot, our gender roles and options shaped by history, culture, and deep divisions across class and color lines.—Nancy Krieger and Elizabeth Fee 1992

Taxonomies are not neutral hatracks for the pristine facts of nature. They are theories that create and reflect the deep structure of science and human culture. A taxonomy is not just a ploy for convenient arrangement, but a hypothetical statement about the nature of things.—Stephen Jay Gould, quoted by Varmus 1989

In contrast to the cacophonous semiosis that I described in chapter 1, the narrative that I have just reviewed derives largely from the official record of epidemic disease in the United States, the *Morbidity and Mortality Weekly Report.* But other voices also contributed to biomedical and public health discourse on AIDS in the United States, including professional scientific and medical organizations, officials, and agencies, influential journals, scholarly books, appointed commissions, conferences, and congressional hearings. If at first these other "regimes of credibility" (Epstein 1996) seemed primarily to reproduce the CDC's reports, ultimately they provided annotation, counterpoint, and challenge to the weekly narrative from Atlanta, in time establishing new nodal points (Laclau and Mouffe 1985) in the epidemic's vast discursive web (virology, immunology, treatments, and so on). I do not intend to explore this intertextual web in any detail; rather, I discuss several articles that explicitly raised "the woman question" in AIDS discourse over this period (1981–88).

Until the virus was isolated and the front shifted to virology, the CDC was the major generator of official AIDS discourse. The CDC's definition of AIDS, with its associated list of clinical manifestations, performed a significant gatekeeping function—as it was intended to. Throughout the epidemic, the CDC had to make continual decisions about the parameters of its definition, seeking to hold some elements constant without blocking out new information. This is, after all, its job. But definitions have great power: they include and exclude, and sometimes they reflect compromise, politics, convenience, guesswork, lobbying efforts, economics, and cultural stereotypes as much as "evidence." In the early years of the epidemic, especially, the catchy "4-H Club" shorthand was hard to beat. Shilts, for example, tells us that, in February 1982, Dr. Arye Rubinstein, a pediatrician at Albert Einstein College of Medicine in the Bronx, was seeing sick babies who seemed to have all the symptoms then considered characteristic of AIDS. He sent a paper on the subject to the *New England Journal of Medicine* but heard nothing; meanwhile, other scientists were calling his hypothesis "improbable if not altogether impossible." "By its very name," writes Shilts (1987, 124), "GRID was a homosexual disease, not a disease of babies or their mothers."[13]

By spring 1983, nearly two years into the epidemic, reports of AIDS in infants were mounting. The CDC had still found no evidence that so-called casual contact contributed to the transmission of the infectious agent believed to cause AIDS. In May 1983, however, a study in the *Journal of the American Medical Association* by James Oleske and his colleagues identified cases of AIDS in infants in families with members who could be considered at risk for AIDS. Both the research paper and the accompanying editorial by Anthony S. Fauci (1983) acknowledged the possibility of "vertical transmission" yet emphasized the alternative possibility of transmission through "routine close contact, as within a household." Fauci's editorial, in particular, as well as the wave of national media coverage that followed, underlined the dire implications of the "routine household contact" scenario. This, of course, departed from the CDC's conclusions a few months earlier; in response to intense pressure from the CDC and other AIDS authorities, the journal issued a disclaimer that downplayed the possibility of household contact in favor of vertical transmission.

Yet the "male disease/gay disease" hypothesis remained firmly in place (Eckholm 1985; L. Altman 1987b, 1987c; CDC 1987a). When evidence of vertical transmission emerged, there was no place to put it. Taking its lead from the CDC categories, AIDS texts and databases evaded (or never entertained) the question of AIDS and HIV infection in women. In one review article on psychological issues in AIDS, for instance, women were mentioned only under such headings as "pediatric AIDS" (Lehman and Russell 1986): that most cases of "pediatric AIDS" presupposed a case of "maternal AIDS," however acquired, was not discussed. The scenario was a familiar one: mothers with AIDS/HIV were bracketed as either transparent transmitters or passive containers (see Bowleg 1992). As the physician Constance Wofsy summed it up in frustration, women came to be seen as a kind of "invisible pass-through" (quoted in Corea 1992, 82), who could transmit HIV without getting it.[14]

The pass-through scenario then took a truly jesuitical turn. While public attention was still riveted on the Rock Hudson case, interpreted by some to mean that "regular guys" were at risk, R. R. Redfield and his colleagues reported in the *Journal of the American Medical Association* a finding of HIV (HTLV-III) infection in U.S. servicemen stationed in Germany who claimed heterosexual contact only—with female prostitutes (Redfield et al. 1985, 2095). The authors suggested that "prostitutes could serve as a reservoir for HTLV-III infection for heterosexually active individuals" (p. 2,095). Attempts to discredit or dismiss the possibility of female-to-male transmission were ingenious. Servicemen, it was argued, would be punished for revealing homosexual behavior or intravenous drug use. So they lied. Or they shaded the truth: that they had really gone to *male* prostitutes. Or, since women were merely passive vessels without the efficient capacities of a projectile penis or syringe for efficiently shooting large quantities of the virus into another organism, the transmission to servicemen from female prostitutes must be only apparent: indeed, perhaps transmission was not really from women to men but was rather "quasi-homosexual": man A, infected with HIV, has sexual intercourse with a prostitute; she, "[performing] no more than perfunctory external cleansing between customers" (quoted in Langone 1985, 49), then has intercourse with man B; he is infected with the virus by way of man A's semen, still in the vagina of the prostitute (Kant 1985). The prostitute's vagina becomes no more than a passive holding tank for infected semen that becomes dangerous only when another penis is dipped into it—like a swamp where mosquitoes come to breed. (In this scenario, one must suppose that the projectile penis now functions as a proboscis or wet/dry vacuum, sucking up virus from the contaminated pool.)

Now, it may be that a man can be infected indirectly from another man's semen. It may also be that a penis can take up HIV-infected semen as well as ejaculate it (through the fragile urethra?). Empirical investigation into precise mechanisms of transmission would seem called for, rather than speculation and prior assumptions about women's "incompetence" and "inefficiency" as transmitters. The efforts of heavyweight researchers to counter the prevailing view that AIDS was predominantly and inherently a gay men's disease often reflected comparable cultural stereotypes. At a congressional hearing, the virologist William Haseltine (successfully testifying in support of increased funding for AIDS research) dismissed exotic explanations of the central African data: "To think that we're so different from people in the Congo is a more comfortable position, but it probably isn't so." So far, so good. Yet, citing the HIV-infected U.S. servicemen in Germany (Redfield et al. 1985), Haseltine invoked a kind of locker-room common sense: "These aren't homosexuals. These aren't drug abusers. These are normal, young guys who visited prostitutes. Half the prostitutes are infected, and these guys got infected." Haseltine distinguished "normal, young guys" from gay men and drug users, shifting in the last clause to a passive construction that reinforced their lack of culpability, representing them as innocent "receivers" of the infection, not problematic "donors."

As cases of AIDS and HIV in women mounted, the dogma that women do not get AIDS required reinforcement. Women do not get AIDS, ran the revamped formula, or, if they do, they are not "women"—at least not "normal women." Given the scenarios that I have already sketched, the women to whom this formula applied will not surprise us. Women not considered "women" included those infected by transfusion, mothers of infants with AIDS/HIV, and lesbians. The categories (of existing "risk groups" and "modes of exposure") to which these "women" were farmed out and thus erased as gendered beings included "transfusion victims," "intravenous drug users," "sex partners of persons with/at risk for AIDS," "minorities," "mothers of infants with AIDS," "spouses of hemophiliacs," those who had had sexual contact with a person in/from a "pattern II country" (i.e., classified by the WHO as countries where "heterosexual transmission" was predominant), and "recipients of artificial insemination." Such classifications reinforced the pass-through scenario: women in risk groups were given that status only by virtue of their sexual or familial attachments—their men and children—and even the country to which they were connected, rather than by virtue of their own activities and identities. This kind of assignment appeared to constitute a return to an earlier system of sociological categorization, one perhaps not fully theorized in the current situation. Finally, most studies of women with AIDS/HIV—however few such studies there were and however they categorized the women they studied—were explicitly justified by arguing that HIV incidence in women provided a general index to the heterosexual spread of the virus and that the purpose of identifying women at risk and preventing "primary" infection in them was to prevent cases of AIDS/HIV in their partners and children. Again, there was no intrinsic concern for women *as women*.

Women considered "not normal" included "prostitutes," "drug abusers," minority and poor women, and women in the Third World. Despite their long-standing professional knowledge of STDs and early activism about AIDS, prostitutes continued to be portrayed as irresponsible or inherently contaminated, their bodies virtual laboratory cultures for viral replication. Cast by history as the canaries of venereal disease, they were equally expendable. Randy Shilts had covered an early case of AIDS in a female prostitute in San Francisco; when she died quietly in 1978 without infecting legions of frightened clients, the story faded away and so, evidently, did Shilts's interest in women. Although he dramatically opened his best-selling *And the Band Played On* (1987) with the death from AIDS of a female Danish surgeon who, he tells us, was a lesbian, women make few subsequent appearances. Devoting only ten pages to heterosexuals, most of that space telling once more the story of the San Francisco prostitute, *Band*'s only index entry for "women" mentions that Larry Kramer wrote the homoerotic screenplay for the film *Women in Love*.[15] CDC methodology required that source of transmission be classified according to a hierarchy of factors, with no dual assignments allowed. At first, the CDC assigned infection in prostitutes to sexual contact with multiple sex partners even though other studies, as well as prostitutes themselves, more readily assigned the source of infection to intravenous drug use. When fear of an AIDS epidemic in prostitutes faded, it was a tidy solution to abandon "heterosexual contact" as a category as well.

Infected female intravenous drug users, or, as they were commonly called, "drug abusers" or "drug addicts" (although it is during *use*, not necessarily *abuse*, that transmission occurs), were given little sympathy or shown little interest. But here is where the categories got really sticky. Statistics for this "risk group" were problematic from the beginning, in part because the group was not a "group," but primarily because, as I have just noted, no clear statistical distinction was made between intravenous drug use and sexual contact as a mode of exposure in women. While AIDS/HIV in prostitutes tended to be attributed to sexual contact with multiple partners (and especially to paying multiple partners), evidence suggested that the sharing of needles in the course of intravenous drug use was the more likely source of exposure. For female intravenous drug users—or partners of male intravenous drug users or men with AIDS—the initial supposition was just the opposite, with drug use identified as the mode of exposure that counted. Minority women were often assumed to be drug users and hence infected through this route, as though sexual activity, let alone sexual diversity, played no role in the lives of non-white women (on this point, see Alonso and Koreck 1989). Janet Mitchell, a physician at Harlem Hospital Center in New York, argued unsuccessfully with the CDC for separate categories (Mitchell 1988, 1993; and see Corea 1992). Although sexual contact had been given precedence early on, the CDC's hierarchical reporting system was reversed in the mid-1980s, shifting drug use over sex as the primary mode of exposure for infected women—which then, because no multiple-mode categories had been established for women, excluded the others.

The "not normal" category also proved useful in explaining the growing evidence from outside the United States of HIV infection and AIDS in women as well as men. In November 1983, the World Health Organization reported from Geneva that AIDS had now been reported in thirty-three countries and on all continents. Lawrence Altman, science and medical correspondent for the *New York Times*, reported "indications that in Africa the disease may be striking heterosexual men and women in equal numbers," noting researchers' puzzlement over its apparently heterosexual nature. Linking this to the small but confirmed number of heterosexually transmitted cases in the United States, Altman described the differing interpretations of the data and disagreements among officials over whether the U.S. public should be informed (L. Altman 1985a, 19). Reports of growing heterosexual transmission in Haiti (L. Altman 1986) coincided with a 1986 paper in the *New England Journal of Medicine* in which Joan Kreiss and her colleagues reported significant prevalence of HIV infection and AIDS among female prostitutes in Nairobi, Kenya, seemingly acquired through heterosexual contact.

Efforts to refute these data paralleled those directed toward Redfield's work. With little conceptual coherence about why a sexually transmitted illness should be homosexual in one region or country and heterosexual in another, speculations about the "Third World" proved even more outlandish than those about U.S. servicemen in Germany. A series of ad hoc explanations proposed that "Third World women" should be understood as yet one more category of "exceptions" ("not normal" women). The reported statistics from central Africa were attributed to—among other things—"quasi-homosexual" transmission (like the servicemen), refusal by African men (or African government officials) to admit to homosexuality or drug use, the practice of anal intercourse as a method of birth control, galloping prostitution and promiscuity (typically treated as identical), the use of unsterilized needles in clinics and hospitals, various practices of "native healers," various "rituals," circumcision in women, lack of circumcision in men, multiple households/marriages, widespread prevalence of disease, malnutrition, and other sexually transmitted infections, daily commerce with green monkeys and other suspect animals, and various additional "unfamiliar practices": in short, explanations based on the whole panoply of stereotyped "differences" summed up by Paul Farmer as "exotica" (see Farmer et al. 1996; and also Shepherd 1987; White 1990; Appleman and Kahn 1988, 1989; Gorna 1996; Bond et al. 1997; Erni 1998; and Abramson and Pinkerton 1993, 1995).

Back in the U.S.A., mothers of babies with AIDS acquired a peculiar duality, both as "not women" and as "not normal." If they acquired the virus "unknowingly" and "innocently," they were seen as passive victims or invisible transmitters. But, if they were found/alleged/believed to have gotten (or stayed) pregnant knowing that they were HIV positive, they acquired instant agency—and sinister agency at that, transformed in a flash from passive receivers to culpable agents invidiously transmitting infected blood to their unborn babies (see Curran 1986). Moreover, testing newborns for HIV constituted a "diagnosis by proxy" of their mothers; this clear violation of childbearing women's civil rights resulted only in further disasters: they would probably lose their children, possibly their jobs, homes, and health care coverage. And AIDS/HIV caretaking and support services were barely getting in gear for the infants, not for the women themselves. Many years later, pregnant women sustained on experimental antiviral treatment to reduce the likelihood of vertical HIV transmission would find their medication withdrawn as soon as they gave birth; their unborn children had been the only real patients.

Lesbians, who figure fitfully, and mostly anecdotally, in the biomedical AIDS narrative, also acquired a dual presence in AIDS/HIV statistics. As a population lesbians have a low incidence of sexually transmitted disease and thus in the abstract appeared to be at relatively low risk for HIV. Moreover, researchers appeared to believe that sex between two women was so gentle and nonejaculatory it really wasn't sex at all; certainly, it seemed much too wholesome to transmit so lethal a virus as HIV. Despite scientific and populist arguments to the contrary (including a women's "kiss-in" staged for scientists at the 1989 International Conference on AIDS in Montreal), no surveillance categories for "female-to-female transmission" or "lesbian" were established, and little thought was given to the educational or social needs of women whose main sexual contacts were with other women. Faced with the factual evidence of HIV-positive lesbians, investigators had three available alternatives: assign the case to one of the "not women" categories (intravenous drug user, etc.); assume that she was not "really" a lesbian and had been infected by a male partner; or assume that she had engaged in "deviant" sexual activities (not wholesome, not gentle) and was therefore "not normal." Confusion over the category "homosexual" had initially led some to believe that male and female homosexuals were at equal risk for AIDS and equally dangerous (hence lesbians, along with gay men, were asked to refrain from giving blood). Moreover, the medical literature periodically produced isolated reports of HIV transmission by way of female-to-female sexual contact (Marmor et al. [1986] and Sabatini et al. [1984] are the obligatory citations), virtually always documenting some element of perceived "deviance": S/M, "rough sex," fisting, or some other activity associated with the most extreme stereotypes of gay male sexual practices.[16] More informed researchers pointed out that "lesbian" was as complicated a category as "homosexual" and that behavior or self-perceived identity could not be predicted from the label "lesbian"; some self-identified lesbians have sex with men, some might be at risk through having chosen to be artificially inseminated, some use drugs, and so on (Shaw and Paleo 1987; see also Reinisch et al. 1988; and Appleman and Kahn 1989).[17]

In sum, then, for all these reasons, women were excluded from the ubiquitous AIDS risk-group pie charts—bracketed as pass-throughs, as individual exceptions or special populations, as always already diseased or blandly uninteresting, or as mere medical surrogates for their male partners, children, and the "general population."[18] Case by case, risk by risk, reason by reason, women's exclusion from the statistics added up to a classic Catch-22 for women as a population: their absence from the AIDS picture could be refuted only with evidence; but their absence meant that no evidence would be gathered. As an issue for women, AIDS unnamed meant AIDS unclaimed.

In sharp contrast to this body of dominant theory and practice, an alternative account of the epidemic was elsewhere under construction, an account that sought to name and claim the epidemic on behalf of women. *Alternative account* may imply too organized a project. Rather, for most of the 1980s, a loose network of researchers, clinicians, social service advocates, women's health practitioners, women with AIDS, AIDS advocates and activists, and writers and journalists focused on "AIDS and the woman question." Described in part by Gena Corea (1992), this "network" represented women concerned about AIDS/HIV and women and dissatisfied with their shadowy presence in the literature as "prostitutes," "mothers of infants with AIDS," "heterosexuals," or "none of the above." The researchers in this network—themselves predominantly women—would continue to study women, including "prostitutes," throughout the decade (and beyond), attempting to sort out the muddle of terms and categories applied, sometimes interchangeably, to women with or at risk for AIDS/HIV, to investigate empirically why and how some women were developing HIV infection and AIDS and others were not, to explore what countermeasures science and medicine could develop, to reconceptualize AIDS as a gendered epidemic, and to call this to the world's attention.[19]

One of the first papers on AIDS and gender did not appear to be about gender at all. Authored by Robin Flam and Zena Stein, "Behavior, Infection, and Immune Response: An Epidemiological Approach" was published in Feldman and Johnson (1986) (the book was conceived in November 1983 and went to press in November 1985). The paper argued that a complex epidemiological model—of the kind characteristically applied to chronic diseases—was more useful for understanding the AIDS epidemic than the simpler single-organism model used for infectious disease. Flam and Stein identify the broad goals of epidemiological studies: "to describe the characteristics of a disease, discover its cause, and eventually interrupt the causal chain to make possible prevention of the disease" (Flam and Stein 1986, 62). The cogent review that follows could have been titled "How to Do Epidemiology in the AIDS Epidemic," so clearly does it present known data (as of mid-1984, to judge by the citations), existing etiological hypotheses, and proposals for testing them analytically. What the paper does not do—what, the authors emphasize, it cannot do—is propose how to "interrupt the causal chain." Why? Too many key issues remain unresolved. With respect to women, they argued, we need to determine the role and weight of cofactors that shape comparative risk of HIV according to gender: How much sexual interaction takes place across "circles of sexual contact"? How robust is the immune system? What is the role of anal intercourse for women? What can cause immune breakdown in the absence of HIV? Until such questions are answered, it is impossible to develop an explicit causal model of AIDS, a project of enormous theoretical and practical importance. "Although biological research relating to a single agent is mandatory, attention must also be given to the other factors in the web of causation." We cannot successfully intervene, they conclude, "until a carefully formulated model, which attributes to each cofactor its own share of input, is derived" (p. 73).

In chapter 5, I say that a similar and much more visible role in the AIDS epidemic has been played by the physician Joseph Sonnabend, who repeatedly inventoried critical issues not yet settled. As time marched on and virology and clinical treatments took center stage, some of these questions were eventually answered through some decent science as well as scientific and technical progress. Other answers emerged through trial and error, lucky guesswork, political and economic expediency, and the sheer accumulation of voices asserting that various questions need not be asked because we already knew the answers. But many of these questions remain unanswered still. (For a sample, see Fujimura and Chou [1994], Katz [1993], and Epstein [1996].) Stein and Flam were arguing that theoretical and conceptual clarity about fundamental questions should guide the plan for answering them. Rereading the paper more than a decade later is sobering, particularly in view of the financial support its authors did not receive. Just as Shilts (1987) cataloged the humiliating experiences of fine scientists like Jay Levy in their early quests for AIDS research funding, Corea (1992) chronicles the failures of women researchers proposing to study AIDS in women. Levy, one of the premier AIDS scientists today, eventually obtained adequate funding for his work. Flam and Stein, repeatedly turned down for even modest grant proposals on AIDS and gender, published the 1986 paper to bring closure to their work and thinking and move on. Other researchers on gender encountered similar difficulties with both funding and publication, often presenting their work at conferences and publishing in specialized collections rather than mainstream biomedical journals.

Of great significance, then, was the April 1987 publication of the first paper on AIDS and women—women explicitly *as* women—in a leading peer-reviewed journal: the *Journal of the American Medical Association* (although the AMA was far from a leading light in the struggle against AIDS at this point [Wolinsky and Brune 1994], publication in *JAMA* was a landmark). In "The Epidemiology of AIDS in Women," coauthors Mary Guinan and Ann Hardy reviewed the 1,819 cases of AIDS in women officially reported in the United States between 1981 and 1986. Within the risk group of *heterosexual contacts of persons at risk*, the percentage of women had increased from 12 to 26 percent between 1982 and 1986 (*heterosexual contact* was the only transmission category at that point in which women outnumbered men). More than 70 percent of women with AIDS were black or Hispanic; more than 80 percent were of childbearing age.

Although they did so in sober academic prose, Guinan and Hardy critiqued the epidemiological model of collecting, representing, and reporting data about risk and prevalence, the problems of categories and classification, the risk-factor hierarchy and exclusion of dual or overlapping categories, problematic terminology about women, and the difficulty of tracking data on women when no tracking mechanisms existed. (Corea's index cites nineteen separate entries under the heading *CDC's refusal to track AIDS and HIV in women* [1992, 346].) Implicitly challenging the Langone-type claim that "a healthy vagina" protected against HIV infection, they argued that knowledge about vaginal health and "portals of entry" was very incomplete; hence, to distinguish between anal and vaginal portals was premature and potentially dangerous. "If the virus can pass through intact mucous membranes," they warned, "the risk of transmission through the vagina or rectum may not be different."[20]

Other voices helped amplify such challenges to conventional assumptions about definition, identity, and representation involving women. At the time the Guinan and Hardy paper appeared, Project AWARE (Association for Women's AIDS Research and Education) in San Francisco had already been carrying out a longitudinal study to assess HIV antibody seroprevalence in high-risk women in California; "high risk" was defined as women reporting five or more sexual partners in the previous five years or sexual contact with a high-risk male, and the study encompassed both prostitutes and nonprostitutes (as identified by the women themselves). Directed by Judith Cohen and Constance Wofsy, the project (invariably called "the prostitute study" by their male colleagues, reports Corea [1992, 44]) included less than one-third of women who defined themselves as prostitutes. In contrast to mainstream research, this community-based project had asked its potential research subjects to participate in the process of designing the research. The researchers learned—as community-based researchers in the AIDS treatment field would later learn—that study participants wanted, among other things, to be interviewed by people like themselves; they wanted anonymity available for those who requested it; they wanted meetings in their own neighborhoods rather than in some distant clinic; they wanted feedback from the study; and, when appropriate, they wanted medical and social service referrals (Cohen 1987; Corea 1992, 87).

Nancy S. Stoller (then Nancy Shaw), a sociologist at the San Francisco AIDS Foundation, carried out a number of studies of AIDS and women, attempting to sort out the various factors that put women at risk of or protected them from HIV. Working with modest institutional resources, Shaw and Lyn Paleo were among the first researchers to challenge the view that prostitution per se necessarily put women at high risk of HIV, citing evidence suggesting that prostitutes were at greater risk not because they had multiple sex partners but because they were likely to use intravenous drugs or have less access to health care. In their preliminary reports, and in later published work, Shaw and Paleo emphasized the importance of considering the two issues as related, but distinct:

> There is no evidence that prostitutes constitute a special risk category.... Some prostitutes do get AIDS. To the extent that researchers have been able to isolate prostitution and/or multiple sexual contacts from such issues as IV drug use, however, neither the number of sexual contacts nor the receipt of money for sex ... seems to put women at a higher risk for getting AIDS. Many women who are in paid sexual activity were concerned about sexually transmitted diseases even before the AIDS epidemic. They protected themselves and continue to protect themselves by being somewhat alert to new medical developments in sexually transmitted diseases and how to avoid them (Shaw and Paleo 1987, 144)

Kreiss and her colleagues (Kreiss et al. 1986) found, similarly, that, among the ninety female prostitutes whom they studied in Nairobi, presence of the HIV antibody was not significantly associated with the number of sexual encounters per year; other nonrelevant factors included age, duration of prostitution, nationality, history of immunizations, injections of medication within the past five years, transfusions, scarification, operations, induced abortions, and dental extractions. Sexual exposure to partners of different nationalities, however, was associated with HIV seropositivity. Other researchers reinforced these data, noting that most prostitute-john encounters are single episodes, with oral rather than vaginal sexual contact predominating (e.g., Center for Women Policy Studies, cited in Corea 1992, 163). Spending as much time as anyone talking with and testing prostitutes on the street, the New York City physician Joyce Wallace confirmed the predominance of oral sex; profiled in the *New Yorker* magazine in 1993, Wallace commented that the nation's move to more economical, gas-efficient cars in the 1970s had an unanticipated payoff in the 1980s: a blow job was a lot easier to manage than sexual intercourse in a small Japanese car (Goldsmith 1993). Service groups like the Women and AIDS Resource Network (WARN) in New York, directed by Marie St. Cyr, were likewise trying to bring attention to the problem of women and AIDS. Women with AIDS were organizing as well: in prisons (for the history of AIDS work in the Bedford Hills Correctional Facility, see Corea [1992]); in brothels (in Nevada, e.g., prostitutes asked in March 1986 that clients be required to wear condoms [Campbell 1991]); and in the development of AIDS policy (see Griffen 1994).

Taken together, these studies, along with the review articles available by the late 1980s (including Schneider 1988a, 1992; Stephens 1988; Cohen and Wofsy 1989; Campbell 1990b), confirm my inventory in this chapter of the cultural stereotypes, unexamined or sloppy language, basic empirical questions left unanswered, and omissions that distorted the representation and role of gender in mainstream research. As I have suggested, when data relevant to women were reported, the word *women* was rarely included in abstracts and indexes: instead, we find *heterosexuals, prostitutes, pediatric AIDS, mothers of pediatric AIDS victims, sexual partners,* and the like. Talk about the worst of both worlds: women had no identities of their own, but, by the almost postfeminist 1980s, U.S. women didn't even rate the old-fashioned chauvinist rhetoric in which innocent womenfolk needed to be protected from the evils of the VD menace. In conference proceedings and edited collections, too, women were usually elsewhere, under some other name—often, one suspects, placed there by the editors rather than the authors. In 1987, I criticized researchers themselves for this tendency—including Guinan and Hardy's (1987) statement that it was important to study women as an index to HIV prevalence in "the general heterosexual population."[21] But, as Corea's (1992) investigation makes clear, the underlying reality was that, like research on so many dimensions of women's health and women's lives, proposed research on women and AIDS was simply not funded; hence, researchers were forced to piggyback their concerns about women onto subjects deemed more legitimate for research funding.

Steven Epstein (1996) argues that the strength of the gay male construction of the AIDS epidemic forced gay men to confront the epidemic; and to confront it was, necessarily, to claim it. One consequence of this claim was that gay men began, early on, to criticize the academic terminology through which they were being represented. Terms like *promiscuous* were forced to give way, at least in regularly scrutinized publications like the *Morbidity and Mortality Weekly Report*, to more neutral terms like *sexually active*. In the representation of women, however, it was as though the women's health movement, with its exhaustive linguistic critique of gender in scientific and medical discourse, had never existed. I return to this point below, suggesting that this critique was alive and well in various activist venues but, like much of the feminist research just mentioned, without the resources fully to override more prominent discourses.[22]

In the last chapter, I noted the conviction of some scientists that AIDS could not be caused by a sexually transmitted agent because homosexual men lacked any appropriate bodily orifice through which an agent could enter. Similar convictions filtered out evidence about women or heterosexual transmission. Although, in interviews and media appearances, the CDC sometimes attempted to counter the commonsense notion of the epidemic and provide more flexible understandings of its definitions and categories and its sound bites performed certain kinds of important cultural work, this did not include educating the public about how epidemiological knowledge is produced. The decree evolved, for example, that "HIV is an equal opportunity virus"—admirably democratic, and in some contexts virologically correct, but for most people neither very enlightening nor descriptive of what they were seeing around them or in the media. How could an equal opportunity epidemic be homosexual in one place and heterosexual in another? If HIV is equal opportunity, why has it not infected sexually active populations like college students, many of whom are doing high-risk things? Basic concepts needed their own sound bites— concepts like *incidence is related to prevalence*, or *it's a virus, and if it isn't around, it won't infect you*, or *behaviors can be placed on a continuum of probabilities for transmission*, or *other STDs aren't so great to have either*, or *the production of knowledge is not the same as the production of certainty*. Instead of preparing the way for the accumulation of knowledge and the gradual elimination of areas of uncertainty, knowledge was doled out in discrete installments and repeated again and again, like the Reagan White House "word of the day," until supplanted.

As Shilts cataloged so persuasively, of course, for much of the 1980s the CDC's AIDS budget was shamefully inadequate and its staff small and overworked. Like other agencies, institutions, and services struggling with the epidemic, the CDC was at the mercy of government funding, and the government had no mercy. Recalling that the jet Rock Hudson chartered to Paris for treatment in 1985 cost more than the total budget for the last four years of the French clinical researcher he was consulting (Shilts 1987,

580), we might turn instead to the private sector, in the form of the U.S. media, and ask what it was doing in the war.

The Media's "AIDS Patient"

AIDS Carrier's Baby Free from Virus, Gov't Confirms.—headline, *Japan Times*, 1987

The article was tricky to write. I could say *homosexual* but I couldn't say *gay*. [I] had to be very coy about sex and about who put what where.—Robin Marantz Henig, on writing about AIDS for the *New York Times* in 1983

While women have never been formally nominated as a "risk group" by epidemiology, they have . . . been nevertheless denied a secure position within the "general population."—Catherine Waldby, *AIDS and the Body Politic*

Media coverage of AIDS offers a barometer of what is considered important at different points in time and illustrates typical strategies for "disambiguating" conflicting information from researchers. As Epstein argues, the media take on special importance in biomedical controversies by creating, through the use of special mediagenic spokespersons, a parallel system of informal credentials: "Media designations of who counts as a spokesperson do not simply *mirror* the internal stratification of a social movement or a scientific community, but can even *construct* such hierarchies" (Epstein 1996, 335). So media coverage cannot be simply taken as a record of the epidemic—although of course it serves this function—but must also be counted as a participant. In the case of AIDS, the U.S. media clearly played a significant role not only in reporting and interpreting biomedical accounts of the epidemic but also in constructing the reality that the public would perceive. As media research makes clear, for example, the sharp spikes of increased coverage in the 1980s mainly represented the media's own ideas of what constituted "a story." The surges in 1983, 1985, and 1987 were precipitated, respectively, by the "routine household contact" scare, Rock Hudson's AIDS, and the "heterosexual spread of AIDS" panic. (The greatest surge of all occurred in 1991, when the basketball star Earvin "Magic" Johnson announced that he had tested positive for HIV and was retiring from the game).[23]

Of all these events, media observers tend to agree with Shilts (1987) that Rock Hudson's illness and death was the event that separated life before AIDS in the United States from everything that came after it (of course, Shilts's judgment could not have taken Magic's 1991 announcement into account, an event that surpassed all others in media coverage of AIDS and that for African Americans certainly marked "life after AIDS" more than Rock Hudson's had). For biomedical science, the Hudson case, in and of itself, did not change prevailing conceptions of AIDS or the AIDS patient. Rock Hudson may have been a movie star, but he was also a canonical person with AIDS: a gay man who had engaged with other gay men in sexual behavior now understood to increase the risk of viral exposure. But, for the media and the public at large, Hudson's illness and death changed their notion of who the AIDS patient was and constituted a critical turning point in the evolution of consciousness about AIDS—increasing the average number of AIDS stories per month in major media outlets from 18 to 111 (Dearing and Rogers 1988) and increasing newspaper coverage by 270 percent (Alwood 1996, 234). For our old friend the general public, the sheer quantity of coverage undoubtedly raised awareness and understanding of the epidemic.

Rock Hudson's announcement was not the only media event of 1985 that shaped coverage and helped build an AIDS media vocabulary. In April, Larry Kramer's play about the epidemic, *The Normal Heart*, opened in New York. Designed to assault and shock its audiences, the production took on the federal government, the New York City and State governments, health care institutions, and the media, especially the *New York Times*, whose drama critic, Frank Rich, called the play "a fiercely polemical drama about the private and public fallout of the AIDS epidemic" (cited by Kinsella 1989, 78). In doing so, Rich joined Kramer in castigating the media in general and the *New York Times* in particular for its failure to cover the epidemic (for further discussion of the *Times*'s coverage, see Kinsella [1989] and Alwood [1996]). But Kramer's play cast women as stereotypically nurturing, a quality that draws only contempt from the play's Kramer-like hero, Ned Weeks, when it is displayed by the gay male characters (whom Weeks denounces as "sissies" and "Florence Nightingales").

In July 1985, *Life* magazine's first cover story on AIDS made a major— some would say notorious—contribution to the iconography of the epidemic. In living color, photographs of people with AIDS stared out at the reader: an African-American soldier in uniform, saluting; the Burks, a white all-American nuclear family (father, mother, daughter, baby son); and an attractive young blonde woman. In bold red letters, the cover warned that "NOW NO ONE IS SAFE FROM AIDS." The story (Barnes and Hollister 1985) reported that the soldier had been infected through a blood transfusion, the family through the blood product given the father to treat his hemophilia, and the young woman through sex with a bisexual man who had since died of AIDS. As in Rock Hudson's case, these examples

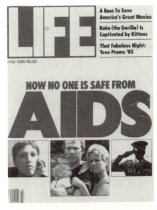

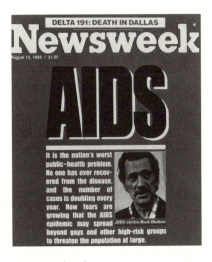

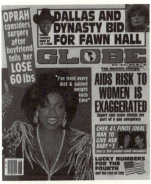

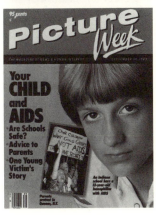

Despite Life's dramatic cover assertion, "Now No One Is Safe from AIDS" (2.1: July 1985), the people pictured with AIDS represented known "risk groups": recipients of blood transfusions, men with hemophilia and their sexual partners, infants born to infected mothers, and sexual partners of bisexual men. Nevertheless, they did not look like the stereotypical "4-H Club" members the public expected. The Burk family, in particular, looked like everything we had been told AIDS was not and never could be. Newsweek's bright red Rock Hudson cover the following month gained overnight fame and infamy (2.2: 12 August 1985). Widely reproduced, it was hailed as AIDS's big break into the media mainstream, reviled as sensationalistic "celebrity AIDS," embraced by network news shows as a seemly graphic icon for the epidemic, and even cast in a cameo role in NBC's An Early Frost (1985): Gena Rowlands shakes the magazine at Ben Gazarra to stress the widespread availability of AIDS information. Throughout the epidemic, media cover stories more typically featured people other than gay men (2.3: Ryan White on cover of Picture Week, 30 September 1985; 2.4: "AIDS Risk to Women Exaggerated," Globe, 30 June 1987).

were not unusual. All represented acknowledged, well-established modes of transmission. Yet the visual shorthand was new. Gone were the pairs of gay men in the Castro, arms entwined, usually photographed from the back; gone was the gay man with AIDS in his apartment, sick, backlit, and alone; gone were the prostitutes working the street at night, usually wearing red. In their place, *Life* showed nuclear families, "innocent victims," and middle-American patriots. Widely criticized for sensationalism and for grossly misrepresenting the actual epidemiology of the epidemic, the *Life* story was framed by a message from Judith Daniels, acting managing editor, explaining the magazine's decision to put AIDS, rather than happy families celebrating the holiday with parades and fireworks, on its July cover. The cover illustration made visual the magazine's position: "AIDS is a problem for all." An effort was made, in other words, to articulate AIDS to important elements of a liberal democracy—we're all equal, we're in this together, we are family—and to freight the "faces of AIDS" on the cover (including, notably, the soldier in uniform) with the patriotic symbolism of the Fourth of July. "I'm sorry we couldn't give you a cheerful cover story," Daniels's editorial column concluded. "I hope you can handle a strong one" (Daniels 1985).

On 11 November 1985, NBC broadcast *An Early Frost*, the first feature-length drama about AIDS on network television. With a well-known cast, a good script, accurate medical information, and unquestionably tasteful policing of desire, *An Early Frost* was widely acclaimed. Promoted as a family drama about a vital public health issue, the movie captured a third of the viewing audience and moved thousands of viewers to call a toll-free information line after the program. In chapters 4 and 6 below, I discuss AIDS in movies and television at greater length. Here, I want to emphasize the choice made by the network and the program's producers to represent AIDS as a public health crisis. Although *An Early Frost* was what could be called an AIDS movie for straight people, its protagonist was nevertheless an appealing gay man whose sympathetic portrayal reinforced the change following Hudson's announcement to more sympathetic portrayals of people with AIDS. This particular made-for-TV movie also carried out the cultural work of narrative television programming, described by Sharf and Freimuth (1993) as dramatizing debates and conflicts over topical issues, offering the audience through a well-choreographed assemblage of characters an array of positions toward AIDS. The movie also illustrated media coverage of media coverage. *Newsweek*'s bold red Hudson cover, for example, was carried in one scene by the Gena Rowlands character to make the point that AIDS was an important public health crisis and that information about it was widely available (in the original script, written before the Rock Hudson announcement, the character was to be shown researching AIDS at the library).

A growing body of media scholarship documents the evolution and implications of AIDS coverage. David C. Colby and Timothy E. Cook (1991, 1992) used nightly television news coverage of AIDS during the 1980s to examine the media's role in public agenda setting, that is, in creating a short list of problems deemed worthy, by the public and by policymakers, of attention and resolution. Colby and Cook usefully distinguish "event-driven" media coverage—news organizations' routine approach to AIDS, which relies largely on authoritative, medical, scientific, or political official sources to identify what is newsworthy—from "topic-driven saturation coverage," in which reporters actively seek stories, showing initiative and covering fresh angles of the epidemic. Although media coverage of AIDS after Rock Hudson's death gradually subsided from saturation to routine, the media blitz, in Colby and Cook's view, had at least five separate but linked effects: (1) although the total number of stories declined, they came earlier in the broadcast, often as leads; (2) once established as newsworthy, AIDS made available story lines for multiple journalists across multiple beats (e.g., medical, science, political, law, foreign, domestic, regional); (3) multiple perspectives meant less consensus about the bottom line, about what AIDS meant; (4) lack of consensus triggered a revival of earlier story lines (e.g., the safety of the blood supply), keeping many dimensions of the epidemic alive at any one time (Dearing and Rogers [1988] identify thirteen distinct subissues within AIDS media coverage, each with its own ebb and flow); and (5) AIDS media coverage became receptive to a different and more diverse range of authoritative sources (see also Perlman 1989). In contrast to 1983 and 1984, when, dominated by medical and political sources, media reports converged on a reassuring narrative of dogged mastery and control, these new sources, including people with AIDS, gay activists, and frontline caretakers, were more likely to express skepticism or pessimism about the course of the epidemic. What might Colby and Cook's inventory mean for women? It might have meant that women's media, by the early 1980s a significant network of outlets, took on the epidemic as an issue for women, covering scientific and medical attention to women, monitoring laws and policy, articulating the experience of women affected by AIDS, and as feminists— like the other more diverse post-Hudson sources noted by Colby and Cook—challenging and disrupting the smooth unfolding of the narrative of biomedical mastery. Instead, women remained a minor blip in the subissue list of several domains but a major issue for virtually no one.

What this centrist reporting meant was that, for most of the 1980s,

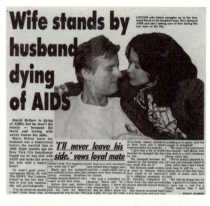

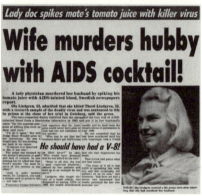

Although cases of women with AIDS were reported early on, media AIDS stories mainly cast women in secondary or traditional roles as mates and caretakers. Maria Hefner was prototypical: she knew her partner, David, was bisexual, but love conquered all. She and David made national news in January 1987 after they learned that he had AIDS and sought to be married in a religious ceremony in St. Patrick's Cathedral. The Weekly World News *(17 February 1987, 17) shows "loving wife Maria" caring for David "during the last days of his life" (2.5). A few months later, the same tabloid (12 May 1987) cast Swedish physician Ola Lindgren as a literal "AIDS carrier" (2.6). Convinced that her husband was holding back her career, the story claimed, this enterprising "lady doc" toted the virus home from a hospital lab and spiked his tomato juice. Unconcerned with whether oral administration of HIV could in fact kill someone, the tabloid shows "sneaky" Lindgren smiling; murdered by an "AIDS cocktail," innocent "hubby" gets the tabloid fate he deserves for marrying an ambitious professional woman: a Madison Avenue epitaph.*

popular and media images of women and AIDS drew their identities from long-familiar narratives: the loyal companion who stands by her man ("AIDS VICTIM TO WED IN ST. PATRICK'S CATHEDRAL"); the scheming carrier who deliberately infects her male victim ("WIFE MURDERS HUBBY WITH AIDS COCKTAIL"); the moral crusader, like former Illinois State Representative Penny Pullen, whose draconian legislative proposals offered her Northshore Chicago constituency the illusion of control; the Madonna (who cured a man with AIDS at Lourdes but made it clear [said the man] that no remission would be granted to nonbelievers); the whore ("CINCY PROSTITUTES FEARED SPREADING AIDS"); the innocent victim (said Kimberly Bergalis's father: "Her sickness would have been easier to accept if she'd been a slut or a drug user. But she had everything right"); the transparent vessel ("BABY BORN TO AIDS CARRIER FREE OF VIRUS, GOV'T CONFIRMS"). Perhaps the predominant image has been of the loving mother, wife, or caretaker whose presence serves to humanize and desexualize the infected (gay) man, a role she shares in photographs with stuffed animals and pets. In general, these stories serve dually as a warning and as a reassurance. Even the rash of "spread-of-AIDS" stories in late 1986 and 1987 managed ultimately to give a reassuring spin to the statistics—largely by replicating the ambiguities and confusions that I have already identified here.

Again, then, with few exceptions, popular images of women and AIDS/ HIV have been marked by the same contradictions as other discourses: stock characters, stereotypes, and exceptions are given unwarranted visibility; real women at risk, real women with HIV and AIDS, are invisible or alibied. These contradictions are particularly obtuse in media images directed explicitly toward "women at risk" and "women with AIDS." Sexually active women of color in urban U.S. settings are perhaps the population most in need of AIDS education, yet they have rarely been written about or pictured except in ways that echo the stereotypes inventoried above. Sex workers are repeatedly represented in photographs, however, almost always wearing red, despite little evidence that their occupation per se puts them at risk or contributes significantly to the spread of HIV. *Newsweek*, for example, showed prostitutes "working the street," bathed in red light; the caption, masterfully hedging its bets, warned, "Some experts fear that prostitutes might turn out to be carriers who could further fuel the epidemic" (12 August 1985, 28). While such images avoid stigmatizing or stereotyping women who do have AIDS and send the important message that, despite stereotypes about the epidemic, many kinds of people are potentially at risk, they also reinforce the incorrect message to women of color and others that they are *not* at risk.

In addition to the images that I have mentioned, other visual contradictions compounded the confusion over gender. Jan Zita Grover and Douglas Crimp, among others, have dissected the tradition of high modernist studio portraits of people with AIDS, Nicholas Nixon's (Nixon and Nixon 1991) photographs a leading example, in which the "AIDS victim," posed in backlit solitude, appears to transcend individual rage, hope, and suffering and contemplates death (see, e.g., Crimp 1992). Another kind of visual

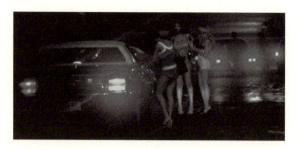

Driven by the discursive burdens of history, early versions of the epidemic targeted female sex workers as likely "reservoirs of contagion." Lacking evidence for this premise, Newsweek *nonetheless ran an ominous, murky photograph of prostitutes "working the streets"; the caption hedged its bets with a string of sub-junctives (2.7: 12 August 1985, 28; courtesy of Ethan Hoffmann Archive).*

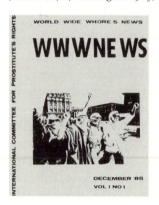
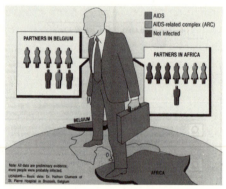

Real-life sex workers, meanwhile, were working both to challenge the premise and to prevent it from coming true. The premier issue of World Wide Whores News *was produced for a 1985 international conference of sex workers in Amsterdam that called on national governments to recognize the threat of* AIDS *to sex workers, pass and enforce strict requirements for condom use by clients, provide adequate health coverage, and involve sex workers in developing* STD *ed-ucation and intervention campaigns (2.8: December 1985). Rarely has the* AIDS *literature targeted a heterosexual male as the "Patient Zero" of a disease cluster. An exception is a case identified by the Belgian scientist Nathan Clumeck and graphically illustrated in* U.S. News and World Report *(2.9: 12 January 1987, 65).*

shorthand linked the person with AIDS to warmer, wholesome, and senti-mental emblems, having him or her appear with a family member (usually the mother), a houseplant, or—most common of all—a pet (dog, cat, bunny) or stuffed animal. Many photographs showed Rock Hudson surrounded by his dogs (manly dogs—in contrast to images of Liberace with his beloved whippets); the reporter George Whitmore's (1988) personal account of his struggle with HIV infection identifies a teddy bear as a recurrent talisman of hope for him (as for many gay men), while a large color photograph shows Whitmore with his cat. Even a "celebrity PWA" like Ryan White was photographed for *Picture Week* (30 September 1985, 36) with a kitten lounging artistically in his hair. Obviously, warm and fuzzy imagery renders the person with AIDS sympathetically and shows up in media representations from *American Medical News* to the tabloids. But such images may also serve to infantilize, desexualize, decriminalize, and prescribe the humanistic embrace of a "beautiful death" (James 1994, xxvii–xxix). (To refuse this linkage—i.e., to disarticulate AIDS from the gentle journey into that good night—the editors of the acidic 1990s PWA publication *Diseased Pariah News* would later commemorate the death of their founding editor by burning mass quantities of teddy bears and photographing the flaming pile for the cover.) But what to do about women with AIDS, already established as interchangeable with teddy bears? Rarely given the stark Everyman role, most women photographed with AIDS were generally more robust than men with AIDS. Teddy bears and stuffed animals did figure in some photographs. Candice Mossop, a Canadian woman with AIDS, was photographed by the newsmagazine *Macleans* (31 August 1986, 34) resting on a sofa in a satin robe surrounded by heaps of teddy bears. For a story on single women dealing with AIDS and safe sex, *People* (14 March 1988, 104) included a photograph of a woman on a bed with her cats; shot from above, the composition could be taken to mean that a pet is the only safe bedroom companion in this dangerous age; at the same time, the text tends to portray AIDS as a nonproblem for postfeminist women or, if a problem, strictly one of individual choice. Still later, a *New York Times* photograph by Sara Krulwich (in L. Altman 1989, 28) shows Della, a woman with AIDS in a New York City hospital, very much at ease in her hospital bed; in this more normalized vision (I think this photograph should have won a prize), the patient smokes a cigarette and talks on the phone, a nurse stands by to take her temperature, and a stuffed animal is propped inconspicuously in the corner.

Oddly, however, the sins attributed to mainstream representations of AIDS in media coverage and popular culture are linked to their virtues. The uniformity of mainstream media coverage (particularly on the three major broadcast networks) made for nearly a decade of safe, clichéd, heterosexist pieties that largely reproduced conventional humanist orthodoxies. But the same centrist uniformity ensured that airtime would mainly be denied to overt extremist hysteria, homophobic quarantine and tattooing schemes, or wild LaRouche-type claims that AIDS was invented by Queen Elizabeth II and the Trilateral Commission. In the years to come, the media would often assert that women were as vulnerable to HIV as men—and just as categorically assert that they were not. (By the mid-1990s, when women began to account for more new infections and AIDS cases than men, authorities asserted that women had long been known to be more vulnerable to HIV.) As I noted in chapter 1 above, John Langone's (1985) article in *Discover* was the most forceful and influential of these efforts; arguing that the virus could penetrate the "vulnerable rectum" but not the "rugged vagina," Langone concluded that "AIDS remains the fatal price of anal intercourse" (p. 52). Other experts played their own version of is she or isn't she, with some espousing Langone's view, others disputing it, others admitting that they didn't know.

All these are isolated instances. As Catherine Warren and I note in our chronological review of media coverage of AIDS and women (Treichler and Warren 1998), media attention to AIDS was steadily increasing (by the end of 1983, the general media had published seventy-seven articles on the epidemic), but evidence of AIDS and AIDS-related conditions in women was almost wholly ignored. In 1984, a total of seventy articles on AIDS appeared, most of them (fifty-two) medical in nature, a focus partially brought about by the isolation of a virus (discussed in chap. 1 above) said to be the agent responsible for AIDS. Although a few titles left open the possibility that both sexes might be affected by AIDS, no articles explicitly focused on women or included them by name (*women*) in the statistics. Although "safe sex" was mentioned and advocated for the first time in 1984, the development of the ELISA test for antibodies to the virus almost immediately deflected attention from sexual behavior and even gender to a view that "anxious heterosexuals" could get regularly tested. In November 1986, the *New York Times* spelled out AIDS's lessons to date. Women were "obliged to take on a new kind of responsibility for their sexuality and to reassess their roles as health professionals, relatives, lovers and friends of people with AIDS." No lesson was offered to men, straight or otherwise. Above all, media coverage represents successive missed opportunities that could have been used to educate, to communicate the epidemic's complications, and to change the terms of the debate from one about dichotomy to one about a continuum of probability.

Nowhere were media recuperation efforts more evident than in the "heterosexual spread of AIDS" stories of 1986 and 1987. "Suddenly," proclaimed the 12 January 1987 issue of *U.S. News and World Report*, "the disease of *them* is the disease of *us*." The magazine's cover graphic represented "us" as a young white urban professional man and woman, a graph

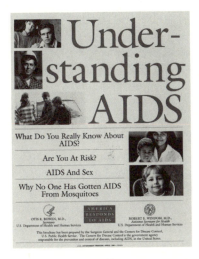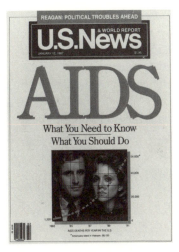

U.S. News and World Report's *cover visually reconstructs the disease of Them as the disease of Us and compares the epidemic's death toll to that of Americans in Vietnam (2.10: 12 January 1987). While the war comparison has remained surprisingly rare in the mainstream media, the "equal opportunity" depiction of the epidemic took hold. The Helms amendment reinforced this emphasis by prohibiting any federally funded AIDS education efforts that might "promote or encourage, directly or indirectly, homosexual sexual activities." As ads, posters, and public service announcements blanketed the country over the years, information was provided to virtually everyone but those most devastated and vulnerable: homosexual men. A case in point was* Understanding AIDS, *the U.S. surgeon general's (1988) last-ditch effort to publicize the epidemic nationwide (2.11). Despite conservative opposition, Helms's constraints, and various glitches, the brochure eventually reached—and was read in—millions of American households. Scrutinizing the publication microscopically for any sign of a gay-friendly subtext, friends of mine finally settled on the guy in the hard hat as the closest they'd get. If gay men infected with HIV today decided to file a class-action lawsuit against Helms and his henchpersons,* Understanding AIDS *could be evidence, for, as Senator Lowell Weicker had predicted in his 1987 opposition to the Helms amendment, "If the knowledge is not transmitted, these people are going to be dead, dead" (*Congressional Record *133 [14 October 1987]: S14209).*

of rising AIDS deaths cutting across their faces. A more interesting and potentially more productive link was less obvious than the us/them symbolism. Accompanying the cover image and graph of rising AIDS deaths (correctly predicted in 1987 to total 54,000 by 1991), a note indicated the total number of Americans killed in Vietnam: 58,135. Ultimately, of course, the death toll of the AIDS epidemic would surpass the number of U.S. combat deaths in Vietnam, Korea, and two world wars combined. As in the *Life* cover story, this powerful link to war and the patriotic effort required to defeat it was never developed in any sustained or productive way in the mainstream media. Rather, the *U.S. News and World Report* story shifted signifieds inside: here, the running total of U.S. AIDS cases was graphed against the New York skyline, seeming to shoot dramatically up through New York City apartment buildings into the sky (McAuliffe et al., 1987). The graphic was confusing and could almost be read as a story about real estate, a possibility fortified by an accompanying box listing "AIDS hot spots"—that is, U.S. cities with a high prevalence of AIDS cases ranging from New York (91 reported AIDS cases per 100,000 population) to Chicago (9 per 100,000). The more obvious reading of these collective representations linked AIDS, urban areas, and the heterosexual yuppies on the cover, and this, indeed, was the meaning that most broadly prevailed in late 1986 and early 1987, when the grave danger to and supposed explosion of AIDS among heterosexuals became big news for virtually all the major U.S. news outlets: stories on the threat to "all of us" appeared in *Newsweek, Time,* and the *Atlantic* as well as *Scientific American* and the *Village Voice.* Stock television footage of "gay street scenes" gave way to footage of heterosexual urban street scenes and nonurban images. A story on ABC (19 March 1987) signaled the change by cutting from a New York street scene to a scene of a man and a woman walking and nuzzling in a rural field. In a four-part series beginning 19 March 1987, the *New York Times* gave front-page coverage to several dimensions of AIDS; in another significant narrative shift, the boilerplate paragraph in each story made no mention of gay men or intravenous drug users. Although these groups were prominently discussed in the stories themselves, they were no longer considered intrinsic to the definition of AIDS (Kinsella 1989; Alwood 1996). During this period, only a few publications discussed the increased cases among minorities and minority women (the *Village Voice* article "Straight Shooters" [Barrett 1985] was an example); minority statistics were generally ignored or used to argue, as I said above, that "real women don't get AIDS." An exception was Richard Goldstein's (1987a) *Village Voice* piece on AIDS and race.

In Chapter 8 below, I return to the problems of identity and its representation in biomedical and media discourses, the long-term logistical morass created by these statistical and definitional practices, and the disastrous structural consequences of leaving women behind. Some closing comments about general media coverage, however, come from a comprehensive review of AIDS coverage in leading print and broadcast media from 1985 to 1996 by the Kaiser Family Foundation and Princeton Survey

Research (Kaiser Family Foundation 1996). The media's major effect in the 1980s, the report concludes, was to inform the public about the epidemic, especially about prevention and transmission. By 1989, this genre of coverage had "topped out," and the media could do little more until the Magic Johnson story in November 1991 recaptured the public's attention. In sheer quantitative terms, Johnson's announcement was the single most significant major news event and crucial turning point in the history of the epidemic, far surpassing Rock Hudson in both immediate surge of stories and lasting influence, opening up AIDS coverage to new beats and new audiences. "After this major news event, AIDS coverage was never the same" (Kaiser Family Foundation 1996, 2). The weekly average over the whole period of study was 30 stories per week; this jumped to 100 stories during weeks of major AIDS news events. In the Magic week, the number surged to an unprecedented 259, with coverage of Arthur Ashe second highest.

The Kaiser study gives the media fairly high marks for its AIDS coverage but notes the overwhelming failure of the U.S. media to cover international dimensions of the epidemic; of all stories studied, only 4 percent carried a non-U.S. dateline, and, of those, the only consistent theme was AIDS/HIV as it figured in the U.S. immigration problem. Another bothersome trend was a significant increase in the 1990s of the "celebrity AIDS" genre—that is, the coverage of celebrities (rather than scientists, say) as major newsmakers. The Kaiser study is exceptionally comprehensive and offers a useful, often counterintuitive, corrective to less systematic impressions. (Of the eight major news events studied, I was surprised to learn, Kimberly Bergalis's testimony to Congress in favor of mandatory testing of health care workers received the least amount of coverage and had the least lasting effect on subsequent coverage.)

But these media surveys take place in a limited universe of discourse and cannot answer questions they do not ask. To conclude that the media successfully educated the public about AIDS/HIV equates "education" with the AIDS 101 info pac: routes of transmission, risk groups, viral etiology, and so on. But more probing questions might tell us how knowledge about AIDS/HIV is understood and used and what this epidemic is teaching us about the world. I would be very interested to know, for example, how the following questions might be answered: How is our knowledge about AIDS produced? What is a virus? How are viruses studied and by whom? What has been the significance of basic research in this epidemic? Whose knowledge is reflected in specific research and treatment discoveries, how it is produced, and why is it uncertain? How do various meanings attributed to AIDS give differential jurisdiction to particular sectors or agencies? How do they make visible some narratives and camouflage others? And so on, for the various domains of the epidemic.[24]

The Feminist Media's "AIDS Patient"

98% of heterosexual transmission of the HIV virus is from men to women; only 2% is from women to men.—*WAC Stats* (1993)

Surely such a pre-eminent twentieth-century condition ought to be a major feminist concern. Yet despite the AIDS activism of many feminists, "mainstream" feminists (with some fine exceptions) have shied away from applying their analyses to the crisis of AIDS. AIDS is about sex, and as such it is an awkward and discomforting battle for feminists battered by the sex wars of the early 1980s.—Robin Gorna, "Feminism and the AIDS Crisis"

Every production of "identity" creates exclusions that reappear at the margins like ghosts to haunt identity-based politics.—Lisa Duggan, in Duggan and Hunter

Questions like those I just listed are more likely to be explored, perhaps, in feminist or other "alternative" media outlets, just as we would expect that these outlets would more readily tackle the epidemic's structural inequalities, discriminatory policies and practices, the experiences of the disenfranchised, and the politics of knowledge. And, indeed, over the course of the epidemic, some alternative outlets have produced coverage that is extraordinary in its quality, depth, and diversity of perspective.

To take just one example, two special issues of *Radical America* (vol. 20, no. 6, in 1987 and vol. 21, no. 2, in 1988), edited by AIDS activist coalitions, brought together important critical writings. Cindy Patton, a lesbian-feminist activist whose commentaries in the *Gay Community News* in Boston and other grassroots papers almost singlehandedly rescued feminist AIDS coverage from statistical nonexistence, contributed a critique of the "professionalization" of the epidemic and specifically safer sex education, arguing that, as AIDS became institutionalized, better funded, and generally routinized in state and federal agencies, many of the successful factors developed by the gay community dropped out: the ethics of "universal precaution" in the use of condoms, creative efforts to eroticize safer sexual strategies, and the goal of changing the culture of a community rather than the behavior of individuals (Patton 1987). Evelynn Hammonds, at that time (according to *Radical America*'s blurb) a "graduate student in the history of science and a black lesbian feminist, scientist, and activist," contributed one of the first commentaries on AIDS in relation to African Americans. Hammonds expressed her shock at a March 1987 article on AIDS and race by Richard Goldstein in the *Village Voice* (Goldstein 1987a), especially the information that "a black woman is thirteen times more likely than a white woman to contract AIDS, says the Centers for Disease Control; a Hispanic woman is at eleven times the risk. Ninety-one percent of infants with AIDS are non-white." Hammonds continued:

> I was stunned to discover the extent and spread of AIDS in the black community, especially given the public mobilization either inside or outside the community. My second reaction was anger. AIDS is a disease that for the time being signals a death notice. I am angry because too many people have died and are going to die of this disease. The gay male community over these last several years has been trans- formed and mobilized to halt transmission and gay men (at least white gay men) with AIDS have been able to live and die with some dignity and self-esteem. People of color need the opportunity to pro- vide education so that the spread of this disease in our communities can be halted, and to provide care so that people of color with AIDS will not live and die as pariahs.
>
> My final reaction was despair. Of course I *knew* why information about AIDS and the black community had been buried—by both the black and white media. (Hammonds 1987, 28–29)

Hammonds went on to charge the white media with ignoring people of color with AIDS as a nonstory for their audiences and as yet one more problematic "race" story best left uncovered. More crucially, the white media positioned people of color as "Other," their otherness compounded if they were also women and HIV positive. But in the black media, too, women with AIDS were Othered. Reviewing coverage in the black wom- en's magazines, Hammonds found no articles until the spring of 1987, and these largely mimicked white media coverage, warning women against the dangers posed by closeted bisexuals in their midst. As for the leading African-American organizations, Hammonds (1987, 31) reports that the *Journal of the National Medical Association* (the National Medical Asso- ciation is the professional organization of black physicians) ran a short edi- torial in late 1986 but nothing else; the NAACP and the Urban League had been silent; and only the Southern Christian Leadership Conference had established an ongoing educational program to address AIDS in the black community. If AIDS coverage for the black community is to change, Ham- monds argued, the social and sexual conservatism of the black media and most black organizations, including the church, must change as well: in the eyes of the black leadership at present, she wrote, black people might be at risk, but AIDS was not "black"; "and most importantly homosexuality and bisexuality were dealt with in a very conservative and problematic fashion." With Margaret Cerullo, Hammonds elaborated her argument in the second *Radical America* issue on AIDS (Cerullo and Hammonds 1988). And in 1992, she wrote that the "impact of HIV infection on African-American women and other women of color has received an odd sort of coverage in the media. On the one hand, when the threat of AIDS to women is discussed, no mention is made of African-American women. When African-American women are discussed, they are relegated to the drug abuser category or partners of drug abusers or bad mother category for passing AIDS on to their children" (Hammonds 1992, 8–9). Using Gross (1987b) as an example, a front-page *New York Times* story headlined "The Bleak and Lonely Lives of Women Who Carry AIDS" (the subhead: "Most Are Poor, Many Are Reckless"), Hammonds (1992, 9) reports, "The women in this article are portrayed as passive victims in abusive relationships with men who are most often drug abusers. Their lives are described as 'unruly,' 'chaotic,' 'despairing.'" Hammonds goes on to place both the silence and the stereotypical judgments in a historical context that includes the Tuskegee syphilis experiment, the common stigmatization (or equation) during STD epidemics of black women as "prostitutes," and the repeated failure of the medical establishment to take seriously and treat STDs in African-American women. Hammonds concludes with a call for a "viable Black feminist movement": "Analysis of gender is desperately needed to frame the discussion of sexual relations in the Black community. Sexism lies behind the disempowerment and lack of control that African-American women experience in the face of AIDS. African-American women are multiply stigmatized in the AIDS epidemic—only a multifaceted African-American feminist analysis can adequately expose the impact of AIDS on our communities and formulate just policies to save women's lives" (Hammonds 1992, 22).

Alternative media is, of course, an enormous catchall category constituted more by its mode of production and size of audience/readership than by its ideology or target constituency—although the latter is perhaps the more accurate key to coverage of AIDS and women. In any case, the coalitions represented by the *Radical America* issues—cutting across minorities, feminists, "the Left," gay men and lesbians, and AIDS activists—were highly unusual. A number of publications, the *Gay Community News*, the *Bay Area Reporter*, and the *New York Native* among them, wrote about the epidemic early and continued to do so, providing a model, as many commentators have certified, for aggressive AIDS coverage.[25] Gay and lesbian (and straight) media activists, too, of whom I say more in chapter 4 below and elsewhere, pioneered AIDS coverage on video, creating their own regular cable programming, independent documentaries, and footage that could be used by more mainstream broadcast outlets. Such media activists as Jean Carlomusto, Amber Hollibaugh, and Alexandra Juhasz were among the first to cover AIDS and women, discrimination against prostitutes, problems for women with children, and medical stereotypes that hindered women's equal access to diagnosis and treatment. Hollibaugh, a feminist and lesbian activist, sex radical, and survivor of the feminist "sex wars," produced the video *The Second Epidemic* (1987) for the AIDS Discrimination Unit of the New York City Commission on Human Rights, a unit that was itself, as Juhasz puts it (1995, 55), simultaneously both "inside and outside the establishment." Carlomusto's videos for Gay Men's Health Crisis and the New York City cable series "Living with AIDS" pioneered community-based AIDS videos that incorporated analysis into their educational project. Juhasz produced a series of AIDS videos in collaboration with members of the HIV-affected communities to which they were addressed. All three brought political, critical, and aesthetic commitments to their AIDS media work that enabled them to take up issues of AIDS and women without essentializing "women" and demonizing "men," including the gay men all around them struggling with the epidemic.

By discussing alternative women's coverage first in this section, I am emphasizing its crucial importance for the AIDS activist movement that it helped generate, other media coverage, and the future directions of the AIDS epidemic. But it is not, sad to say, representative. When we examine AIDS coverage in feminist outlets, we find the influence not of activism or grassroots gay and lesbian analysis but of entirely conventional mainstream medical and media sources. Moreover, as Catherine Warren and I argue elsewhere (Treichler and Warren 1998), the glossy centrist women's magazines did, overall, a better job of covering AIDS than their feminist sisters.

Although the glossy women's magazines (*Ladies Home Journal, Vogue*, etc.) published no articles on AIDS during 1981 and 1982, by the second half of the 1980s most had published at least one "what women need to know about AIDS" article. In addition to "the facts," these publications presented AIDS as a personal health issue for women, as an epidemic involving families and children, as a human interest story, and as a topic associated with benefit fund-raising events. A 1983 article in the *Ladies Home Journal* by Bibi Weinhouse, for example, presented AIDS as an epidemic still confined to the familiar "high-risk groups" but nevertheless as news and as a potential personal health issue for women. "AIDS: What It Does to a Family" (1983), by K. Barret, was a sympathetic profile of the widow of a bisexual man who died of AIDS. "People need to understand that there are children involved," the widow tells the author, "and wives and mothers. . . . I'm tired of hearing about AIDS as a gay disease. It doesn't matter how it's transmitted. What matters is how much AIDS victims suffer and how their families suffer."

Health-related stories appeared regularly. As early as 1984, such magazines as *Glamour, Mademoiselle,* and the *Ladies' Home Journal* were warning women that they might be at risk for AIDS. Sources included researchers and health practitioners concerned with women, including some of those mentioned above. A 1985 *Mademoiselle* story entitled "AIDS Is Not for Men Only," for example, was written by Chris Norwood, whose book on women and AIDS would appear in 1987. "AIDS: What Women Must Know Now!" cited the Project AWARE study; the 1985 *Good Housekeeping* story warned readers that antibody testing should not replace safer sex precautions and provided the phone number of the twenty-four-hour CDC hotline. A *Vogue* story by Ellen Switzer (1986), titled "AIDS: What Women Can Do," introduced a theme echoed in biomedical, popular, and feminist discourse: "The killer disease called acquired immune deficiency syndrome (AIDS) not only has begun to strike women, but its control and eventual conquest are probably in their hands." Switzer quoted AIDS researcher Michael Gottlieb: "In such battles, women have historically been our best allies. They want to protect their families and themselves, so they pay attention to what science can tell them about any new threat, and act accordingly." Switzer concluded: "Saving ourselves and our families from this deadly disease depends on facts and action, responding to warnings without giving in to panic" (see also Avery 1988a, 1988b; Norwood 1986, 1988).

In contrast to these relatively neutral reports, coverage by explicitly feminist writers was often horrendous. In April 1986, Erica Jong addressed the readers of *New Woman.* For some women, she wrote, the AIDS crisis is a good "excuse to turn away from casual sex" (46). And, she suggested playfully, "Think of the time saved for working, for playing, for family, for gardening, for needlepoint!" (42). AIDS was not even an issue two years ago, she continued, so the current flood of information on heterosexual transmission was sudden, overwhelming—and hard to assimilate. Given the "plague mentality" of the media, "what's the informed woman to think—and beyond that, to do—about AIDS?" (44) She continued: "By far the sanest and most detailed discussion of the disease I have read was published in *Discover* magazine's December 1985 issue. Its message to women was for the most part reassuring. *Discover* concluded that AIDS is 'the largely fatal price one can pay for anal intercourse'; that the virus 'is only borne in the blood and semen'; that AIDS is a difficult disease to catch; and that vaginal intercourse is much less likely than anal intercourse to spread the disease because of the ruggedness of the vaginal lining and its relatively few exposed blood vessels" (44).

So here, without a shard of further evidence, was Langone's (1985) article, with all its problematic certainties reproduced intact to reassure women. To make matters worse, Jong highlighted a set of boxed "facts" captioned "good news (for women) about AIDS" (1986, 46). After contrasting our old friends the vulnerable rectum and the rugged vagina (e.g., "the tissue in the vagina has fewer blood vessels than the rectum, and natural lubrication during intercourse lessens the chances of tears"), she repeated the familiar alibis to explain why women would not get HIV from ordinary sexual intercourse with men: women with AIDS in Africa actually get it from anal intercourse, contact with bisexuals, or needles used in clinics and "in certain tribal customs"; the AIDS virus is fragile and cannot be easily transmitted (especially if "simple sexual precautions like not exchanging bodily fluids" and "the use of condoms" [44] are followed); women in the United States with AIDS attributed to heterosexual transmission are also long-term partners of intravenous drug users; even if a woman does become infected, "researchers estimate that only 5 to 20 percent of those who test positive for the virus will develop the disease"; "men haven't been very good to their immune systems" and therefore appear to be more susceptible to AIDS. Though fear of AIDS is scaring women into chastity, like the terror of kitchen-table abortions in the 1950s, this is OK because it will make sex "a little more mysterious and precious again" (46).

As Edward Alwood has indicated in tracking AIDS coverage in the press, it was the centrist gay media and centrist publications like the *Village Voice* that did the best overall job of covering the epidemic, not the self-identified radical media. In comparison to the centrist "women's magazines" like *Vogue*, the self-identified feminist media were compiling a dismal record on AIDS. Longtime feminist writer Barbara Grizzuti Harrison (1986) contributed an article to *Mademoiselle* called "It's Okay to Be Angry about AIDS." This was not, as you might expect, a call to arms in the fight against AIDS but an attack on gay men for spoiling things for the rest of us. Specifically, wrote Harrison, it's OK to be angry that some gay men have had as many as fifty sexual partners a week: "Is that normal? I don't think promiscuous gay men have a right to demand that we think the way they live is fine and dandy; their business is now our business, and we are under no obligation to find it lovely. . . . Even, however, if we acknowledge our anger—and/or our aesthetic and moral revulsion—does it follow that we don't extend succor and compassion to AIDS victims? Of course not. They suffer; they must be helped" (p. 96). Harrison's article exemplified the kind of feminist coverage earlier critiqued by Marea Murray. In a 1985 letter to *Sojourner*, Murray challenged the view held by some women, including lesbians, that AIDS was a problem that "the boys" had brought on themselves—while heterosexual women were still tending to see AIDS as nothing to do with them or as something that "self-help" procedures would guard them against.

In April 1987, one year after Jong's "good news," AIDS appeared in a *Ms.* magazine special issue "The Beauty of Health." On the cover, an attractive woman in an orange shirt was shown eating an orange and smiling. "Wake up and be healthy!" the cover blurb commanded, listing what we should wake up to:

Skin Problems
RU-486 the Unpregnancy Pill
Exercises You Can Do in Bed
Guarding against AIDS
Why Doncha Smile, Honey?

The two-page story by Lindsy Van Gelder attempted to bring the topic of condoms to *Ms.* readers. Van Gelder had earlier written for *Ms.* one of the only "politics of AIDS" stories to appear in a glossy women's publication (Van Gelder 1983). Although it assumed that "a good many lesbians are monogamous" and therefore not at risk for AIDS—odd logic two years into the epidemic—the article examined the politics of funding and the problems of racism and homophobia. Not until the end of the decade would *Ms.*, the most visible feminist journal, return to this theme. Van Gelder had also coauthored a competent overview of the problems of AIDS on campus for *Rolling Stone* (Van Gelder and Brandt 1986). But this 1987 story for *Ms.* was just a little too cute. It began with an anecdote in which she asked a sexually active woman friend whether she had asked her male friend to begin using condoms: "*Rubbers??*" said the friend. "Yuck!!" But, Van Gelder wrote, "You sleep not just with him but with all his sex partners." Should you trust him? she then asked her readers, slipping uncharacteristically into the voice of *Seventeen* magazine in the old days: "This is a toughie." She offers some straight talk: "Brace yourself for a shocker: men *lie* to get laid." Van Gelder emphasized some important (if not precisely accurate) points: the term *heterosexuals* is misleading because "most people who contract AIDS heterosexually are women"; she also argued that "safe sex with many different men is less risky than unprotected sex with one [infected] man," a logical deduction, but one that many writers were failing to make. But the article ended with a breezy reinscription of conventional sexual division—that outdated staple of *Ms.* magazine's version of feminism—us against them, women against men: "How much do you want to bet that if female-to-male transmission begins to be documented in great numbers, *men* will be demanding safe sex—with no wimpy worries about turning women off?"

Also addressing women as a quasi feminist was the sex therapist Helen Singer Kaplan, whose 1987 book *The Real Truth about Women and AIDS* warned women that their government was selling them a bill of goods. Geared toward heterosexual middle-class women and their "unborn babies," the book retrogressively asserted, in the name of saving women from a fate synonymous with death, that AIDS was caused by who you are, not by what you do. Kaplan revisited the mucous membrane and found it anything but rugged: "the moist vulnerable mucous membranes" (p. 78) make the female genital organs a welcoming harbor for HIV. The advice to "avoid unsafe practices," said Kaplan, is "nonsense!" Rather, "avoid infected partners." The only way to "avoid sexual exposure to high-risk males," unless you want to move to North Dakota, is to (1) make your candidate take the ELISA test; (2) wait; (3) make him get tested again. If he's clean and you still want to, (4) go ahead and have sex. And then, I guess, (5) handcuff him to you for the rest of your life. The book also called on women to be the conscience of the nation, using their monogamy to contain the infection and preserve relationships from the tides of men's sexual rampages: "We women form the 'bridge' that is virtually the only avenue by which the AIDS virus can escape from its current confinement to the small, highly concentrated pool of infected high-risk men and spread out to the general population, which is still largely uncontaminated. . . . We can close the bridge if, like Lysistrata's union of women, we do not have sex with infected males. We must form an impenetrable barrier. We must not let the virus use our sexual organs, which were meant to bring forth life, to kill our children, our families, and ultimately everyone." (Kaplan 1987, 145).

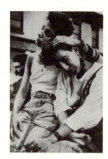
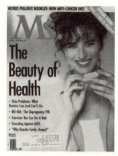
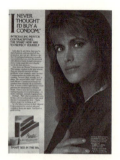

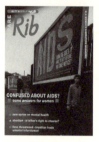
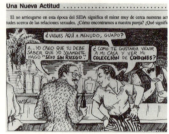

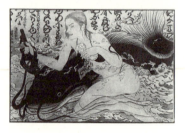

Throughout the 1980s, Ms. magazine, the leading U.S. feminist glossy, failed to recognize the AIDS epidemic as a feminist issue—that is, as a broad social crisis with serious gendered dimensions. With a few exceptions (e.g., the photo essay by Gypsy Ray and Jane Rosett in Ms., September 1987, including 2.12, Ann and Juliette at New York City annual AIDS vigil in 1985), Ms. covered the epidemic primarily as an unfortunate health risk for sex-obsessed men, best addressed by women through prudent individual self-help measures (2.13: "Guarding against AIDS," Ms., April 1987). Middle-class women were the target market for Mentor contraceptives, promoted in spring 1987 as "smart sex" and packaged to look like yoghurt (2.14). But don't lose the 800 number in the lower right: when you try to follow the complicated directions on the microscopic package insert, you may need it. Some women activists grasped the social nature of the AIDS crisis, calling for collective action, AIDS information for women, solidarity with gay men, and innovative approaches to sex and sexuality (2.15: U.K. AIDS education campaign billboard; 2:16: illus. by Allison Bechtel for Patton and Kelly's Making It [1987] 1990). Technological solutions, however, have been slow in coming. The sensuous "female condom" envisioned by artist Masami Teraoka (2:17: New Wave Series, watercolor, 1992) bears little resemblance to the actual 1990s market product—a good idea that costs too much, should work better, and, according to some U.S. sex workers, looks like a colostomy bag.

Until 1988, which was a turning point of sorts for the mainstream feminist media, three premises remained fairly constant in these feminist magazines, echoing Kaplan's message: (1) women prefer monogamy; (2) men are duplicitous; (3) getting tested—"the only way to know for sure"—is the answer to your prayers (Van Gelder 1987, 64, 71). Such a perspective reinforced the dominant message that AIDS, "a gay men's disease," was a direct consequence of men's hedonistic and destructive promiscuity. It failed to articulate the social and political aspects of the epidemic. Indeed, not only did feminist journals offer no effective counternarrative, but they often repeated, endorsed, and even magnified the standard account. The discourse of mainstream feminism even amplified Jong's take on AIDS as a "good news, bad news" disease. The bad news was that hundreds of thousands of people worldwide were dying, with no end in sight, and this was scary. But the good news, repeated in magazines from *Ms.* to *New Woman*, was that "women don't get AIDS."

Women and AIDS: Toward a Feminist Analysis

This is what the study of gender, class, and race is really about: how subordinated sectors accommodate to and resist the power of privileged sectors, how privilege (like resistance) is camouflaged, how power is earned, learned, and occasionally spurned. Just as the reality of male privilege affects the lives of every woman, whether she is conscious of it or not, the concept of power is by definition a factor in every feminist's research.—Margery Wolf, *A Thrice-Told Tale*

I want the words *sex* and *condoms* to go together like cereal and milk or peanut butter and jelly.—Young woman infected with HIV, quoted by Patton (1995)

The role of a dissident intellectual is not to teach "theory" to the nontheoretical classes or masses, but to find ways for theories and activisms to learn from each other in the joint effort to re-form the institutions and practices that shape and constrain us all.—Lisa Duggan (1995)

What should biomedical scientists have known about women and AIDS, and when should they have known it? Although somewhat ambiguous, data on women were available from the very early years of the epidemic. What scientists and physicians failed to do was duplicated by the mainstream media, who took little leadership in exploring AIDS's potential threat to women and women's interests. Feminist publications, too, took little leadership in the epidemic: they largely failed to challenge the mainstream neglect of women, to disambiguate the data on gender, to articulate for their constituencies "women's interests" in relation to the epidemic, and to counter the conservative forces that were aggressively constructing the social meaning of AIDS.

It is important to be alive to recycled incarnations of gender, identity, and cultural authority in commentary on the AIDS epidemic and to challenge and disrupt them through research, caretaking, and activism focused on women. This means refusing the appeal of any binary division. If we, as women, are to cope with AIDS and HIV in any reasonable and intelligent way as well as with the other health crises that we face, we must unequivocally see ourselves connected to them and refuse the lie that our own identities and gender offer magical protection against the invasions of some alien Other. As evidence of women's potential risk began to emerge, it should have warned us to rethink our current conceptualizations, and it should have fundamentally challenged, once and for all, the value of dividing "the disease of them" from "the disease of us." Yet most discourse about—and by—women continued to embrace the division, simply rearranging the contents of the categories to match the latest bulletins from Washington, Atlanta, Paris, or Nairobi, and advising "us" (women) to protect ourselves from "them" (men). What was reinforced was the notion that "them" (whoever they were) was an expendable category of people, while "us" was a category of people worth saving. Despite all that we had learned about the social construction of sexual difference and how it had been used against women in the past, the categorization process was given scant scrutiny in the case of AIDS.

AIDS is complex, in part, because it exposes the artificiality of the categories and divisions that govern our views of social life and sexual difference. It challenges the existence of *women* as a monolithic sisterhood and as a meaningful linguistic entity. But feminist theory also suggests why a woman-centered analysis remains imperative, for women are both linguistic and material subjects who exist within language and history. Even as we work to deconstruct and perhaps finally to dissolve the linguistic subject, we must nonetheless keep our attention fixed relentlessly on the inequities still embodied in the material one.

By the end of the 1980s, such work was beginning to take place. A growing body of writing, research, performance, and media production took up the issue of women and AIDS and carried out a diverse series of interventions in the name of women: not "Woman," or even "Women," but women. Here are a selection of them.

During the parliamentary debate on Clause 28 in the United Kingdom, a measure like the Helms amendment in the United States to prohibit educational materials that might be seen as "promoting homosexuality" (what Nan Hunter [see Duggan and Hunter 1995, 124] calls "no promo homo" initiatives), lesbian activists infiltrated the visitors gallery of the House of Lords. At the peak of the debate, they tied ropes to the gallery railings and, in protest and solidarity, abseiled onto the House floor. (It was reported that some of the honourable lords woke for the first time in decades.)[26]

An international network was forming to monitor, report, and remedy the situation of women in the global epidemic. Such authorities as Jonathan Mann, then the influential director of the WHO Global Programme on AIDS in Geneva, took up the call for attention to women—significantly, linking their vulnerability, in country after country, to structural inequalities.

In Australia, sex workers, working with the nation's health ministry, developed a comprehensive educational intervention program for sex workers and other sexual minorities at risk for HIV (Saunders 1997). An Australian documentary, *Suzi's Story* (I. Gillespie 1987), was filmed in Sydney in March and April 1987 and shown on Australian television (it was shown in the United States in late 1987 on *America Undercover*). Representing "women," Suzi Lovegrove talks to the camera and to her family in the last two months of her life; family members talk about caring for her and combating ignorance. Although the source of her infection (a man she knew before she met and married Vince Lovegrove) is mentioned, the film chooses to emphasize points less familiar to the public. Vince says, "Knowing I'm not infected with AIDS often makes me feel guilty in a strange sort of way. The doctors say it's easier for a man to pass the virus to a woman than from the female partner to the male partner, and I guess we're proof of that." (Australia isn't perfect. Although feminists lobbied for years to have AIDS education provided to straight men, the one program finally funded in 1992 was discontinued after six months [Waldby 1996, 148].)[27]

In the United States, a group of women in the New York chapter of ACT UP mobilized to protest the 1988 publication in *Cosmopolitan* of an article reassuring women that "ordinary sexual intercourse" would not put them at risk for AIDS/HIV. They picketed the offices of *Cosmo*'s publisher, staged a number of related actions communicating the statistics of cases among women, produced a video about the *Cosmo* action, and developed a handbook later published as the book *Women, AIDS, and Activism* (ACT UP New York Women and AIDS Book Group 1992). In 1991, even *Ms.* magazine produced a special issue on AIDS relying on AIDS activists as sources rather than famous feminists or women's health experts uninformed about AIDS.

Finally, as John D'Emilio (1992) emphasizes, gay and lesbian activism was booming. Contrary to predictions that AIDS would be the death knell of gay liberation, the AIDS crisis instead created new solidarities across generations, genders and sexualities, political commitments, and cultures and helped galvanize the formation of queer theory and sustain, despite the constant presence of illness and death, the AIDS activist movement.

In this chapter, I have reviewed the role of gender in biomedical and public health discourse on AIDS during the 1980s, arguing that the theoretical and chronological accounts produced during these crucial years relied on culture and history as well as scientific evidence. Moreover, although explicitly provisional, these accounts significantly shaped our conceptions of the role of gender in AIDS and HIV transmission well into the 1990s, a fact perhaps better explained by the sociology of science, cultural studies, and feminist theory than by science and medicine. I then showed how these biomedical narratives reverberated (if often faintly) in other discourses of the period, including news and science reporting for general audiences, glossy women's magazines, and the alternative press (left, minority, gay, lesbian, and feminist). Indeed, over this same period, media coverage took on a life of its own, developing its own routines and experts not wholly dependent on AIDS experts in biomedicine and government agencies. Although, in time, media reports goaded biomedical and public health authorities explicitly and sometimes aggressively to refute them, these powerful early narratives have had a number of consequences and continue to influence our understanding of the epidemic as well as our failure to ask—much less to answer—significant biological, social, and epidemiological questions about women, HIV, and AIDS. I concluded this chapter with the year 1988, when, I argued, conceptions of gender and AIDS underwent a significant and sustained change as women began to toss out the scripts handed to them and, through research, media production, and direct political action, break the silence and rewrite the AIDS plot. In chapter 8 below, I bring the story up to date, exploring more fully the specific impediments to women's involvement in the AIDS crisis as well as the evolution of policy, research, and activism in the 1990s. In that chapter, too, I look at the long-term effect of AIDS on the feminist movement and on feminism's possible futures.

3

AIDS and HIV Infection
in the Third World:
A First World Chronicle

Understanding the AIDS epidemic as a medical phenomenon involves understanding it as a cultural phenomenon. Yet excessively positivist or commonsensical notions of *culture* may limit our ability to recognize that AIDS is also a complex and contradictory *construction* of culture. This is particularly true of AIDS in developing countries. In the developed world (the "First World" and, to a lesser extent, the "Second World"), AIDS is now routinely characterized as a social as well as a medical epidemic, as a challenge to conflicting values, and as an unprecedentedly complex cultural phenomenon; in contrast, in the developing world—the "Third World"—AIDS is believed to lead a much simpler life.[1] Even when these cultures themselves are seen as mysterious, AIDS is seen as a scientifically understood infectious disease that, without our help, will devastate whole countries, whose passive citizens struggle against it in vain.

This vision is well intentioned and perhaps even necessary to marshal external resources. But it obscures the fact that diverse interests are articulated around AIDS in the developing world in ways that are socially and culturally localized and specific. Deeply entrenched institutional agendas and cultural precedents in the First World prevent us from hearing the story of AIDS in the Third World as a complex narrative. One consequence of this inadvertent cultural imperialism is that very simple generalizations about the epidemic may be accepted as "the truth about AIDS," with few efforts made to unravel their diverse and often contradictory claims.

This chapter does not seek to determine "the truth about AIDS." Rather, I look closely at how selected First and Third World publications have attempted to chronicle and conceptualize the epidemic. To show a typical discursive construction of "Third World AIDS," I begin with a discussion about AIDS in Haiti. I then contrast the familiar statistical chronicle of the global epidemic with other accounts, suggesting how differing conceptualizations, different "truths," work to promote differing material consequences. I examine contradictory accounts of the epidemic in Kenya in the late 1980s to suggest the value of acknowledging rather than resolving contradictions; selecting a given account too readily as the definitive truth short-circuits efforts to better understand how truth is situated—and how it is produced, legitimated, sustained, and interpreted. I argue that understanding the discursive production of the AIDS crisis—the production, that is, of these differing narratives and how they function—is necessary, if not sufficient, if we are to understand its conceptual and material complexity. In turn, such understanding provides grounding for fresh approaches to cooperation between the developed and the developing worlds.

A U.S. Doctor Unmasks Truth in Haiti: Third World AIDS in First World Media

We had come near the end of a long line of anthropologists working in these remote villages. . . . Coming at the end gave us certain advantages. . . . But as time passed we became aware that we had also inherited serious problems. The !Kung had been observing anthropologists for almost six years and had learned quite a bit about them. Precedents had been set that the !Kung expected us to follow.—Marjorie Shostak, *Nisa*

The very activity of ethnographic *writing*—seen as inscription or textualization—enacts a redemptive Western allegory.—James Clifford, "On Ethnographic Allegory"

Accounts of the AIDS epidemic in the Third World, whether they are medical reports, patient testimony, media observations, investigative journalism, World Health Organization news bulletins, or government reports, are at some level linguistic constructions. These diverse representations of AIDS in the Third World draw their authority from many sources, including the credentials and persuasive powers of individual authors and organizations, consistency with accepted beliefs and knowledge about AIDS and about the Third World, compatibility with our own social and political perspectives, and resonance with familiar traditions of discourse. Although often covert, the influence of discourse is powerful and pervasive in establishing and legitimating a given representation.

Discourse about AIDS, for example, draws on widely accepted narratives of past epidemics. Although these histories may be employed to supply a variety of arguments and moral conclusions about today's epidemic, they share the premise that any infectious disease is a knowable biological phenomenon whose strange and seemingly contradictory aspects are ultimately illusory: decoded by experts, its mysteries will one by one become controllable material realities. Discourse about AIDS in the Third World shares but exaggerates this premise, first equating the Third World (especially Africa, "the dark continent") with the savage, the alien, or the incomprehensible, then asserting the importance and achievability of reason and control. Although these two features may seem to be in conflict, they exist in fact in a relation of discursive symbiosis: the metaphors of mystery and otherness produce the desire for control, which is in turn fulfilled and justified by the metaphors of otherness and mystery.[2]

A highly visible story, for example, was written for *Life* magazine by the physician-author Richard Selzer (1987), who visited Haiti in the mid-1980s in an effort to learn the truth about AIDS behind the government's apparent attempts to downplay its prevalence. The metaphor of the article's title, "A Mask on the Face of Death," invokes the government's denials in the language of exotic tropical rituals such as carnival and voodoo. The subtitle is "As AIDS Ravages Haiti, a U.S. Doctor Finds a Taboo against Truth"; although these probably are not Selzer's words, they suggest to the reader not only that official denials mask the brutality of the epidemic but also that Selzer, the expert medical observer, can perceive the reality beneath the mask. Selzer's article is in the tradition of the privileged First World informant of conventional anthropological, ethnographic, and travel literature, the stranger in a strange land whose representation of AIDS in the Third World is legitimated by its claim to be an objective, scientific account of phenomena observed or experienced firsthand. As Mary Louise Pratt (1986) has observed, travel writing has provided ethnographic description with a discursive legacy, despite the ethnographer's desire to repudiate it; both, in turn, permeate representations in other genres.[3] Thus, Selzer's article opens with the conventional arrival scene of this dual legacy: "It is 10 o'clock at night as we drive up to the Copacabana, a dilapidated brothel on the rue Dessalines in the red-light district of Port-au-Prince" (p. 59). Outside the bar, Selzer is importuned by men and women offering a variety of sexual pleasures; inside, he interviews three female prostitutes from the Dominican Republic, who describe AIDS as an economic problem for them, not a health problem. The direct interrogation of the native informant is another staple of privileged observer accounts; in AIDS narratives, it is often prostitutes who are interviewed. The following day, Selzer talks with physicians and examines a large number of patients with apparent HIV-related illnesses for whom little in the way of treatment is available.

Selzer is carefully nonjudgmental with respect to street life and, indeed, speculates that the virus may have entered Haiti as an accidental feature of First World exploitation: "Could it have come from the American and Canadian homosexual tourists, and, yes, even some U.S. diplomats who have traveled to the island to have sex with impoverished Haitian men all too willing to sell themselves to feed their families? Throughout the international gay community Haiti was known as a good place to go for sex" (1987, 64). Selzer pursues this characterization of Haiti as sexual victim ravaged by Western capitalists. Acting on "a private tip from an official at the Ministry of Tourism," Selzer and guide drive to a once luxurious hotel fifty miles from Port-au-Prince that was a prime vacation spot for gay men. Because the two Frenchmen who own the hotel are out of the country, Selzer and his guide are shown around by a staff member, a man of about thirty who clearly "is desperately ill. Tottering, short of breath, he shows us about the empty hotel. The furnishings are opulent and extreme—tiger skins on the wall, a live leopard in the garden, a bedroom containing a giant bathtub with gold faucets. Is it the heat of the day or the heat of my imagination that makes these walls echo with the painful cries of pederasty?" (p. 64). Ill at ease among the tiger skins of a hotel in Haiti, the Western travel writer goes to work on "Third World AIDS." Ultimately, for Selzer, AIDS in Haiti is an unambiguous mor(t)ality tale about the evils of sexual excess: as Northern homosexual men ravaged Haitian boys, so does AIDS ravage Haiti. Nostalgia for the observed culture's original innocence gives way to regret at its exploitation by decadent foreigners and speculation about the deadly effect of exotic customs and sexual practices. Selzer's account therefore tells us something about his concrete daily activities, his heated imagination, and his strategies for transforming selected experiences into prose, but his desire to bring the country's plight to world attention is as much about language as about AIDS in Haiti.

The status of Selzer's article as a firsthand report of observed phenomena does not rest on our firsthand knowledge about AIDS, the Third World, or Haiti. In certain concrete ways, just as cinematic convention represents scenes viewed through binoculars as two intersecting circles, Western AIDS discourse transforms a culture so that it ceases to recognize itself but paradoxically becomes recognizable in the West. What is needed is to sort out the multiple voices, texts, and subtexts of the AIDS epidemic—which has in part evolved, as Jan Zita Grover puts it, as a "creature of language" (1988b, 3; see also Watney 1989).

Several elements of Selzer's account of AIDS in Haiti are now virtually obligatory in First World chronicles of Third World AIDS. First, the opening arrival scene, as I have noted, situates the First World observer in relation to the Third World culture—a culture that, in AIDS chronicles, almost always belongs to the fallen world of postcolonial development. Indeed, the term *Third World* grew out of the perceived confrontation between capitalist and Communist interests and hence presupposes an analysis dependent on such concepts as *colonialism, industrialization, modernity,* and *development.* Second, the statistics provided by Haitian physicians function in at least two ways: to anchor in objective fact Selzer's more personal observations about the prevalence of AIDS and to demonstrate the specialized knowledge of expert native informants whose on-the-scene experience equips them to reveal the truth behind the official mask. (In Selzer's story, the inside informants assert that AIDS is more widespread than officials admit; but, in other AIDS stories, insiders also function to accuse the government and the media of exaggerating the AIDS crisis for political gains.) Another element is provided by "the reigning American pastor," a nonnative informant whose unreliability as a cultural informant is demonstrated by his moralistic condemnation of voodoo—a system of practices believed by some to facilitate the spread of HIV. Voodoo, he tells Selzer, is "a demonic religion, a cancer on Haiti" that is "worse than AIDS" (1987, 62). In positioning himself against his fellow American, "a tall, handsome Midwesterner with an ecclesiastical smile," Selzer secures his own reliability, much as ethnographers quote descriptions of a given culture by earlier travel writers to repudiate the bias of such unscientific observations. Selzer's visits to health-care settings constitute another element, revealing a devastated health-care system—part of the economic fallen world that parallels his image elsewhere of Haiti as the victim of First World sexual exploitation. A further familiar feature of AIDS stories is "the view from the street," represented by Selzer's talk with the three healthy Dominican prostitutes. Their remarks seem designed to underscore the ignorance and dangerous false security engendered by the government's official silence. One of them, Carmen, scoffs at Selzer's suggestion that prostitutes as a population are sick with AIDS: "'AIDS!' Her lips curl about the syllable. 'There is no such thing. It is a false disease invented by the American government to take advantage of the poor countries. The American President hates poor people, so now he makes up AIDS to take away the little we have.' The others nod vehemently" (p. 60). The notion that AIDS is an American invention is, like so-called conspiracy theories, a recurrent element of the international AIDS story. It is one not easily incorporated within a Western positivist frame—in part, perhaps, because it often reveals an unwelcome narrative about colonialism in a postcolonial world. The West accordingly attributes such theories to ignorance, state propaganda, or psychological denial, or it interprets them as some new global version of an urban legend, like alligators in the New York City sewer system.[4]

But Carmen's theory of AIDS invokes two further narratives that reinforce the notion of a global economy changing in ways the West cannot fully control. One is a tale of postmodern scholarship about the difficulty of finding good native informants these days. As Marjorie Shostak's introduction to her ethnographic study *Nisa* (1983) makes clear, native informants are quite likely to be already wise in the ways of Western inquisitors. Discussing *Nisa*, Pratt (1986) convincingly argues that Shostak is nevertheless able ultimately to transcend the "degraded" ethnographic culture of too-knowing informants and achieve a redemptive resolution for her story. Selzer's framing of Carmen accomplishes something similar, together with a second narrative, to which I have already alluded, concerning the construction of the subject in a fallen world. Pratt suggests that ethnographic characterizations of the !Kung changed in the course of foreign colonization. Precolonial ethnographers rendered them as sly, bloodthirsty, untrustworthy, appetitive, manipulative; after colonization, they came to be represented as helpful, friendly, innocent, good, and vulnerable. Carmen's speech takes place at a pivotal moment in the global AIDS drama, and this context encourages us to hear her emphatic denial of AIDS as a prelude to tragedy—perhaps as we hear Violetta in the first act of *La Traviata*.[5]

Selzer finally sums up: "This evening I leave Haiti. For two weeks I have fastened myself to this lovely fragile land like an ear pressed to the ground. It is a country to break a traveler's heart. . . . Perhaps one day the plague will be rendered in poetry, music, painting. But not now, not now" (1987, 64). Here, the stance of physician as ethnographer is clearer, the physician's ear pressed to the body of Haiti as he might press it to the body of a patient. But, although the diagnosis is grim, the language is utopian: the First World AIDS narrative successfully repels the threat of postmodern disruption to deliver a message of transcendent, universal humanism.

What are we to make of this? I am suggesting neither that Selzer's account is not "true" nor that we should exonerate the government of Haiti for its AIDS policies. I wish rather to point out how narrative conventions establish and sustain our *sense* of what is true, "our" referring at the least to the American readership of *Life* and perhaps to most U.S. citizens as well. Visual representations reinforce the illusion of truth, in part because they reproduce familiar representations of the Third World and reinforce what we think we already know about AIDS in those regions. Thus, the color photographs in Selzer's *Life* story show us frail, wasting bodies in gloomy clinics; small children in rickety cribs; the prostitutes, who always seem to be wearing red. One of the Dominican prostitutes, for example, is glamorously photographed, the full skirt of her red dress fanned out across a bed. Similarly, a May 1988 news account of the fear of AIDS in Mombasa, Kenya, reports an exchange between a U.S. sailor and a prostitute, a "23-year-old Ugandan woman in red shorts" (Schmemann 1988). A *Newsweek* photograph of a woman in red leggings and skirt is captioned: "'Avoid promiscuity': Prostitute with men in Zaire" (Nordland et al. 1986). Other photographs in the *Newsweek* story, which is about AIDS in central Africa, depict the "Third Worldness" of health care: in Tanzania, a man with AIDS lies hospitalized on a plain cot with none of the high-tech paraphernalia of U.S. representations; a widely reprinted photograph shows six "emaciated patients in a Uganda AIDS ward," two in cots, four on mats on the floor; rarely are physicians shown. A story on Brazil carries similar low-tech images. In contrast, publications originating in these countries do not omit technical images: African publications often show African scientists and physicians, and, among the photographs in a 10 August 1988 story on AIDS in *Veja*, the Brazilian equivalent of *Newsweek*, are those of an enormous, fully equipped modern hospital and masked and gowned physicians and nurses.[6]

A different problem occurs in a 1988 *National Geographic* story called "Uganda: Land beyond Sorrow" (Caputo 1988), where the story's portrait of unrelieved despair is challenged by the magazine's characteristically stunning photographs. A young woman with AIDS in a long flowing dress, for example, stands supported by her mother, who is wearing vivid pink; the caption tells us that the woman, Jane Namirimu, is pregnant and already too weak to stand alone (Caputo 1988, 470). Yet the beauty of the composition, even the adjacent photograph of Jane's grave taken when the photographer returned three months later, transforms the text's bleak assertions into an almost utopian narrative of elegiac fatefulness in which aesthetic universality redeems individual suffering. (On the fallen post-colonial world of ethnographic writing and the trope of utopian universality, see Pratt [1986, 40, 45].)

A final problem that I will note is the literal appropriation of images. J. B. Diederich's photographs for the Selzer story were at least original, but some AIDS photographs are familiar not simply because they invoke a familiar tradition but because precisely the same images circulate among diverse publications. In one of Diederich's photographs, a large, striking study in brown and white, an emaciated Haitian woman in a white dress

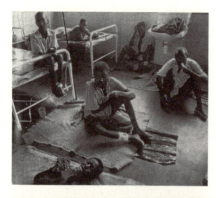

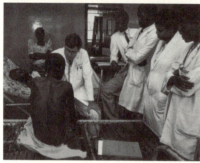

First World representations of the AIDS epidemic in less-developed regions usually fulfill our expectations of what "Third World AIDS" should look like. A Newsweek *photograph (3.1: photo by Chris Steele Perkins-Magnum, 24 November 1986) shows patients in an AIDS ward in a Ugandan hospital—abandoned, passive, waiting for death. But a story by Lisa Krieger about global AIDS activism (*San Francisco Examiner, *17 June 1990, 9) shows that it can be done differently. In one photo, a hospitalized Ugandan patient talks with a group of physicians (3.2: photo by Joanna B. Pinneo/Blackstar). Such examples press us to examine the many kinds of cultural work that visual representations do.*

sits gracefully on a wooden bench and looks out at the camera. The caption reads: "Tuberculosis is but one of the wasting infections of what Haitians call *maladi-a*" (Selzer 1987, 62). Selzer's article does not define *maladi-a* or tell us whether tuberculosis is counted in Haiti as a disease that signals AIDS or whether, like AIDS, it is simply one of many wasting diseases; nor is it clear that the woman in the photograph has actually been diagnosed with AIDS. But, reproduced months later in the Canadian newsmagazine *Maclean's* (31 August 1987), the identical photograph, no longer ambiguous, is captioned "Haitian AIDS victim: a former playground for holidayers" (p. 37).[7] The *Newsweek* photographs accompanying Nordland et al. (1986) have also been widely reprinted. One (p. 44) shows an emaciated woman framed in the doorway of her home, holding a small, thin baby on her lap. The *Newsweek* print is captioned "Two victims: Ugandan barmaid and son" and is credited to Ed Hooper–Picture Search. Appearing on the cover of the 24 May 1988 issue of the *Washington Post*'s weekly

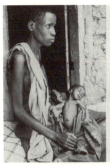

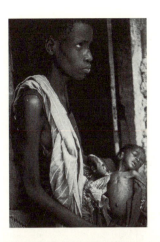

Florence and Ssengabi, sitting outside their hut in Gwanda. Florence died one month after this photograph was taken; her baby, Ssengabi, died four months later

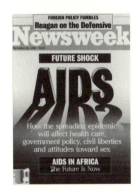

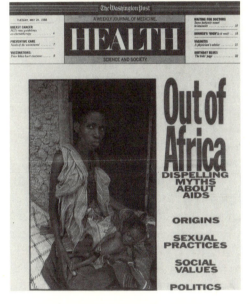

*Describing the "AIDS photo opportunity" arranged for journalists in Uganda, photographer Ed Hooper expressed discomfort with the orchestrated conditions that yielded these photo-*graphs. Although Hooper pragmatically accepts the photo as "the dinosaur's egg" his profession requires as proof of authenticity, his 1990 memoir, Slim (3.3: Florence and Ssengabi), takes pains to contextualize and individualize its human subjects. But, as Hooper's photographs circulated internationally, their captions became increasingly generic: "Ugandan barmaid and son," "Ugandan AIDS victims," and so on. And, while Newsweek (Morganthau 1986) took an alarmist approach (3.4: "AIDS: Future Shock") and used the photograph to represent the epidemic's gravity (3.5: "AIDS in Africa: The Future Is Now," 24 November 1986), the Washington Post's journal Health employed the photograph for a cover story arguing that in fact Western media were exaggerating the severity of AIDS in Africa (3.6: 24 May 1988).

journal *Health* is a photograph of the identical woman shot at a slightly different angle; accompanying Philip J. Hilts's featured story, "Out of Africa," the photograph is now captioned "In the Ugandan village of Kinyiga, Florence Masaka, 22, and her 2-month-old daughter have both tested positive for the AIDS virus." Incorrectly credited to "Al Hooper," the photograph is used here to illustrate an article arguing that claims about AIDS in Africa are greatly exaggerated. Hilts's article and the photographs were reprinted in *Africa Report* ("AIDS and Africa" 1988, 26–31) to accompany an article titled "Dispelling Myths about AIDS in Africa"; the photographs were captioned with pull quotes from the story. The Hooper photographs also accompanied Catharine Watson's "Africa's AIDS Time Bomb: Region Scrambles to Fight Epidemic" (1987); and the 24 June 1988 *Weekly Review* (Nairobi) reprinted the mother-and-child photograph with the caption "Ugandan AIDS victims" and no picture credit (p. 18). The photograph also appears in Hooper's memoir *Slim: A Reporter's Own Story of AIDS in East Africa* (1990), where the caption reads: "Florence and Ssengabi, sitting outside their hut in Gwanda. Florence died one month after this picture was taken; her baby, Ssengabi, died four months later" (p. 170). In the text of *Slim*, Hooper expresses numerous misgivings (confirmed by Matthew Little [1994] in an interview with Hooper) about the photograph and the occasion on which it was taken.

Hence, our understanding of the AIDS situation in Haiti—in central Africa or in some other elsewhere—is based on a series of filtering devices, a layering of representational elements, narrative voices, and replicating images. These mediating processes are not, of course, a simple function of high-tech Western representation. Firsthand experience is not unmediated either, so one cannot get off a plane in Port-au-Prince or Nairobi, look around, and determine who is correct. Within these countries, there are also differing constructions: there are people who agree with the Western media's account that AIDS is devastating the whole region; there are people like Carmen who believe that the disease is largely imaginary, the latest Western trick to reduce the Third World's population in the wake of failed birth control strategies in the past; there are others, including scientific investigators, who believe that the disease exists but is a "white man's disease"; and there are still others who point to serious flaws in most existing data about the prevalence, incidence, epidemiology, chronology, and social history of AIDS and HIV infection in the Third World.[8]

Discrepancies between doomsday predictions by the Western media and official denials by Third World governments introduce another complicating factor: every state has a "social imaginary," something it dreams itself to be, and its explicit declarations and official statistics are likely to be pervaded by this implicit social dream (Anagnost 1988). The dream of controlling the AIDS epidemic—whether controlling the blood supply, statistical and epidemiological knowledge, media coverage, biotechnology, or moral and sexual behavior—may well declare itself in a Western tongue. The photograph of the Brazilian hospital may accurately document the existence in Brazil of sophisticated medical capabilities (see n. 6 above). But, as a representation of "the AIDS epidemic," it may be as bogus as the "Haitian AIDS victim" or "Toronto sidewalk traffic." Symbiosis is self-perpetuating: while Third World representations function as elegiac icons that can be seamlessly decontextualized and appropriated by the First World narrative voice, the Third World media, dependent in varying degrees on First World sources and technology, recontextualize these images as their own. As Edward Said argues, modern representation in the decolonized world depends increasingly on a concentration of media power in metropolitan centers; this contributes to the monolithic nature of Third World representations, which are in turn a major source of information about Third World populations not only for the "outside world" but also for those populations themselves (Said 1985, 5; see also Valdivia 1996).

There is, however, another way of confronting the epidemic. If we relinquish the compulsion to separate true representations of AIDS from false ones and concentrate instead on representation and discursive production, we can begin to sort out how particular versions of truth are produced and sustained and what cultural work they do in given contexts. Such an approach illuminates the construction of AIDS as a complex narrative and raises questions not so much about truth as about power and representation. Richard Selzer's essay on AIDS in Haiti provides useful information—not necessarily about the true nature of AIDS in the Third World, but about the power of individual authors and the Western mass print media to produce and transmit particular representations of AIDS according to certain conventions and, in doing so, to sustain their acceptance as true.[9] Other forms of representation, drawing on different conventions, different rules, may make claims to truth in different ways.

The Country and the City: Dreams of Third World AIDS

It is not impossible that in the future, as in the past, effective steps in the prevention of disease will be motivated by an emotional revolt against some of the inadequacies of the modern world. . . . Knowledge and power may arise from dreams as well as from facts and logic.—René Dubos, *Mirage of Health*

A régime of truth is that circular relation which truth has to the systems of power that produce and sustain it, and to the effects of power which it induces and which redirect it.—John Tagg, *The Burden of Representation*

You'd be surprised: They're all individual countries.—Ronald Reagan, after returning from Latin American trip, 1987

"The statistical mode of analysis," argued Raymond Williams in *The Country and the City* (1973), was "devised in response to the impossibility of understanding contemporary society from experience." Characterizing preindustrial English society as knowable through experience (if only partially so), Williams contrasted this "knowable community" with the "new sense of the darkly unknowable" produced by urbanization and industrialization. The metaphor of darkness was routinely invoked in discussions of the rise of cities: the East End, for instance, was called "Darkest London." Statistical analysis was one of the new forms of knowledge "devised to penetrate what was rightly perceived to be to a large extent obscure."[10]

Given this historical mission, it is not surprising that statistical analysis is widely seen as a powerful way to understand the latest incarnation of the "darkly unknowable": AIDS in the Third World. Statistical data, at the least, are seen as the necessary foundation for other knowledge. The ability to produce statistical information is used to measure a nation's degree of development, predict its ability to cope with the AIDS crisis, and in some cases determine its eligibility for external aid.[11] Even if a country cannot produce its own statistics internally, it can demonstrate its ability to cope by cooperating with external studies.[12] But, more obviously, the international discourse on AIDS and HIV infection in the Third World is shaped on a day-to-day basis by statistical findings and projections. Once numbers are generated and publicized, they take on a life of their own. Because they may generate calls for action (and therefore time, money, and organization), AIDS estimates may be initially resisted. But, although specific numbers may be questioned and even denounced in given instances, the use of numbers as a fundamental measure of the reality of AIDS is not.

Data with regard to AIDS/HIV in Third World countries are regularly generated by several sources, including the U.S. Public Health Service Centers for Disease Control and the World Health Organization's Global AIDS Program (GPA); the GPA's AIDS Surveillance Unit is widely regarded as a legitimate producer, synthesizer, and interpreter of international numbers. By 31 January 1989, the number of countries reporting to the GPA was 177, of which 144 had reported one or more cases of AIDS (up from 175 and 138, respectively, in three months): a total of 139,886 cases worldwide had been reported to WHO, although WHO considered a more realistic total to be 250,000–500,000; WHO at this point estimated that 5 million were infected worldwide, with 1 million or more infected in Africa alone. These totals meant that at least 1 new case of AIDS was being reported somewhere in the world every minute, or 60 new cases every hour and 1,440 each day. Projections about the worldwide distribution and future prospects of AIDS and HIV infection led Jonathan Mann, director of the GPA, to conclude, "The global situation will get much worse before it can be brought under control" (Mann et al. 1988b, 82; see also L. Altman 1988a).

WHO did not officially acknowledge AIDS as a global health problem until late 1986—some five years into the epidemic for some countries. By the end of 1987, however, WHO's surveillance reports and seroprevalence data were sufficient to suggest three broad global patterns of AIDS (Mann et al. 1988b, 84; Piot et al. 1988, 576). According to this scheme (subsequently revised, as I note in later chapters), *Pattern I* is considered typical of industrialized countries with large numbers of reported cases (the "First World," roughly, including the United States, Canada, Western Europe, Australia, and New Zealand); it is characterized by the initial appearance of HIV infection in the late 1970s and rapid spread primarily among gay and bisexual men, intravenous drug users in urban coastal centers, and recipients of blood products. HIV infection and illness are at present slowly increasing in the heterosexual population but at highly variable rates, with perinatal transmission (from mother to infant) likewise increasing but not uniformly widespread; infection in the overall population is estimated to be less than 1 percent. In *Pattern II* countries (typically in sub-Saharan central Africa, the Caribbean, and Latin America), HIV infection may have appeared in the late 1970s but was not widely identified as AIDS related until 1983; heterosexual transmission is the norm, with males and females often equally infected and perinatal transmission therefore common; transmission via gay sexual contact or intravenous drug use is asserted to be low or absent. A *Pattern III* profile is attributed to the Second World countries of the then Soviet bloc as well as to much of North Africa, the Middle East, Asia, and the Pacific (excluding Australia and New Zealand): HIV is judged to have appeared in the early to mid-1980s, and only a small number of cases have been identified, primarily in people who have traveled to and engaged in some form of high-risk involvement with infected persons in Pattern I or II areas (Mann et al. 1988b, 84; see also Mann 1988a and Piot et al. 1984, 1988).[13]

What will be the material effects of the global epidemic? Again, we can identify a widely accepted set of predictions. In developed countries such as the United States, where 13 percent of the gross national product is spent on health care, AIDS and HIV-related illnesses place considerable stress on the health-care system. In many developing countries, where annual expenditures on health care are often less than five dollars per person and grossly inadequate for health needs prior to AIDS, future prospects are grim. The epidemic has further jeopardized the World Health Organization's ambitious global goal of health for all by the year 2000. Further, despite the widespread stereotype of people with AIDS as the disadvantaged of society, the twenty-to-forty age group is the most vulnerable worldwide—the age group most central to the labor force, to childbearing, to caring for the dependent young and old, and, ironically, to marshaling and managing the resources for addressing the AIDS epidemic. Synthesizing many studies of AIDS in Africa, in 1988 Miller and Rockwell spelled out the demographic, economic, and medical consequences of the epidemic. Education and prevention, they accurately predicted, still the best resources for controlling the spread of the virus, are difficult enough in media-rich Western countries; the task of communicating complex health messages to the diverse populations and geographic sites of Third World countries will remain even more formidable (Miller and Rockwell 1988, xiv–xxiv). The breakup of the former Soviet Union and dismantling of the Berlin Wall pose a new series of problems, as do the rising numbers of AIDS/HIV cases in the Far East. These predictions have combined to bring about widespread international agreement about the significance of the epidemic, and, as experience increasingly documented the futility of closing boundaries to the virus, so also have many global leaders come to agree with the WHO doctrine that "AIDS cannot be stopped in any country until it is stopped in all countries" (quoted in Chase 1988a, 4). Despite the open borders trumpeted by its current free trade agenda, the United States remains equivocal in its endorsement of the WHO doctrine.[14]

   In chapter 7 below, I talk about the ethical and economic crisis posed by the cost and distribution of new HIV treatments. But here I want to talk about knowledge and how we come to know what we think we know about "AIDS in the Third World." The power of numbers and their centrality to this knowledge are obvious. Without the sophistication and authority of statistical methods, the epidemic as a global issue could never have been articulated at all. Yet, while this First World numerical chronicle of global AIDS may have appeared to be unfolding smoothly as our knowledge grew, in fact it is problematic. Consider the following judgments about Africa, all published in 1987 or 1988:

1. "The continent hardest hit by the AIDS pandemic is Africa where all three infection patterns can be found" (WHO) (Mann et al. 1988b, 84).
2. "Medical experts consider the epidemic an accelerating catastrophe that, in the words of one, 'will make the Ethiopian famine look like a picnic'" (Congressional Research Service, cited in Copson 1987, 9).
3. In many urban centers of Congo, Rwanda, Tanzania, Uganda, Zaire, and Zambia, "from 5 to 20 percent of the sexually active age-group has already been infected with HIV. Rates of infection among some prostitute groups range from 27 percent in Kinshasa, Zaire, to 66 percent in Nairobi, Kenya, and 88 percent in Butare, Rwanda. Close to half of all patients in the medical wards of hospitals in those cities are currently infected with HIV. By the early 1990s the total adult mortality rate in these urban areas will have been doubled or tripled by AIDS" (WHO) (Mann et al. 1988b, 84).
4. "A *Newsweek* cover story claimed one Rakai village [in Uganda] had seven discos and 'sex orgies.' In reality it has 20 mud huts, a handful of fishing boats, and no electricity" (*Guardian*) (Watson 1987, 10).
5. "The tale of AIDS in Africa is not one of widespread devastation and the collapse of nations. There are 53 countries in Africa and AIDS exists substantially in only a few of them" (*Washington Post*) (Hilts 1988, 12).
6. "Like the tenacious theories put forward as explanations for the heterosexual spread of HIV in Africa, the whole AIDS pandemic is shrouded in mystery and uncertainty. There is no reliable information on AIDS and by the time one message has percolated its way down to the general population, it is out of date and a new one is already on its way to replace it" (*West Africa*) (Harper 1988, 2072).

Given the statistics cited above and the reality of global AIDS as widely accepted today, how can it be that the most fundamental meanings of the narrative have all along been contested?

Using these quotations as representative of larger discourses in conflict, several sources of confusion and contradiction can be identified. Estimates of infection and actual cases of AIDS for entire populations may be derived from inadequate data: too few studies, studies of too small a sample size, nonrepresentative samples, and so on. Rates estimated for all Africans in a given country (or even "Africa") are often based on small studies in urban areas; studies of "prostitutes" may in fact classify all sexually active single women as prostitutes.[15] Chronological claims (about when AIDS first appeared) are primarily based on flawed blood-testing procedures and other problems of diagnostic method. In Africa, "underreporting" is taken for granted and estimates corrected upward; at the same time, the number of positive cases actually diagnosed may be too high or too low, depending on the procedure used. Research cited as evidence may be unpublished, based on conference papers unavailable for detailed scrutiny, or sloppily interpreted, and many published papers do not report important data. Moreover, interpretations of the epidemic may be based on divergent and not mutually understood paradigms and forms of evidence. Testing blood samples in a laboratory involves different practical operations and generates knowledge different from that produced by a clinician examining patients or a journalist interviewing people on the street. Experienced medical experts in Africa, who tend to make lower estimates of cases, claim that their knowledge is discounted as clinical and experiential by Western and European academic scientists.[16]

Rumor and fantasy play their part as well. Cultural practices are taken out of context, exaggerated, distorted, or invented. Voodoo continues to animate accounts of HIV in Haiti, with grizzly descriptions of voodoo sorcerers biting off the heads of infected chickens and sucking the bloody stumps. African tales often involve the notorious African green monkey, whose photograph keeps circulating long after his role in AIDS has been discounted. Africans are said to have sexual contact with these monkeys, or eat them, or eat other animals they have infected (Haitian chickens?), or give their children dead monkeys as toys. Purporting to explain why HIV transmission is heterosexual in Africa, reports hypothesize radical differences between African and Western bodies based on physiological, behavioral, cultural, moral, and/or biological factors. As Sander Gilman (1988b) has comprehensively documented, these rumors are tirelessly fueled by historically entrenched myths of the exotic.[17]

While increased international scientific dialogue has answered some questions about global AIDS and HIV, it has confirmed the difficulty of answering others and underscored the need for thick description—complex, multilayered, interdisciplinary research. Jay A. Levy's (1989) outstanding collection on AIDS, for example, includes detailed review chapters on AIDS in Haiti and in Africa. Both demonstrate the diverse and very different clinical manifestations of HIV infection in those settings and emphasize the need for revised diagnostic and reporting systems. Treated at length in the Haiti chapter (Johnson and Pape 1989) is the complex interaction of HIV infection with tuberculosis (alluded to by Selzer), while the African chapter (Clumeck 1989) reviews controversial origin questions as well as various explanations for the high rate of heterosexual transmission; both chapters emphasize remaining questions and the need for continuing investigation. Mirko Grmek's 1990 history moves toward a multi-layered analysis of origins by drawing on epidemiological, virological, clinical, and social data and analyzing them systematically over time. What is striking, however, is that, even as specific questions appear to be answered for one intellectual or social community, they often live on for other communities. Thus, the resurgence of questions about "African AIDS" in the HIV–Duesberg–*Sunday Times*–*Nature* standoff of the 1990s was not altogether surprising (see Fujimura and Chou 1994; and Epstein 1996).

The overwhelming difficulty of even characterizing the diversity of the epidemic, let alone containing it, suggests that statistical measures—numbers—may once again be functioning as Williams says they did in the late nineteenth century: to offer us the illusion of control. As these numbers are taken up and deployed for various urgent purposes, however, they may take on a life of their own and reinforce a view of HIV disease as an unmediated epidemiological phenomenon in which cultural differences (such as differences in sexual practices) can simply be factored into a universal equation. But the local interacts with the global, AIDS continually escapes the boundaries placed on it by positivist medical science, and its meanings mutate on a parallel with the virus itself. Added to the medical, epidemiological, social, economic, and educational challenges of the AIDS crisis is its inevitably political subtext. AIDS is not a precious national resource; it is something nobody wants. Wherever it appears, AIDS discourse quickly becomes political as it is articulated to preexisting local concerns. To begin to identify these, it may be useful to retreat from the power of numbers and see what other forms of knowledge tell us.

In Africa, analysis of AIDS must inevitably confront questions of decolonization, urbanization, modernization, poverty, endemic disease, and development: in Uganda, for example, the legacy of civil war has been significant in assessing the AIDS situation, as has the influence of the church in discussions of health education; in Kenya, for the independent press at any rate, AIDS was used during the 1980s as an ongoing test of the central government's ability to acknowledge and resolve conflict (Caputo 1988; Timberlake 1986; and Ng'weno 1987). Feldman (1988) found in interviews that, for French AIDS researchers, the AIDS epidemic revealed the impact that France's colonial past and present African immigration have on French life (see also Pollack 1988). In his ethnographic study of AIDS in urban Brazil, Richard Parker placed the epidemic in the context of "the social and cultural construction of sexual ideology," or what he called the "cultural grammar" of the Brazilian sexual universe (1987, 158, 159). In both the United States and Great Britain, AIDS has intensified stress on health-care systems already in crisis (although in different ways). In South Africa, apartheid was seen to reproduce itself in the government's public health campaign: a postcampaign survey of black attitudes in the Johannesburg area found that many believed that there were "two totally different kinds of AIDS. The one that only affected blacks was acquired through sexual and ritual contact with baboons in central Africa. The other was acquired by sexual contact with homosexuals—white AIDS" (Seftel 1988, 21). In Cuba, mandatory HIV testing of the general population identified a small number of infected people, who were placed under indefinite quarantine. Placed in AIDS sanitoriums, they have received air-conditioning, color television, regular health checkups, and other amenities not generally available to the population at large. This treatment has been variously interpreted by Western commentators as a manifestation of Cuba's progressive health-care policies (one can certainly argue that Cuba has provided more support and resources for its infected citizens than many other countries) or as totalitarian and homophobic repression in a police state.[18]

These examples and others suggest that the reproduction in AIDS discourse of existing social divisions appears to be virtually universal, whether it is white or black AIDS, gay or straight AIDS, European or African AIDS, wet or hot AIDS, East or West German AIDS, central or west African AIDS, foreign or native AIDS, or guilty or innocent AIDS.[19] The First World/Third World dichotomy took diverse forms in the 1980s. In Africa, people with AIDS were initially described by those in their own countries as having sexual practices as strange as those of gay white men in San Francisco.[20] In Japan, officials believed initially that transfusion-related HIV infection among Japanese would not be a threat thanks to procedures for sequestering the national blood supply; while this Japanese/foreign division remained an animating feature of AIDS discussion and policy, statistics soon made clear that this safeguard was not magic (Haberman 1987). Richard Parker identified a similar dichotomy in the Brazilian medical community's transition from conceptualizing AIDS as a "foreign import" to accepting it (from 1985 on) as a disease that has "taken root" (1987, 157; see also Riding 1987, 8). Great Britain's announcement that HIV-positive applicants for visas from high-risk countries would be denied entry provoked accusations of racial imperialism when central African countries were classified as "high risk" but the United States was not (Sabatier 1988, 106–7; see also Pear 1987b; Masland 1988; and Schmemann 1988).

These divisions were, and are, at least in part, produced by what Dubos

([1959] 1987) calls "the inadequacies of the modern world"—that is, by a set of historically produced social arrangements. When AIDS in sub-Saharan Africa or Brazil is termed *a disease of development*, it is precisely the intractable social topography of recent history that is invoked, the problematic contours of development—environmental devastation, malnutrition, war, social upheaval, poverty, debt, endemic disease, movement toward democracy—now unavoidably illuminated and scrutinized in the international light of the AIDS crisis. As Rudolph Virchow wrote in 1948, "Epidemics correspond to large signs of warning which tell the true statesman that a disturbance has occurred in the development of his people which even a policy of unconcern can no longer overlook" (quoted in Dubos [1959] 1987, 218; see also Epstein and Packard 1987; and Dawson 1988).

Even the seemingly simple message to "use a condom" is actually a complicated drama that must incorporate competing scripts, play to hostile audiences, and ultimately raise as many questions as it answers. Already it has returned to the world stage such stock characters as the Ugly American, who, in the guise of the U.S. Agency for International Development, distributed in central Africa condoms that were too small and inelastic (Schoepf et al. 1988, 218). But in addition, as Brooke Grundfest Schoepf and her colleagues argue, the adoption of condoms involves "much more than a simple transfer of material culture" (Schoepf et al. 1988, 228).[21] Describing their experience with Project CONAISSIDA (an AIDS education and research program in Zaire), these researchers identify myriad ways that the condom question puts stress on the entire fabric of social relations. They point out, too, that the AIDS crisis is embedded in a continuing economic crisis that affects men and women differently: married women in traditional plural households may take up prostitution as a means of economic existence when their husbands can no longer support the household. Women's groups with which CONAISSIDA has contact express interest in information about AIDS and about condoms, but they also articulate resistance to the view that information and condoms offer a total solution, emphasizing the role of deepening poverty and the need for income-generating activities for women to provide alternatives to multiple-partner sex.

A different sort of complication is raised in Africa by the important role of nongovernmental organizations (NGOs). While these organizations may be reluctant to shift their agendas for AIDS or ally their already fragile causes with a yet more stigmatized one, they nevertheless often have excellent international and community networks. The International Family Planning Agency has prepared and distributed a well-received manual on AIDS for local as well as national use (Gordon and Klouda 1988; the manual is reviewed in Harper 1988); such efforts are likely to bring about increased U.S. aid for family planning. But, as Schoepf and her colleagues point out, "Ideological issues also need to be addressed. In Zaire nationalist sentiment currently links contraception and condom use to western population control strategies, which are viewed as a form of imperialism. Some husbands also view contraception as an encouragement for wives' extra-marital sexual relations. . . . These considerations suggest that it may be preferable to separate AIDS prevention from birth control efforts, rather than to place responsibility for AIDS interventions with family planning programs" (Schoepf et al. 1988, 219).

Fruitful acknowledgment of division is not accomplished by formula. To take one final example, the system of sexual classification that dominates discussions of AIDS internationally—heterosexual, homosexual, bisexual—is not universal. Criticisms of this system applied to AIDS discourse in Western industrialized countries are all the more valid in other cultures, for not only is sexuality complicated for individuals, with no fixed correspondence among the components of sexual desire, actual practice, self-perceived identity, and official definition, but it is culturally complicated as well. Richard Parker (1987, 161) argues that the hetero/homo/bi classification is seriously, conceptually, at odds with "the fluidity of sexual desire" in contemporary Brazil. While the medical model's distinctions clearly exist in Brazilian society and are increasingly familiar as a result of media dissemination, they remain largely part of an elite discourse introduced to Brazil in the mid-twentieth century. The traditional classification relates sexual practices to gender *roles*, with both gender and sex constructed by a fundamental division between a masculine *atividade* (activity) and a feminine *passividade* (passivity). Two males engaged in anal intercourse would be distinguished by who was the active masculine penetrator, who the passive feminine penetrated. Neither would necessarily perceive their activity as *homosexual*, nor would everyday language furnish them with the lexicon to do so. As Parker warns, this different perception of same-sex behavior has obvious and dismaying implications for conventional notions of "risk-group" identification and "safer sex" education (pp. 160–63).[22]

Parker's work, like other projects cited in this book, demonstrates the contributions of interpretive cultural analysis. The provisional nature of science is very difficult for policy and funding agencies to live with. Rather, there is pressure to produce a coherent narrative in which, if qualifications and ambiguities must be mentioned, they become simply routinized features of the story, to be quickly forgotten; problems of data are perceived to be mere temporary impediments to a refined and comprehensive analysis. Western medical science is conceived as a transhistorical, transcultural model of reality; when cultural differences among human communities are taken into account, they tend to be enlisted in the service of this reality, but their status remains utilitarian. This utilization may effectively accomplish specific goals: it was reported in the 1980s that some native practitioners (e.g., of voodoo) successfully overcame men's traditional resistance to the use of condoms by describing AIDS as the work of an evil spirit who uses sexual desire and the virus as secret weapons; condoms were presented as a means to trick the spirit and escape its lethal designs (Sabatier 1988, 134).

One can certainly support a global anti-AIDS strategy that mobilizes the scientific model of AIDS in culturally specific ways yet acknowledge imperialist aspects of a strategy that valorizes itself as universal rather than as culturally produced. As the foregoing examples suggest, ethnography and other forms of interpretive research are neither better nor less mediated than statistical approaches or other "objective" ways of knowing a culture, but they are different and produce unique insights. Nor are they incompatible with theoretical sophistication.

Research of this kind is not, however, the currency of the First World/Third World transaction. Expert advising is now a major Third World industry: more than half the $7–$8 billion spent yearly on aid to Africa in the 1980s went to European and North American professionals trained to provide expertise to the Third World (Timberlake 1986, 8). Gathering information, reporting facts, and advising the Third World are also mediated activities, permeated by history and convention. In *Blaming Others*, the Panos Institute's immensely useful 1988 sequel to and self-critique of its 1986 dossier *AIDS and the Third World*, Renée Sabatier observes how ironic it is that, in the information age, information should be such an elusive resource (1988, 4; and see also Panos 1990). But a second irony explains the first. It is not, precisely, a question of obtaining and disseminating "information" but, rather, one of acknowledging what information entails: acknowledging how language works in culture, how stories contradict each other, how narratives perform as well as inform, how information constructs reality. Cultural analysts in many fields are acknowledging the inevitability and indeed even the necessity of such multiple and contradictory stories. Yet, having recognized the theoretical complexity of communication, we continue to press communication into a purely pragmatic role that subordinates complication and contradiction to unequivocal assertion and scientific harmony.

Different accounts of truth produce differing material consequences. Tracing the historical relation between the "country" and the "city" and their evolution in English literature and social thought, Raymond Williams argued that, in the course of nineteenth-century imperialism, these two ideas became a model for the world, dividing not only rural from urban within a single state but the undeveloped world from the developed one as well. Underlying this model is the notion of universal industrialization, underdeveloped countries always on their way toward becoming developed, just as the poor man is always assumed to be striving to become rich. "All the 'country' will become 'city': that is the logic of its development" (Williams 1973, 284). Although this linear progression is largely a myth of late capitalism, that does not impede its deployment as an agenda item for the Third World.

For the new possibilities arising out of the AIDS epidemic, the "country" is a very fertile field. As early as 1986, according to a reference work called *Emerging AIDS Markets* (1986), 1,119 companies and other organizations were involved in AIDS-related activities: only 20–30 of them at that point were based in Third World countries, but at least 200 were engaged in research on AIDS in Africa and other projects likely to entail the use of Third World populations as trial subjects in the development of diagnostic products and vaccines (see Glaser 1988; and Ratafia and Scott 1987).[23] Subsequent reports about vaccine trials have made explicit the need for test populations that are "pharmacologically virgin" and, further, are still becoming infected at high rates. Gay men and intravenous drug users in the First World do not fulfill these criteria, not only because infection is leveling off in the first group and pharmacological virginity is not characteristic of the second, but also because *any* First World population is too educated, too exposed to the media, and too likely to take steps (including alternative treatments) to avoid infection or reduce clinical illness. In the mind of the city, only the country can furnish the unspoiled virgin material that the market needs, the naive informant still too ignorant to contradict instructions.[24]

First and Third World Chronicles

History is a legend, an invention of the present.—V. Y. Mudimbe, *The Invention of Africa*

The ethnographer's trials in working to know another people now become the reader's trials in making sense of the text.—Mary Louise Pratt, "Fieldwork in Common Places" (40)

But there is always another story, and a continuing one in the AIDS epidemic involves the untrustworthiness of other stories—their sources, motives, data, presuppositions, methodology, and conclusions. Media coverage in Africa of AIDS offers an alternative chronicle. In January 1985, for example, the *Nairobi Standard* publicly reported the presence of AIDS in Kenya for the first time in stories headlined "Killer disease in Kenya" (15 January) and "Horror sex disease in Kakamenga" (18 January). Subsequent accounts in state-owned newspapers repudiated the reports, claiming that the deaths were from skin cancer rather than AIDS, but Western press accounts speculated increasingly on the frightening implications of the presence of AIDS in central Africa. Then, in November 1985, Lawrence K. Altman's multipart series on AIDS in Africa in the *New York Times* reported not only that the epidemic was spreading rapidly in Africa but also that prominent U.S. researchers were convinced that the disease started there. Altman's opening sentence dramatically presented the thesis that was to become most controversial: "Tantalizing but sketchy clues pointing to Africa as the origin of AIDS have unleashed one of the bitterest disputes in the recent annals of medicine." Altman went on to say that these "sketchy clues," including blood samples, "have led to what has now emerged as the prevailing thesis in American and European medical circles that the worldwide spread of acquired immune deficiency syndrome began in Central Africa, the home of several other recently recognized diseases." As Altman conceded, however, not everyone accepts this designation of the virus's homeland: "The Africans vigorously disagree, and there is some criticism of the validity of the studies on which the theories are predicated. Indeed, controversial new results point both to and against AIDS originating in Africa, a fact that is fueling the international furor" (1985b, 1).

Two effects in the West of the *Times* series were to establish AIDS in Africa as an important scientific question and to place Africa on the U.S. agenda for AIDS media coverage, culminating in the journalistic frenzy of late 1986, which represented Africa as "devastated" by AIDS and AIDS-related illnesses. But stories about Africa were designed primarily to warn Western readers about themselves. "FUTURE SHOCK," proclaimed the cover of *Newsweek* on 24 December 1986, citing new worrisome projections of AIDS increases in the United States; one sub-head was titled "AFRICA: THE FUTURE IS NOW." (Recall the finding of the 1996 Kaiser Family Foundation media study, mentioned in chapter 2 above, that stories in U.S. media outlets about AIDS internationally virtually always concern the domestic implications of the epidemic.) In African countries, the effect was different. When Altman's series began to run

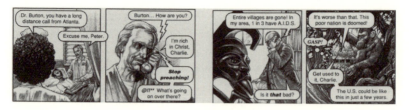

Like AIDS *in the First World,* AIDS *in the Third World is readily articulated to pre-existing interests and agendas. In* Going Home, *a 1991 evangelical comic book by Jack T. Chick (3.7), medical missionaries in an African nation attempt to communicate the apocalyptic nature of the epidemic to the "outside world," later in the comic persuading their* AIDS *patients to accept Christ ("home"=heaven).*

in the *International Herald Tribune* in November 1985, for example, outraged Kenyan officials confiscated the entire shipment of the paper. The African offensive against the "African origin" theory was launched with an editorial in *Medicus,* the official publication of the Kenya Medical Association, which hypothesized that tourists from around the world had introduced AIDS into Africa.

At this point, the Kenyan newsmagazine *Weekly Review,* published and edited in Nairobi by Hilary Ng'weno and widely considered one of the best newsmagazines in Africa, took on the responsibility of keeping the public informed about AIDS reports in the African and international press. In the face of increasingly vocal controversy and government silence, the magazine took the general position that developing adequate health care measures was more important than countering Western propaganda. Thus, the *Weekly Review* began providing summaries and analyses of scientific and press reports printed in the West, citing the numbers of AIDS patients reported in Zaire, Rwanda, Uganda, and Kenya. Although itself often critical of the Kenyan government's mode of responding to the AIDS epidemic, the *Weekly Review* was also critical of Western reporting. What Africa needed, Ng'weno told the Panos Institute, was concrete assistance, not "a never ending siren recounting a litany of disasters about to engulf the continent" (quoted in Sabatier 1988, 97).

An insightful analysis of the AIDS situation in Kenya (predating, of course, the instability that changed Kenya's politics in the 1990s) was provided by the political scientist Alfred J. Fortin (1987). Although Fortin criticized the actions of African governments, he was primarily critical of what he elsewhere (Fortin 1988) called the "aggressive bureaucratic and careerist politics" of the "development establishment"; unless development agencies remain under fire, he argued, the AIDS epidemic would allow them to reproduce the power relations of dominance and dependency already in place. In "The Politics of AIDS in Kenya," Fortin argued further that the dominance-dependency relation of development guaranteed English as the international language of AIDS discourse, a language that is necessarily "blind to the African world of meaning." He concluded that, despite Kenya's "comparatively well-developed medical infrastructure and working coterie of Western scientists, its efforts have fallen short of even the minimum requirements suggested by its statistics" (Fortin 1987, 907).

However much the *Weekly Review* might itself have been skeptical of "the development establishment" as well as Kenya's response to the AIDS epidemic, it did not buy Fortin's position either. Calling his paper "a hard-hitting and indicative, if lopsided, criticism of the Kenyan government, the ministry of health and the local press," the editor went on to contest a number of points of Fortin's analysis—for example, Fortin's point about language:

> [Fortin's] paper questions the language of discourse at discussions on AIDS in Africa. It argues that Africans have chosen to use the Western language when talking about the disease and since the language is transplanted, Africa is dependent on the West for its meaning and its continued development. Since the language is not indigenous to Africa, Fortin says, it is "blind to the African world of meaning."
>
> Students of African history have long argued that most of the diseases prevalent in Africa today were first witnessed with the advent of the foreigners on the continent and most of the terminology used by the medical practitioners in Africa [is] also borrowed from the developed world.
>
> African governments and researchers have also been emphatic that the AIDS virus was first diagnosed in the United States and, therefore, it would follow automatically that the language used in reference to the disease should be that developed by those who diagnosed it first. (Ng'weno 1987, 11–13)

As I understand it, Fortin's argument about discourse was intended to challenge—as Parker's was with regard to Brazil—the entire discursive formation of international AIDS discussions applied unthinkingly and hence in some sense imperialistically to diverse cultures; it is a position that most discourse analysts would share. Ng'weno, however, rejected the corollary implication of this view: that English is somehow "foreign" to Kenya and Kenyan leaders. Although English is indeed a colonial legacy, it plays many roles in Kenyan activities today. Hence, the Zairean philosopher V. Y. Mudimbe (1988) argues that Western discourse has contributed to but not monopolized what he calls "the invention of Africa"; rather, the objects of that discourse are also subjects who have produced an intricate interweaving of European and African commentary, rendering the notion of a "purely African discourse" an impossible dream. At the same time, Ng'weno made the political point that language marks nationality and origin: to use English with regard to AIDS helps sustain its identity as a Western disease. Ng'weno's position acknowledges the power of linguistic constructions of reality and demands the right of Africans to participate in that construction process. This resistance to adopting AIDS, to giving it—in the words of the Altman story—a home, was reflected elsewhere in the *Weekly Review*, where supposedly indigenous African terms for AIDS and AIDS-related diseases (like *slim disease* and *AIDS belt*) were placed in quotation marks and often explicitly rejected; the term *magada*, cited by Fortin as the name for AIDS in Swahili, was never used in the *Review*.[25]

The juxtaposition of these two complex and interlocking analyses makes clear that the chronicle of AIDS in the Third World cannot be understood monolithically. It must be understood not only in terms of the "rich history and complex political chemistry" (Miller and Rockwell 1988, xxiii) of each affected country but also as a heteroglossic series of conflicted, shifting, and contradictory positions. Even "AIDS" and "the AIDS epidemic" and "HIV disease" must be understood this way. We are talking, after all, about an epidemic disease with more than forty distinct clinical manifestations, some of which consist of the absence of manifestation, some of which are unique to particular regions of the world, and some of which apparently have nothing to do with a deficiency of the immune system. When we talk about the Third World, we are talking about more than a hundred countries of the world. In Africa alone, we are talking about a continent four times as large as the United States, which has more than fifty countries, nine hundred ethnic groups, and three hundred language families (Zambia alone has more than seventy languages). As Miller and Rockwell argue, it is absurd to talk about "the AIDS problem in Africa" (1988, xxiii) except for specific and well-defined purposes.

The international AIDS narrative is hence neither complete nor fully accessible. The present invents the past, but the present itself has not yet been invented; accordingly, this is a narrative necessarily in process, which we must read with all our critical faculties at work. A crisis serves as a point of articulation for multiple voices and interests, and the AIDS crisis in the Third World is no different. My goal has been to demonstrate (1) that, as in the First World, diverse interests are articulated around AIDS in ways that are socially and culturally localized and specific; (2) that institutional forces and cultural precedents in the First World prevent us from hearing the story of AIDS in the Third World as a complex narrative; (3) that understanding this complexity is a necessary, if not sufficient, condition for identifying the material and conceptual nature of the epidemic; and (4) that such an identification is necessary in order effectively to mobilize resources and programs in a given country or region.

In the course of this chapter, I have identified several analytic strategies through which we may explore these questions and tried to suggest areas of discourse where better understandings may be particularly valuable: the conventions of mass media stories, the discursive traditions and modes of representation that figure in the AIDS narrative of the sciences and social sciences (including tropes, stereotypes, linguistic structures, and pervasive metaphors); the emergence of a dominant international AIDS narrative and its role in the linguistic and professional management of the epidemic; the processes through which AIDS is conceptualized within given institutions for everyday use; and the very terms through which we identify what chronicle we think we are telling. The checks and balances provided by the warring voices at each of these multiple discursive points render it impossible to refuse contradiction—that is, to argue that any single unchallenged account of AIDS exists in the Third World, any more than it does in the First World.

To hear the story "AIDS in the Third World," we must confront familiar problems in the human sciences: How do we know what we know? What cultural work will we ask that knowledge to perform? What are our own stakes in the success or failure of that performance? How do we document history as it unfolds? In concrete terms, we certainly need to forsake, at least part of the time, the coherent AIDS narrative of the Western professional and technological agencies and listen instead to multiple sources about and within the Third World (Schmidt 1990). When we do so, we may find it less instructive to determine whether a given account is true or false than to identify the diverse rules and conventions that govern whether and where a particular account is received as true or false, by whom, and with what material consequences.

The performative work that such narrative structures do can be identified, challenged, recuperated, reassigned; it cannot be eradicated. Language about AIDS, illness, and epidemics is already informed with metaphor (influenza got its name because illnesses were believed to be under

the *influence* of the stars; *infect* means "to contaminate," "to communicate," and "to stain or dye," a connotative web even the most vigilant
housekeeping cannot sweep away). To believe that information and communication about AIDS will separate fact from fiction and reality from
metaphor is to suppress the linguistic complexity of everyday life. Further, to inform is also to perform; to communicate is also to construct and
interpret. Information does not simply exist; it issues from and in turn
sustains a way of looking at and behaving toward the world; it shapes
programmatic agendas and even guides capital investments.

Diverse voices, then, represent not diverse accounts of reality but significant points of articulation for ongoing social and cultural struggles.
Further, once we adopt the view that reality is inevitably mediated, we
become ourselves participants in the mediation process; such voices may
then provide important models for challenging existing regimes of truth
and disrupting their effects—in the Third World as in the First.

4

Seduced and Terrorized:

AIDS in the Media

We had no such thing as printed newspapers in those days to spread rumors and reports of things, and to improve them by the invention of men. . . . Such things as these were . . . handed about by word of mouth only; so that things did not spread instantly over the whole nation, as they do now.—Daniel Defoe, *A Journal of the Plague Year, 1722*

It is journalism's responsibility to comfort the afflicted and afflict the comfortable.—Media maxim

If it bleeds, it leads.—Media maxim

There is a particular breed of monkey that, like other monkeys, is curious by nature; it is also, even in captivity, terrified of green snakes, its evolutionary enemy. If you put a green snake in a paper bag on the floor of the monkey's cage, the monkey, irrepressibly curious, will slowly approach the bag, open it, and look in: a green snake!!! The monkey will fly to the top of the cage and cling there, terrorized. But, as its panic gradually subsides, its eyes will fall again on the paper bag. What could be in it? Slowly the monkey descends, approaches the bag, opens it: a green snake!!! To the top of the cage again, clinging and terrorized.[1]

Like the monkey confronting the green snake, many of us recoil in terror when we encounter media representations of the AIDS epidemic, especially representations on the major television networks; yet we are also aware of the medium's seductive power and indeed experience it anew with every return to the brown bag.

But should we care? Why analyze network television, an industry proclaimed to be increasingly corporate and uniform? Patterns of AIDS coverage on the networks seem at times so identical that one imagines their representatives all at the same AIDS workshop—learning how to give events the same conventional interpretations, select the same AIDS experts, use the same misleading terminology, and recite the same pieties about scientific progress. Yet television, including the three major networks and PBS, is not monolithic. Rather, like every cultural form, it offers openings and opportunities for intervention. Further, television's unique power to shape public opinion means that, in the current crisis, we cannot afford to dismiss it as unsalvageable. A brief inventory of the problematic approaches to the AIDS epidemic in the 1980s suggests, in turn, how television could more intelligently engage, educate, and galvanize its audience.[2] A look at the 1990s explores, in turn, whether the brown bag holds anything new.

The 1980s

What Kind of Story? The AIDS Narrative as Always Already Written.
Whereas the *Los Angeles Times* and the *San Francisco Chronicle* printed stories about a rare pneumonia among gay men within days of the CDC's first official report in June 1981, television network news did not cover AIDS until June 1982. Television coverage of the epidemic has remained largely passive, relying on an inherited as-told-to narrative format that does not encourage careful, complex, and original reporting or analysis. The AIDS epidemic, by contrast, is unprecedentedly complex and a prototypical challenge to current social systems. Some media organizations have accordingly assigned a "point person" to coordinate AIDS coverage, but this remains the exception rather than the rule. Media specialists say that the AIDS epidemic has generated twelve or more official subissues for the mainstream media (Dearing and Rogers 1988). These are the "pegs" that reporters require to hang stories on. This narrative division of labor has the advantage of keeping AIDS and HIV in the news because each issue (children, virology, blood, drugs, etc.) has its own narrative trajectory, its crises and dead periods. But, if a story does not fit one of the established pegs, it is typically doctored or dropped. Of course, what is not covered as news may be carried elsewhere: an "L.A. Law" (NBC) episode addressed ethical questions of euthanasia; "The AIDS Connection" was a viewer call-in show; and "Nightline" (ABC) has staged several debates over controversial AIDS issues. But individual components of the epidemic are always part of the larger story, and it is this larger story that network television, addicted to simplicity and convention, hardly ever gets right. Stories begin portentously: *AIDS is the plague of our times. AIDS continues its deadly spread. The Third World is devastated by AIDS. AIDS: Is a cure at hand?* They end predictably: *Will the plague be stopped? Only time will tell. We may be closer to a cure, but it will not come in time for people like John Smith.* Although often undermined or even contradicted

by the story they surround, these rhetorical bookends promote an illusion of containment. Even stories *about* controversy get packaged in a univocal way.

One could argue that this is not bad. The physician and writer Marshall Goldberg (1987) asserts that, although flawed by sensationalism, melodrama, inaccuracy, and a desire to entertain, television nonetheless succeeds in controlling hysteria by teaching the basics: AIDS is believed to be caused by a virus, the virus is not transmitted by casual contact, and so on.[3] But the problem is that AIDS 101—AIDS by the book—is always an already written narrative. Although treatment experience was suggesting by the mid-1980s that people with AIDS might live many years beyond their diagnosis, perhaps indefinitely (and see L. Altman 1987a), in 1989 PBS's "The AIDS Quarterly" was still calling AIDS "finally fatal." Apart from the fact that life itself is finally fatal, actual footage within these reports often challenged their doomsday judgment. In a spring 1989 segment, a number of experts characterized AIDS as a chronic, manageable condition; people with AIDS were shown living their lives, taking considerable responsibility for treatment choices; and a group of physicians emphasized the importance of refusing the orthodox scenario, of "not looking down the end of the film." Yet the program's prior declaration of inevitable doom had already been established by the opening signature: an electronic green image of the human immunodeficiency virus (HIV) invades white cells and fills the television screen; a *Jaws*-like soundtrack pounds inexorably; and a weeping female intravenous drug user cries to the camera, "I'm breaking out in sores all over my body—open sores."

As I noted in chapter 2 above, the media's failure to challenge or subvert dominant accounts of AIDS reduces subsequent contradictions to mere errata slips tucked discreetly into the formula narrative. A 1987 "Nova" (PBS) program on AIDS vaccines said nothing about government inaction in testing drugs, nor did it challenge the FDA's single-minded focus on AZT. Such programs on the epidemic conform to the formula attributed by Dorothy Nelkin to television science documentaries in general: "In an effort to personalize science, the scientist is made a star; the tweed and turtleneck chic of Carl Sagan and Jonathan Miller represents a contrast with the eccentric and dangerous figures on entertainment programs, but these scientists are equally idealized. Many documentaries, such as those produced by NOVA, are thick with awe and reverence; while explaining science carefully, with elegant visual images, they . . . perpetuate the images of science as arcane" (Nelkin 1987b, 74–75).

A 1984 "Nova" documentary titled *AIDS: Chapter One* clearly struggled to keep science idealized even as its scientific protagonists engaged in bitter debate over the discovery of the virus believed to cause AIDS. The film's title draws on the conventional conceit that scientific progress is an unfolding story, yet it can also be interpreted to suggest that scientific progress itself is a story, a novelistic fiction. The documentary displays many of the requisite features that Nelkin identifies: viral images enhanced and magnified, background music that telegraphs significance, the AIDS crisis presented as a "puzzle" being solved by an interdisciplinary detective team, laboratory footage shot and edited to simulate key moments in the chronology of AIDS (Robert Gallo telephones the CDC), interviews with participants, schematic drawings of the immune system. As viewers, we take these sequences in stride, hardly thinking twice about what we are actually being shown or why. Anne Karpf's (1988) study of media coverage of medicine provides a more reflective framework for analysis. Karpf identifies four basic approaches or frames for media representations of medicine and health: the medical, the consumer, the self-help, and the environmental. *AIDS: Chapter One* exemplifies the medical frame, featuring the test tubes and white coats of the biomedical lab, clinicians examining patients, an authoritative omniscient voice-over, metaphors of mystery and puzzles, and the theme (despite setbacks, dead ends, unanswered questions) of scientific progress triumphant. Uncertainties and contradictions are contained within the progress narrative, and patients are shown in relation to scientists and physicians. As Bertin and Beck (1996) contend, when science is presented as news, it is largely stripped of the context we need to make sense of it. This enables scientific facts to float free, attaching to whatever context presents itself. No wonder such effort is made to present AIDS 101 as a package deal.

In 1989, Peter Jennings ended an "AIDS Quarterly" piece on treatment options with an upbeat comment: "So, for a change, at least all the news about AIDS is not all bad—in part because we have the financial resources in America, and also because there has been enormous pressure to mobilize those resources." The grammatical structure of Jennings's "there has been" disguises the facts concerning just who has exerted the pressure and how long they have been doing it. Outstanding exceptions, such as a "MacNeil/Lehrer News Hour" segment of 2 May 1989 entitled "AIDS: Drug Dilemma," demonstrate that television coverage can be bolder—and effective. Leading off the "News Hour," Spencer Michaels of station KQED in San Francisco chronicled the enormous pressure that gay activists had placed on the FDA and some of the successes and failures that activism had produced; the segment opened and closed with shots of the familiar SILENCE = DEATH button of the AIDS activist group ACT UP.

Public Broadcasting: The Nonalternative Alternative. These last examples suggest that public broadcasting could challenge the commercial networks' AIDS coverage. In fact, it rarely does so. "PBS?" asked the independent video artist John Greyson in the late 1980s,

> Don't get me started. After nearly a decade characterized by benign neglect and not-so-benignly horrendous coverage . . . their big contribution to America's number one health priority is . . . a 2.5 million-dollar quarterly newsmagazine, that will update viewers on the "facts" . . . interview "experts" . . . and feature profiles of AIDS "heroes." . . . In other words, over $12,000 per minute to replicate what the commercial networks do so offensively already as a matter of course. . . . This, from the same network that has a Congressional mandate to buy substantial amounts of independent work, but has so far aired only one of the over 100 independent works produced on AIDS to date. (Greyson 1989a, 23)[4]

Public television's role could be to provide critical and interpretive commentary on the prevailing stereotypes of the commercial networks; instead, it reiterates professional wisdom, merely performing such tasks as translating scientific language into baby talk and generally reproducing the most conventional views about the function and role of "art." Douglas Crimp writes that "AIDS and the Arts," a July 1987 feature aired on "MacNeil/Lehrer," reinforces the stereotypical equation of AIDS with homosexuality, suggests that gay people have a natural inclination toward the arts, and "implies that some gay people 'redeem' themselves by being artists, and therefore that the deaths of other gay people are less tragic" (Crimp 1988c, 4). In treating "the arts" as universal as well as omitting mention of the wide range of artistic responses to AIDS, PBS was depriving its viewing audience of some of the most exciting video works around. Examples from this era include Greyson's *The ADS Epidemic* (1987), *The World Is Sick (Sic)* (1990), and *The Pink Pimpernel* (1989b), Marshall's *Bright Eyes* (1984), Huestis and Dallas's *Chuck Solomon: Coming of Age* (1986), Julien's *This Is Not an AIDS Advertisement* (1987), Hammer's *Snow Job* (1986), Kybartas's *Danny* (1987), Kalin's *They Are Lost to Vision Altogether* (1988), and Parmar's *Reframing AIDS* (1987).[5]

What's Wrong with This Picture? Television and Representation. Network television consistently doles out orthodox blocks of AIDS-related content like a series of bricks:

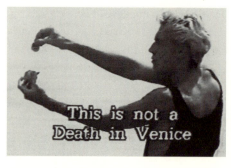

Toronto artist John Greyson's brilliant "music video" The ADS Epidemic (1987) reworked the plot and imagery of the film Death in Venice to argue that the AIDS epidemic need not spell the death of love, sex, joy, life, or gay liberation (4.1). In just over three minutes, the video's parodic reenactments, hilarious lyrics, and zippy musical soundtrack skewered the clichéd modernist link between sex and death, rejected the tradition of moral judgment in epidemics, and called for collective resistance: social, political, and biomedical.

AIDS is caused by HIV, or "the AIDS virus."
AIDS is spread by those infected with HIV, or "AIDS carriers."
Those infected with HIV will develop AIDS.
Those with AIDS (or "AIDS victims") will die.
AIDS is a gay disease.
AIDS is everybody's problem.
Fear of AIDS is worse than AIDS itself.
Science is conquering AIDS.
Conquering AIDS may be impossible.
The face of AIDS is changing.
The general population is still safe.

From such shabby bricks is network AIDS news built; no wonder the structure totters whenever a novel spread-of-AIDS rumor comes along. As Alexandra Juhasz (1995) puts it, network television invokes tried and true strategies for producing "pleasure and power" (120), as much in science reporting as in other domains (see *AIDS: Chapter One* 1984, for example—an early "NOVA" documentary on the epidemic). Instead of these truisms, or catechisms, television could be providing state-of-the-art bricks; better yet, it could provide knowledge and analysis about the construction process. It is nonsense to think that such knowledge is too complicated for television audiences or too hard to communicate visually. True, network news is an expensive and fast-paced operation with little room for experimentation. Yet many models and resources are available that could be adapted to news formats. For example, Coleman Jones's 1987–89 radio series "The AIDS Campaigns" for the Canadian Broadcasting Corporation's "Ideas" series explored such sophisticated notions as the social construction of reality, representational icons, and discursive strategies that disguise homophobia. *Will Sex Ever Be the Same Again?* produced in 1990 by Jane Ryan and Helen Thomas for ABC Radio National in Sydney, addressed equally difficult questions of representation and reality. Such examinations of the construction of knowledge are not beyond the grasp of the average American listener; nor are such independent video documentaries as Jean Carlomusto and Maria Maggenti's *Doctors, Liars, and Women: AIDS Activists Say No to Cosmo* (1988) and the several productions since 1987 of the Testing the Limits Collective (see, e.g., Testing the Limits 1987). In *All of Us and AIDS*, a 1987 educational video produced by Catherine V. Jordan, high school students make a video about AIDS; the film-within-a-film device effectively raises questions about representation. In contrast, the networks appear to believe that the real world, simple and accessible, is out there waiting for prime time; processes and decisions about representation—what the Brazilian writer Herbert Daniel (1989) calls the "staging of the epidemic"—are ignored.

Instead, television's analysis of representation might graphically demonstrate and deconstruct its own recurrent conventions in representing persons with AIDS: the emaciated gay man in a hospital bed; the "innocent" transfusion victim surrounded by loving family; the Third World prostitute, in red. Counter-examples to these canonical AIDS victims were for many years systematically excluded from media reports, just as some people with AIDS were rejected by photographers because they did not look sick enough (Crimp 1992). Such an analysis could examine how disjunctions between text and image affect AIDS stories. For example, while Mervyn Silverman argued on "Nightline" in the early 1980s that AIDS was not "caused" by gay men, the television audience saw shots, not visible to Silverman, of gay men kissing (Steve Rabin, personal communication). Timothy E. Cook (1989) cites an early NBC report that "homosexuals say that AIDS victims are being discriminated against, evicted by landlords, and feared by health workers," but the accompanying visual footage showed gay men in bikinis sporting in the sun on Fire Island (see also Shilts 1987; Silverman 1989; and Alwood 1996). In another case that Cook identified, a local news station hinted, in contradiction to all existing scientific evidence, that mosquitoes transmit AIDS, illustrating the story with footage of virologist Robert Gallo lecturing on a completely different subject.

It is not that network television is incapable of illustrating its own representational processes. The cable network C-Span regularly describes the conditions of media production, and, even in such highly charged contexts as U.S. presidential campaigns, television has been willing to devote time to the way candidates are packaged for the mass media. Perhaps this coverage is neither as complex nor as politically inclusive as we might wish, but it shows clearly that the networks grasp the concept of representation, have indeed put it to work in representing their own operations, and believe that viewers will get the point.

What's Wrong with This Picture? The Representation of Gay Identity.
The human interest of an individual's story can capture viewers and challenge stereotypes about the epidemic. Television often does this well. What is more difficult is linking these individual stories to the collective social crisis and showing accurately the complexity and contradictions of individual and social identity. *An Early Frost*, the first feature-length drama about AIDS on network television, which premiered on NBC in November 1985, features an appealing yuppie attorney with an attractive gay lover; but, when the attorney finds out that he has AIDS (possibly infected by his lover, who turns out to have had occasional "promiscuous" episodes), he returns to the bosom of his nuclear family to die, with limited signs of the gay community or its support. *An Early Frost* demonstrates television's tendency to dissolve the gayness of the gay person with AIDS into a homogenized and universalized person facing death. Without denying that this universalizing process may sometimes be valuable, I would suggest that it enables television both to dramatize death and to escape a fate worse than death: showing gay people being gay. *TV Guide*'s story on lead actor Aidan Quinn was entitled "Why This Young Hunk Risked Playing an AIDS Victim." The story spells out what the "risk" is: "Back in Chicago, Quinn's home town, acquaintances couldn't understand why their gruff friend wanted to play someone so . . . unmanly, an outcast with such a vile disease. 'You gotta be courageous to play a fag, Aidan,' one told him" (Leahy 1986, 34–38).[6]

In retrospect, despite its unsatisfactory emphasis and resolution, *An Early Frost* seems downright benign compared to the March 1986 "Frontline" (PBS) program *AIDS: A Public Inquiry*, which includes within its two-hour framework the crashingly homophobic film *Fabian's Story*, or the infamous December 1988 episode of "Midnight Caller" on NBC. Both programs present gay men as dangerous "AIDS carriers," pathological and sadistic "Patient Zero" figures who continue to have unsafe sex even after they are diagnosed and warned. Both the documentary and the drama kill off their villains by the end. And neither clearly distinguishes HIV infection from the multiple clinical conditions that warrant a diagnosis of AIDS.[7]

Television could provide a great service by finding ways to convey the relation between self-identified identity, perceived identity, fantasy, desire, and actual behavior—as well as between one's identity in acquiring HIV infection, transmitting it, and experiencing its consequences. Interestingly, television soap operas, which thrive on the paradoxes and complications of identity, have easily incorporated the AIDS epidemic into ongoing narratives. The video *Ojos que no ven* (Eyes that fail to see) (Gutierrez-Gomez and Vergelin 1987), produced primarily for Spanish-speaking communities, although also available in English, uses the popular telenovela format to weave together several different themes about AIDS embedded within the story of an extended Latino family. Given the many confusions about gender that I outlined in chapter 2 above, such a clarification of identity would have been especially useful for women. As I said, despite various educational efforts, many women continue to believe that they are not at risk; nor are most AIDS agencies set up to provide treatment or social services for women. Further, many women, "at risk" or not, are still unaware that the epidemic indirectly threatens all women's rights (routine testing of all pregnant women and so on)—a threat spelled out clearly in Parmar's *Reframing AIDS* (1987) and Amber Hollibaugh's *The Second Epidemic* (1987). Finally, a different kind of media coverage could show people speaking for themselves, thus acknowledging political, sexual, cultural, social, ethnic, gender, and class identities as something more than "special interests."

Divisions of gender, sexuality, race, and class are only the most common of the us/them divisions that AIDS seems universally to generate wherever it appears. Many projects throughout the world have tried to address the problems created by this division. A film called *Se met ko* (Benoit 1989) was produced by the Haitian Women's Program to educate heterosexual people in Haiti about AIDS and HIV. Taking as its starting point the division between the middle class and the stigmatized populations associated with AIDS and HIV transmission, the film opens with an extended middle-class family sitting around the kitchen table talking about a neighbor who's in the hospital with AIDS. The husband walks in: "You still talking about AIDS?" He's sick of the topic; moreover, it makes him very uncomfortable. The film deliberately downplays the "homosexual connection" to concentrate instead on the division between straight women and straight men, taking on issues of denial, communication, condoms, and the double standard. To get away from the talk about AIDS, the husband storms away to go hang out and play cards with his buddies at the barbershop. As they sit around bullshitting and trading macho misconceptions about AIDS, they are gently interrupted by their friend Pierre, who challenges their stereotypes. How surprising, too, when he insists that AIDS is very serious, that they must protect themselves from becoming infected, and that, above all, they must take responsibility for not infecting their partners. "Come on, Pierre! Lighten up!" they say, trying to change the subject, but instead they receive a careful demonstration of how to use a condom.

The decision in *Se met ko* to downplay homosexuality is not unusual in targeted educational vehicles and raises important questions. To call such a decision "homophobic" may obscure important information about a cultural text's context and the cultural work that it is meant to perform. This does not mean that every AIDS film, television show, or educational video must be judged solely on its own terms and given two thumbs up for subcultural authenticity—no matter how rigid and conservative its message. Rather, a standardized checklist of loaded categories (race, class, sexuality, gender) may miss the salient issues that the text embodies. To take one example, Maria V. Ruiz examined the video *Alicia*, an educational AIDS video in Spanish targeted at Latino populations, especially women. Using a dramatic narrative format, *Alicia* explicitly communicates the message that AIDS (SIDA) is serious and incurable, that—contrary to stereotypes— HIV is not confined to groups of "others," and that a woman may contract HIV from her husband, whose life outside the home may bring him in contact with the virus. Clearly, and perhaps predictably, a double standard is built into this scenario, yet one can also argue that, realistically, that double standard is part of what does put women at risk for HIV. Through her careful analysis of the juxtaposition of images, settings, and language (e.g., use of medical terminology, selective use of English and Spanish words), Ruiz also reveals *Alicia*'s dubious subtext: that the major source of HIV risk for Latinos is assimilation with Anglo culture (Ruiz 1996).

Safe Sex, Safe Texts, and the Market. Although many individual television stations readily accepted ads and public service announcements on both birth control and AIDS, the commercial networks initially refused to do so on the grounds that accepting them would violate their First Amendment rights of free speech. Their refusal exemplified what Greyson (1987) calls "the ADS epidemic": acquired dread of sex, which you can get from worrying about AIDS or watching too much television. Embodying a

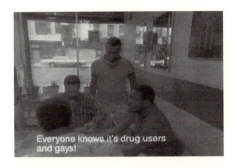

Everyone knows it's drug users and gays!

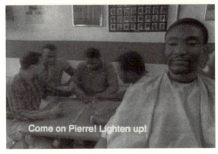

Come on Pierre! Lighten up!

Creative responses to AIDS/HIV throughout the world draw on diverse traditions and formats: social realist drama, avant-garde video, postmodern animation, black-and-white documentary, No theatre, reggae rhythms, oral histories, soap operas, grafitti, and sandwich boards. Se met ko (Benoit 1989) uses a "telenovella" format to tell the story of an extended middle-class family in Haiti and how its various members come to terms with the realities and risks of HIV. When a male neighbor is hospitalized with AIDS, the straight male husband character will have none of it—AIDS is what "other people" get—and storms off to find solace and shared denial among his barbershop buddies. There, however, they unexpectedly receive an enlightening if unwelcome lecture from their friend Pierre on the severity of the epidemic and necessity of using condoms—to protect both oneself and one's partners (4.2: the usual suspects; 4.3: Pierre lectures on condoms).

formidable array of AIDS-related phobias, including homophobia, erotophobia, fear of the exotic and unknown, fear of death, and fear of conservative retribution, the networks' uncharacteristic prudery is pathetically portrayed as "nonpolitical"—as though something called *neutrality* can actually be achieved. One irony is that the networks spend vast sums developing ways to commodify people, products, events, and phenomena for the viewing public. To an industry equipped for the market, condoms should not have presented a major challenge. A second irony is that, back in 1989, before Newt's rise and fall in the 1990s, he and Henry Waxman—congressional champion of progressive approaches to AIDS—participated in a PBS town meeting on the epidemic. For at least one frozen minute of television time, the two actually agreed that a bipar-

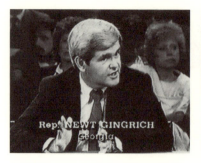
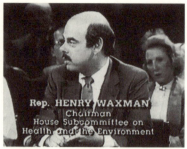

Although public television was criticized for waffling on whether to show such powerful independent videos as Tongues Untied, *PBS achieved some memorable moments. In this 1989 installment of the Frontline series* Managing Our Miracles *(4.4), Henry Waxman once again called for an aggressive, progressive public health assault on AIDS and criticized the networks for refusing to advertise condoms on television. Somewhat surprisingly, Newt Gingrich responded that Congress and the president could quite likely persuade the networks to cooperate (not that they ever actually tried).*

tisan federal effort could successfully convince the American public, and the television networks, to accept condoms as a critical public health measure.[8]

In part, individual television journalists have created their own reporting problems. The first network story on AIDS, by NBC in June 1982, took the line that "homosexual lifestyles" had triggered an epidemic. This angle on AIDS endured, presenting reporters with the ongoing problems of talking about a group—gay men—not usually covered on the nightly news. They had to find suitable language to communicate the facts of transmission and prevention and educate viewers about potential risk without causing panic. Accordingly, television coverage evolved a kind of visual and verbal shorthand that allows "the facts" to be telegraphed: two men together in an urban setting, in shops or among crowds; phrases like *the exchange of bodily fluids, homosexual acts, safe sex.* The dreaded phrase *anal intercourse* was finally uttered only after the way had been paved by detailed broadcasts about Ronald Reagan's 1985 colon surgery.[9] The problem of conveying information without causing panic was handled through messages that mixed fear with reassurance—the "bookends" around the story that I mentioned above. Thus, ever-popular "spread-of-AIDS" stories were quick to reassure viewers that the epidemic's spread remained confined to isolated groups and locales: in other words, people newly identified with AIDS were efficiently relegated to the (still) growing category of contaminated Other, while the "general population," the presumed category of the viewer, although (still) shrinking, remained pristine and pure.

By the time network television finally broke down and told viewers to "use a condom," this once explicit piece of advice had itself become a euphemism, a symbolic stand-in for the difficulty of talking frankly about AIDS and sex, a piece of technical information to be moved from group to group, culture to culture, in isolation from the social, political, economic, cultural, and moral understandings and commitments of those to whom the advice was given.[10]

Spectacles of AIDS, Regimes of Truth. Michel Foucault (1977) uses the term *régime of truth* to describe the circular relation between truth, the systems of power that produce and sustain it, and the effects of power that it induces and that it in turn reconfigures. Truth, in this sense, is already power: we can forget the fight for or against a particular truth and instead interrogate the rules at work in a society that distinguishes "true" representations from "false" ones. Media accounts of AIDS conform to such regimes; they come to seem familiar, true, because they simultaneously reinforce prior representations and prepare us for similar representations to come. Media research often contributes to these regimes, for example, by studying media coverage of the epidemic without examining gay or alternative media or, as I said in chapter 2 above, by evaluating media effects in simplified terms. These studies often plot the quantity of media coverage in relation to some "real-world" variable like the number of AIDS cases or scientific findings. That Rock Hudson's illness and death provoked a dramatic increase in coverage is then deplored, as though it revealed a deep moral weakness in the American psyche. But the Hudson case was more than simply the first major case of celebrity AIDS: it provided significant evidence that the media and "the masses" alike will pay attention if something interests them.

The networks excuse their haphazard, reactive response to the AIDS epidemic with direct appeals to the market. "The public is sick of AIDS," said the director of research at one of the major networks at a conference a few years ago. "It has lost its market value." If we think that we can overcome that reality, "we exaggerate our own importance" (Stipp 1989). This newfound humility camouflages a fair degree of cultural and institutional imperialism. Moreover, the statement "The public is sick of AIDS" depends on the tedious us/them dichotomy embedded in AIDS's social construction; "the public," of course, is "the general population," here constructed as a media market assumed to be heterosexual and to be (or to want to be) white, middle class, and securely enmeshed in the nuclear family. The networks could aggressively examine how to present televisually the complex aspects of this epidemic, seeking advice from more creative and knowledgeable videomakers than themselves. Instead, caught in the production and reproduction of overdetermined images, journalists reflexively phone predictable requests to the nearest AIDS service organization: "Can you get me a black prostitute with two kids who shoots drugs and is still on the street spreading AIDS?"

The 1990s

So where are we now? By the end of the 1980s, more people in the United States knew what AIDS was than knew that George Bush was president. Meanings and theories continue to proliferate, and virtually every media outlet has by now contributed to the inventory. Total media stories on AIDS outnumber those on cancer, on Saddam Hussein, on the fall of the Soviet Union. AIDS routinely shows up on television dramas, soaps, sitcoms, and talk shows. Resources on the Internet are vast. Recent writings about AIDS as harbinger of viral apocalypse fuel fascination with the virology and immunology of human life, while sinister pop culture narratives about viral warfare will probably help the Pentagon secure its funding far into the next millennium.

As I suggested in chapter 2 above, the networks have not dramatically changed their coverage of the epidemic in the 1990s. Yet change has come, primarily through the explosive diversification of outlets and formats and the flexibility with which audiences can gain access to them. On the networks, some specific improvements can be identified. Most noticeable, perhaps, is the introduction of alternative viewpoints into regular news coverage—for example, in the use of AIDS activists and critics of federal policy as sources. This was especially evident at the Sixth International Conference on AIDS in San Francisco in June 1990, when many media outlets assigned reporters to cover the activists as well as scheduled conference activities. A model of AIDS programming during the conference was provided by San Francisco network affiliates, encompassing live interviews and commentaries on the conference, regular "town meetings," and independent documentaries and feature videos on a range of topics. Although such efforts may not alter the format or authoritative stance of network coverage, their sheer volume allows diverse voices to be heard. Similarly, several segments of "The AIDS Quarterly" moved toward a more critical and investigative stance; one, for example, demon-

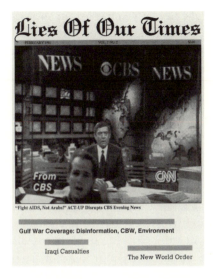

Lies Of Our Times

"Fight AIDS, Not Arabs!" ACT-UP Disrupts CBS Evening News

Gulf War Coverage: Disinformation, CBW, Environment

Iraqi Casualties

The New World Order

Bob Huff's satiric video Rockville Is Burning *chronicled the takeover by* AIDS *activists of a network news broadcast. During the Persian Gulf War,* ACT UP *members really did infiltrate the "CBS Evening News" broadcast studio and even appeared briefly on camera, before surprised anchor Dan Rather cut to a commercial* (4.5: cover, Lies of Our Times, *February 1991*).

strated how federal AIDS funds are actually spent and, in some cases, misspent at the state and local level.

International reporting and programming have slightly improved. "The AIDS Quarterly" examined the epidemic in Poland and Eastern Europe, a story that required resources unavailable to many videomakers, and also offered *Born in Africa* (Lutaaya 1990; Bayles 1992; Koehler 1990), a documentary of events after Ugandan rock star Philly Lutaaya announced that he had AIDS. But international coverage that moves beyond familiar American perspectives is still rare on the networks. To its credit, *Born in Africa* included information about the conditions of and constraints on its own production, provoked in part by prior sensationalistic coverage of AIDS in Africa by the Western press. An excellent BBC program on AIDS and art moved far beyond the humanist perspective familiar in U.S. reporting. Programs from the United Kingdom include the series "Out on Tuesday," independently produced by Mandy Merck for Channel Four; unfortunately, these are rarely accessible in the United States outside film festivals.

In the 1989 mock documentary *Rockville Is Burning* (Bob Huff and Wave 3), AIDS activists take over a CBS-like television station and—with the help of "live uplinks" from the people who were *really* there—begin broadcasting a radically different version of the epidemic. In January 1991, shortly after the United States declared war on Iraq, AIDS activists from ACT UP disrupted the start of the "CBS Evening News with Dan Rather" and the "MacNeil/Lehrer News Hour" on PBS. "Fight AIDS, not Arabs!" shouted the protestors at CBS as the network cut hastily to a commercial; at PBS, the group carried a sign reading "Act up, fight back! Fight AIDS, not Iraq!" (Associated Press 1991). The takeover, however brief, enacted *Rockville Is Burning* in real life, reminding us that, on occasion, the mass media can be induced to deliver the unexpected.

Another example is suggested by CNN's live coverage of the events in Tiananmen Square in China, C-Span's live coverage of various AIDS events, and the popularity of alternative and resistant films and videos at the Fifth and Sixth International AIDS Conferences.[11] Television's coverage of the Persian Gulf War, particularly by CNN and C-Span, was, we now know, highly centralized and controlled. At the same time, the near-saturation coverage also (if not always intentionally) educated viewers about the conditions of televisual production. We also glimpsed the potential, via satellite access, for global perspectives that are still, at this point, virtually unavailable to the average U.S. viewer.[12] Rather than accept hopeless judgments from research and marketing departments that "AIDS is a dead issue" or that "We can't say *condom* on television," network executives and individual reporters can look at what interests people, what they watch, what they find compelling. They can repeatedly communicate the simple and undisputed messages about AIDS and HIV infection that are still widely misunderstood. They can find clear ways to dramatize the fact that you cannot get HIV infection or AIDS from giving blood. They can aggressively seek international and alternative perspectives. They can be courageous enough to do what network television has thus far failed so dismally to do—provide programming and public service announcements directed at the general population in its *true* diversity, including gay men and women, poor people, old people, middle-class and working-class people of color, drug users, sexually active adolescents, and so on.

The proliferation of AIDS media discourses in the 1990s radically diversifies sources of knowledge and takes some of the burden off any particular cultural product to do it all. Again, studies of media coverage and media effects measure only the most important outlets (the *New York Times*, the "CBS Evening News," and so on). Williams and Mathery (1995) tell us, however, that an extraordinarily diverse and eclectic range of media sources is actually used by people to gain information, form attitudes, and learn the terms of public debate. Although we cannot yet precisely track the diversification of AIDS discourse through every viewing format, specialized print outlet, cable channel, independent video, radio talk show, or website, we can sketch some of the terrain.

The massive coverage of Magic Johnson's announcement in 1991 that he was HIV positive took AIDS media messages into almost every conceivable media venue—notably, into the African-American media and into sports media. I tracked a lot of this—not very systematically, but enough to say that the story showed up all over the world within twenty-four hours; that it ran under various headings, including breaking news, sports, style, business, and health; and that Johnson's announcement—a decade into the epidemic—triggered thousands of calls to hotlines and hospitals from people—especially young men—seeking information about the risk and prevention of heterosexual transmission. As sports reporters scrambled to learn AIDS 101 and find the right language and tone for the Magic story, they also assumed that "guys all over the country are running to get tested." They didn't say, "Hey guys, use condoms." One spin-off was Magic's appearance on "The Arsenio Hall Show," the consciousness-raising potential of Arsenio's visible modeling of anti-AIDSphobia (hugging Magic, treating him as your everyday superstar, not a sick or disabled one) offset, unfortunately, by the audience applause that followed the emphasis on *hetero*sexual as opposed to *homo*sexual transmission. One would like to have ethnographic data to see what real television audiences made of this.

To digress on this subject of real audience response, I would also be curious to know reactions, from audiences or focus groups or whatever, to the series of radio and television public service announcements released with great fanfare in early 1994 by Donna Shalala and the Clinton administration as "hipper, hotter" messages about AIDS and safer sex. I found incomprehensible the one in which the speaker puts a condom on a microphone and it muffles the sound. In another, cute but hardly "hipper" or "hotter," a condom sneaks by a cat and jumps into bed; the message is that, until condoms are automatic, we have to put them on ourselves. But I am most curious about the one in which a young white man speaks directly to the camera, supposedly to his beloved (him, her, or us, the viewers): "I'll never hurt you, I'll never lie to you, I'll never put you in danger. There's a time for us to be lovers. We will wait until that time comes." When Shalala was criticized by some AIDS education groups for once more producing ads that ignored the target population still hardest hit—gay men—she pointed to this ad as counterevidence because the gender of the person addressed is unknown; therefore the sexuality of the guy speaking is equally unknown. But, as I see it, the guy speaks in the idiom of romantic heterosexual love, and he's saying that we—well, he and his beloved; I don't feel like he's speaking to me personally—will wait until. . . . Until what? Until we're married? Until we've had our HIV tests? Until we can get to a drugstore? Others have reacted differently to this PSA; "World News Tonight" correspondent Phil Greenwood stated simply that it promoted abstinence, while students in my classes have read it in various and sometimes contradictory ways. So I would like to know more. But perhaps at this point only well-designed, multimedia, and carefully targeted intervention programs can provide that knowledge.

This would seem to be the conclusion of recent research. AIDS media campaigns to date largely reflect the assumptions and methods of traditional mass media. Yet, in their comprehensive review of AIDS/HIV mass communication education and prevention efforts, Flora et al. (1995) concluded that the cumulative state of knowledge and research is "dismal." Although the ubiquitous behavioral change model in AIDS/HIV campaigns (with its progression, e.g., from changes in information to attitude to behavior) is widely assumed to be valid and used repeatedly, few campaigns actually reflect a sound understanding of media research and evaluation, and no campaign to date reflects what could be called state-of-the-art knowledge. Hence, after more than a decade, we still do not know precisely what we know, whom we have reached, what they have learned, how they have changed, or even how and whether the "mass media" and "mass communication" had anything to do with the claimed effects—let alone what should be done in the future. This conclusion seriously challenges the existing and accepted knowledge base of the social and behavioral sciences (positivist behavioral theory with its rational action model, the biomedical model of disease, and quantitative methodological principles).

So, in one sense, the versions of AIDS and AIDS education in specialized media outlets provide information about what more successful campaigns might look like. Reoriented toward specific communities, toward social and cultural values as well as medical information, and toward collective as well as individual behavior, they also suggest how contemporary media—news, entertainment television, talk shows, MTV, CMTV, and so on—can supplement structured educational campaigns by accomplishing specific kinds of cultural work. A 1996–97 story arc on the prime-time NBC dramatic series "ER" is a good example. Although previous AIDS episodes had included a range of topics, this story line featured Jeanie Boulet, a regular ensemble character who contracted HIV from her former husband. In addition to addressing personal relations in the context of this revelation, the program addressed issues raised by Jeanie's HIV status for the hospital and the ER and took the audience through the process of developing policy concerning infected health professionals. As the chief of staff charged his attendings with drafting a policy, he handed them stacks of documents, studies, briefing books, and policy guidelines; in a print behind him, a raven overlooked the process. Throughout the subsequent discussion, the camera continually circled the two attendings—going "round and round," in mimicry of their conversation.

The two prototypical made-for-television movies about AIDS, *An Early Frost* and *Our Sons* (which I discuss in detail in chap. 6 below), have been joined by other prime-time television movies (e.g., *In the Gloaming*, 1997) and by ambitious cable films like HBO's *And the Band Played On*, *Longtime Companion*, a theatrical release that then aired on PBS's American Playhouse series, and *Philadelphia*, a box-office success later shown on network television. Problematic as each of these films is, in its own unique way each accomplished important cultural work. One unusual theme of *Longime Companion* was its self-conscious use of media for character and plot development. The opening scene uses the first story about the epidemic in the *New York Times* as a device to introduce the cast of characters (who are shown at work and at home reading successive paragraphs to each other), "the facts" of the epidemic at that point, and divergent interpretations of these facts by the characters. One of these is an actor in a daytime serial drama, another is the scriptwriter, and a high point of the film shows the scriptwriter gathered with his friends to watch and cheer his career triumph: the first gay kiss on daytime television.

And the Band Played On, hugely annoying though it was to many expert AIDS communities (see, e.g., "Playing It Safe" [1994], a review symposium on the film to which I contributed a partial defense), was the first screen drama to communicate the history and international scope of the epidemic, tie together the work of various scientific and clinical fields, emphasize politics and policy, and, in short, go beyond stories of individual suffering. It is flawed by playing down sex and homosexuality—no surprise there—and by reproducing Shilts's moralistic positions and blockbuster certainties; but, to many who watched it, it remains a revelation (on the film's history, see Cathcart 1987). When I saw *Philadelphia* in theatrical release, a group of African-American adolescent guys were sitting behind me; they were attentive, especially after Denzel Washington appeared, and did not treat me to any of those overheard student zingers that academics love to turn into teaching points; when the movie ended, one of them broke the silence to say, simply, "I had no idea." So I hated the opera scene: big deal. "Saturday Night Live" capitalized on the film's unexpected hit status with a hilarious "*Philadelphia* action figures" commercial parody, complete with courtroom and ejector seat ("sold separately") for those who discriminate against people with AIDS. An equally funny and even more tasteless AIDS-related sketch portrayed "Saturday Night Live" regular Ellen Cleghorne as former Surgeon General Jocelyn Elders teaching grade school kids to recite "C is for condom." "Tomorrow, children," she concludes, "we do D is for dental dam."

Let me conclude with a final concrete example. In April 1995, the soap opera "General Hospital" (ABC) introduced an AIDS story line that itself received considerable media coverage. Although other soaps had featured characters with HIV or AIDS in recent years, "General Hospital" was the first to make AIDS a central story line rather than a mere plot device and use it to educate and explore the meanings of AIDS. (In an excellent overview of the soaps' treatment of illness and disease, including the "General Hospital" story line, Jones [1997] notes how well suited the topic is to the soap opera format, where doctors and nurses as characters are so plentiful they outnumber the patients by about eleven to one.) The person stricken with AIDS was adolescent Stone Cates, a relative newcomer to "General Hospital" but already popular as the love interest of longtime favorite character Robin Scorpio. Stone was a former street kid who did "bad things" and hence was not a classic "innocent victim" (although, in the soap world, *bad* covers everything from premarital sex—Stone's source of HIV—to murder). His mysterious symptoms dragged on for months, creating pain and anxiety for him, Robin, their loved ones, the Port Charles community, and the show's many fans. Finally, in April 1995, he was diagnosed with AIDS (the long period of undiagnosed symptoms enabling the scriptwriters to dispense with years of "asymptomatic HIV infection"). The revelation sparked widespread media coverage as well as lively debate and speculation among "General Hospital" newsgroup fans on the Internet, who in the first few weeks after Stone's diagnosis addressed such topics as the following:

the difference between HIV and AIDS;
deaths of friends with AIDS;
other shows with AIDS themes;
how well Stone's physician broke the bad news;
how well the actor playing Stone's physician handled the scene;
whether the cast of "General Hospital" was in general up to such a demanding and serious story line;
what the actors in real life think about AIDS, safe sex, drugs, etc.;
whether a physician would be required to tell Robin, Stone's sexual

partner, that he is HIV positive—or whether, alternatively, he or she would be required *not* to tell Robin (doctors and lawyers contributed to this series of exchanges);
confidentiality in doctor-patient relationships in general;
physician options, treatment options;
state-by-state differences in and exceptions to confidentiality and reporting requirements;
whether the "General Hospital" writers and producers would really kill off a beloved character; or, worse, *two* beloved characters; or, even worse, all of Port Charles.

Some of these topics point to the connectedness of characters on soaps and the audience members' intimate knowledge of those connections. The last point, in particular, reminds us of the common truism about sexually transmitted diseases: You're not having sex with just one partner; you're also having sex with all the people your partner has ever had sex with, and all the people those partners have had sex with, and so on. When any longtime fan can actually put a face and name to all those partners, a soap like "General Hospital" offers a potent and vivid representation of the mystery and messiness of sexual contact.

One message (or post) on the Internet spoke directly to this intimacy with the characters (I have slightly edited these posts): "If GH is going to allow Stone—and maybe Robin—to contract the disease, they are taking this opportunity to show that AIDS/HIV can truly strike anyone—namely, the people we love." This led to speculation about the various tasks the story line could accomplish. Another participant wrote, "It may be painful and scary to lose these friends. As a young gay man I know what it feels like. If GH can evoke all these feelings, maybe it will contribute to the eradication of this disease. A lot to ask of a soap opera, I know, but we all have our responsibilities, and GH seems to be accepting theirs." Another fan replied, "I agree that that's an important message. But I hope they can do it without infecting Robin. Did you ever see a now-defunct show called "Life Goes On"? The story line that made me watch was one in which a teenage girl's boyfriend had AIDS and she stuck with him through the course of the illness. I thought it was outstanding, and I'd like them to do the same with Robin." Of particular interest was the possibility that suspense over Robin's HIV status would play itself out in real time, providing "six months of uncertainty as everyone waits to see if Robin has been infected while simultaneously dealing with the progression of the disease in Stone." Another post was about media coverage and audience response:

"I just saw a piece on 'Good Morning America' on the Robin/Stone/AIDS story and also on the local news here in Raleigh NC that talked about the National AIDS Hotline nearby in Research Triangle Park. I was sorting papers at the time so I may have missed something, but apparently the hotline is getting a lot of calls as a result of people watching GH. It surprised me how many had not known until now that AIDS had anything to do with them."

With Stone's death that November came the bad news that Robin, whose first HIV assay had been negative, now tested positive for HIV. Having used Stone's character to educate viewers about AIDS in its many manifestations, the importance of tolerance and social support, and the ups and downs of treatment, the show used Robin to exemplify "long-term nonprogression" and regularly update viewers about treatment advances, including protease inhibitors.

All these examples contribute to AIDS media discourse. They may not embody the imagination, political acuity, or pizazz of John Greyson's wonderful music video *The ADS Epidemic* (1987), but now, ten years later, I would take them over a green snake any day.

5

AIDS, HIV, and the Cultural Construction of Reality

Scientific activity is not "about nature," it is a fierce fight to construct reality.
—Bruno Latour and Steve Woolgar, *Laboratory Life*

You don't have 500 dollars for the operation? For 50 bucks I'll touch up the X-ray.
—Groucho Marx

As the AIDS epidemic entered its second decade, its importance as a social and cultural as well as a biomedical crisis was widely acknowledged. The Fifth International AIDS Conference in Montreal in 1989, for example, was titled "AIDS: The Scientific and Social Challenge" and featured more social and cultural presentations than in past years. Richard A. Morisset, M.D., chair of the program committee, wrote in the official program that the conference was expected to be "an extraordinary one" not only for its scope but also for "the profoundly humanistic philosophy guiding it." He continued: "Anyone who has kept a close watch on the series of International Conferences on AIDS that began in Atlanta in 1985 will have noticed how these encounters have gradually opened up. Originally, you will recall, the meetings dealt almost exclusively with biomedical topics. Yet scientists soon had to admit that AIDS is not simply a medical problem, but also a human drama" (Morisset 1989, 6).[1] With nearly one-third of the panels and papers devoted to "social aspects of the epidemic," the commitment of the Montreal conference was clear.

What is less clear is precisely what it means to describe AIDS as a social or cultural phenomenon or, in a phrase becoming common, *a cultural construction*. To call AIDS *cultural* may mean simply that—like any great event or crisis—AIDS significantly affects social life and symbolic expression. But to call it *culturally constructed* invokes long-standing debates about human knowledge and the nature of the world. This is far from evident in Morisset's opening statement, which characterizes the *problem* as medical, the *drama* as human, and links the recognition of AIDS's *social*

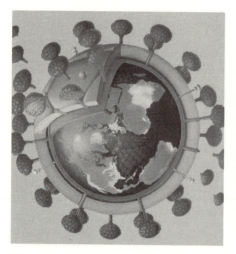
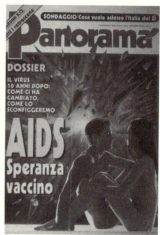

This image of HIV *appears on the cover of* AIDS: A Global Crisis, *a handsome spiral bound booklet produced and distributed by the Wellcome Foundation (1989); inside, a more technical image of* HIV *appears. In contrast to most representations that fill the scholarly, popular, and marketing literature, this image is labeled "Artist's Impression of* HIV I*" (5.1: copyright Graphico Hamburg, Hans Ulrich Osterwalder). The virus is very differently stylized on the cover of the Italian newsmagazine* Panorama *(23 June 1991), an issue highlighting the 1991 International* AIDS *Conference then under way in Florence (5.2).*

challenge to a humanistic philosophy. The anchoring tradition remains biomedical: "Naturally, we all know that the ultimate solution will eventually come to light in a laboratory. But meanwhile, what can the virologist or microbiologist offer an AIDS victim and his or her loved ones to ease the burden? To help them combat the ignorance and intolerance they face, which are growing day by day?" (Morisset 1989, 6). Here, the human sciences, handmaiden to the biomedical sciences, do their best to ease the suffering and combat ignorance until the laboratory can find the "ultimate solution." The "social challenge," primarily a matter of helping individuals cope with pain and death, is what happens "meanwhile."

The biomedical vision embodied in this conference statement is widely shared and deeply embedded in Western postindustrial culture. The discourses of virology, molecular biology, and immunology permeate the ways we think and talk about the AIDS epidemic. "We report here," wrote the Pasteur Institute research group in *Science* in 1983, "the isolation of a novel retrovirus from a lymph node of a homosexual patient with multiple lymphadenopathies" (Barré-Sinoussi et al. 1983, in Kulstad 1986, 49).

Just seven years later, the sprawling exhibitors' area at the 1990 Sixth International Conference on AIDS in San Francisco was dominated by an immense three-dimensional glass model of the human immunodeficiency virus (HIV). Not only aesthetically stunning, HIV had become an intensely personal experience as well. Andrea Walton, for example, "one of the one thousand people with HIV who attended this week's conference," was profiled by a San Francisco television station; the camera followed Walton as she wandered through the exhibit hall and paused to scrutinize the model glass virus: "That's my enemy—that's what I fight every day. I'm feeling overwhelmed because it's killing me—and it's actually pretty. There are a lot of things in nature that are deadly and pretty and I guess that's what I'm dealing with" (Saiz 1990).

Elsewhere in the world, the virus is also experienced and represented in many ways. In a Central African Republic pamphlet on AIDS written in Sango (c. 1988), the immune system is shown surrounding the human figure like a rope; viruses, pictured as beaked and bat-like birds, are eating through the protective boundary. In the Brazilian magazine *Veja* (10 August 1988), HIV is pictured attacking cells that look like Caspar the Friendly Ghost, a popular way of illustrating the immune system in 1950s medical textbooks (see Haraway 1989a). Paul Farmer (1990) shows that understandings of AIDS (SIDA) among villagers in rural Haiti were diverse until 1987, when accumulated knowledge and firsthand experience of the disease led to a shared model based on tuberculosis and, therefore, believed to be caused by a microbe. Writing about the cultural construction of AIDS in Botswana, Benedicte Ingstad (1990) notes that, with incidence still low, people sometimes talk about AIDS ironically as the "radio disease"—widely publicized but not yet experienced. Although associated with violation of sexual proprieties, the disease will need to become more common before traditional healers can decide whether it should be diagnosed as a traditional (*Tswana*) disease or as a "modern" disease.

If we think of cultural construction as a symbolic model of reality, these formulations of HIV raise several questions. What kind of correspondence do we presume to exist between the representation of a virus and its reality? Is this reality universal and unchanging? What features of culture determine the form in which reality is constructed? What is the role of language in articulating and popularizing a particular construction? Is any articulation a construction? Do different representations make a difference? Three general takes on these questions are familiar. First, the virus is a stable, discoverable entity in nature whose reality is certified and accurately represented by scientific research; a high degree of correspondence is assumed between reality and biomedical models. Second, the virus is a stable, discoverable entity in nature but is assigned different names and meanings within the signifying systems of different cultures; all are equally valid, although not all are equally correct. Third, our knowledge of the virus and other natural phenomena is inevitably mediated through our symbolic constructions of them; biomedicine (including germ theory) is only one of many, but one with currently privileged status. While none of these views is purely realist ("HIV is an autonomous physical reality that we merely label") or purely idealist ("HIV is an abstraction that exists only in the mind"), the first—despite the provisional nature of much scientific inquiry—is characteristic of science and medicine, the second of a nonjudgmental cultural relativism that nonetheless often assumes the fundamental correctness of Western biomedicine, and the third of a radical constructionism that foregrounds such mediating processes as language and makes few claims about universal truth.

Professionally allied to both the first and the third positions, medical anthropologists have tended, by default perhaps, to take the middle ground on this epistemological and ontological continuum: most seem more comfortable with the notion of a single, stable, underlying biological reality to which different cultures assign different meanings than with the view that everything that we know about reality is ultimately a cultural construction. Ingstad, for example, argues that health officials in Botswana should recognize traditional healers' knowledge and influence over villagers' health-seeking behavior. Yet, ultimately, she privileges a Western biomedical account of HIV infection, noting that some healers are cooperative and receptive to modern health information while "others are skeptical, prefer to keep a distance, and may promote behavior that is counterproductive to prevention. Considering the seriousness of the AIDS epidemic and the likelihood that the incidence of the disease will increase in Botswana in the near future, it is important that healers be made to feel that they have a role to play in the prevention of this disease" (Ingstad 1990, 38). The "be made to feel" of this conclusion suggests, perhaps, the moral and intellectual burden of carrying out ethnographic fieldwork driven in part by the threat of a particularly vicious and terrifying infectious disease for which Western health intervention strategies seemingly remain the best form of prevention. As new cases of AIDS around the world continue to escalate, many researchers engaged in cultural analysis are having to develop theory under crisis conditions and, at the same time, efficiently produce data to guide prevention programs. Our growing knowledge of cultural difference and specificity does not make this easy. Pedagogy across culture involves more than translating prescriptions for behavior change into different languages; inevitably, we need to know more about the meaning of given practices and conceptions, their place in a community's social and cultural life, the political economy that frames them, and the contingencies that sustain or discourage them.

There are pressing reasons for attempting to clarify the concept *cultural construction*. In the face of the epidemic's growing toll, the moral and technical limitations of a facile constructionism are obvious. To paraphrase Pauline Bart, everything is cultural construction, but cultural construction isn't everything.[2] "Culture," moreover, figures so insignificantly in the crude realism of most discussions about AIDS that cultural scholars hardly have time to do more than lobby for its inclusion somewhere in the big picture. Yet, with its long-term influence over the direction of policy, research, education, and legislation, the AIDS crisis makes it all the more imperative to take seriously the conceptual clashes between different symbolic models and the ways in which biomedicine is itself culturally constructed. Because the question of culture is central to interdisciplinary work on AIDS and to wider struggles against the epidemic, this chapter explores relations between AIDS and culture and seeks to refine our understanding of how AIDS can plausibly be characterized as a cultural construction. The epidemic demonstrates the unique value of the concept *cultural construction* and, at the same time, highlights the danger of using it.

Cultural Construction and Mannheim's Paradox

If we are asked: "How can a logical construct like culture explain anything?" we would reply that other logical constructs and abstractions like "electromagnetic field" or "gene"—which no one has ever seen—have been found serviceable in scientific understanding.—A. L. Kroeber and Clyde Kluckhohn, *Culture*

"Culture," writes Raymond Williams, "is one of the two or three most complicated words in the English language" ([1976] 1983, 87). As Williams shows, *culture*'s historical legacy encompasses both material and non-material meanings—for example, both the concrete objects that a cultural community produces (pots, books, television sets, glass models of HIV) and the complex of practices, attitudes, beliefs, and ideas that make up its way of life. This is a duality on which ethnography rests and the reason for the elaborate fieldwork practices aimed at helping the investigator reconstruct the signifying or symbolic system underlying another culture's everyday life. At once useful and problematic in examining the AIDS epidemic, it is one of several dichotomies that the term *culture* invokes: Williams notes that *culture* has served to distinguish *material* from *spiritual* development yet also to distinguish *human* from *material* development. In American anthropology, A. L. Kroeber and Clyde Kluckhohn's (1952) exemplary and instructive semantic history of the word and concept was instrumental in institutionalizing ethnographic, relativist definitions of *culture* over older elitist and chauvinist uses of the term to mean progress toward the practices and values of European civilization. (In his appendixes to Kroeber and Kluckhohn [1952], Alfred G. Meyers notes that anthropologists tend, in contrast, to hold up other cultures as a "didactic mirror" [p. 208] that reflects unfavorably on modern society.) Their review demonstrates, too, that the term continues to embrace both specialist and nonspecialist meanings.[3]

The term *cultural construction* derives less from the field of anthropology than from the sociology of knowledge. Our current understandings are informed by a number of sources, including Karl Mannheim's *Ideology and Utopia* ([1936] 1985), a study in the sociology of knowledge that examines the way in which knowledge is bound up with being. For Mannheim, although all knowledge of the world is finally indirect and partial, any object of knowledge becomes clearer with the systematic and cumulative analysis of different ways of seeing it (from Dilthey: "situational determination" or "seat in life"). These ways of seeing are existentially determined, not mere perspectives but fully naturalized worldviews; identifying them is the task of the scholar or researcher (the "socially unattached intelligentsia"). Political and historical change comes about, in part, through the clash between two ways of seeing the world that Mannheim terms *ideology* and *utopia.* For Mannheim, *ideology* is not the politically tainted doctrine of conventional usage but a serious worldview; it is a position that constructs the world as situationally congruent—that is, so that the status quo is reinforced. *Utopia* constructs the world as situationally transcendent—so that the status quo is challenged. "The world," the same material object, is rendered by ideology and utopia as two very different realities, each of which the world's material data appear to support. Particularly useful is Mannheim's emphasis on the hermeneutical activities that produce different constructions. Both ideology and utopia produce distorted determinations of reality, but ideology works to maintain what is (as ideology renders it), while utopia works to transform reality into its own image. When ideological and utopian visions become locked in sustained opposition over time, proponents of the two camps inevitably become intimately familiar with each other's positions and, therefore, symbiotically and ironically, perfectly situated to engage in a sophisticated exchange of critiques. I return to this symbiosis below.

That Mannheim treated ideology as a subject for serious investigation was important for Peter Berger and Thomas Luckman's influential work *The Social Construction of Reality* (1967), originally formulated as a project for sociology, although ultimately taken up more vigorously by other fields. Drawing on Dilthey, Mannheim, Weber, and others, Berger and Luckman argue that we routinely experience the world in the form of multiple realities. Given the constraints of environment and biology on the human animal (i.e., human beings have no species-specific environment), the worlds that we inhabit are largely socially—not physically—constructed. We work to create meaning, to achieve and maintain a cognitive coherence, because our ability to be in the world at all is at stake (no habitat will do it for us). When problematic sectors of experience threaten to disrupt the totality, we work to integrate them, often by marking them as "finite provinces of meaning" (Berger and Luckman 1967, 25) through explicit linguistic transitions. Although anchored in its specific set of social determinations, each of these multiple realities is nevertheless experienced as total, nontrivial, and inescapable. The commonsense reality of everyday life occupies a privileged position for Berger and Luckman; although it is but one reality among many, it offers a realm where our subjective experience of the world seems trustworthy and meanings seem to be unproblematically shared with others. The object of sociological analysis is the self as it goes about creating meaning in everyday life.[4]

Originating in a phenomenological analysis, *The Social Construction of Reality* had immediate resonance throughout the social sciences. The book's very title, its insistence on the validity of multiple socially determined realities, and its analysis of ideology's function in deploying what we think we know to resolve knowledge that has been rendered problematic—all provided a way of thinking about the production of knowledge that moved away from the pervasive realism and totalizing determinism of postwar social science. But, in the United States, Thomas Kuhn had in 1962 published *The Structure of Scientific Revolutions*, a sociology of knowledge in the natural sciences; although more or less cleansed of its Continental and phenomenological influences, Kuhn's analysis treated scientific theories as social constructions rather than assigning them (as even Althusser did) to a realm of truer discourse that transcends social history. True, Kuhn ultimately pulled back from the precipice of radical constructivism (in the enlarged 1970 edition), yet, as a compelling and socially situated account of scientific change, the book's influence and liberatory potential were enormous, in some respects preempting and even superseding the project of Berger and Luckman.

On such works is founded a dialectical view of the intersections between the real material world and human consciousness—*dialectical* because the known world is determined neither by "reality" nor by the perceiving mind but is rather a product of the interaction of the two, a product continually modified first by one, then by the other. Such works also provide a foundation for self-reflexivity in the social sciences, enabling social and cultural critics to characterize positivist accounts (of social life or scientific progress, say) as themselves "social constructions." Making this argument in *The Interpretation of Cultures*, Clifford Geertz charges that positivist social science is not qualified to analyze symbolic action adequately; it is the ethnographer who is best equipped to attempt "the perfection of a conceptual apparatus capable of dealing more adroitly with meaning." Geertz insisted that the cultural be inserted into the study of sociology of knowledge, challenging the widespread view that science is radically different from ideology—that, in the recurrent simile of the literature, thought determined by fact is like a crystal clear stream while ideological thought is like a dirty river. That the study of ideology itself repeatedly and inevitably becomes ideological is what Geetz labels "Mannheim's paradox." Geertz continues: "Where, if anywhere, ideology leaves off and science begins has been the Sphinx's Riddle of much of modern sociological thought and the rustless weapon of its enemies" (Geertz 1973, 194).

The Sphinx's riddle can be read more broadly as the problem of any constructionist approach, for where, if anywhere, does construction leave off and reality begin? That cultural constructionism is itself culturally constructed, the product of particular intellectual interests at a particular point in history, creates the potential for theoretical paralysis or relativism, which may in turn inspire impatience, the embrace of a reliable realism, and charges of idealism, mentalism, armchair speculation, or semantics. But there are differences between the kind of dialectic embodied in cultural constructionism and the conventional realist-idealist dualism. This is made clear by more radical versions of constructionism in which ideas have a life and logic of their own yet are in intimate dialogue with the material data—including the discursive data—of a real world (*a real world*). The point is that these data always engage with an already constructed perceptual and interpretive apparatus, albeit one designed to mitigate or erase its own effects (e.g., scientific method). A construction-ist view must, therefore, encompass the apparatus as well as the data. The Sphinx's riddle is answered then, or at least finessed, by such studies as Karin D. Knorr-Cetina's (1981) application of a rigorous ethnography to the sociology of knowledge; setting out to examine the production of scientific knowledge in a laboratory setting as an anthropologist would study a strange culture, Knorr-Cetina moves away from social explana-tions for scientific research, in Kuhn's sense, to an emphasis on meaning, discourse, and the discursive construction of knowledge within a given disciplinary culture. Insisting on the manufactured, *made* nature of sci-ence, Knorr-Cetina concludes that science must be seen as radically con-structive rather than descriptive and that scientific discourse is not quali-tatively different from other discourse. Noting the laboratory's concern with "making things work," she emphasizes the etymological connection between *fact* and *fabrication*. One can compare Ludvik Fleck's earlier definition of a scientific fact not as an entity with established ontological autonomy but as that which constrains subsequent scientific discourse: "a stylized signal of resistance in thinking" (Fleck [1935] 1979, 98).

Crucial insights here are the recognition of the role of discourse and the insistence that discourse entails concrete practices. Like Foucault's sys-tem in which entities are products of the discourse that embodies them, Knorr-Cetina's detailed analysis dissolves any strict dichotomy between material and nonmaterial elements of scientific research (e.g., laboratory apparatus vs. "ideas"), between objects and discourse, and between sci-ence and ideology. Scientific laboratory operations, she argues, are consti-tuted by the exegeses and symbolic manipulations in the laboratory itself; these construct an argument primarily designed to make sense within the field. Written communication—mainly in the form of scientific journal publications—crystallizes the laboratory's entire argument and stakes its claim. As a discursive field of interaction, science is directed at and sus-tained by the arguments of others; writing is, therefore, at the heart of its social and symbolic foundation. But writing is in no simple correspon-dence with natural reality, and Knorr-Cetina reminds us of Pierce's asser-tion that manifestation in writing reveals the presence not of an object but of a sign (i.e., not of a referent but of a symbol).

Knorr-Cetina also asserts, quoting Dorothy L. Sayers ([1927] 1987, 70), "Facts are like cows—look them in the face long enough and they gener-ally run away." But the observer must get close enough to phenomena to glimpse their true character: getting a good hard look requires uncovering the rules of everyday practice and attempting to capture the meanings in the culture being observed. In short, one must go beyond simply the desire to understand or even to describe the other culture; one must let it speak and then give voice to the story it tells. This approach does not guarantee an unconstructed account, indeed cannot, for this is impossible; but it does enable us to achieve a "decentered constructivity." Finally, scientific inquiry and the study of science always take place within a given context, a context that includes the community of one's peers. Departing from conventional notions of peer review as a rational and authoritative evaluation by a scientific elite, Knorr-Cetina argues that a scientific laboratory does not simply enter its product—its publications—into open competition in the scientific marketplace; rather, the publication is shaped from the beginning by the gatekeeping operations of scientific peer review. Gatekeeping thus influences the entire research process, including which research project is selected and how it is pursued. Gerald Geison's (1995) compelling study of Pasteur's laboratory notebooks argues this same point in detail, tracing the interaction of the lab work with the broader social and scientific worlds in which it took place as well as the discursive conversion of everyday notes and records into public science, specifically into the format of the scientific journal paper. Geison argues not that the notebook science is more "true" or "real" than its public representations but rather that the relation is interesting and far from transparent (involving, e.g., what Geison calls "formulaic discrepancies").

For Knorr-Cetina, the constructed nature of science is defined through concrete practices situated within the culture of a discipline. Bruno Latour and Steve Woolgar, whose study *Laboratory Life* ([1979] 1986) builds on Knorr-Cetina's work, further sketch this cultural domain. Observing that *fact* means simultaneously what *is* fabricated and what is *not* fabricated, they maintain that scientific accounts are necessarily provisional and uncertain; this is their essential character, whether explicitly articulated or not. They define the construction of scientific facts as "the slow, practical craftwork by which inscriptions are superimposed and accounts are backed up or dismissed." "It is through practical operations," they continue, "that a statement can be transformed into an object or a fact into an artifact" (Latour and Woolgar [1979] 1986, 236). There is no inherent or persistent difference between material and intellectual dimensions of construction: what is the subject of today's intellectual dispute is incorporated into tomorrow's laboratory furniture. (Compare Antonio Gramsci's rejection, so influential in the development of cultural studies, of the classic Marxist dichotomy between materialism and idealism [Laclau and Mouffe 1985], Stuart Hall's [1980a, 1980b] discussion of the mediations between discourse and material practice that mass communication routinely produces, or Donna Haraway's [1989b] characterization of Harlow's primate research as the transformation of metaphor into hardware.) Those accounts of phenomena that have come to be taken for granted as reified autonomous objects—"black-boxed," as Bruno Latour (1987) puts it—constitute what is referred to as *reality*. Characterizing the social study of science as "the construction of fictions about fiction construction," they also define *reality* discursively as the set of statements considered too costly to modify.[5]

What does this mean in terms of human disease or a "natural" entity like a virus? Where the object of knowledge is a living human being—or even a living host environment for a virus—symbiosis is even more intense. A virus—any virus—is a constructed entity, a representation, whose legitimacy is established and legitimized through a whole series of operations and representations, all highly stylized. Each of these must be critically analyzed on its own terms rather than accepted as though a scientific assertion about a virus stood for a referent rather than a sign. Yet we encounter peculiar difficulties in the cultural analysis of medicine. On the one hand, the biomedical model shares qualities with physics or molecular biology, appearing to describe entities and phenomena that are transcultural and natural. On the other hand, it is the human body—and the perceiving self—that gives the virus its host environment, experiences and reports its effects, and undergoes treatments (and cognitive and affective events) that may change both the environment and the virus.[6]

It is said of Western medicine that the patient comes to the physician's office with an illness but leaves with a disease. Disease is thus taken to represent the medical model, illness the patient's subjective experience or, in anthropological terms, the native's point of view. Current conventional wisdom is that the patient's view must be honored; the physician is, therefore, urged to understand the patient's construction of reality, to read the native's text. This fits nicely into current ethnographic theory. George Marcus and Michael Fischer (1986), for example, argue that *dialogue* is the primary underlying metaphor for ethnography today. This has a pleasing and contemporary ring to it and seems in one sense perfect: the social in dialogue with the physical, the cultural with the natural. Yet, as Atwood Gaines and Robert Hahn observe, "for many anthropologists, Biomedicine is *the* reality through the lens of which the rest of the world's cultural versions are seen, compared, and judged" (1985, 4). And, as Arthur Kleinman notes (in the introduction to Gaines and Hahn [1985]), the entry of the social sciences into medicine has for the most part prompted not dialogue but "an enriched biomedical monologue" characterized by the subversion of social science to medicine's aims. As a model for research or clinical practice, the notion of dialogue breaks down, for in whose words does the body speak?

This question lies at the heart of Michael Taussig's germinal essay "Reification and the Consciousness of the Patient" (1980), which addresses at once the moral foundations of the physician-patient encounter and the particular social and historical conditions that cause moral questions to emerge *now* as problematic. Taussig forcefully challenges the recommendation that physicians learn to understand what constitutes illness for people of diverse cultural backgrounds—to understand, that is, the "cultural construction of clinical reality": "Like so much of the humanistic reform-mongering propounded in recent times, in which a concern with the natives' point of view comes to the fore, there lurks the danger that the experts will avail themselves of that knowledge only to make the science of human management all the more powerful and coercive. For indeed there will be irreconcilable conflicts of interest and these will be 'negotiated' by those who hold the upper hand, albeit in terms of a language and a practice which denies such manipulation and the existence of unequal control." "It is a strange 'alliance,'" writes Taussig, "in which one party avails itself of the other's private understandings in order to manipulate them all the more successfully." The issue, he argues, is not "the cultural construction of clinical reality" but the "clinical construction of culture" (p. 12). In this view, Western medicine must be seen as an ideological system (in the sense of Mannheim, Berger and Luckman, and Geertz): it is experienced by its practitioners as inescapably natural, as what *is*, and whatever data they collect will sustain a vision of biomedical knowledge as true. Taken for granted as reality, the underlying system of biomedicine is precisely what need not be examined.

The unfolding journal literature on HIV reads like a case study on this point, documenting, on the one hand, the instability of linguistic signs and their presumed referents and, on the other, the efficient ways in which instability is repaired. The compilation of papers published in *Science* from 1982 to 1985 (Kulstad 1986), for example, illustrates several ways in which the research laboratory of the virologist Robert C. Gallo at the National Cancer Institute (NCI)—"codiscoverer" of HIV with Luc Montagnier of the Pasteur Institute in Paris—was able to stake out fairly ambitious territory: by repeatedly citing each other's work, members of a small group of scientists quickly established a dense citation network, thus gaining early (if ultimately only partial) control over nomenclature, publication, invitation to conferences, and history. The "Introduction and Overview" chapter of the *Science* collection—written, quite appropriately, by a leading AIDS researcher who is, however, within the NCI network (Max Essex)—serves to stabilize the scientific narrative up to that point: reinforcing some lines of thinking, omitting untidy anomalies, cleaning up terminology. Subsequent articles in journals like *Scientific American* by Gallo and others accomplished the same kind of textual cleansing and fortification. As we would expect, the journal literature on AIDS journal literature (e.g., Small and Greenlee 1989) documents the increasing reality of "the AIDS virus" as a legitimate object of scientific study and shows that citation evolves an intertextual life of its own. As the *Science* collection suggests, one group of influential papers can significantly shape subsequent citation patterns, fix nomenclature, and stimulate or close off particular avenues of research. But it also suggests that density of signification may tell us as much about a given laboratory's authority in the field to produce statements as about the concrete operations by which it claims to transform statements into scientific objects. This may include the power to influence acceptance or rejection of papers for publication, to shape the language of someone else's publication, to determine the speakers and formats of conference sessions, and to interpret the significance of research for other scientists and the media; the effect is not only to help or hurt individual scientists but to set a gold standard for future discourse. Using the Freedom of Information Act to trace the history of the identifying names given by various laboratories to the AIDS-related viruses and viral strains that ultimately emerged as *HIV*, John Crewdson (1989) found that records of Gallo's lab created a chaotic trail of signifiers that often simply disappeared. While much of this may not be rare in scientific investigation and publication, questions and controversies in this case continue to call attention to the apparatus of production, to the practices through which facts are fabricated, and to the tenuous correspondence between objects and signs.

No wonder, then, that *the cultural* becomes precisely what must be repeatedly transcended (or jettisoned) in order to identify and maintain a sense of what is real and universal. In addition, as Philip Setel writes, "Medical literature virtually creates 'culture' as a reservoir of unhealthy practices to be stamped out" (1990, 18). Such observations inevitably challenge medicine's narration of the real.[7]

AIDS and HIV in Montreal

The evidence for HIV is overwhelming. There is a primary etiologic agent, the sine qua non. Take it away, and you don't have an epidemic.—Robert C. Gallo (1989)

We are 10 years into this epidemic and the HIV picture remains foggy and blurry. —Nicholas Regush (1989a)

AIDS and HIV are now taken for granted as stable, observable entities, fully institutionalized through scientific journals, funding incentives, clinical regimens, health practices, educational brochures, books and poems, personal testimonies, and corporate investments. One sees this clearly at the annual international AIDS conferences that have been held since 1985. At rare moments, however, medicine's narration of the real is interrupted long enough to glimpse other narratives. Such a moment occurred at the Fifth International AIDS Conference in Montreal in June 1989. This was by far the largest conference yet: over ten thousand delegates, one thousand media representatives, one thousand corporate and organizational delegates, and—uninvited—a few hundred AIDS activists. Quite unexpectedly, several factors converged to challenge biomedical control over the epidemic, specifically, the accepted view that AIDS is caused by HIV and that HIV acts alone—in Robert Gallo's words, as the "Mack truck" of AIDS. Although the participants in the debate never articulated it in quite these terms, their questions about HIV—how it works, how it does damage, how it can be the sole cause of AIDS—inevitably opened the black box of what had been considered settled and wholly routinized within the apparatus of scientific investigation and reporting. Even as the conference overwhelmingly confirmed (in hundreds of scholarly presentations as well as in the conspicuous presence throughout a huge exhibition hall of the one thousand corporate and organizational delegates) that this particular virus had probably become a reality too costly to give up, questions about HIV called attention to the cultural construction of AIDS and, specifically, its construction within the culture of biomedical science.

It is germane to my account to say that most people who do cultural research on the AIDS epidemic have at least a rudimentary theoretical grasp of virology and immunology. The same cannot be said of most scientists' grasp of social and cultural theory. At a press briefing on 8 June, for example, Robert Gallo was asked whether he thought the Montreal conference's unusual emphasis on social challenges was overshadowing the science and whether he would come to these annual conferences in the future. He replied that, while his decision to come the next year would depend on the final conference program, "I must have heard fifty or one hundred scientists yesterday say there wasn't enough time for science." He continued: "I appreciate women's rights, but I would like a chance to make a choice. We didn't expect this amount of diversity. People from Third World nations need a chance to get together, but is here the best place? You can't even find the people you want to talk to here."[8] For Gallo, the term *social* seems to invoke a range of issues: the amount of conference time allotted to social issues and social sciences as opposed to "science," the visible presence of AIDS activists (whose agenda is apparently what Gallo means by "women's rights"), the "diversity" represented by "people from Third World nations," and the social congestion caused by conference crowds. These characterizations, including the conflation of conventional academic social science with political activism, cropped up elsewhere. Indeed, one could say that, in general, *the cultural* in AIDS discourse is collapsed with *the social* into an amorphous undifferentiated domain containing sociology, anthropology, other cultures, other countries, humanism, the humanities, art, linguistics, economics, the media, morality, ethics, religion, popular culture, politics, political activism, the quilt, and anything else that is not paradigmatic biomedical science or clinical medicine.[9]

Yet, by June 1989, social and cultural questions were periodically disrupting the tidy biomedical narrative. A number of questions about HIV had accumulated and not been fully answered by leading AIDS scientists, at least to the satisfaction of the challengers. Most prominent was the bitter struggle between the NCI and the Pasteur Institute over the name, genesis, paternity, and mechanism of the virus and credit for discovering it. As early as 1983, according to Crewdson (1989), when the Pasteur group submitted a paper to *Nature* that was at odds with Gallo's more well-known representations of the virus, one American reviewer wrote that, if what the French were saying was true, it would be an important paper— but it was not true. The paper was rejected; indeed, it ultimately required a patent battle and the threat of an international lawsuit by the French to get the true significance and legitimacy of their findings recognized. Many American scientists supported the French, believing that Gallo's laboratory had done sloppy work and perhaps even stolen the Pasteur virus; although their support was often expressed in code or in private, it ultimately spurred international compromises that took into account the interests of the French.

A different challenge came in 1988, when Peter Duesberg, a retrovirologist at the University of California, Berkeley, contended that no retrovirus could cause the kind of damage being ascribed to HIV. While other scientists' grumblings about "the AIDS Mafia" are to some degree discounted as professional sour grapes, Duesberg's relentlessness has led him to be treated as a monomaniacal eccentric whose charges drain time from valuable research. Another long-standing critic has been Joseph Sonnabend, a New York City physician who has repeatedly argued that AIDS research has too narrow a focus: although a number of factors may be involved in the epidemic, he has charged, the government has based all its financing on the assumption that HIV is the sole cause of AIDS. "The HIV hypothesis has consumed all our resources," Sonnabend argues, "and yet hasn't saved a single life." Whether or not HIV is a causal factor, the epidemic in his view is most likely the product of immune suppression caused by dramatic social and environmental changes during the 1970s and the action of other widespread viruses. He has wanted to see these factors investigated as well as the potential role of syphilis, malnutrition, malaria, repeated sexually transmitted diseases (STDs), and drug use; he founded the *Journal of AIDS Research* to provide a forum for nonviral research. When it became clear that the viral etiology of AIDS was emerging as triumphant, the journal's editorship was transferred to a virologist and (ironically, in view of Sonnabend's original intent) renamed the *Journal of AIDS Research and Human Retroviruses*. At Montreal, Sonnabend participated in a press briefing to announce that a range of community research initiatives was being established to explore many causal factors in AIDS and test a wide array of treatments, including nonviral drugs. Meanwhile, the gay journal the *New York Native* published weekly assemblages of counterevidence, charging that a virtual conspiracy was functioning to champion HIV as the sole cause of AIDS and suppress alternative evidence that would implicate syphilis and/or suggest the role of other viruses.

A common effect of criticism has been to isolate the critics from the scientific establishment, from other journals and science writers, and from many people with AIDS—most of whom have been increasingly inclined to take HIV as an established fact and shift attention to issues of treatment and cure (see Treichler 1991b; and also chap. 9 below). But, at the Montreal conference, media criticism of HIV orthodoxy went more mainstream.[10] Nicholas Regush, an experienced Canadian science writer, has contended for some time that AIDS research is dominated by a small coterie of U.S. government scientists who endorse HIV as the cause of AIDS. Regush argued on a Canadian Broadcasting Corporation radio series in 1987–89 that few journalists (American or Canadian) had critically examined the processes by which the virus theory was constructed and maintained and that even fewer understood or reported the "escalating debate about the actual role of the so-called AIDS virus." As early as 1984, Regush himself had come to challenge the orthodox scientific argument on principle: "I felt that a reasonable argument that HIV could be the cause—*could* be the cause of AIDS—was being translated all too quickly by science and the media as *the* cause of AIDS, and no one seemed to give a damn about really questioning whether in fact that was true or not." Most U.S. science journalists, Regush argued, "are basically fan clubs of certain scientists who believe that HIV is the cause of AIDS. [The coverage of AIDS] is one of the most disgraceful performances by science writers that I've ever come across" ("The AIDS Campaign," 12–13 January 1988).

Covering a major basic science session at the Montreal conference, in his column of 6 June Regush (1989a) used the foggy slides produced by a defective projector as a metaphor for the current state of AIDS theory: "We are 10 years into this epidemic and the HIV picture remains foggy and blurry." Pursuing the same theme, his column of 8 June took the form of an open letter to Robert Gallo. Titled "OK, Bob! Are You Going to Talk Turkey about HIV or Not?" the column opened by noting that, although Gallo had not arrived in Montreal in time to deliver his listed conference paper, he had nevertheless reassured Regush by phone that the mechanism of HIV's action was well understood:

> I admit [writes Regush] I smiled when you said your lab was researching a dozen ways that HIV could somehow indirectly cause AIDS—considering that you once argued forcefully that direct action of the virus on key immune-system cells was all that was required. You summed up your position by saying that given the right strain of the virus, the right dose and enough time, a person will develop AIDS.
>
> But then you added that it was quite possible that a person could live to a ripe old age with HIV infection and not get AIDS.
>
> Look, Bob, we both know this may sound authoritative to a lot of people, but it really isn't convincing. And frankly, it is getting quite confusing. We really need the scientific details of how this all works. (Regush 1989b)

In refusing to grant unchallenged authority to scientific assertions and suggesting central contradictions in Gallo's account, Regush is not denying the value of orthodox science. Like the other challengers cited above, however, he emphasizes that scientific accounts are constructed versions of reality rather than simply transparent discoveries. Science writers, accordingly, must not merely act as scribes, reproducing or translating scientific representations into discourse for the general public, but must also oversee the signification process, examining and cross-checking the discourse at multiple points on the assumption that, if the statements in the literature do not hold up, the objects that they purport to establish will not either. Examining the structure of language—exposing the seams in the apparent seamlessness of scientific accounts—is the writer's check on reality, carried out on behalf of the public. Thus, Regush urges Gallo to present his findings at Montreal: "Bob, we really need you. The HIV-theory side of the conference is in worse shape than I expected." In conclusion, Regush mentions that Peter Duesberg has called him to say that he is convinced that Gallo does not have the data that he claims to have: "Prove him wrong, Bob."

Gallo tried to prove him wrong that afternoon, at the press briefing from which I quoted above. In response to a packed house and some rather sharp questions, he reasserted his position that HIV was not simply a factor in a "multifactorial" explanation of AIDS. "Look," he finally said to his questioners, "I'm in one laboratory. The world is free to find what it wants. Peer reviews do the decision making, not us." He continued: "Pasteur, NIH, WHO, NCI—these are not stupid people. The evidence for HIV is overwhelming. There is a primary etiologic agent, the sine qua non. Take it away, and you don't have an epidemic. This particular epidemic has as its cause HIV. . . . We cannot demonstrate or explain every aspect of the way the virus causes disease. We don't *have* to explain everything to agree upon an agent. We have more evidence about *this* disease, and this agent, than any other in history." Gallo was asked whether he was sufficiently convinced that HIV is the sole cause of AIDS that other sources of pathogenicity should no longer be explored. "Absolutely," responded Gallo, "they should no longer be explored." When Regush arrived, Gallo broke off his comments to address him: "Mr. Regush," he said, "I'm sorry you were late—I opened my remarks in response to your open letter." From the back of the room, Regush responded, "You were the one who phoned me in the first place." The next day Regush's column did not even bother to discuss Gallo's assertions about HIV, focusing instead on the alternative theories of Sonnabend and others.[11]

I cite these exchanges in some detail to show how dialogue at this conference between scientists and their critics called attention to and at times even disrupted the machinery by which scientific discourse is produced and accepted. The disruption of media machinery was evident as well. The physical setup of television monitors in the media center enabled reporters, individually or in groups, to follow any major conference paper via closed-circuit television without being physically present at the session; at the same time, the media center was closed to all conference participants except credentialed media representatives, with their official green badges, and their individual "interview subjects." In theory, at least, a reporter could cover the entire conference without ever leaving the media center or encountering a single nonmedia person (see chap. 7 below). The chants and actions of AIDS activists were prominent at the conference, however, delaying the opening plenary session by more than an hour and in the process garnering much of the coverage by giving the media what they wanted: the visual, the quotable, and the unexpected. By the third day of the conference, activists had color xeroxed multiple copies of the official green badges and were regularly attending the closed press briefings inside the media center, including those organized by their friends and colleagues. This "artificial" crowd in turn drew a "real" crowd of "real" media representatives, whose coverage generated more crowd and more coverage, with the consequence of more fully communicating and legitimating nonestablishment perspectives and projects.

This orchestration of simulated identity and its transformation into the real parallels the construction of HIV's own reality. Recall Knorr-Cetina's claim that peer review is not a detached postresearch evaluation process but a continual gatekeeping operation. When, at his famous 1983 press conference, Gallo announced the discovery of "the AIDS virus," he provided it with a proper name—*human T-cell leukemia virus, type III (HTLV-III)*. This name for the virus was subsequently challenged, even down to what the *L* would stand for; the Pasteur Institute—whose published findings appeared in the same issue of *Science* that Gallo's did—called its virus *LAV*, for *lymphadenopathy virus*, marking its association with lymph gland phenomena rather than leukemia. John Crewdson's book-length analysis in the *Chicago Tribune* in November 1989 reported that Gallo not only peer reviewed grant proposals and manuscripts of close competitors but, in at least one case, changed the wording of a manuscript to bring it into conformity with his own hypothesis that the virus acted like a leukemia virus. While Gallo's network of colleagues at the National Institutes of Health and elsewhere consistently used the name *HTLV-III* in their publications and the French used *LAV* in theirs, during this period a number of other scientists and journals used the name *HTLV-III/LAV* (or *LAV/HTLV-III*) to give recognition to both the NIH and the Pasteur Institute or even to express skepticism about Gallo's claims. The slash helped mark the virus's identity as culturally constructed and disputed. The compromise name, *HIV*, recommended in 1986 by the Human Retrovirus Subcommittee of the International Committee on the Taxonomy of Viruses and adopted in the 1987 settlement of the NIH-Pasteur dispute, was a consequence of this turmoil. As Latour and Woolgar conclude from their study of scientific contestation, reality is often "the *consequence* of a dispute rather than its *cause*" ([1979] 1986, 236).

Names play a crucial role in the construction of scientific entities; they function as coherent and unified signifiers for what is often complex, inchoate, or incompletely understood. In turn, names establish entities for the public as both socially significant and conceptually real.[12] The existence of multiple signifiers for the virus, even within the pages of the same journal, reproduced the competition among several laboratories and kept alive a tension over just what the signified consisted of and how it was being constructed. It is in this context that the names *HIV* and *AIDS* are still interesting as one legacy of battles in AIDS research for authority, power, and control over resources, including control over the discourses of the field. Many questions remain about the various signifieds represented by the original array of names, but the existence of *HIV* and *AIDS* as unifying signifiers now makes it possible to proceed *in discourse* as though the questions have been resolved. It takes capital to make capital: as the adoption and acceptance of these terms become increasingly widespread, their linguistic capital continues to accrue.

Montreal did not change AIDS science or science writing, but it did call attention to disjunctures in signification, to "the AIDS virus" as a constructed entity across multiple discourses, to the function of metaphors in shoring up favored versions of reality, and to the substantial investment in the notion that reality exists out there to be discovered. In terms of HIV's market currency, the debates over HIV at Montreal did not bring about market failure or anything close to it. But they did bring about scrutiny of the market and, at least in some cases, a more critical examination of individual investment portfolios.

The Reality of HIV and the Apparatus of Production

In metaphor one has, of course, a stratification of meaning, in which an incongruity of sense on one level produces an influx of significance on another.—Clifford Geertz, *The Interpretation of Cultures*

First umpire: I calls 'em as I sees 'em.
Second umpire: I calls 'em as they are.
Third umpire: They ain't nothin till I calls 'em.
—Baseball saying

We can construct a set of statements about HIV, varying the points and the degree of transparency to vary the visibility of fabrication and cultural constructedness:

1. HIV causes AIDS.
2. *HIV* is the name that scientific culture gives the virus widely believed to cause AIDS.

3. *HIV* is the compromise name proposed by an international commission to resolve the bitter international dispute over the "discovery" of a virus judged by many to be a causative factor in the infection and immune deficiency that can lead to the specific clinical conditions diagnosed as AIDS.

4. *HIV* is the acronym adopted in 1986 by the international scientific community to name the virus hypothesized to cause immune deficiency in humans and eventually AIDS, another acronym, adopted in 1982 to designate a collection of more than fifty widely diverse clinical conditions believed to be given the opportunity to develop as the result of a severely deficient immune system.

5. *HIV* is a hypothesized microscopic entity called a *virus* (from Latin *virus*, "poison") invented by scientists in the nineteenth century as a way to conceptualize the technical cause and consequences of specific types of infectious disease. A virus cannot reproduce outside living cells: it enters into another organism's host cell and uses that cell's biochemical machinery to replicate itself (in the case of HIV, often years after initial entry), at which point the cell's DNA, with which the virus is integrated, is transcribed to RNA, which in turn becomes protein. Our knowledge of this "life history" has been produced by an intense national research effort focused both on HIV and on drugs designed to disrupt its life history at various points; as the major subject of scientific investigation and pharmaceutical research efforts and the major recipient of AIDS research funding, HIV is, therefore, also, as Joseph Sonnabend puts it, "metaphorically representative of other interests."[13]

This comparative exercise illustrates some of the tools of "fiction construction": it suggests that reality is always contextual, always to be read and understood in relation to specific discourse practices, specific metaphors, and the representations and claims (e.g., based on its mechanical operations) in which a specific discipline or subdiscipline specializes. HIV cannot, therefore, be read and understood as "the same" entity in each of the foregoing statements.

In these five statements, we see a move away from the apodictic free-floating assertion of statement 1 toward the explicit linguistic markers that assign statements about reality to specific provinces of meaning—for example, to those of virology and immunology. Different realities are signaled by these differently constructed accounts of viruses. At the same time, the set of statements shows how realities come to be merged and muddled through discursive collapses. Thus, statement 1 involves the collapse of *HIV* with two other signifiers: *the AIDS virus* and *the cause of*

AIDS. The interchangeability of these three terms—precisely what Regush was questioning in his open letter to Gallo—here goes far beyond the discourses of virology and molecular biology. That the universe of scientific investigation and clinical practice with respect to AIDS is now primarily determined by the simple acronym *HIV* and that HIV has come to seem natural, inevitable, and taken for granted as the cause of AIDS mark this construction of reality as the hegemonic position from which AIDS research and treatment are typically understood.

The set of statements suggests that "facts are like cows" and in some sense dissolve in the face of close scrutiny, only to reemerge as soon as one shifts one's focus. As Foucault writes, "A statement always has borders peopled by other statements" (1972, 97), and, as Fleck observes, when scientific terms are broken down to show their underlying assumptions, those assumptions must then be broken down to show *their* assumptions, and so on, in an infinite regress, with each definition growing larger and more unwieldy ([1935] 1979, 114–15). In place of these semantic pyramids, scientific discourse is a form of shorthand in which facts, once admitted, need no longer retain the history of their fabrication.

The statements also reveal that metaphors do important work. Communication and coding metaphors like *transcription* as a vehicle to describe viral replication, for example, import significant elements into the reality claimed about what viruses do. As I. A. Richards (1936) put it, where tenor meets vehicle, the transaction between the two produces a meaning that cannot be attained without the metaphor because the vehicle brings with it a range of associations that cannot be suppressed or excluded in its new context (a proposition further developed by Max Black [1962]). This gives metaphors a special kind of cognitive power—including the power to shape cognitive processes.[14] In science, Knorr-Cetina (1981, 84) observes that some conceptions, including metaphors, may be seen as interesting or useful because they generate puzzles in new ways, represent resources perceived as unrealized, or mobilize various cognitive interests. In contrast to Gallo's Mack truck metaphor, we see in statement 5 a different set of metaphors drawn from the terminology of communication, computers, and high-tech postmodern warfare. Donna Haraway (1989a) argues that it was the move away from the military/industrial complex of metaphors to the postindustrial information age metaphors of coding and communication that enabled immunology to claim its current high-theoretical status.

Evident in this discussion is the metaphoric and connotative richness of both *HIV* and *AIDS*; indeed, AIDS metaphors are now routinely compared and critiqued to refine their effectiveness and usefulness. For example, Allan M. Brandt (1988a, 415) describes AIDS (like other epidemic diseases) as a "natural experiment" in how societies respond to disability, dependence, fear, and death; society's response reveals its most fundamental cultural, social, and moral values. Using an earthquake as an even more specific vehicle for the idea that a sudden serious calamity like a natural disaster at once reveals the stresses and vulnerabilities of a society, Mary Catherine Bateson and Richard Goldsby (1988) write that AIDS reveals the "fault lines" in our society. But, speaking on the "MacNeil/Lehrer Newshour" (7 December 1989), June Osborn argued that the AIDS epidemic is *not* like an earthquake, which happens all at once and brings normal life to a standstill, but is drawn out over a period of time, never creating for a broad mass of people enough sense of urgency to address it effectively. Note that there are political implications here as well: if an earthquake— or an epidemic like AIDS—is conceptualized as a natural disaster, an act of God, people in some cultures are less likely to expect or demand government assistance than if it is seen as a massive social or public health crisis (in other cultures, the opposite might be true). At the same time, this metaphoric richness is reciprocal, with HIV and AIDS exported to explain other concepts just as other concepts are imported to explain them; indeed, there is no lingua rasa to be found. As Nancy Scheper-Hughes and Margaret Lock (1986) so eloquently argue, an illness always constructs its metaphoric double, which speaks truth as faithfully as any biomedical diagnosis. If a term is being used in the culture with increasing breadth and frequency, what I have elsewhere called an "epidemic of signification" is inevitable: no matter how literal and denotative a linguistic form may at first appear, it will develop new meanings almost as fast as we can identify old ones. This makes it difficult to predict what a particular metaphor will actually do. The plague metaphor for AIDS, for example, is now so routine that we cannot really say how meaningful it is unless we can examine exactly how and where it is deployed, how it is understood, and how it is acted on. The apocalypse metaphor functions very differently in the history of formulations about AIDS in Africa, in contrast to formulations about AIDS in the West or to formulations about AIDS by Africans. To attribute a particular effect to a metaphor too readily closes off inquiry into contradictory senses of metaphors operating in the culture and inquiry into the legacy of diverse historical tropes.

The Montreal conference also introduced and strengthened a way of thinking about AIDS itself as no longer inevitably fatal but as a chronic, manageable condition. Although arising from several different discourses (scholarly papers, activist press releases, social issues debates), this view achieved currency only when these discourses coalesced at the conference. The term *AIDS discourse* is not simply descriptive but entails an examination of the context—the entire apparatus—through which utterances about AIDS are produced and interpreted and speaking positions made possible. The issue is not whether HIV "exists" or whether a "cultural construction" is pure discourse. The issue is what the grounds and consequences are in a given context for positing HIV and AIDS as realities and embedding them within various networks of signification and what body of "craftwork" this represents. Discourses are also in some sense always oppositional. Any given discourse or context, that is, can always be characterized in relation to some other discourse or context as representing a dominant, negotiated, or oppositional position (see Hall 1980a).

Yet the Montreal conference also makes clear the impossibility of strictly separating a "dominant discourse" from an "oppositional discourse." No discourse is autonomous; rather, discourse is shaped in the light of ongoing day-to-day struggles for survival and legitimacy, in the light of processes of signification, and in the light of what happens when edges touch. Here, Mannheim is especially useful: when ideological and utopian visions become locked in sustained opposition over time, proponents of the two camps become intimately familiar with each other's positions—symbiotically dependent on each other for continuing self-definition but also for continuing critique. Through this symbolism, knowledge, differently produced, has come to be shared to such a degree that a range of collaborative research initiatives has been created. One of the reasons for examining AIDS discourse, and the construction of HIV within it, is to see language in the process of formation—terms and concepts entering and reshaping the discursive field. The scientific culture that constructed the virus is now what most effectively disguises its existence as a cultural construction. Thus reified, HIV exhibits a number of predictable characteristics: it is referred to by a universally agreed-on signifier; conventional representations for it have been developed in journals, the media, three-dimensional glass models, and elsewhere; and its reality continues to be verified through ongoing laboratory and clinical operations (e.g., its structure and life cycle can be described). In addition, HIV is now a taken-for-granted reality in discussions and plans across many social and cultural institutions and in the lives of many individuals (scientists, people with AIDS, health-care professionals, others). Pervasive in discourse, HIV is used as a weapon both to defend and to attack the current state of science, as a metaphor to explain other phenomena, and as an entity through which further research will be generated. Widely identifiable on computer databases and indexes, HIV now exists across the discourses of the culture. Both fabrication and fact, HIV has become, in short, a reality that is too costly to give up.

This is all the more reason to keep track of these costs by asking such questions as, What is the range of existing discourses in which HIV is mentioned? How is HIV articulated to the preexisting issues and codes in those discourses? How do discourses empower people and people empower discourses? To what extent does a "dominant" discourse on HIV continue to be identifiable, under what circumstances and under whose auspices did it emerge, and what kind of resources have been required to sustain its authority? How are authoritative definitions constructed and deployed? Conversely, how are they challenged, evaded, disrupted, or redefined? How does discourse, in other words, work to articulate, codify, maintain, or challenge various forms of authority, power, and control over material resources? And what difference does it make?

Conclusion

The concept of cultural construction can be understood as follows. It is a way of talking about how knowledge is produced and sustained within specific contexts, discourses, and cultural communities; it takes for granted metaphor and other forms of linguistic representation; it presupposes that ideas are produced out of concrete contexts and have concrete effects; it takes for granted hermeneutical activity; it is a complex of ideas and operations sustained over time within a given community; hence, it is institutionalized. Although often confused with idealism or more recently with a view that "everything is discourse," the notion of cultural construction is not a matter of arbitrarily envisioning an unknowable material reality but one of engaging in highly *non*arbitrary ways with the material world. Although meaning is indeed arbitrary and fluid, this does not mean that it is arbitrary and fluid within a given signifying system. The predictability and stability provided by a given history, society, culture, and set of disciplinary conventions are anything but arbitrary. This point is often misunderstood when a given meaning or idea is termed a *cultural construction.* Within the signifying system, that *is* the meaning. No wonder, then, that we expend great effort to preserve belief in a given system where meaning appears stable, indeed, even universal. Recognition that reality is culturally constructed makes such belief impossible.

Why does the concept of cultural construction emerge so strongly now?

Asking what precisely it is that language tells us about material reality, the philosopher Hilary Putnam (1975) posits a "division of linguistic labor," whereby we cede particular realms of reality to acknowledged experts, and suggests that problems and contradictions presented by human disease phenomena may be disguised by the denotative power of medical experts. During a period like the current one in which medical authority is widely challenged, the existing division of linguistic and conceptual labor is inevitably challenged as well. In Montreal and elsewhere, we are seeing a challenge to the "clinical construction of culture" in which "the natives" talk back, articulating their own interests and writing their own texts.

As a crisis named and interpreted through culture, the AIDS epidemic demonstrates the argument that the concepts *culture* and *cultural construction* encompass both material and nonmaterial phenomena and that analysis must emphasize the ongoing interaction and mutual influence between the two. This task presents two difficulties: the first is that the claims of any analysis always press at the boundaries of their established context, dissolving the evidence of origins and disclaimers as they are taken up, with the force of powerful metaphors, in new discourses. The second is that the material and the nonmaterial cohabit much more intimately and inseparably than we usually suppose. If we take Saussure's famous image of linguistic duality as a sheet of paper with the material on one side and the conceptual on the other, we can also always flip the sheet of paper over, with the result that what we thought was the material entity is seen also to have a conceptual life and the conception a material life: metaphor into hardware, but hardware into metaphor, too. Although ideas and conceptions emerge from material reality, that reality has itself been named and interpreted according to the rules and understandings of scientific culture. That scientific findings are overdetermined by culture, however, does not mean that they are not deeply engaged with the story that material reality has to tell. Cultural constructions are not lies, as the touched-up X-ray of Groucho Marx is a lie. To be sustained, a lie requires the invention of an alternative universe: hence, to be sustained, the touched-up X-ray requires the falsification of medical records, the murder of the radiologist, or perhaps the development of new interpretive conventions that redefine what a "bad" X-ray looks like.

With numbers of new cases continuing to escalate and other emerging infectious diseases posing new threats to human health, the moral limitations of a facile constructionism are evident. Even if we will never know reality, specific tasks, goals, and crises may require us to go with our best shot as though it were real. Yet the enormity of the AIDS crisis should not force us back toward the complacent imperialism of a transparent realism, for this equally abuses the multiple ways in which the AIDS epidemic is experienced, interpreted, confronted. Resisting realism means abandoning, not the real world, but faith in transparency. This raises a third difficulty, however, another version of Mannheim's paradox: an analysis aimed at revealing the cultural constructedness of a body of theory can hardly avoid acknowledging its own cultural constructedness as well. This certainly complicates the voice with which social scientists are to enter these discussions about AIDS and culture. Features so crucial to scholarly projects in the last two decades—features like irony, satire, self-reflexiveness, and the desire to understand how different groups construct and represent reality—do not compete well in an international crisis against the certainties that anchor other discourses, some of which have been noted here.

Although it is useful to characterize AIDS and HIV as cultural constructions, this by no means liberates us from taking responsibility for the existence of a real, material world and analyzing its intersection with our conceptions and interventions; indeed, so long as the analysis is local, provisional, and contextualized in terms of specific purposes, a serious commitment to a constructionist model undermines rather than reinforces relativism or pluralism. Likewise, the use of the concept *cultural construction* intensifies the responsibility to make choices. But, if we take seriously the contradictions built into the term *culture* from its earliest days, we can work more seriously with the dialectic that these contradictions offer. It is the contradictions that mark the pleasure and danger of cultural theory.

6

AIDS Narratives on Television:

Whose Story?

Another friend of Molly's died. . . . She tried to think of something else, something calming. But there was nothing else. It wasn't like turning to another channel on the TV because AIDS was on all of them, but only in the most idiotic terms. Everyone on television who died of AIDS got it from a blood transfusion. Or else it was a beautiful young white male professional with "everything to live for," and even then the show focused on his parents and not him.—Sarah Schulman, *People in Trouble*

The AIDS epidemic poses problems of representation, identity, and narrative convention for network television. *An Early Frost* and *Our Sons*, two prime-time network television dramas that centrally address issues of AIDS in gay men, offer several lessons about narrative form and function provided by television in general and the AIDS epidemic in particular. It is by no means simple to determine whether, to what extent, in which contexts, and, above all, for whom a particular cultural production embodies or undermines "dominant" cultural values and positions.

An Early Frost *and* Our Sons: *Made-for-TV Movie*
Meets Medical Melodrama

Production creates not only an object for the subject but also a subject for the object.—Karl Marx

An Early Frost, a made-for-TV movie originally broadcast on NBC on 11 November 1985, was the first feature-length drama about AIDS on network television.[1] Its protagonist is Michael Pierson, an appealing and successful young Chicago attorney whose surprise visit home for his parents' wedding anniversary opens the story and establishes the rhythms of life that AIDS will disrupt. Significantly, before we meet Michael's lover, we meet his family: his parents, Nick and Kay; his grandmother, Bea; and his sister, Susan, with her husband and little boy. This scene also introduces us to the dramatic rendering on television of Michael's first symptom of immunodeficiency: weight loss. At the dinner table, Michael is describing a momentous meeting with the head of his law firm when his grandmother passes him the potatoes:

Michael: No, thanks.
Bea: You look awfully thin to me.
Nick: Everyone looks thin to you!
Bea: *You* could lose a couple of pounds.
Kay: Children, children—
Michael: Anyway—

Resuming his story, Michael announces that he has been made partner in the law firm. Amid the general congratulations, Kay says that she hopes that he will leave a little time for "relaxation":

Nick: What your mother wants to know is: are you shackin' up?
Michael: [*Very seriously.*] Well, I have something to tell you. [*He pauses, then with a charming smile.*] I'm not a monk.
Kay: What I was trying to say is—if there's anyone you ever want to bring home, she's always welcome.
Nick: She can sleep in my room.

What is absent or unspoken in these two interactions is what fills the next two hours: Michael's gayness and his illness. This is a domestic drama, a familial coming-out story, and an illness story—what television calls a "disease-of-the-week" story. *An Early Frost's* text is marked by these genres. But it is teledrama as well as melodrama, thus marked also by television's well-established narrative conventions and uniquely overt commercial context; this format has special significance in the representation of illness because, unlike television in general, television movies are able to focus on problems that are complex, controversial, and difficult to solve.[2]

An Early Frost is of particular interest because it was the first television drama about AIDS: in development for some time before Rock Hudson disclosed that he had AIDS, the movie aired within weeks of Hudson's death, when AIDS was just beginning to generate its own narrative conventions and televisual agenda. AIDS was widely believed to pose great problems for coverage on television: the problem of depicting a "homosexual lifestyle," of representing homosexuality and other transgressive practices associated with HIV transmission, the bleak prognosis of AIDS, the stigma and blame attached to persons with AIDS, the baffling role of sexual difference, and the rapidly changing and often nondefinitive nature of medical information. Because actual experience was limited in 1985, *An Early Frost* provides a useful case study of the representational challenges of AIDS and how at this relatively early point in the epidemic they were handled.[3]

I should emphasize that prime-time network television, my primary focus in this chapter, by no means offers the only, the best, or the most interesting video representations of the AIDS epidemic. At this point, as I mentioned in chapter 4 above, several hundred films and videos have been produced by independent film and video artists, cable stations, and educational and health-care agencies; many of these can be called alternative or oppositional in form or politics to mainstream television.[4] But different kinds of productions do different kinds of cultural work. A range of research establishes that, internationally, television is the single most important source of information about AIDS and HIV.[5] My interest here is thus in the cultural work of the popular medical drama on prime-time network television, a form characterized by a straightforward narrative, conventional chronology, and "classic" form. With its stunning cast, good script, accurate medical information, and unquestionably tasteful policing of desire, *An Early Frost* was widely acclaimed and not unreasonably hailed as the prototypical AIDS narrative. The *Los Angeles Times* critic Howard Rosenberg wrote: "You hesitate to use 'landmark' in connection with two hours of TV. But if NBC's *Adam* marked a turning point in a campaign to alert the nation about missing children, *An Early Frost* may just as effectively define the AIDS peril for millions of Americans who inexplicably may still remain apathetic and ignorant of reality" (1985, 1). Promoting the film's subject as a vital public health issue, NBC mailed advance information to more than 200,000 health, educational, and social organizations, and NBC news anchor Tom Brokaw hosted a special AIDS information program afterward. The night of its premiere, *An Early Frost* captured a third of the viewing audience, beating out a controversial "Cagney and Lacey" episode as well as ABC's "Monday Night Football," and moving thousands of viewers across the United States to call a toll-free information line after the program (Gendel 1985). Despite its critics on both the Left and the Right, *An Early Frost* became the gold standard for the representation of AIDS on television, a standard that most critics predicted would not be sustained: "You can bet that this will not be prime time's last word on AIDS, and that few succeeding stories on the same subject will travel such a high road" (Rosenberg 1985, 9).

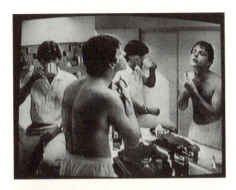

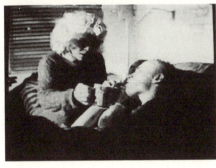

An Early Frost *(1985) and* Our Sons *(1991) were for a decade the only made-for-TV AIDS movies centered on gay men. Each paid a price for prime time, focusing on the families of the men involved, largely deleting evidence of a wider gay community, and replicating conventional understandings of sexual difference. As Michael shaves for work in* An Early Frost, *he admits to Peter that he has once again failed to tell his family about their relationship, also noting that they're almost out of shaving cream; Michael's is the masculine, breadwinning role, Peter's the domestic (6.1). In a final scene in* Our Sons, *as Donald lays dying in his lover's mother's house, his own more conservative mother at last learns to show compassion, even though he is "one of them" (6.2). Despite warnings about Hollywood homophobia and AIDS-phobia, all four male actors in these films have had steady work (Aidan Quinn, D. W. Moffet, Želcko Ivanek, Hugh Grant).*

As it turned out, television studios did not flock to produce movies on AIDS. Although a few television movies did address the epidemic, they were, as Schulman's character charges, about people who "got it from a blood transfusion"—people, as John O'Connor (1991c) puts it, with "straight AIDS." Not until ABC's *Our Sons* in April 1991 did the networks try again to tell the story of a gay man with AIDS.[6] Even now, AIDS is hardly a topic that television takes for granted. Warren Littlefield, president of NBC entertainment, commented as follows about a repeatedly postponed AIDS episode on the medical drama series "Lifestories": "There are few things in broadcasting that we know for sure, and one of those is that when you do an episode of any series that deals with AIDS, there is going to be advertiser sensitivity to it. And if you choose to do it anyway, you better count on losing money" (quoted in Weinstein 1990b, 1). In his study of AIDS on broadcast television, Buxton (1992) confirms this. Despite its glowing ratings and reviews, *An Early Frost* did lose money, both at its premiere broadcast and at its rerun. Buxton also notes that the made-for-TV movie is different in format from, say, sitcoms in its tendency to copy prior programming: the fact that *An Early Frost* did establish the gold standard probably discouraged imitators. Describing the decision by PBS not to air Robert Hilferty's 1991 AIDS documentary *Stop the Church* on the series "P.O.V.," Monica Collins (1991) wrote in *TV Guide*, "Television has been dealing with the issues and realities of AIDS since the airing of the landmark NBC drama *An Early Frost* several years ago. But clearly the subject is still risky and potentially controversial for the medium."[7]

This is confirmed by comparing *An Early Frost* with *Our Sons.* Like the earlier film, *Our Sons* has an excellent cast, which includes Hugh Grant and Željko Ivanek as James Grant and Donald Barnes, the central male characters, and Julie Andrews and Ann-Margret as Audrey Grant and Luanne Barnes, their mothers. As the film opens, Donald has become too sick to be cared for at home and is being taken by paramedics to the hospital; we assume that this is not the first crisis because James knows his way around the hospital, embraces Donald without a glance at the intensive-care equipment, and falls easily into caretaking routines. Donald's first words to James, however, signal his understanding that this crisis breaks the routine: "Toto, I have the feeling we're not in Kansas anymore." The film is verbally and visually franker about the relationship between Donald and James and more explicit about their "gayness" (the closest thing to a Judy Garland reference in *An Early Frost* is Patti Page's voice singing "How Much Is That Doggie in the Window?"). It also conveys more matter-of-factly what living with AIDS entails. As James and Audrey visit Donald in the hospital, Audrey remarks that she has not encountered death since her husband died; James says, "Donald and I have been to fourteen funerals in the last eighteen months." At least some members of the audience will share Audrey's shock as the casual statistic makes her stare at him, aghast, suddenly understanding something of the epidemic's impact. At the same time, the very title *Our Sons* contains its volatile topics within familial bonds (even if maternal rather than paternal), striving to domesticate not only homosexuality and AIDS but the class difference between the two mothers as well: when James charges Audrey with "tap-dancing"—using surface charm to evade her real feelings about the reality of his homosexuality—he might be talking about the film's own tap-dancing. Like *An Early Frost*, *Our Sons* strongly urges compassion, medical rationality, intelligence, and tolerance; it also, like *An Early Frost*, offers viewers the family's perspectives, treats homosexuality as a central—and legitimate—problem for the straight characters, makes little reference to AIDS as a national health-care crisis, and renders the rage and political mobilization of activist groups invisible, indeed, incomprehensible.

During the 1980s, the conservative political climate produced increasingly vehement and vocal attacks on progressive, controversial television dramas. Conservative advocacy groups organized letter-writing campaigns, product boycotts, and other protest actions. By 1991, however, radical and progressive advocacy groups had also organized; spurred by the AIDS epidemic, gay and lesbian organizations were finding increasingly sophisticated ways to protest what they deemed negative representations of homosexuality in film and television.[8] These protests often take up Vito Russo's (1987) critique of "gay movies for straight people," which focus on "coming out as a family problem [and] subtly say that there are no homosexuals, only a homosexual problem" (p. 227). ("In *Consenting Adults*," he writes, "we see how a handsome young jock's coming out of the closet affects his mother, his father, his sister, and his college roommate. When the latter learns of his buddy's homosexuality, he says, 'I don't believe this is happening to me!' Such films are about the real people in our society, the straight people. Gays are the problem they have" [p. 227].) Or, as the *New York Times* television critic John O'Connor put it, many homosexuals today "are fed up with seeing their very existences viewed primarily as 'controversial.' Even the occasionally more sensitive films use distancing ploys, exploring not the lives of homosexuals but the anguished fretting of their parents or friends" (O'Connor 1991b, 32).

On the one hand, then, television can hardly be considered a vanguard medium with respect to AIDS. On the other hand, television looks good compared to Hollywood cinema, increasingly berated for its failure to develop films about AIDS: as of 1991, *Longtime Companion* was the only U.S. feature film on AIDS shown in theaters (I am not including films like Bill Sherwood's extraordinary *Parting Glances* of 1987 because, although AIDS is woven into its fabric, it is not "about" AIDS). Julie Lew argued in the *New York Times* that "AIDS offers everything a scriptwriter could wish for: drama, medical intrigue, sex, death, heroism, pathos, social conflict and immediacy. Yet to date only television has approached the topic" (Lew 1991). Lew lists several possible reasons why "the movies are ignoring

AIDS": the identification of AIDS with homosexuality; the homophobia of actors, agents, producers, and audiences; Hollywood's addiction to the bottom line and therefore to upbeat endings; presumed audience intolerance for anything about AIDS; the physical unattractiveness of AIDS as a disease; and the entrenched nature of gay caricatures in Hollywood. That Randy Shilts's bestseller *And the Band Played On* so clearly displayed these ingredients perhaps explains its problematic and ultimately failed transition to theatrical film (Cathcart 1987). Above all, said Shilts himself, was Hollywood's continuing perception that "AIDS is spelled g-a-y" (quoted in Lew 1991).[9]

But an added or alternative explanation is surely not just the topic per se (AIDS, homosexuality, death) but the changes in form, genre, and ideology needed to tell the AIDS story fully—to politicize disease, to make it social and collective, to show the intrigues and bureaucratic failures of medicine, science, and public health. In American films and television, this is simply not done. Of the elements of the AIDS story that Lew identifies, medical television dramas are equipped to deal with a very few indeed; only drama, death, pathos, and social conflict are staples (and social conflict only when it means interpersonal conflict). As Joseph Turow and Lisa Coe (1985) argue, it is the systemic, structural dimension of health care that figures in crises today and causes such need for a shared national agenda; yet, as their study demonstrates, disease on television is virtually always something that happens to individuals—it is not socially produced and does not demand social action or policy. The television medical drama, it would seem, is not *All the President's Men*; it is not even "Dallas."[10]

Medical dramas on television are typically credited with serving a number of cultural functions: they give disease a "human face"; they portray the world of medicine and disease realistically; they educate viewers; they allow the television industry to claim that entertainment has a serious social edge; and they engage the viewer imaginatively in contemporary social and ethical issues. Like most commentary on fictional medicine in general, criticism and commentary on television medicine treats it as a representation, even a reflection, of social reality and "real" medicine. It is accordingly judged by the realism of its images of patients and healers, its medical accuracy, its authenticity, its real-life therapeutic efficacy (medical dramas often provide toll-free numbers for further information), its ability to heal the wounds of ignorance, prejudice, silence. Given its concern with the real, it is ironic that such criticism continues to privilege the individual to the exclusion of the social and political. The human face of disease, even a gay face, may ultimately be more tolerable for television than a political face.[11]

In this chapter, I examine AIDS narrative drama on television less strictly as a representation of reality than as, following Buxton in his analysis of the controversial "AIDS episode" of the series "Midnight Caller," "a discursive universe that constructs a hierarchy of meaning" (Buxton 1991, 46). I want also, as Mary Poovey puts it, to "interrogate the boundary between medicine and literature" on the grounds that narratives—all narratives—always and inevitably do more than "reflect" and "depict" (Poovey 1991, 292). Even mainstream prime-time television medical narratives do not simply reinforce traditional dichotomies between the real and the fictional, the objective and the subjective, the scientific and the entertaining. Rather, to quote Poovey again, medical narratives are also "laboratories in which one can observe and learn to interpret the dynamics of meaning production" (Poovey 1991, 292). Understanding their representational struggles and strategies helps us understand the same dynamics in the construction and deployment of medical meaning, including the meaning of AIDS.[12] In doing so, I take account of Buxton's positioning of these made-for-TV AIDS movies as family melodramas, but melodramas that—because of the depth of the AIDS crisis and its disruptive effects—can never fully achieve their goal of restoring the stability of the nuclear family.

An Early Frost and *Our Sons* illuminate many of the problems of creating an AIDS narrative for television. As a starting point, I use a generic definition of *narrative* provided by J. Hillis Miller (1990). For Miller, a narrative—a story—requires three elements: formal structure (plot), character, and linguistic patterning.[13] In terms of form, character, and language, a number of concrete questions relate directly to the exploration of AIDS on television: How do these two films serve as prototypical AIDS dramas, and what are the differences between them? How does narrative representation facilitate or discourage identification with characters and with which characters? What makes a given representation "positive" or "negative," and can interpretation be fully determined? What kind of cultural work do these narratives do? How do they use television codes and conventions as well as the unique constraints, possibilities, and pleasures of television? How do they display complexity, or what Turow and Coe (1985) call "texture"? How is AIDS constructed? As a medical problem, a social issue? As controversial, sympathetic, interesting? As a viewing experience? Through what mechanisms do these television narratives reinforce prevailing cultural values—or criticize, police, disrupt, or challenge them? Do these narratives enable us to explore alternative assumptions about the world and reality? Do these illness stories function therapeutically? Whose story do they tell?

An Early Frost: Domesticating AIDS for Broadcast Television

We tried to make a movie that hopefully we wouldn't be ashamed of in five years. We tried to make an honest depiction, something where people would say, "Hey, that's real. That's not phony, that's not TV."—Steve White, NBC vice president for movies and miniseries

In development for two years before NBC gave permission to begin production in June 1985, *An Early Frost* "was a movie whose time almost didn't come"; it went through at least thirteen script rewrites, "some due to changing medical knowledge about AIDS, others to the network's fears about giving the appearance of either endorsing or condemning homosexuality" (Hall 1985).[14] As one producer told Jane Hall, "We wanted neither to romanticize the homosexual relationship nor hit it with a sledgehammer"; or, to put it another way, in the words of *Atlanta Journal/Constitution* editor Bill King, "the phrase 'family drama' gets quite a workout from network executives discussing *An Early Frost*. While the film is quite open in its depiction of [Aidan] Quinn's character as a homosexual, NBC is anxious that it not be seen as a 'gay' story" (King 1985, 4).

The scene that introduces Michael's lover, Peter, illustrates this balancing act. We know that Michael is back in Chicago by the exterior shot of an urban high-rise—in itself an already standard piece of televisual AIDS shorthand (Colby 1989). A close-up shows him asleep in a dark bedroom. Someone enters, and a hand reaches down to tickle his ear; he swats at it:

> *Peter:* Are you gonna stay in bed all day or what?
> *Michael:* What time is it?
> *Peter:* It's eight o'clock.
> *Michael:* Why didn't you wake me?
> *Peter:* [*Sits on bed, putting on socks.*] Well, I've been trying for the last half hour.
> *Michael:* I'm gonna be late. I'm exhausted. [*Sits up.*] Ohhh.
> *Peter:* Well, you better start saving your strength for falling asleep on one of those beaches in Maui. [*Michael begins coughing.*]
> *Peter:* Hey, you OK? I'll tell you what—why don't you stay home today?
> *Michael:* I can't. Meetings . . . back to back.

We learn from this scene that Michael and Peter live together, have a domestic routine together, and indeed share the same bed, but we do not see them in it at the same time. We also learn that Michael is experiencing new symptoms, coughing and exhaustion. As he gets up and heads for the bathroom, Peter says that he has found a travel agent who has made hotel reservations in Maui. Michael now breaks the news that he cannot leave because he has a trial coming up:

> Peter: Michael, I've made arrangements to close the store.
> Michael: Well, what can I do? They just made me a partner.
> Peter: [Throwing his shoe in the air and catching it.] OK! Here we go again!

If, as feminist literary critics have suggested, the real protagonist of Victorian novels like *Jane Eyre* is the house that the heroine gets at the end, we could argue that the real protagonist of *An Early Frost* is the American nuclear family. The scenes between Michael and Peter largely do not challenge a mom-and-pop division of labor but reproduce it, even to Peter's culinary expertise, expressive emotional life, and desire for a more open, communicative relationship. Despite the surprise element of the bedroom scene that introduces Peter as Michael's lover and the erotic symbolism of beaches on Maui, the following scene restores the interpersonal economy of a conventional heterosexual marriage. Michael is shaving at the bathroom mirror when Peter comes in with a plate of toast:

> Peter: Breakfast is served.
> Michael: Thanks. We're almost out of shaving cream.
> Peter: Oh—OK. [Sits on bathroom counter.] So—how'd it go with your folks?
> Michael: Great! I really surprised my mom.
> Peter: Mmmm. That's not what I meant.
> Michael: [With slightly sarcastic emphasis.] Well, what did you mean?
> Peter: You didn't tell 'em.
> Michael: [Still sarcastic.] Yeah I told 'em—they were thrilled. Come on—I was there less than twenty-four hours.
> Peter: How long does it take?
> Michael: Look, I don't have the same relationship with my parents that you do with yours. I don't talk about sex with them, they don't talk about sex with me.
> Peter: Who's talking about *sex*? I'm talking about us.

As Michael silently continues to shave, Peter comes over to him and plucks something from Michael's head: "Grey hair," he says, smiling. "Time's running out." The scene invokes the formal figure of time and untimely death repeated throughout the film and embodied in the elliptical phrase *an early frost*. Here, it is we, the viewers, who are able to give the phrase *time's running out* ironic resonance and link it to the temporal trajectory of medical melodrama. As Judith Pastore observes, Shilts's chronology of the epidemic, using a similar strategy, "combines new journalism techniques with the bitter irony of formal tragedy. Like watching Oedipus, we cannot escape the knowledge eluding the characters, which makes all they say and do reverberate with ominous prescience" (Pastore 1993, 9). As the film unfolds, Michael does become sick and is hospitalized and diagnosed with AIDS; when Peter confesses that he has not been strictly monogamous during their two years together and therefore may be the source of the virus, Michael is angry and kicks him out of the house; Michael goes home to break the news to his family and to deal with their pain, anger, and denial. When he is hospitalized again, he makes friends with Victor (played by John Glover), a rather flamboyant gay man with AIDS. After the crisis, Michael is back home with the folks when Peter visits and they resolve their conflict, knowing now that Michael could well have been infected before he met Peter (nothing is said about Peter's health). When Victor dies and Michael reads into the death his own fate, he tries to commit suicide; he is rescued by his father and reconciled with him. In tidying the loose ends, the story is not unconventional, but there is no deathbed scene, and, indeed, the movie ends with Michael returning to resume his life with Peter.

This bathroom scene helps establish Michael and Peter's characters and their relationship—one is closeted, the other is not; one holds a "real job," the other manages domestic arrangements (making travel arrangements, cooking, buying shaving cream); one has AIDS, the other (like women in general in AIDS discourse) is positioned as the infector whose own health as infectee is not our concern. Significantly, their limited physical contact occurs as teasing (when Peter tickles Michael's ear, a Disney-like soundtrack invokes the innocent flirtation of a bunny with a butterfly). The negation of sexuality appears to have been accomplished fairly effortlessly, yet it is actually quite skillfully orchestrated through many small moments. (Buxton's [1992] interviews with the movie's writers provide many telling examples.) The larger question is precisely what is happening with sexual difference here. With Peter placed so consistently in the feminine/wife position, are conventional sexual roles reproduced and possibilities for oppositional representation negated?

While many commentators, including gay activists, can find solid evidence for answering yes and calling this yet one more gay movie for straight people, this judgment assumes that we fully understand the nature of the viewing subject, how identification occurs, and how people engage with television. Surely, scenes like this one require us to acknowledge the existence of several linked but not equivalent subject positions. And, surely, it is important that two men in a love relationship, no matter how "straight," no matter how conventional, are being shown without too much fanfare on prime-time television. Part of the pleasure of formula fiction is its manipulation of its own conventional elements; here, Ozzie and Harriet are two gay men. The politics of the relationship, its ideological conservatism, and its ultimate fate are, of course, the price paid for the relationship's prime-time existence; yet, whether or not one is willing to call this scenario progressive, the price needs to be separated from the sheer fact of representation and what it may offer different viewers. This shaving scene is shot to complicate any unitary perspective. In the previous family scenes, we have seen Michael primarily from his mother's point of view: he first appears—to her, to the camera, and to us—when she opens the door and finds him on the front stoop with a bouquet of roses. We are the mother; he is the other. In the shaving scene, we begin to see from Michael's point of view, the camera behind him looking toward Peter. Yet the mirror complicates this, showing us Michael and Peter and their reflections—their relationship turned around, as it were. Drawing on long-standing visual codes, we can also see this mirrored glimpse of Michael's hidden life as a figure for his constricted vision, his concern for his image. It also, perhaps, figures the clearer vision and understanding that he will ultimately (and obligatorily in such a movie) attain. Finally, the shot plays off the image—repeated with various permutations throughout the film and highlighted in promotional stills—of various family members looking out windows (notably, only the nuclear family, never Peter, appears in these publicity pictures). These window shots, paralleling the framing action of the television screen itself, also underline the metaphoric and literal importance of entrances and exits, doors, entryways, stairs, porch and patio, garden and garage, reminding us of television's theatrical—perhaps more than cinematic—origin as well as the ongoing interaction between the stage and the space of the television within the home (Spiegel 1988).

When Michael subsequently repents and shows up at Peter's store to surprise him with airplane tickets to Maui, we learn that Peter sells restored objects, specializing in wholesome and innocent stuff from the 1950s—a jukebox, a carousel horse. When Peter asks, "But what about your case?" and Michael responds, "It can wait a week: I am a partner!" any television fan knows that optimism like this is heading for a fall. And, sure enough, as Michael is working late at his office to prepare for the trial, he collapses and wakes up in the hospital.

I want to talk about this first hospital scene in some detail. We hear only the doctor's voice at first: "Michael? I'm Dr. Redding." Michael sits up, coughing, as the physician examines his lungs; Peter is sitting beside him:

> *Peter:* What's wrong with him?
> *Redding:* The tests we did show that you have pneumonia.
> *Peter:* Pneumonia? I thought it was flu or something.
> *Redding:* Are you two lovers? [*Michael and Peter exchange looks.*] There are a lot of gay men in my practice.
> *Michael:* [*Answering question.*] Yes.
> *Redding:* How long have you been together?
> *Peter:* Two years. I'm Peter Hill. [*Stands, shakes hands with physician.*]
> *Redding:* I'm glad you're here—you should be a part of this. Michael, the type of infection you have—*pneumocystis carinii*—doesn't usually attack someone who's otherwise healthy. So we ran some very specific tests to see if your immune system was functioning normally. The results indicate a disorder. I'm sure you've heard of acquired immune deficiency syndrome.
> *Michael:* AIDS? Are you telling me I have AIDS?
> *Redding:* We only make this diagnosis when there's the presence of an opportunistic infection like this pneumonia.
> *Michael:* I couldn't have AIDS—it's not possible.
> *Redding:* I know this is difficult.

The doctor sits on Michael's bed and provides 1985 AIDS boilerplate: "We know a lot more than we did. . . . We've isolated the virus. . . . We're working on experimental drugs. . . ." The immediate treatment plan: "We'll leave you on the IV for a week—if you're still doing well, we'll send you home on oral medication. Now try and get some rest. I'll come back and see you in a while. [*Nods to Peter.*] Peter." Left alone, Michael and Peter are silent. Film music begins:

> *Peter:* I thought—I don't know what I thought. [*Stands.*] I'm gonna go talk to that doctor.
> *Michael:* Peter. Don't leave me.

As he says this, Michael is staring out the window to our right—Peter is in the foreground on his way out the door with his profile looking left. The shot is held as Michael says "Don't leave me." It is ambiguous whether Michael is talking about this moment or in general. Peter pauses, then returns and sits down, taking Michael's hand in his two hands; Michael curls toward him into a fetal position. Now comes a dark screen, and then the title *An Early Frost* appears, superimposed on the signature image: in the background, a pastoral village with a white church steeple visible among wooded hills; in the foreground, a tree branch on which green leaves are beginning to change color. There have been no commercials throughout this long opening sequence of the film; thus, we are fairly caught up in the drama before the dreaded word AIDS occurs at last.

One goal of the medical teledrama is to entertain, but, as a number of scholars demonstrate, another long-standing mission is to educate (see Turow 1990a, 1990b; and Kalisch and Kalisch 1985). *An Early Frost* is unusually conscientious in carrying out its pedagogical functions (as critic Howard Rosenberg commented, "This is integrity time" [1985, 1]). Certainly, *An Early Frost* escapes the charge leveled at other television dramas of using AIDS simply as a "plot thickener"—in other words, as just another issue that the genre absorbs without particularizing. A noted and well-publicized feature of the production was its "hot sets," in which the hospital setups were maintained almost up to airtime so that the scenes could be reshot with absolutely up-to-date information. Medical consultants greatly affected ongoing script revisions—changes were made not just to incorporate changing medical information but also to reflect growing public knowledge of the epidemic (an early version had Kay going to the library to research AIDS; the final version merely has her holding the issue of *Newsweek* with Rock Hudson and AIDS on the cover).[15]

The film's take-home messages about AIDS attempt to set the record straight on contamination and casual contact, give basic biomedical AIDS information, and suggest the risks of sexual contact. The fear of contamination and its groundlessness are first presented visually. A close-up shot shows a tray of food sitting in the corridor outside Michael's hospital room. Two nurses stand in the background, looking at the tray. As Dr. Redding approaches, we hear one of them whisper, "I don't want to go in there." As Redding picks up the tray and carries it into Michael's room, we see the "ISOLATION" sticker on the door. Redding looks back toward the nurses, his expression grim. As he tells Michael with exasperation, "You can't get AIDS just by being around someone who has it. It's only transmissible through intimate sexual contact or blood."

In interviews about his role, Aidan Quinn expressed particular outrage about the fear of people with AIDS and their isolation: "The real concern around AIDS patients is that you might give *them* something because their immune system is so low" (he donated part of his earnings from the movie to an AIDS foundation that assisted him in researching the part [Hill 1985, 9]). A number of scenes reinforce this theme. When Michael returns home, Peter stands at the sink holding a cup from which Michael has been drinking coffee. Staring out the window, he begins to take a sip, then suddenly realizes what he is doing, dumps out the coffee, and rinses the cup. When friends of Michael and Peter learn of Michael's illness, they give their excuses for not coming to dinner. When Michael goes home to break the bad news, physical revulsion is his father's first negative reaction. His sister, too, will not let her son touch him and will not visit him herself because she is pregnant. Meanwhile, his mother reads up on AIDS, his grandmother provides understanding and love, and, in the hospital, Michael gradually, if at first reluctantly, makes friends and gains support from a group of other men with AIDS, including Victor, a former chef who lost his job and was evicted by his roommates when he got sick. These multiple perspectives and examples provide not only a textured representation of AIDS, in Turow and Coe's sense, but also a series of lessons in the facts of transmission.[16] When Michael collapses with seizure, ambulance attendants refuse to transport him once they suspect what he has. Paul Volberding, one of the physicians consulted on the script, commented that he feared that "the viewer will think that scene was made up. It's not. This has happened in San Francisco, where we pride ourselves as a model for the care of patients with AIDS" (quoted in Steinbrook 1985, 1).

Boilerplate biomedical AIDS information constitutes a second take-home message. Here, *An Early Frost* represents Western liberal humanism doing what it does best: arguing for compassion, reason, compliance with scientific authority, common sense. No one could argue that, with respect to AIDS, this is not crucial cultural work: "It's not a gay disease, Michael," Redding says. "It never was. The virus doesn't know or care what your sexual preference is. Gay men have been the first to get it in this country, but there have been others—hemophiliacs, intravenous drug users—and it hasn't stopped there." Further, the film even acknowledges that a number of unanswered questions remain:

> *Michael:* [How] did I get it? I haven't had any blood transfusions lately and haven't been with anyone except Peter.
> *Redding:* Has he?
> *Michael:* Of course not. We have a *relationship*.
> *Redding:* I'm only asking because we've discovered it's possible to be a carrier of the disease without actually showing any of the symptoms himself.

Michael: You mean you can pass it on without actually getting it?

Redding: [Nods.] Michael, I'm not judging you. It's important that we know [*your sexual history*] because the number of contacts would increase your chances of being exposed to someone who—

Michael: [Interrupting.] It was years ago! Before anyone knew about this!

Redding: The problem is, Michael, that we don't know how long the incubation period for the disease is—it might be 5 years, it could be longer. We're just not sure.

Michael: You're not sure of very much, are you?

The formula for medical dramas dictates that physicians be shown to be in control, and scriptwriters usually accede to the dictate, a practice that downplays uncertainties, ambiguities, and incorrect interpretations. According to Howard Stein (1990, 213–27), control and containment are also at work in accounts of "real" medical cases. Stein's medical ethnographies, functioning to excavate what he calls the "story behind the story" of conventional biomedical narratives, show that the everyday discourse of practicing physicians works precisely to disguise its own self-questioning. The prime-time movie on American television is likewise poorly equipped to display subtleties, suggest ambiguities, draw fine distinctions, pose problems. Take the statement, for example, that someone can "pass it on without actually getting it." Since one does not transmit AIDS itself but rather a virus that destroys the immune system, and since one does not transmit the virus without carrying it oneself, this statement is accurate only if *it* in *pass it on* means the virus and *it* in *not getting it* means full-blown AIDS. Granted, this is a subtle point compared to the crucial proved distinction between justified prudence about established modes of transmission (sexual contact, contaminated blood) and groundless fears about "casual contact." Yet blurring the difference between the virus and its later clinical manifestations makes it hard to understand the subsequent statement that "we don't know how long the incubation period . . . is." The message intended to be communicated here is no doubt that an infected person may not look sick or be sick but is still infectious to others.[17]

The take-home message about sex is even murkier, reflecting the decision "neither to romanticize the homosexual relationship nor hit it with a sledgehammer." Predictably, the movie was attacked by conservatives because it was soft on homosexuality and by activists because it was desexualized. Certainly, sex is handled delicately, to say the least. In what must have been one of the most controversial and negotiated exchanges in the movie, the language is almost Victorian:

Michael: What about Peter? I mean . . . when I get home?
Redding: Touching is fine. Hugging. But I'd be careful about being more intimate than that.

Well, we do not see much touching, let alone hugging. Indeed, when Michael comes home, he makes up a bed in the study. Peter is surprised: "But Dr. Redding said—" and Michael replies, "I know what he said. I just don't think we should take any chances." What do these cryptic exchanges mean? That Michael thinks that even touching and hugging are risky? That "Dr. Redding said" something different to Peter off camera? That when he said "I'd be careful about being more intimate" he really meant "use condoms"? That he really meant abstention so that sharing a bed is dangerous because it might lead to some kind of erotic contact? Or that it is simply a device to keep the two men out of bed together? Later, after Michael has told his family that he is sick, his grandmother begins to kiss him, and he stops her; but she says, "It's a disease, not a disgrace— Come on, give your old grandmother a kiss." This kiss was controversial, too, but the medical consensus that friendly kissing is safe prevailed.[18]

By conventional critical (although not monetary) standards, *An Early Frost* was a success. Jane Hall (1985) in *People* hailed it as "a shattering AIDS TV movie [that] mirrors a family's pain," a "landmark" in dealing with the "feelings" associated with AIDS. But whose feelings? Vito Russo writes that in "*An Early Frost* we see how AIDS affects a young man's mother, father, sister, brother-in-law, and grandmother. There is no consideration given to the fact that this is happening to him—not them" (Russo 1987, 276–77). And Jan Zita Grover writes: "NBC's *An Early Frost* enforced existing prejudices by returning its PWA protagonist to the bosom of his family. Evidently he lacked long-term, close-knit friends back in Manhattan [Chicago, actually]; it was only after being shorn of his sexuality and his identity as a gay man that he could be returned, neutered, to his mother and father, enfolded once again within the nuclear family, and die in peace" (Grover 1989b, 13).[19]

These critiques, uncompromisingly argued from a gay and lesbian activist position, cannot be denied. Yet it seems to me that the film may offer points of identification and perspective that require further exploration. Most obviously, *An Early Frost* deliberately avoids the traditional ending of the disease-of-the-week films, a genre that, as Howard Rosenberg describes it, is designed to produce "a torrent of teary movies about illness, each usually climaxing with a manipulative deathbed finale intended to leave viewers limp but uplifted"; it is "apparently impossible," he adds, "to be terminally afflicted these days without also being inspirational" (Rosenberg 1985, 1). The producer of *An Early Frost* said that this was precisely what he wanted to avoid, and Quinn, as Michael, said that, as he learned more about real people living with AIDS, he appreciated the ending, which, without implying that Michael will get well, does not kill him off on-screen. I would suggest, too, that the narrative structure does other kinds of work at the ending. For example, in the scene where Michael attempts to commit suicide, he goes before dawn to the garage, closes the door, and turns on the ignition. Meanwhile, his father wakes up to work out, as he does every morning. With carbon monoxide filling the garage and Nick running on his treadmill, the camera cuts back and forth between the two settings, building suspense as Michael coughs more and more, the smoke gets thicker, and Nick keeps jogging. Finally, Nick goes to the kitchen, at last sees the light under the garage door, and gets Michael out in time—keeping him alive and acknowledging that he *wants* to keep him alive.

This narrative structure is such that the practiced viewer of American film and television cannot *not* want Michael to be saved. Indeed, the viewer's knowledge creates a responsibility for Michael that, for many viewers, may not have existed before and, indeed, may even now exist against their will. The narrative code, in other words, dissolves the particulars and, in this instance, virtually requires the viewer to take up an engaged subject position. As in the earlier scene between Michael and Peter, one may quarrel with the ideological values embedded in the scene (father saving son, active saving passive, straight saving gay), not to mention the macho scene that follows the rescue—first Nick sends Kay away ("Go back to the house. . . . This is between me and my son"), then goads Michael into losing his temper ("Well, I don't give a damn what you think anymore," yells Michael, "because I'm more of a man than you'll ever be, you son of a bitch!" "That's right, that's right," croons Nick. "You go on, you call me anything you want—you hit me if you want to, as long as you don't give up!"). And, despite Michael's return to Chicago and to Peter, heterosexuality gets the finale, with the final credits rolling against a family photograph of Michael, his parents, his sister, and Bea. Nevertheless, numerous points of the narrative enable, even require, the viewer to "identify" in rather fluid and unpredictable ways. As we look more closely at the apparently conventional surface of the television movie, we need to consider the ways that subject positioning, critical viewing, and the legibility of television texts generate meaning for viewers at different points in their psychic, erotic, chronological, and cultural lives.

Our Sons *and Their Moms*

[*Our Sons*] is a very carefully constructed and classy production. . . . [It might,] then, be expected to leave the gay community reasonably pleased. Perhaps even a little gratitude would be in store. Don't count on it. Many homosexuals today are not about to be satisfied with occasional crumbs from the groaning board of popular culture. They are fed up with seeing their very existences viewed primarily as "controversial." Even the occasionally more sensitive films use distancing ploys, exploring not the lives of homosexuals but the anguished fretting of their parents or friends.—John O'Connor, *New York Times*

Our Sons was broadcast as an "ABC Movie of the Week" on Sunday, 19 May 1991.[20] It is the story of two gay men, one on the verge of dying of AIDS, and how they and their mothers face and are changed by this crisis. The movie's opening credits appear against the background of the California coast, accompanied by tranquil piano music. The ocean image dissolves to a luxurious pool and a light, open, California house. An alarm clock rings; it is early. Julie Andrews as Audrey Grant reaches to turn it off, picks up her dictaphone, and begins cutting deals. This is no pastoral hometown with a white church steeple but "the Coast," immediately a more urbane and sophisticated setting. And, where the central metaphor of *An Early Frost* was natural, that of *Our Sons* is familial.[21]

We next see Audrey at the office making high-powered phone calls. Last on her list of tasks is "Call James." As she dials and the phone rings, we hear the prerecorded message on her son's answering machine: "Hi, you've reached James and Donald. Leave a message for either of us—we don't have secrets from each other—well, maybe one or two." In *An Early Frost*, Kay's voice on Michael's answering machine serves mainly to reinforce how little she knows about his life. *Our Sons*, aired six years later, uses the prerecorded message as a simple device to introduce "the gay relationship" and establish its openness—to all listeners, including Audrey, and us. AIDS is introduced at the outset, too: as we hear Audrey leave her message, we see, in sharp contrast, the crisis taking place at James's end; rushing to get Donald into an ambulance, he simply has no time to pick up the phone. As in *An Early Frost* when Peter tells Michael teasingly, "Time's running out," our knowledge here that Donald is already seriously ill gives a twist to Audrey's closing plea that James call as soon as he can: "It's Monday the twenty-third and counting. Have a heart."[22]

Our Sons is a coming-out story, or, rather, it is a road movie embedded in a medical movie embedded in a coming-out movie embedded in a family melodrama. Donald has little inclination to tell Luanne Barnes, his mother in Fayetteville, Arkansas, that he is dying: she kicked him out eleven years earlier because he was gay, and now, even if he wanted to, he is too sick to attempt a reconciliation. So, unknown to Donald, James persuades Audrey to go to Fayetteville and bring Luanne back to Donald before he dies. Luanne's refusal to fly makes the road movie necessary, giving the two women an extended opportunity to identify their class differences: in music (country western vs. classical), in personal habits (smoking vs. nonsmoking), in ideology (intolerance vs. tolerance of homosexuals), in hair color (blonde vs. brown, a tip-off that Luanne and Audrey are the couple the film is interested in, not James and Donald).[23] Ultimately, for the sake of their sons, Audrey and Luanne not only transcend their differences but also acknowledge their similarities (e.g., they find that they both love jazz and that neither has a boyfriend at the moment). This in turn makes harmony possible between Luanne and Donald, who are reconciled by the time of Donald's death; between Donald and James, who have disagreed about Donald's desire to die at home (James resisting Donald's wishes as part of his own denial); and between Audrey and James, who mutually agree to try for a more honest relationship. In *An Early Frost*, Michael Pierson wrestles with his father's rage and perpetual injunctions to "be a man"; in *Our Sons*, fathers are virtually erased.

So what's new? In the vision of *Our Sons*, AIDS has become habitual, pervasive, and less mysterious. James is familiar with the hospital and its routines. No doctors explain "the facts of AIDS"; they simply go about their business in the background, hooking up respirators, IVs, etc. Funerals are old hat. When Audrey breaks the news to Luanne about Donald and starts patiently to explain what AIDS is, Luanne interrupts drily: "I mean I watch TV." Whereas the producers of *An Early Frost* decided not to show Michael's health deteriorate seriously, here Donald looks very sick, very weak, and his Karposi's sarcoma lesions are visible.[24] Donald telling James, "Toto, I have a feeling we're not in Kansas anymore," allows him to acknowledge that he is seriously ill and also signals another important difference in the two movies: Michael's character was made sympathetic to a "general audience" in part by "de-gaying him"; Donald's more interesting character is self-aware, relatively campy and unconventional, and extremely funny. All three character traits—which are permitted perhaps because progress has been made or perhaps because Donald dies before the movie ends—are evident as he makes offhand conversation in the hospital with Audrey: "I gave up smoking for my health. The insurance companies should come up with a whole new concept: irony insurance. There's a fortune to be made." "What's wrong with this picture?" Donald asks when his mother appears in his room after eleven years' estrangement. "How you been, Donnie?" asks Luanne. "I guess that's startin' out stupid." As she comes toward his bed, Donald replies, "I've been fine prior to this current nuisance." Then, "I like your outfit—très chic, Ma." Everyone gets good lines in *Our Sons*, and all get their share of irony, even when it is dark. Audrey, intensely uncomfortable with her mission in Fayetteville, obviously wishes that she were anywhere but in Luanne's trailer:

> *Luanne:* Want a drink?
> *Audrey:* I'd *kill* for a drink.

Luanne, waiting tables after Audrey's visit and repeatedly queried about the mysterious limousine that arrived at her door, finally says, "I won a contest, OK?" "What for?" she is asked. She replies bitterly: "mother of the year."

While some reviewers complained that Luanne's Archie Bunker role was overwritten, the scriptwriters may have been trying to make her reactions complex, as Nick's, in *An Early Frost*, were not; or perhaps the critics are insulated in Los Angeles from the range of American views about AIDS. She gets other lines as well, however: "I feel like I'm in 'Dynasty,'" she says, looking around Audrey's house, the house that Donald designed. And, although in some sense the straightest of the characters, James also gets opportunities to be sardonic (Hugh Grant in training, perhaps, for his subsequent roles on the big screen). After Donald has been hospitalized, Audrey suggests that his mother "should be told . . . about Donald, what's happening." James bluntly interrupts: "Mother, try to stop saying that, would you—'about Donald,' 'what's happening.' Donald has AIDS. He's dying. Would you stop tap-dancing?"

Our Sons has little of the medical boilerplate that was centrally featured in *An Early Frost*. There is no lecture on the high-risk groups: Donald's hospital roommate is another man with AIDS; the woman caring for him tells James, "He's my husband. I've got it, too." Virtually nothing is said about how Donald became infected (indeed, the line most explicit about sex is Luanne's response to hearing that, when James was younger, he had sexual relationships with women: "I can't understand how someone could jump the fence after tastin' normal"). In any case, the screenwriters seem more comfortable with the topic, with their own knowledge and authority. James, for example, says "Donald's dying," not "Donald's doctor says he's dying," and "He's much too sick to travel," not "They say he can't travel." He speaks with his own authority.[25]

Neither movie makes much of AIDS treatment, but there are differences. *An Early Frost* provides explicit information about the course of the disease, emphasizing the inevitability of death and the futility of treatment. After the emergency room doctor tells Kay that, "in my experience, I've never known anyone with AIDS to survive," she cries, "But there must be something you can do! You're a *doctor!*" Although in 1985 health care professionals were becoming more skillful at treating the symptoms of AIDS, and although people with AIDS and HIV infection were already trying out various experimental treatments, *An Early Frost* accurately represented conventional medical wisdom: asked about a cure for AIDS, the physician replies, "I wish there were. We're trying to find one. But it may take years." By 1991, many physicians had shifted their views to favor treatment, including early intervention with AZT and other drugs.

In the face of divided medical opinion in 1991, *Our Sons* is pretty fuzzy on the treatment issue, as in the scene where Donald and James are playing cards and Donald tries to persuade James to be tested for HIV (a term the film does not use):

> *Donald:* When are you gonna be sensible?
> *James:* You said you wouldn't bring that up again.
> *Donald:* I lied. It just isn't rational not to be tested.
> *James:* If I promise to do it, will you leave me alone?
> *Donald:* It could be negative, James.
> *James:* Yeah, and what are the astronomical odds of that being true; let's find the nearest computer.
> *Donald:* Michael Roby died two years ago, and Peter's still testing negative.
> *James:* Peter wants to *know*, Donald.
> *Donald:* Yes, and if God forbid he does go positive, he will have had the earliest treatment possible—as I might have had when I was still in denial mode— "*Me*—it can't happen to *me.*"
> *James:* It's my choice, Donald.
> *Donald:* [*Looking at his cards.*] I think I'm gonna win, and I haven't even started cheating yet.

This scene suggests accurately that early treatment helps. Although it does not get into the changing science and politics of testing, it does skillfully show the kind of discussion and speculation through which many people at risk have gone and also shows, in James, the psychological and conversational mechanisms of what Donald calls "denial mode." The implication that treatment helps, however, is contradicted elsewhere, first by Donald's puzzling implication that seroconversion (as opposed to the appearance of symptoms) can happen even years after exposure to HIV, and again toward the end of the film, after Audrey admits that she *has* been evading—"tap-dancing"—the issue of James's sexuality, not communicating her resentment that, as she tells him, "you would not be marrying the girl of my dreams." She asks for a second chance at honesty between them: "I want you to be tested. Because then we'll know how much time we have to try again." Perhaps the ambiguity is for dramatic effect; perhaps it is because treatment and the prognosis for long-term management are not yet taken for granted; perhaps it attempts to reflect genuine disagreements among people working with AIDS. But, still, a positive test for HIV is not a death sentence, nor will it tell Audrey how much time they have.

After Donald's funeral, Audrey and James accompany Luanne (and Donald's coffin) to the airport. As they leave, Audrey gives James Donald's childhood drawing of a castle that he used to tell Luanne he would build for the two of them to live in. "She wanted you to have it," says Audrey. The final shot is of Luanne's plane flying home, against the sunset. Then a white-on-black dedication appears: "This film is dedicated to the memory of the 108,731 people in the United States who have died of complications from AIDS."

Critics were divided over *Our Sons*. Stephen Farber (1991) saw the disparity between the film's grim subject matter and its "glossy soap operaish format" as evidence of the extreme nervousness with which television still approaches AIDS. Howard Rosenberg (1991) called it ironic that an AIDS story should take the form of "a buddy movie"—"Except that the bickering buddies in this case are not the two male companions directly touched by AIDS but their mothers . . . [who] have nothing in common beyond motherhood." His review stung *Our Sons* coproducer Micki Dickoff to respond that he had "missed the point" in saying that the film played "peekaboo with AIDS." "If the issue of AIDS has to be approached from around the corner," she writes, quoting Rosenberg, "or through the back door, better that way than not at all." And why assume, she continues, that "the network's motive was to avoid the negative backlash of conservative pressure groups? ABC's approach to the story, by directly confronting homophobia, is more likely to offend those conservative media watchdogs and advertisers" (1991, 3). Although many gay viewers and AIDS activists disliked *Our Sons* for its focus on the mothers, Dickoff was correct that conservatives were the group most totally and vocally outraged.

But, although the broadcast of *Our Sons* was certainly a political event, the text itself does not present collective, political, policy dimensions of the epidemic—only the closing dedication hints at such a possibility. At the same time, the narrative's conclusion reverberates with the sense that AIDS is a disease experienced by individuals and that homosexuality, inevitably, inescapably, and underlined by the absence of fathers and other straight men, has something to do with mothers. The event that most clearly resurrects and recycles this chestnut is Luanne's gift of the castle drawing to James, a gift, loaded with psychoanalytic implications, that brings almost too many meanings to the end of the film: Donald's identity, literally salvaged (outed?) from Luanne's closet, is passed on to James; Luanne's defense structure is relinquished; the world of "Dynasty" is restored to those who already inhabit it; and Donald's impossible dream—to live in a castle with his mother—is transferred to his lover, who is now free to live in Donald's castle with *his* mother. In the final scene, the plane bearing Donald's casket flies off into the sunset.

To some degree, both *An Early Frost* and *Our Sons* fulfill the goal of the family melodrama: to restore stability to the nuclear family and reinforce the traditions of a patriarchal order. In *An Early Frost*, this restoration is signaled by Michael's sister coming to terms with his illness; by the end of the film, she invites Michael to touch her pregnant abdomen and feel her unborn child inside—in contrast to her earlier act of pulling her young son away from him. In one of the final scenes of *Our Sons*, Luanne—who has earlier described herself sarcastically as "mother of the year"—takes care of Donald as a good mother should. Perhaps the more important point, however, is that in *Our Sons*, as in *An Early Frost*, the seemingly conventional and seamless television-movie surface gives way to a more interesting array of subject positions potentially available to the viewer. Together, the two films suggest some useful ways of thinking about the format of network television dramas, the complex nature of those hypothesized figures *the character*, *the viewer*, and *the audience*, and the legibility and intertextuality of television texts.

Whose Story? Identification without Guarantees

"There are eight million stories in the Naked City, but [ours] will not be one of them."—Donald, in *Our Sons*

In this chapter, I have raised and attempted to explore several questions: the characteristics of these two films as prototypical AIDS dramas spaced six years apart, *An Early Frost* treating AIDS as a classic disease of the week, *Our Sons* treating it as a pervasive, even routine condition experienced by many; the interesting and not fully readable ways that narrative representation facilitates or discourages the viewer's identification with characters on the screen, above all challenging any simple notion of identification on the basis of demographic similarity; the specific contexts in which a given representation of gay men or people with AIDS can be—even must be—evaluated as "positive" or "negative," for example, in the context of political efforts to influence television "images" or of public health efforts to make viewers sympathetic toward people with AIDS; the problematic assumption, underlying many of these efforts, that unmediated representation can be achieved; the diverse kinds of cultural work that different AIDS narratives perform; the cultural work of these mainstream, conventional dramas (in contrast to alternative and experimental videos) in creating points of identification and concern even among resistant viewers, in part by treating AIDS, despite its controversial, volatile nature and enormous social impact in the real world, in the tradition of medical television dramas (i.e., as a disease experienced by individuals) and by chronicling it in the established conventions of television realism; and, finally, the manipulation of television codes to tell stories about AIDS from seemingly acceptable perspectives, at the same time offering occasionally transgressive perspectives, a range of attitudes toward prevailing cultural values, and a complex and textured account of AIDS. Do these narratives enable us to explore alternative assumptions about the world and reality? Only the most subtle of footholds is offered for such an exploration. Whose story do these stories tell? This remains a difficult question.

The process of identification with a video representation is not passive, with the spectator holding a checklist on which certain features are relevant and others are not. Take, for example, the following exchange from the first scene between Donald and Luanne:

> *Luanne:* You've got no accent anymore.
> *Donald:* No.
> *Luanne:* Well, maybe just a smidgeon here and there—you can hardly hear it. [*Long silence.*] I hear you've got real successful.
> *Donald:* Yes, I've done pretty well. Would you care for a chocolate? [*Luanne refuses.*]
> *Luanne:* From drawin', more or less?
> *Donald:* Sorry?
> *Luanne:* I mean you got successful just from drawin'?
> *Donald:* More or less.
> *Luanne:* You was always drawin' when you was a kid.

In contrast to many scripts about AIDS, here the scriptwriters deliberately work to avoid heavy-handed moral judgments. This casually clever and compact exchange shows its participants in mild verbal combat, its light touch camouflaging Luanne's refusing the chocolate, thus failing a basic fear-of-contamination test. (Donald afterward tells James, "She wouldn't touch me, you know," and James responds, "Of course.") In television conventions, Luanne's behavior is not inevitably "negative," in part because the conversational exchange that surrounds it does not force the viewer to give it a negative interpretation, in part because it is contained by Donald and James's resigned lack of outrage. Likewise, recall the exchange between Michael and Peter in *An Early Frost*:

> *Michael:* We're almost out of shaving cream.
> *Peter:* Oh—OK.

Who does this exchange "represent"? Is it "negative"? If so, in what way, and for whom? I suggested above that it reproduces heterosexual marriage roles, with Peter the "wife" who manages the domestic space. Is this then a "positive" representation in the eyes of middle America? Does the straight man watching say, "I wish I had a partner like that, who'd get the shaving cream when I told him to and not give me a lot of shit like my wife does"? Defending *Our Sons*, Micki Dickoff argues that such films have brought about "real-life reconciliations" (1991, 3); meanwhile, a colleague tells me with dismay that her two sons (aged ten and twelve) made vomiting sounds during a gentle hugging scene between two gay men in *Longtime Companion*. So much for the "promotion of homosexuality" claimed by the Right! Who knows what "real audiences" really do? ("If 'the media' were so powerful, I'd be heterosexual," says Harvey Milk in the documentary about his life, *The Times of Harvey Milk* [Epstein 1984].) And what, in any case, is the relation supposed to be between television drama and real life? Does Donald's physical appearance mean that he is portrayed realistically? Is his love of and quotation from old movies a stereotype? An accurate reflection of the aesthetic preferences of some gay men (although not all, including James, Michael, and Peter)? A genre-specific convention for establishing intertextuality? A gay in-joke? Moreover, a narrative's potential for indeterminability is perhaps strengthened by network television, where commercials may address a different persona than the programs do, where one can always walk out, and where the picture on the screen often resembles the viewer's own living room (Hay 1990).

The AIDS teledrama embodies a tangled legacy of cinematic and televisual codes, familial and sexual metaphoric displacements, and gender and genre conventions—to the point that real life is virtually irrecoverable. At the same time, television exists within real social and historical contexts that also shape its discursive universe. As Lynn Spigel (1988) demonstrates in her wonderful essay on television in the 1950s, there was intense concern with television's potential role as an invader of the private domestic space of the home (the doors on console television sets were originally designed to provide privacy—from the television set!). Given this legacy, one could argue plausibly that, if AIDS has been so profoundly stigmatized, television should have been less hospitable to the epidemic than movies—which enable people to encounter it in the already contaminated space of public theaters rather than the sanctity of the home. Yet perhaps the privacy of the home is precisely where some people would prefer to learn about AIDS—not in a public theater, where they might be seen, might be identified as homosexual, might share the space with homosexuals or people with AIDS, and where they cannot just change the channel if they do not like it.[26] But what does this legacy really mean in the 1990s?

Rock Hudson's announcement in the summer of 1985 that he was being treated for AIDS was a turning point in the public's perception and in media coverage of the epidemic. As people talked about Hudson and AIDS, they created an interested community that had not existed before, a community that thought about AIDS as something that could happen to them or to people they knew. This was true of women as well as men: Hudson's illness was the point at which, ironically, the epidemic ceased to be seen strictly as "a gay disease." This suggests a powerful lesson about identification: we may identify with other persons not because they are demographically "like" us but because we feel that we have something in common, because we have shared their experience and knowledge, laughed with them, talked with them, walked in their shoes. The narrative structures of film and television can provide this sense of shared experience; indeed, in the case of major film stars like Hudson, we may feel that we know them, have even "been" them. We must therefore think carefully about narrative form, identity, and textuality, for ultimately these elements may be more significant determiners of viewer response than whether a given representation is "demographically correct."[27]

In summary, questions of identity and identification appear to involve memory, the nervous system, present goals and activities, life experience, familiarity with and pleasure in the conventions of a given narrative genre, demographic and circumstantial characteristics of the human figures (including their physical appearance, political perspective, values, real-life similarities and differences [class, gender], etc.), emotional and political connections to the text, and psychic commitments. Identification can obviously also be partial, can shift in the course of a performance or text, and can piggyback on formal elements of a dramatic work: formal or technical points of identification thus include the trajectory of the drama; the structure and angle of camera shots; our knowledge; our knowledge of the characters' knowledge; characters' function in the drama (i.e., their classic dramatic positioning as protagonist, antagonist, commentator, learner); their role in producing irony, laughter, and pathos; and their ability to mark difference, to offend, to charm. Finally, the text can draw us in by virtue of its own structure and its relation to other texts: through language, linguistic patterning, dramatic and emotive associations, use of the visual and verbal codes of television and television genres, allusion, metaphor, conversational inventiveness, and other elements of discourse.

It is in this detailed, technical sense that we can use television texts as, to recall Poovey's phrase, "laboratories in which one can observe and learn to interpret the dynamics of meaning production" (1991, 292). It remains to be seen whether such laboratory findings will prove directly useful in formulating our various agendas—intellectual, medical, political, cultural—for AIDS on television; but they will certainly arm us with a more intelligent and nuanced understanding of all the ways that television texts produce meaning and of the diverse kinds of cultural work that television narratives can do.

But this conclusion must *not* forestall critique. Yes, these made-for-TV movies can be taken up and used in more diverse and progressive ways than their makers or critics may have imagined; yes, they do important cultural work for many viewers despite their limited utility for gay and AIDS activist sensibilities; yes, our critique should not be based on simplistic and unsupported assumptions about how identity and narrative form function; and, yes, these cautious movies could have been much, much worse. Given the continuing urgency of the AIDS/HIV crisis in America, however, a radically different vision must accompany any generosity toward mainstream television narratives. Think, for example, of the stories that might have been told, that should have been told, about gay men and this epidemic. Instead, we have two bland, humanistic, made-for-TV movies. Created with better-than-average production values, resources, and good intentions, ultimately these movies are a pathetic legacy. By the time *Our Sons* appeared, more than 200,000 Americans were diagnosed with AIDS, and more than 100,000 had died. In this second decade, infection among women and young people has been growing faster than preventive behavior, people of color and gay men are continuing to become infected, the manifestations of the disease are still not fully known, the provision of drugs and treatment is still enmeshed in politics and bureaucracy, and the health-care system is a disaster. Having identified the success of these two modest movies, I am even more outraged at their failure: their failure to exploit the enormous resources of narrativity demonstrated in activist and independent work, to represent the courage and dedication of the AIDS activist community, to mention the words *condom* or *safe sex* or *gay community*, to show gay men and lesbians being gay, to make manifest the shabby politics surrounding the epidemic, and to challenge the systemic inequities of the health-care system. Whose story? Almost two decades into the epidemic, the story of AIDS remains untold. Instead, AIDS narratives on television tell the story of network television, still on its fearful, cautious path to self-destruction.

7

AIDS, Africa, and Cultural Theory

An ambitious 1990 *New York Times* series on the AIDS epidemic in Africa undoubtedly played a significant role in underlining the continuing AIDS crisis in Africa and ensuring its place on the public agenda.[1] On successive days, the four lead articles addressed the scope of the epidemic, its effect on the African family, "social marketing" education and prevention strategies, and Uganda's fight against AIDS. Even readers reasonably familiar with the crisis probably found themselves overwhelmed by the estimates of prevalence: noting that "hundreds of valid studies confirm experts' worst fears," the first article placed the number of infected adults at a staggering 5 million (out of 8–10 million estimated to be infected worldwide). Because 80–85 percent of the cases are believed to be the result of heterosexual contact among infected men and women, hundreds of thousands of infants are expected to die of HIV disease over the next decade. Infection afflicts professionals, working-class, and poor people and, because of interlocking extended networks of relations (Dr. Samuel Okware, director of the AIDS Control Programme in Uganda, says, "Here, nobody is born an individual"), sometimes strikes whole families. If geographic boundaries once contained the virus's spread, a map accompanying the article, captioned "an atlas of spreading tragedy," suggests that this is no longer true. James Chin, chief of AIDS surveillance at the World Health Organization, says that the 1990s will bring "an avalanche" of cases: "The worst lies ahead."

Based on weeks of reporting by Erik Eckholm and John Tierney in seven sub-Saharan countries, the series overcame many of the problems that had characterized U.S. media coverage of "Third World AIDS." The series cites African as well as Western and European "experts"; broadens the category *expert* to include traditional healers and frontline community service workers, not only directors of state agencies and conventionally trained biomedical physicians and scientists; interviews a variety of women (not just the token prostitute, a naive and inevitably doomed informant); represents diverse positions *within* African communities; resists facile speculations about the "African origin of AIDS"; and attempts to avoid the all-or-nothing tendency of previous reports either to exaggerate or underplay AIDS's existence and effect. The series also avoids the stark linguistic contrasts between the First World and Third World epidemics: populations in the industrialized world are "affected" by HIV and locations "infected"; their developing world counterparts are "devastated" and "infested." Although titled "A Continent's Agony," invoking once more the doomsday theme that overwhelmingly dominates U.S. AIDS coverage in developing countries, the series generally shows Africans actively and creatively *responding* to the epidemic, not simply waiting passively for the apocalypse.[2]

And yet . . . and yet . . . as the more egregious and hyperbolic writing about HIV disease in Africa diminishes, fundamental issues involving the burden of representation remain. If we look at the *Times* articles closely, we find, despite explicit disclaimers, some predictable rhetorical signals.

As I argued in chapter 3 above, the familiar statistical chronicle of the epidemic is a specific kind of narrative based on a specific kind of knowledge. Not only does it leave certain important questions unanswered; it cannot even ask them. Statistics in the *Times* series are presented with great authority and claim to be based only on "studies that used accepted HIV antibody testing methods." Previous reports on the epidemic have carried similar assurances, only to be called into question by subsequent investigation. Included also is the caution that "the figures may be understated"; in past reports, this statement has often served as a coded allusion to the unsophisticated testing and surveillance procedures of ("primitive") Third World countries. It is important to keep in mind that the possibility of "underestimation" is virtually universal in AIDS surveillance and certainly not confined to developing countries; at the same time, documented instances of "overdiagnosis" have occurred in African countries, often by Western and European physicians not entirely familiar with the somewhat different spectrum of HIV's clinical presentation in central Africa or its similarities to common endemic diseases.

Although the profile of seven countries localizes the epidemic, the recurring series title "A Continent's Agony" reinstates *Africa* as an undifferentiated mass of disease. The map (Eckholm with Tierney 1990) shows that, of the more than forty-five countries in Africa, only three are shaded to categorize them as "most severely affected." Further, although the map is labeled "AIDS in Africa: an atlas of spreading tragedy," the legend indicates that the percentages represent estimated HIV infection, not reported AIDS cases, and are based primarily on studies of sexually active adults in urban areas. I am not claiming that the map exaggerates the scope of the epidemic; certainly, however, it obscures details of degree and specificity.

Perhaps most telling is Erik Eckholm's article accompanying the opening of the series, "What Makes the Two Sexes So Vulnerable to the Epidemic" (1990a). Here, Eckholm reviews the "host of medical, cultural, and economic factors that make Africans especially vulnerable to the heterosexual spread of AIDS." This is the latest chapter in the continuing search for the elusive "cofactors" that facilitate HIV transmission, infection, and/or disease progression. In this article, five are cited: "rampant sexually-transmitted diseases," "lack of male circumcision," "little-known sexual practices," "promiscuity," and, finally, prostitution, which, "always an engine of sexually transmitted diseases, has played a major role in African AIDS." The search for links among the diverse populations affected by HIV has typically led to outrageous generalizations—for example, in a 1988 piece in *Vanity Fair*, Alex Shoumatoff claimed that "Africans, Haitians, and many Western homosexual men are riddled with amoebas" (p. 95).[3] The displacement of difference and pathology onto the Other is, in prior reports and in this one, most obvious in discussions of sexuality. "Researchers," writes Eckholm, "are just now turning their attention to little-known sexual practices that might also raise transmission odds." In fact, the attention to "little-known sexual practices" is a long-standing obsession with Western observers of Africa and other "exotic" cultures. The practice claimed as a potential cofactor in this instance is "dry sex," women's drying of the vagina with herbs; but it is only the latest in a speculative series, offered without research findings or disclaimers to certainty. Gone, in this instance, is female (as opposed to male) circumcision, sexual contact with monkeys, anal intercourse, violent intercourse, and so on. Again, not only have these notions, images, and theories been recycled throughout the last decade, but they go back centuries to origin theories of other infectious diseases (see Gilman 1985, 1988b).[4]

This chapter revisits themes introduced in chapter 3, reflecting further on how chronicles of AIDS make claims to truth and what kind of critical interventions and interpretive strategies might enable us to read the story of AIDS in Africa as a complex but necessarily partial narrative.

Maternal-Child Health Care in Africa Conference

Several conferences and related events during the summer of 1990 provide food for reflection. On 4–6 May 1990, an AIDS conference on maternal and child health care was organized by Dr. Ibulaimu Kakoma, one of my colleagues at the University of Illinois at Urbana-Champaign. Sponsored by the African Studies Center and numerous other academic units of the university, this was originally planned as a working conference but ended up with an audience of fifty to seventy-five people. Kakoma, a Ugandan virologist who holds D.V.M. and Ph.D. degrees and specializes in veterinary pathobiology and tropical medicine, had pulled together representatives of several national and international agencies, including the World Health Organization and the U.S. Agency for International Development, and faculty from both U.S. and African medical schools and universities.

This conference was immensely informative and useful on the subject of the AIDS epidemic in Africa, specifically its effect on women and children—a topic of growing urgency in the United States as well. Like most AIDS conferences, this one, too, presented AIDS policy, research, and service in the form of several distinct narratives: the biomedical chronicle of the virus and its behavior; the statistical chronicle of incidence, prevalence, and geographic spread; the public health chronicle of education and prevention; the social science chronicle of socioeconomic variables, attitudes, and behavioral change; and the discursive chronicle of language, meaning, and representation.

Most speakers at the conference were scientists, physicians, and policy experts, so it was unusual and refreshing to find several papers directed toward this last chronicle. Alma Gottlieb (1990), a cultural anthropologist, talked about the importance of meaning in understanding the epidemic's cross-cultural similarities and differences. As one example, she cited the documentation of rumors connecting AIDS to vampires; while such "conspiracy theories" can be dismissed as ignorant misconceptions, they often offer insightful metaphors about colonialism and other geopolitical realities—in this case, colonialism as sucking the lifeblood of African societies. She noted, too, that, despite virtually uniform agreement that the sexual transmission of HIV in Africa is predominantly heterosexual, there has in fact been "extraordinarily little research" on homosexuality. (On this topic, a difficult one, other speakers were largely silent, reproducing a silence that has systematically fallen over community after community when AIDS appears.)[5]

William A. Check (1990), a scientist who has reported on the epidemic since 1982 and coauthored *The Truth about AIDS* (Fettner and Check 1985), identified four obstacles to competent Western coverage of AIDS and HIV in Africa: the magnitude of the crisis, political obstacles, cultural differences, and existing media conventions. Magnitude causes both downplaying and exaggeration, which both represent attempts to gain at least the illusion of control or understanding; children with AIDS are found particularly difficult. Cultural and geographical differences include language, travel distance, and unfamiliar myths and customs (e.g., rumored sexual contacts between people and monkeys—Check speculated that ultimately polygamy probably presented a greater cultural gap for U.S. journalists than gay sexuality). As for politics, American reporters do not use available services like the All African News Service in part because they resent the new information order coming out of Africa. Media conventions include the perennial fascination with high-tech medicine, of which Africa has less to offer than industrialized settings.

Nancy Schmidt (1990), in contrast, provided an overview of AIDS coverage within Africa. Her survey of all African publications on the AIDS epidemic except the African-language press has yielded a bibliography of more than a thousand citations (as she noted, this would be larger had she included oral media like radio, conferences, and performances, but these are hard for Western observers to monitor). Within the Eurocentric, biased, doomsday mode of reporting typical of Western AIDS coverage, afflicted African people appear as the passive recipients of internal and external help, while Africans at large are charged with failing to address the epidemic, even failing to be aware of it; but these judgments are based on a virtually universal ignorance of the African press. A very different view emerges in African publications, which catalog multiple efforts to fight the epidemic by governments, women's organizations, church groups, school authorities, nongovernmental organizations, artists, prostitutes' groups, and so on. In African publications, Western AIDS coverage is criticized. Traditional African medicine is discussed with respect; although it is sometimes criticized, it is not, as in the West, treated as a curiosity or with derision.

It is perhaps fair to say that most speakers were committed to a positivist worldview and, in addition, tended to articulate positions that seemed directly related to their official position, scientific discipline, or agency affiliation. Within the frame of the conference as a public event, little uncertainty or skepticism was expressed (or at least not in any way that I, with limited understanding of international health policy debates, was able to decode). For example, several of the male speakers (who predominated) expressed definite views on the roles and behaviors characteristic of *women* and *mothers* and *prostitutes* without the kind of challenge or controversy that these terms and attributions would predictably generate in comparable discussions of AIDS in the First World. Likewise, statistics were regularly cited, but contradictory statistics were usually not challenged unless some official territorial clash was at stake. Widespread male resistance to condom use (as reflected, e.g., in such sayings, frequently quoted by conference speakers, as "No one eats candy wrapped in paper" and "No one takes a shower in a raincoat") was in fairly absolute terms condoned as "tradition" or deplored as "backwardness," just as the existence of myths and conspiracy theories and representations of cultural practices were judged correct or not, with little interest expressed in how or why such phenomena would exist. "We will not dwell on the misconceptions," said Kakoma in his opening remarks, "because we need to get on with the practical solutions." The production of knowledge and the ability to distinguish it as correct or incorrect were in this sense taken for granted.

What is obvious is the depth to which the AIDS epidemic in these central African countries has become politicized, like AIDS everywhere, but also so easily appropriated by outsiders into the preexisting and dangerous stereotypes to which I referred earlier. For example, as I argued in chapter 3, the stereotype that "Third World peoples" are passive, compliant, and incapable of understanding complex messages is what partially underlies proposals by Western scientists, U.S. State Department officials, and pharmaceutical manufacturers to test anti-HIV vaccines in central Africa. The reasoning is that testing such vaccines requires a critical mass of people who are (a) "pharmacologically virgin" and (b) continuing to get infected at high rates. Western people of color and intravenous drug users are, according to a related stereotype, too pharmacologically promiscuous (to use the term that typical AIDS discourse counterposes to *virgin*), and probably too unreliable as well, to include in official clinical trials; gay men, in contrast, are seen as too sophisticated to obey their masters' voices, may be using experimental treatments covertly, and in any case are no longer getting infected at rates high enough for good science. Only in the Third World, the logic continues, can sufficient numbers of subjects who meet these criteria be assembled for testing: too ignorant (or mired in "tradition") to change their behavioral practices (and thus lower rates of infection), too poor and unsophisticated to seek alternative treatments, compliant and dependent enough to follow orders, Third World people are definitely a promising population.

For good reason, then, representatives of African countries seek to close off the hyperbolic flights of fancy that feed the stereotypes and promote unilateral agendas; one strategy is to conduct public discourse in language regarded as neutral and scientific. The necessity for being careful, conservative, and protective was underlined at this conference by the presence not only of funding and policy agencies but also at least a hint of the vested economic interests of the North that make nations of the South wary. This note of intrigue was supplied by the attendance of an immensely tall American man from the East Coast whom nobody seemed to know; he wore no name tag and, whenever he was asked what he did, replied in elliptical euphemisms or mumbled double-talk (like Chevy Chase in the *Fletch* movies). Rumors of shadowy political and entrepreneurial dealings were further fueled by a conference speaker whose research had at an early stage been partially funded by the Central Intelligence Agency and whose presence on the program provoked a protest by a group of university students and faculty. The controversy inescapably raised, as so many AIDS controversies do, the question of how, why, and for whom knowledge is produced and who has the right to talk about it.[6] It provides some context, too, for Tierney's quotation in the *Times* series of Joseph Conrad's charge that the colonization of the Congo represented "the vilest scramble for loot ever to disfigure the history of human conscience" (1990b).

The Sixth International Conference on AIDS

The Sixth International Conference on AIDS opened on 21 June 1990 in San Francisco. With ten thousand delegates, hundreds of media representatives, and daily demonstrations by AIDS activists outside the Moscone Center, the conference is beyond easy summary. I attended as a media representative (for *Transition* and *Art in America*), having found the year before in Montreal that this made the immense conference more manageable; in addition, events within the media center in Montreal were as interesting as the conference itself. Some participants (rightly, I think) have come to see these conferences as opportunities for theater as much as for academic exchange. As I mentioned in chapter 5 above, this was nowhere more evident than at the informal press briefings within the media center in Montreal where famous figures in AIDS research and treatment addressed the press up close and personal. The power of these briefings to garner media coverage was quickly discovered by AIDS activists, who, having duplicated the official green media badges on a color Xerox machine, infiltrated the center in large numbers and began skillfully orchestrating briefings and interviews to get their own messages across. Because all the media representatives shared the same space, there was a real sense of who was there, from the *New York Times* to Swedish television, *Africa Reports*, National Public Radio, and *Rolling Stone*.

The mix of politics, outlets, and nations was less evident in San Francisco than in Montreal. In part, this was because many organizations and nations—including many activist and community groups—participated in an international boycott of the conference to protest U.S. immigration policy restricting the entry of people with HIV disease (at least eighty-five to one hundred groups participated in the boycott). Delegates' widespread display of red armbands in solidarity with those who could not or would not attend was dramatic. Yet equally striking was the absence of people of color. At the opening news conference, I saw a handful of Asians and no black media representatives and heard that successful efforts the previous year among journalists from richer countries to cover costs for those from poorer countries had fallen apart as a result of the boycott.

At the opening briefing, moderated by Media Director James Bunn, we heard talk of openness, glasnost, global representation, and great science. But glasnost was not exactly on the docket. In San Francisco, security was tight and the media setup totally orchestrated—almost, one might suspect, so that nothing unexpected *could* happen. Indeed, as Robert Wachter's (1991) account of organizing the conference tells us, deliberate decisions were made to minimize disruptions and uncontrolled access to conference events. To begin with, the badges were hard three-dimensional plastic objects in several colors, much harder to duplicate (it took activists a whole day to figure out how). Next, the various media were stratified, with the big networks all in one room, big print outlets in another, small print outlets in another, and so on, down to miscellaneous independents like myself. Official terms were also established: *press* meant print media, *media* meant everybody, and *news conferences*, not *press conferences*, would be held. Many services were available to make the media's job easier: selected footage would be supplied each morning for broadcast, and every evening Bunn would preside over a three-hour cable recap of the day's highlights, accessible on television monitors in all the conference hotel rooms. In fact, the only sour note involved the excellent espresso coffee supplied free to the media in Montreal; only two conference-sized espresso machines exist in the entire world, we were told; they cost $15,000 each, and Montreal has both of them. The announcement that only regular coffee would be supplied led to some grumbling among the media and talk of their own boycott. But otherwise the orchestration seemed to be working: as I left the briefing (or, rather, news conference), I overheard an ABC television reporter working out the evening news clip with his camera crew: "I would use glasnost and AIDS, some global bits, and wind up with the science."

Of course, good organization was imperative, given the massive media attendance. At this point, the AIDS epidemic was not merely *a* media issue but at least twenty-five separable media subissues, each with a life of its own, and each likely to want its own conference coverage—whether the blood-banking industry, pediatric AIDS, gay politics, Wall Street, the pharmaceutical industry, hard science, clinical medicine, Latin America, legal policy, and so on. Given all this and all that has been written about media coverage of AIDS, a special session called "AIDS and the Media" turned out to be a bit surprising. Organized by the energetic James Bunn, the panel included several experienced AIDS journalists and strategically placed agency officials who had all agreed to participate as themselves in a "media scenario." In the scenario, an American journalist gets a tip that an American serviceman, previously stationed in Uganda and now in the Philippines, is rumored to have infected forty female prostitutes in Subic Bay. In a sense, the panel did help illustrate how the media really work. Agreeing that "nothing normal is news," they all said that it probably was not a story, and Bunn had to slog hard to get them to play along. Allen White, a journalist with the *San Francisco Bay Area Reporter*, said that he would absolutely reject the "Patient Zero" angle, which would only reinforce the fruitless search for and stigmatization of supposed "carriers" of the virus; rather, if he had to cover the story, he would probably examine the rumor's effect on the status of U.S. military bases in the Philippines. Dr. Samuel Okware, director of the AIDS Control Programme in Uganda, dismissed as "trivial" a report of forty cases of AIDS in a site where and among a population in which AIDS is known to exist. "This would only be interesting to the West," he said, charging, too, that the scenario exemplified the West's propaganda campaign about "African AIDS" in implicating Uganda as the source of the serviceman's infection; it was indeed more likely, he observed, that the serviceman imported the virus to Uganda, rather than exporting it from there. James Curran, director of the AIDS/HIV Division of the Centers for Disease Control in Atlanta, concurred. Toward the end of the session, Laurie Garrett, then of *Long Island Newsday*—who in the scenario had gotten the original tip but as a panel member steadfastly resisted Bunn's encouragement to produce a sensational story—astutely observed that there is no such thing as genuine "neutrality" in journalism. Although American newspapers are not like Italian newspapers in which each has its own explicit political agenda, numerous aspects of coverage are determined by the nature of the outlet. Implicit ground rules exist among experienced AIDS reporters for establishing background, separating real breakthroughs from recycled press releases, checking reliability of sources, and so on; while these do not guarantee "objectivity," they do produce consistency in how journalists determine "facts." All news is inevitably a distortion; the journalist's task is to decide the nature and direction of the distortion and, perhaps, who will have to be offended. (One thinks of Todd Gitlin's [1977, 1980] definition of news as the exercise of power over the interpretation of reality.) This was one of the few self-conscious statements at the conference about the nature of representation.

Representation in its other sense was more in evidence, for a great effort had gone into making the large sessions "representative"—of science, medicine, the East and West Coasts, America and France, North and South, orthodoxy and activism. (On the travails of conference planners in achieving broadly based representation, see Wachter [1991].) Among the speakers at the opening plenary session was Peter Staley, an AIDS activist from New York who gave a rousing call to arms complete with graphics, flyers, and audience participation. He invited delegates to stand and join him in an anti–George Bush chant: "One hundred thousand dead from AIDS—where was George?" Not just his activist colleagues gathered around the stage but much of the audience packed into the Moscone Center accepted his invitation and chanted away enthusiastically. Another plenary speaker was Eunice Muringo Kiereini, a midwife with the World Health Organization, who talked about the effect of AIDS on women in Africa. The African welfare system is the extended family, she said, but this family may fail the woman with AIDS by rejecting her; further, "entire families are about to become extinct." This was a straightforward and moving talk, but one largely devoid of politics. Media coverage subsequently treated political activism as the province of the developed world, limiting the Third World's rhetorical powers to a simple catalog of troubles and pleas for assistance.[7]

Just as the media setup and conference program encouraged certain kinds of coverage over others, the selection criteria for scholarly papers encouraged certain kinds of academic research. Most painful were the conventional social science panels. For example, against all odds, a panel on "Human Sexuality and Issues of Sex Workers" was so boring that it was hard to sit through. I had hopes for the paper on gay male identity: I was not exactly expecting a postmodern account of the fragmented subject, but I was expecting something interesting. Nope. After laboriously describing her method of statistical analysis, the researcher tentatively suggested that there are sometimes discrepancies between a man's self-identified sexuality and the actual gender of his sexual partners: that is, a man who labels himself *heterosexual* may in fact have sexual contact with men. As you would imagine, this hardly produced gasps of shock throughout the audience. It was typical of the entire conference that, with rare exceptions, the problems of identity, sexuality, and representation were, to put it mildly, inadequately theorized.

A Digression

Nor was identity addressed consistently by the activist groups present in San Francisco. The day before the 1990 conference began, a series of pre-conference workshops had been put together by a number of AIDS activist and service groups. I attended the workshop "Racism, Drugs, and the AIDS Crisis." Despite a promising composition of people from many cities in the United States and Canada, the workshop was trying. It opened with a lengthy monologue by the group facilitator, who called for an international workers party, a worker-client-owned health-care system, and, oh yes, the complete overthrow of capitalism as we know it—events that seemed even more remote than they had before the Berlin Wall fell, Eastern Europe turned upside down, and the Soviet Union threw in the towel. An organizer interrupted briefly to deliver a message from an NBC News crew requesting to come in and get some footage. It sounded great to me, but purer politics prevailed, and the messenger was sent briskly on his way. This did interrupt the monologue, however, and several participants, including people with AIDS, now broke in to say that in this *particular* workshop they were more interested in talking about AIDS than reviving the dream of world communism ("Get real!" is how they put it). But it was too late, and possibilities for fruitful discussion trailed off. Few connections were made to AIDS and racism elsewhere in the world. In other ways, the event seemed very California. At the point that a Bay Area woman referred to class-based inequities of the American health-care system as "the two-tiered dignity thing," I decided to throw in the towel myself.

With considerable relief I fled to "Rules of Attraction," a conference held in conjunction with the annual San Francisco Gay and Lesbian Film Festival, in time to hear several filmmakers talk about their work. This was what the moderator, Cornelius Moore, called "the colored folks panel," and the speakers included Susana Muñoz, Silvia Rhue, Pratibha Parmar, and Richard Fung. At last, identity, sexuality, and representation were addressed. Muñoz, an Argentine filmmaker living in San Francisco, described her frustration with what the historian Lisa Duggan (1991) calls "the Balkanized territory of feminist identity politics"; at a feminist music festival some years ago, Muñoz had found herself racing from the Women of Color Caucus to the Jewish Caucus to the Middle-Class Caucus to the Lesbian Caucus, and so on, trying to get her many identities represented. "We are not only one thing," she said. The all-or-none version of identity divides and conquers: "It keeps us apart and thus serves the interests of the empire." Rhue observed that the film *The Color Purple* had reduced a twenty-year love relationship between two women to one twenty-second-long kiss. "I call this 'cousinism' rather than 'lesbianism,'" she said, "because it's what I do with my cousin." Parmar (who said she had made her first film, *Sari Red*, for $400) addressed the problem of multiple identities when, during particular periods of history, events require that one dimension of identity take precedence: national identity, for example, takes on powerful meaning when deportation laws are passed. Filmmakers who belong to strong ethnic, national, or social communities, she said, may encounter great pressure to create *positive* representations; in order to find their own voice, they probably need to resist this pressure. For Richard Fung, a "fourth-generation Trinidadian Chinese gay man who lives in Canada and speaks English as a first language," history may also require particular representational strategies at a particular time. The AIDS epidemic is an example. On the one hand, Fung praised an experimental film by Colin Campbell in which men are interviewed about their experiences with HIV disease; the film's revelation when the credits roll that the men are actors disrupts the convention by which first-person stories of sickness are accepted automatically as unmediated accounts of true experience. On the other hand, wishing to educate Asian men about HIV disease, Fung decided that it was crucial to show real Asian men with real HIV infection; the decision dictated his use of a more traditional realism.

Back at the Moscone Center

Between sessions, I was able to talk with Samuel Okware; I thought that, since he had participated in the "AIDS and Media" scenario (and was to be extensively quoted in the *Times* series), he might be able to answer some of the questions that had come up at the maternal and child health conference at Urbana in May. He confirmed some of the difficulties of diagnosing HIV disease in Africa, particularly in infants; no official definition of pediatric AIDS existed yet, so only retrospective diagnosis based on the condition of the mother was possible; and HIV infection is easy to miss because it can mimic so many other conditions.

I was curious about how *prostitute* was officially defined in AIDS research and prevention. This turned out to be a fairly complicated question, involving not only diverse languages but a disjuncture between legal and lived reality that reminded me of Queen Victoria's supposed insistence that reference to *lesbianism* be deleted from an 1885 bill criminalizing homosexuality on the grounds that women were incapable of such perversion. There is evidently no legal term for *prostitute* in Uganda, although the Swahili word *malaya* is sometimes used in nonlegal contexts; because there is no legal word, there can be no legal offense, so prostitutes can be charged only with being "idle and disorderly," a mild felony. This was one of several areas in which efforts to reduce the risk of HIV transmission were creating pressure to modify the existing legal system. Prohibitions against incest were being expanded to include a brother's wife; attempts were being made to strengthen laws against the defilement of minors, who, perceived as being disease-free, were becoming more attractive as sexual partners. Only women could be penalized for adultery, so the goal was to extend this to men. Despite the prohibition of behavior "against the order of nature," said Dr. Okware, there is no prohibition of homosexuality per se because (unlike Victorian England) there is no word for it; the only word available is *kiarabu*, meaning "of Arab culture"—another example, presumably, of the us/them divisions that so consistently mark AIDS discourse throughout the world.

Prevention and education continue to be called our primary resources against AIDS in less-developed countries, with little emphasis on the treatment alternatives being explored and tested in the United States and other industrialized countries. I asked Okware how he felt about the experimental drugs advocated by Project Inform and other groups in the United States and the United Kingdom. He said that these were inappropriate for Africa; until they had been fully tested under scientific conditions, they must not be made available. Since few African countries can afford AZT (or the drugs that have followed), the harsh reality is that, unless tested alternatives become available, most Africans with HIV disease will die.[8]

I reflected on this as I wandered through the huge exhibition area, housing hundreds of publishers, service organizations, and representatives of pharmaceutical companies. At the booth of the Burroughs-Wellcome Company, makers of the AIDS drug AZT, delegates could pick up a handsome, slickly produced spiral bound booklet called *AIDS: A Global Crisis*. Fourteen color diagrams, each unfolding to a size of eleven by sixteen inches, illustrate the human immunodeficiency virus, its epidemiology, supposed routes of origin, geographic prevalence, mechanism of replication, routes of transmission, the clinical presentation of HIV infection and of AIDS, and the role of the immune system, diagnosis, and clinical management. The illustrations were originally prepared as a poster display for an international conference on AIDS in Africa. So many delegates requested reproductions or slides that the booklet was produced; especially in settings where educational resources are scarce, the illustrations can be hung up, used for slides, or torn out to create poster displays. The booklet is produced by the Wellcome Foundation, a nonprofit agency supported largely by profits from Burroughs-Wellcome. The cover graphic shows the human immunodeficiency virus encircling the world. Given the multiple economic and political interests at this point bound up in AIDS in developing nations, it is not unreasonable to imagine that the graphic's subtext involves the role of AZT in saving the world from HIV. But who will pay for it? And, if nobody does, is it then arrogant or only fair to give African people the opportunity to have vaccines and other drugs tested on them? Certainly, complex cultural questions are bound up along with the Wellcome booklet's spirals.

The Wenner-Gren Symposium, 1990

A presentation on AIDS given by Gilbert Herdt, a professor at the University of Chicago, in a plenary session at the American Anthropological Association's 1987 annual meeting led to a Wenner-Gren Symposium, "AIDS Research: Issues for Anthropological Theory, Method, and Practice," held 25 June–1 July 1990 in Estes Park, Colorado. The twenty or so participants, primarily cultural anthropologists, were gathered together to think about what AIDS research could or should contribute to theory and practice in anthropology. For most participants, however, the question quickly became what anthropology could and should contribute to the fight against AIDS—a question that would explode just a few years later in a larger and more public setting.[9]

In 1990, a decade's experience with the epidemic seemed to reinforce the conclusions of ethnographers that the "risk-group" categories produced by epidemiology often have little to do with the lived realities of human experience. Stephanie Kane talked about the category "sex partners of intravenous drug users," the target population for a Chicago project in which she participated; in terms of sorting out the precise sources and probabilities of "risk," the category presents a "logistical nightmare." Furthermore, it does not exist as a "group" with a self-defined identity at all; rather, it is a collection of individuals who happen to have a single characteristic in common—indeed, a characteristic of which they may not even be aware. Experimental ethnography, she argued, has repeatedly shown that epidemiological categories, methods, and assumptions are problematic. In suggesting the limits of the epidemiological narrative, such a critique is essential; yet as responses to the crisis are routinized, as practical concerns (like obtaining research funding) grow more pressing, as the political and economic stakes increase, it becomes virtually impossible to insert this critique into the established discourses on AIDS.

By this I mean that the power and authority of quantitative research—from epidemiology to survey research to computer modeling—have been theoretically challenged from many perspectives in the human sciences over the last two decades. Ethnographic research, for example, reveals how deeply the concept *sexual intercourse* is enmeshed in meaning and social experience—that is, in complicated signifying systems where language, behavioral practices, cultural institutions, and self-identification regularly produce contradictions. But the ongoing dependence of international agencies and policymakers on quantitative evidence requires the use of standard surveys and other crude but quantifiable measures. The meaning and social reality of sexuality will be subordinated to measures of "frequency and direction" and identities and social networks to "risk groups." The assumption that these are somehow "neutral scientific categories" goes unquestioned. Likewise, the imperative toward providing "information" in short order to diverse regions of the world translates virtually by default into the deployment of the health promotion model in which people are given answers but not questions and in which AIDS education is systematically counterposed to the erotic.

Another set of problems in relation to the AIDS epidemic emerged at the symposium around the conception *the Third World*. Like other generic signifiers emerging out of postwar modernization and development theory, the term obscures salient features specific to given regions. While a country's overall economic resources are obviously significant to its ability to fight the AIDS epidemic, so are such other variables as the way all its resources are distributed. What are a nation's (region's, community's) attitudes toward sexuality, free expression, sexual diversity? What are its religious commitments and practices in relation to, for example, birth control policy? What are the government's policies regarding candor versus secrecy about HIV disease? Who controls the press? What are the social interactions among different groups and communities? To what extent has a country preserved or forged workable ties to the First World (e.g., do cooperative scientific projects exist)? What languages are spoken? What social infrastructures already exist through which education about HIV and health care could take place? Anthropologists, often well placed to answer such questions, have traditionally been reluctant to leave the universe of ethnographic inquiry for such mundane political economic scutwork. AIDS, however, mandates the shift. Only then can anthropologists begin to relate symbolic phenomena to their concrete political and historical context and determine why—for example—when significant external change creates widespread cultural change, AIDS inquiries continue to focus, repeatedly and obsessively, on "exotic sexual practices."

So-called conspiracy theories of AIDS pose special problems. As I have noted, conspiracy theories of blame and causation circulate geographically with astonishing ease, serving as templates readily adapted to the charged social divisions and power inequalities of the epidemic's latest home. For anthropologists, these theories can pose pressing conflicts. On the one hand, fieldwork training requires that the worldview of "the native informant" be honored, even if it is implausible, incomprehensible, exasperating, or appalling (e.g., Shostak 1983; Wolf 1992; Whitehead 1992; and White 1993). Indeed, strongly held beliefs about motive and method may provide important information about historical and current social arrangements and perceptions (Farmer et al. 1996; Schoepf 1991, 1992b; Waite 1988; and Parker 1992). Moreover, conspiracy theories have sometimes turned out to be true. At the same time, anthropologists at work during a serious health crisis may feel professionally and morally obligated to take on public health responsibilities, correcting the "misconceptions" of their informants and seeking to control their dissemination. They may have considerable biomedical knowledge about the disease and may even be funded by agencies charged with improving health within particular communities and populations. There is little conflict in exploring what beliefs about AIDS prevail: how people come to understand AIDS and HIV, after all, affects their responses to education, prevention, and treatment. But what to do next? On the one hand, people's understandings are shaped by the resources they bring to the epidemic as well as by the scientific information they receive, and there are theoretical and practical reasons for learning what their resources are—a process that may be cut short by the didactic assertion of biomedical "facts." On the other hand, an epidemic disease would seem to justify privileging facts and clear-cut behavioral guidelines over accounts that do not encourage effective preventive behaviors.

A pilot project in Haiti, reported at one of the earlier international AIDS conferences, sought a pragmatic compromise between the honoring of "native" theories of AIDS as a spirit curse and the assertion of an STD model: voodoo priests were enlisted to rework the curse theory by telling people that the spirits accomplished their evil magic through sex and that the use of condoms would trap them and make them harmless. Such compromises are common in the medical anthropology literature and rarely interpreted as patronizing or imperialistic.

But we can do other things with theories of AIDS than seek to eradicate them or, more pragmatically, circumvent them. As we look over the meanings that AIDS has generated as it moves among subcultures and around the globe, we can ask different kinds of questions. Who are cast as villains in a particular account of AIDS? How does a given account resonate with different constituencies? What's in it for its adherents? The widespread belief that AIDS is a deliberate experiment conducted on vulnerable populations is an example. In sub-Saharan Africa, the idea is common that AIDS is the latest effort by a white global elite to control the reproduction of people of color.

Moreover, segments of this same vulnerable population are now put forward as subjects for drug and vaccine testing by Western biomedicine; studies under way by 1997 compared AZT with various cheaper treatments believed to be "within the means" of developing countries. Given that AZT is not affordable at its current prices, the study really sought to determine how much worse people would fare on more affordable regimens—on the only regimens, I should say, that would be available to them no matter how ineffective the study found them to be. Well, say the directors of the study, at least they'll be getting something; without us, nothing would be available. Such a view is consistent with a history of colonialism in which the interests of empire take precedence over those of the colonized; empire in this case has apparently nothing to gain by paying for AZT. Many black Americans, similarly, hold the belief that people of color are especially vulnerable to the projects of science, a belief consistent with such events in U.S. history as the Tuskegee syphilis study (Hammonds 1992). Antigovernment beliefs about AIDS have been celebrated, lamented, denounced, and trivialized by scientific authorities. Several scholarly commentators have argued that, at the least, it must be treated as a historical reality and taken seriously (see, e.g., Guinan 1993 and Richardson 1997). A somewhat different tack is taken by David Gilbert (1996), a white 1960s leftist serving time in prison for the Brinks robbery; examining the popularity in men's prisons of accounts that cast AIDS as part of a deliberate campaign to exterminate communities of color, Gilbert argues persuasively that such theories are appealing for two reasons: they offer a political analysis of racism and disempowerment and, in doing so, provide male inmates with a "seemingly militant rationale for not confronting their own dangerous practices" (p. 57). Gilbert ultimately argues against AIDS-as-racist-conspiracy theories because they "divert energy from the work that must be done in the trenches if marginalized communities are to survive this epidemic" (p. 57), but not before giving serious attention to their claims from the perspective of their adherents.[10]

Some of the idiosyncratic, unreasonable, apparently demented meanings attributed to AIDS provide important insights into how people make sense of the world, collectively and individually, and how language works in culture. They reveal sources of mistrust, resistance, fear, and disempowerment. In her ethnographic analysis of vampire narratives in postcolonial Kenya and Uganda, Luise White (1993) likewise insists that the perception of the participants must contribute to the investigator's process of data collection and interpretation: "vampires" cannot simply be read by liberal Western anthropologists as a transparent metaphor for the ravages of colonialism (sucking the blood of indigenous people) but must be understood as an effort by people to explain novel phenomena at a particular historical moment—in this case, the introduction of new technologies and the rearrangement of labor inequities under colonial and postcolonial regimes.

Nor are these meanings and accounts of AIDS inevitably narratives of powerlessness. As vehicles that convert "science" into "popular science," many conspiracy theories offer their proponents exciting possibilities for empowerment as well as for the exercise of considerable prowess in original research. For people who find "real" scientific accounts of the material world the most thrilling of all possible narratives (and I am, more than 51 percent of the time, one of those people), the proliferation of quasi-scientific conspiracy theories about AIDS can be heard as a serious wake-up call about the sorry state of scientific literacy. But it can also be seen in other ways: as a stimulus for critical thinking, as evidence of enthusiasm for science and continued belief in scientific authority, as testament to excitement about and passionate interest in how the world works.

A final set of concerns involved the production of knowledge and how that knowledge is used in the world. As participants in the conference, we acknowledged that, despite the international diversity of our research sites and our largely progressive politics, we were all "First World" representatives. Further, our discussion had in many ways reproduced a persistent bifurcation in AIDS writing in which sexuality is generally not at the forefront for researchers in poor postcolonial settings like Haiti and Zaire while class and poverty are not primary concerns for researchers working in gay communities in the West. We acknowledged our privilege in being able to spend six days engaged in concentrated intellectual work; there was little of the customary acrimony on this point, perhaps because most participants were also engaged in various forms of day-to-day political activity, perhaps also because we did believe (sincerely, if predictably) that intellectual work and scholarly analysis can contribute vitally to the fight against the epidemic.

Action and Activism in the 1990s

The worldwide AIDS epidemic raises new questions in both developing and developed nations and at the same time revisits old and familiar cultural stereotypes. Because HIV infection and AIDS cannot yet be cured, prevented through vaccination, or—for most of the world's population—effectively treated, the epidemic must still primarily be addressed through education and prevention efforts aimed, in the end, at bringing about individual behavioral change and, at the level of groups and communities, slowing the spread of the virus. These efforts entail interventions based on language, education, information, representation, communication, and interpretation. According to some approaches, this is essentially a matter of translating the knowledge and findings of Western biomedical science and medicine in ways that are meaningful to those in other cultures. The handsome Wellcome Foundation portrait of HIV (mentioned above and reproduced in chap. 5 above) is a prime example. Such representations are familiar to those of us educated in Western, postindustrial university settings: many of us grew up with images like this, and we get the idea, even if we don't know the technicalities of glycoprotein structures, or why the virus is drawn to look like a tennis ball with golf tees sticking into it, or what the purple beehive is. If we wanted to know, we would have the technological resources to find out.

But should this virus and its representations be treated as universal, as a truth to be exported anywhere in the world? As I said above, this particular representation was designed, literally, for export purposes. Yet, as I have been asserting, the AIDS epidemic is cultural and linguistic as well as biological and biomedical. This proposition entails, among other things, more than translation. It means making sense of AIDS and HIV in context. And context, in turn, entails a corollary proposition: *culture* and *discourse* acquire meaning and have consequences within specific material circumstances. Although the usefulness of both terms is their dual alliance with formal texts and with material phenomena, they can easily divert us (into either the apparent autonomous power of texts or their seemingly

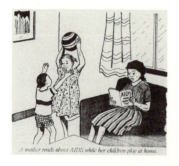

A mother reads about AIDS while her children play at home.

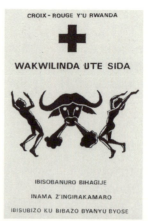

CROIX - ROUGE Y'U RWANDA

WAKWILINDA UTE SIDA

IBISOBANURO BIHAGIJE

INAMA Z'INGIRAKAMARO

IBISUBIZO KU BIBAZO BYANYU BYOSE

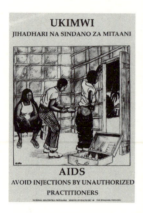

UKIMWI

JIHADHARI NA SINDANO ZA MITAANI

AIDS

AVOID INJECTIONS BY UNAUTHORIZED
PRACTITIONERS

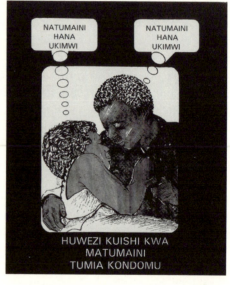

NATUMAINI HANA UKIMWI

NATUMAINI HANA UKIMWI

HUWEZI KUISHI KWA MATUMAINI TUMIA KONDOMU

An educational AIDS booklet shows a housewife reading an educational AIDS booklet (7.1: educational pamphlet, Kenya). Maternal and child health is a priority of AIDS/HIV intervention strategies in less-developed countries, starkly highlighting the vast North/South differences in the distribution of resources as well as women's global vulnerability. As in the United States and elsewhere, individual health ministries and nongovernmental organizations have developed their own priorities, artistic conventions, slogans, and visual icons to fight the epidemic (7.2: SIDA as water buffalo, from pamphlet prepared by Rwandan Red Cross; 7.3: "I hope he/she doesn't have AIDS": "You can't live on hopes. Use a condom"; 7.4: Ministry of Health poster, Tanzania, 1988).

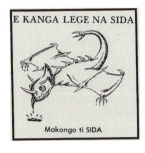

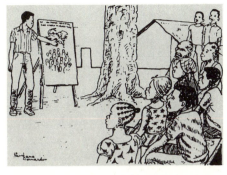

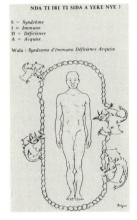

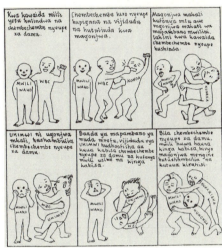

The visual representation of
AIDS *and* HIV *is subject to many*
influences and often takes shape as a hybrid compromise. The creature created
for an educational booklet (ca. 1988) in the Central African Republic to encapsu-
late graphically the key features of SIDA, is—with the talons of a hawk, the adapt-
ability of a chameleon, the stealth of a bat, etc.—a hybrid par excellence (7.5).
Deployed pedagogically in village education sessions, however, the creature is
taken as a literal rather than a symbolic figure: "I've never seen such a horrible
thing—thank goodness there's no SIDA here" (7.6). In figure 7.7, the viral creature
is shown destroying the immune system, represented as a protective chain encircling the human body. Figure 7.8 (Tanzanian Ministry of Health brochure, with
UNICEF) employs the image of defensive battle, with the white blood cell protecting the body from many dangerous microbes, then succumbing to HIV and leaving the body defenseless.

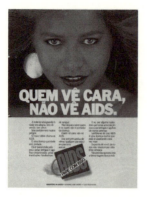

Despite local adaptations, it sometimes seems as though public health campaigns draw ideas and images from some secret central vault, so similarly are they structured over time and space. These examples draw metaphorically or literally on earlier themes: the warning that beauty is no guarantee of health (7.9: condom promotion from Brazilian ministry of health, ca. 1992; compare the "She may look clean" catchphrase mentioned in chap. 2 above), the Scriptographic citizens morphed into speakers of Spanish (7.10: SIDA as Tupperware party, booklet

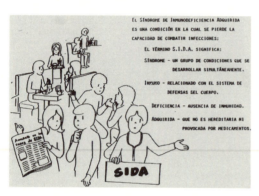
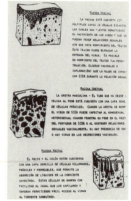

transparent correlation with the material world) from examining the crucial codependencies of signification. In any case, keeping in mind my interest in an epidemiology of meanings, I document some of the meanings and attributions that AIDS has acquired across time and space and briefly suggest some kinds of cultural work that these meanings perform.

What follow, of course, are only examples. A systematic account of global AIDS can be found in *AIDS in the World*, a remarkable book first published in 1992 and revised in 1996 (Mann and Tarantola 1996). Developed under the auspices of the Global AIDS Policy Coalition and the International AIDS Center of the Harvard AIDS Institute under the direction of Jonathan Mann, the book addresses multiple dimensions of the global epidemic more intelligently and comprehensively than any other single publication. Committed to influencing theory, policy, and practice, the book deploys a range of analytic approaches and draws from the grounded experience of hundreds of AIDS intervention projects worldwide.

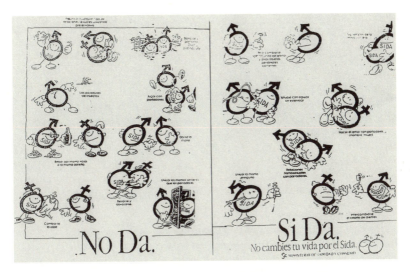

by Channing L. Bete, ca. 1990), and the rugged vagina now a global form of protection (7.11: Puerto Rican educational materials on SIDA, ca. 1990). Although
the SiDa/NoDa poster in figure 7.12 (Puerto Rican educational materials on
SIDA, ca. 1990) looks similarly generic, unexpected features include the play on
"Si" and "SiDa," the back-to-back flip format (high-risk behaviors are on one side
of the flyer, safer behaviors on the other), the potentially confusing linkage of si
(yes) with negative behaviors (i.e., those that put you at risk for SIDA) and no
with positive ones, the festive decoration, and the very unusual depiction, amid
an apparent heterosexual universe of possibilities, of two male biological symbols having anal intercourse.

Within sub-Saharan Africa, many AIDS initiatives have been undertaken by both governmental and nongovernmental organizations. Booklets designed for the public and for health extension workers address
transmission, prevention, compassion, and tolerance. Others address the
science of AIDS/HIV. Still others venture to talk about touchier subjects:
conflicts in moral values between urban and rural areas; the need for men
to take more responsibility for the household when their wives or partners become ill; the importance of changing sexual practices; the importance of economic restructuring; tensions between church and state; the
realities and pitfalls of Westernization; the potential risk of familiar customs and rituals; and so on.

A pamphlet from the Central African Republic, circa 1988 I'd judge,
illustrates some of these points. Sent to me by Colin Garrett, then a Peace
Corps volunteer there, it is written in Sango, a lingua franca throughout
this part of Africa, only recently given written form. The country's liter-

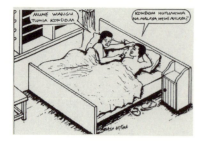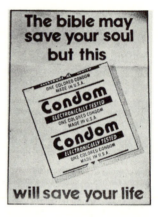

Safer sex campaigns pioneered within urban gay communities lowered incidence rates for STDs among those populations. Not until condoms were widely institutionalized in formal AIDS intervention campaigns and sent out to protect diverse populations around the world did their various and often deeply problematic meanings fully emerge. Differences in gender equality, legal protections, religious dictates, and cultural norms surrounding practices like male circumcision can all influence denotations as well as connotations of condom promotion messages. In time, condom messages have been increasingly adapted according to a strategy that could be called "think globally, fuck locally." Although health campaigns still rely on generic templates, initiatives developed on the ground are more likely to work through local groups and organizations, employ local artists, and incorporate cultural norms and nuances. "Use a condom, my husband,"

acy rate is low: about 35 percent among French speakers (the postcolonial and most widely used common language) and about 1 percent among Sango speakers. The pamphlet is not widely available and is intended primarily for health educators in the villages. The creature that appears in the pamphlet (and on posters and other materials) represents the virus that causes AIDS. It is a composite of various creatures, explained Colin, and "there is a little history that goes with it":

> The creature that symbolizes the AIDS/SIDA virus is a composite of various other creatures. . . . The tail is the tail of a scorpion; a scorpion's sting hurts a lot, as does AIDS. The body and eyes are those of a chameleon; like the chameleon, AIDS adapts, and may look different in different people. The spines are those of the porcupine: would you pick that up? It would hurt you. Wings of a bat: bats fly at night, and you can't see them. Thieves also come in the night and steal your

urges the wife in 7.13 (educational booklet, Zaire; drawing by Abass Mtema); he counters with a stereotypical prejudice that the narrative proceeds to challenge: "Prostitutes use condoms—Are you a prostitute?" Compromises between public health and religious groups have taken many forms. A condom promotion slogan from Zaire appears in 7.14; in Uganda, bookmarks containing information about safer sex were inserted into Bibles and the two together were distributed to 3 million schoolchildren. The instructions for condom use in figure 7.15 are designed as a pocket-size foldout booklet.

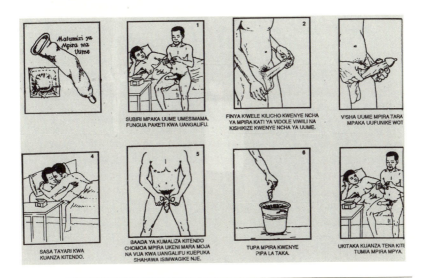

clothes, as AIDS comes and steals your health, and you don't even know what has happened. Claws like a hawk or eagle: when a hawk swoops down and steals a chick, they never let go; AIDS is the same. Horns of a rhino: you sure wouldn't want to get near that. Beak like a parrot: also hurts a lot. The blood on the creature's beak is to remind you that it likes blood and thus to beware of blood.

This imaginative representation of the dimensions of HIV and AIDS follows a long tradition in village health education among nonliterate people. The same booklet depicts such a village teaching scene, even down to the HIV creature on the easel. We can readily identify differences between Wellcome's HIV and this creature. While we are likely to grant considerable authority to the Wellcome image, we are also likely to regard the CAR representation as imaginative, culturally specific, and quite complex in its symbolic condensation of the characteristics of AIDS. Yet Colin continued:

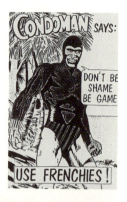

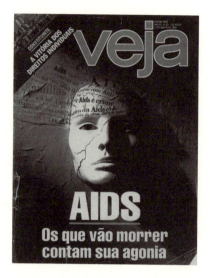

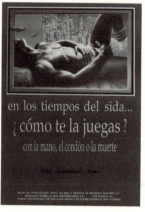

Amateur and professional artists have contributed to the struggle against the epidemic, creating educational messages specifically for their own communities, producing striking visual images that challenge the studio portrait tradition of dying AIDS *victims, and enfolding wildly diverse icons and artifacts of the epidemic into ongoing art projects (7.16: "Condoman," a poster and comic book designed primarily by Aboriginal health care workers in Queensland, Australia; 7.17:* AIDS *cover story in* Veja *[Brazil], 10 August 1988; 7:18: "In the time of* AIDS . . . *[Taller de Documentación Visual, offset print, 1992, in* Mexican Art: Images in the Age of AIDS, *30 September—5 November 1994, University of Colorado, Boulder]).*

Village health extensionists run through this explanation for their AIDS education presentations. But there have been a lot of problems trying to explain to people that this creature is only a *symbol* of the virus, and despite grand efforts, villagers will often come away from an education session saying something like "Did you see that horrible creature? I've never seen anything like that around here—I'm sure glad there's no SIDA here." Because of this, many of the health extension people want to get rid of the creature, but it is the brainchild of the director, so that whole issue has been turned into a huge battle of egos.[11]

Like those from other countries, these central African materials show intersecting codes and influences. Some employ specifically local emblems and conventions: a water buffalo symbolizes AIDS; a particular setting or style of dress, as in the sketch of women protesting Western media claims, signals location, occupation, or class; or a cultural product like the *Condoman* comic is created by the aboriginal communities to whom it is targeted. Two Tanzanian calendars produced to raise funds for AIDS efforts communicate cultural information of this kind. The village health extension worker shown in the 1991 calendar scene is marked as a professional woman by the dress she is wearing, but her corn rows and traditional wrap mark her as "respectable." The rural men and women listening are being warned about adultery and prostitutes and encouraged to honor marriage and use condoms. In the upper left, an educator urges a barber to use new razors, while, on the upper right, two bar women and their escorts are shown how to use condoms. In the 1992 scene, representatives of many walks of life journey collectively to conquer AIDS; shown left to right are a woman worker, priest, businessman, student, policeman, nurse, schoolgirl, Zanzibari woman, and military man.

Other examples, including most of the condom promotions, suggest the priorities and trade-offs guiding campaigns in various settings (just as the Helms amendment left its mark in the United States through the glaring absence of homosexual men from a whole generation of anti-AIDS materials). A Brazilian condom promotion poster featuring a beautiful woman's face, in another example, clearly carries forward the legacy of the U.S. wartime anti-VD campaigns that I cited in chapter 2 above. "She may look clean," ran the caption of one I quoted there. A U.S. AIDS poster showed a similar woman's face: "Does she or doesn't she [have HIV]?" the caption asked. The Brazilian caption reads, "He who sees the face does not see AIDS." Other materials represent literal copies, like the ubiquitous Scriptographic booklets that apparently adapt effortlessly to every country, every language, and every human problem from AIDS to traffic accidents to fear of public speaking. A Puerto Rican educational brochure shows the "rugged vagina/vulnerable rectum" (discussed in chaps. 1 and 2 above and 8 below), indeed seems to have traced it from the Lewis Calvert illustrations for Langone's 1985 *Discover* article. Another poster contrasts safe with unsafe activities; making a pun on *SIDA*, the Spanish term for *AIDS*, one side of the poster shows "NoDa" (activities that will not give you AIDS), and the flip side shows "SiDa" (activities that might transmit SIDA). The SiDa group includes a rare image of two male cartoon symbols having anal intercourse.

Triumphing over a lack of resources and infrastructure, the Tanzanian Media Women's Association CHAWAHATA produced a special AIDS issue of their journal *Sauti ya siti*. Brought to me and translated by Stacie Col-

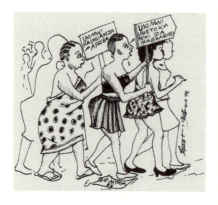
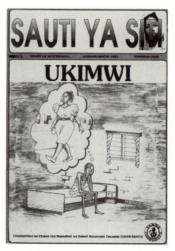

While, like "local community standards," "cultural specificity" is no guarantee of progressive, democratic, or effective approaches to public health interventions, materials produced within specific communities tell us more about social differences and salient issues than imported materials simply translated into local vernaculars. Sauti ya Siti *is a journal written and produced entirely—and with minimal resources—by a women's media organization in Tanzania; this special issue on* AIDS *(*UKIMWI*) departs from the predominant family theme of most* AIDS *campaigns aimed at African women; it shows concern for women as individual beings who can think and act and whose vulnerability to* HIV *and other health problems is gendered (7.19: "*AIDS *did not begin in Africa": women protest*

---

well, whose dissertation research was carried out in Tanzania, this journal issue is unusual in its focus. While growing attention is paid to the vulnerability to AIDS/HIV of women in central African countries, the emphasis on family in this discourse is overwhelming. In contrast, from the moment one sees the cover of *Sauti ya siti*, one perceives its concern with women as individuals and as *gendered* members of larger communities. The Western feminist may automatically read the cover as a punitive bad girl/good girl message, but, in the context of more conventional admonishments to "love faithfully," the contrast is articulated to a more complex constellation of issues: rural versus urban life, independence versus family, and oblivion versus self-awareness.

What Can Cultural Theory Do?

In the face of the AIDS epidemic's global impact, scholars, writers, and intellectuals may feel impotent, as though only material intervention is

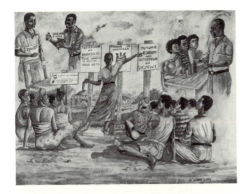

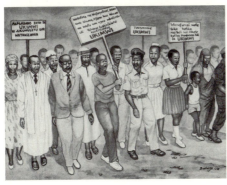

Western media assumptions, drawing by E. Mtaya, 1992; 7.20: cover of Sauti ya Siti; *both from issue of January–March 1992). Original artwork for two Tanzanian calendars (designed to raise funds for* AIDS *interventions) similarly captures internal differences of—for example—social status, locale, occupation, commitment to tradition, age, ethnicity, and gender. The 1991 calendar shows extension workers carrying out* AIDS *education in the field (7.21: illus. by Walter Lema), while the 1992 calendar shows diverse populations in unity against the epidemic (7.22: illus. by R. Mbago).*

useful. But, as the second decade nears its end, the epidemic has become a symbolic arena for other struggles, many seemingly far from health care. Pervasive across social and cultural institutions, the epidemic has come to be connected to and to have far-reaching effects on labor patterns, courtship, erotic life, marriage, childbearing and child raising, family life, health care, cultural production, and the national and international economy. Precedents established today with respect to legislation, the appropriation of resources, political alliances, discursive conventions, freedom of expression and censorship, the permeability of borders, the nature of erotic life, the diversity of structural household arrangements available, and the embrace of tolerance or discrimination will affect much more than AIDS.

The epidemic is at a particularly crucial point. As Margaret Connors and Janet McGrath emphasize, AIDS is "far from being under control in any part of the world" (1997, 1). Particularly needed is the construction of sound, compelling, and politically progressive cultural theory that can challenge the unquestioned supremacy of other chronicles of the epidemic. The conferences that I have briefly discussed here offer several lessons:

Cultural knowledge relevant to the AIDS epidemic is being produced at a variety of geographic and cultural sites, but few opportunities exist for international discussion. Rather, *culture* is typically understood within conventional AIDS discourse in the narrowest and most old-fashioned sense: enrichment, civilization, uplifting art, which fork to use. The sensibility of liberal humanism predominates, while vital contributions of feminist, postmodern, and postcolonial writing and theory may be absent.

The production of knowledge is, as it must be, a fragmented enterprise. But, with regard to the AIDS epidemic, this sequestration of culture from both scientific and social discourse has especially negative effects on international dialogue. Statistical knowledge travels well; cultural knowledge does not.

To judge from some recent writings, a backlash against *culture* as an explanatory concept is probably inevitable. But this backlash consists of several distinct critiques, and only one of them deserves attention. This is the charge, best articulated by Farmer et al. (1996), that *culture* is now being taken up wholesale to explain, justify, and excuse nonexistent, inadequate, or failed intervention campaigns and the research base that spawns them. *Culture* is becoming a favored invocation of such projects, which are usually grounded in traditional social science theory focused on individual behavioral change or in information campaigns developed in pristine ignorance of structural forces and the myriad material environments in which behavior acquires shape, meaning, and consequence.

A social scientist at the maternal-child health conference asked whether the politics and policies of the AIDS epidemic must inevitably be based on inadequate data. Without "data" about meaning and representation, the answer is inescapably yes. But, without the participation of artists, intellectuals, and cultural theorists, no one will be equipped to produce or contribute such knowledge or even to recognize it is not there.

8

Beyond *Cosmo*: AIDS, Identity,

and Inscriptions of Gender

"In its simplest form," writes philosopher Avrum Stroll, the problem of identity "may be thought of as the problem of trying to give a true explanation of those features of the world which account for its sameness, on the one hand, and for its diversity and change, on the other. . . . Difficulties about identity lie at the heart of a vast corpus of seemingly unrelated problems" (1967, 121). Certainly, our understanding of the AIDS epidemic requires us to sort out an extraordinary number of difficulties about identity. These have serious implications for women: perhaps no arena of AIDS commentary has been more consistently confusing and problematic than gender—for AIDS experts, AIDS educators, clinicians, and media commentators as well as for women themselves.

Let me put this another way. An effective response to an epidemic (as to any widespread cultural crisis) depends on the existence of identities for whom that epidemic is meaningful—and stories in which those identities are taken up and animated. As I argued in chapter 2 above, many identities and narratives for women were readily available in relation to AIDS, indeed, were ready and waiting when the epidemic began: loving helpmate/ swinging single, madonna/whore, good mother/bad mother, and so on. But these have rarely been meaningful or useful in changing women's own awareness or bringing about social change. Even today, facts about the epidemic, scientific data, and stories of sickness serve, sometimes inadvertently, to discourage the formation and mobilization of meaningful identities for women. Representation significantly limits access not only to "data," in other words, but also to the subject positions, narratives, and identities that could make sense of information and act on it. And, if women themselves cannot make sense of the epidemic, articulate its influence on their lives, and shape interventions that embody their interests and perspectives, historical precedent holds out little promise that anyone else—whether scientists, physicians, policymakers, media professionals, or politicians—will do it for them. Feminism, too, has failed to influence the direction of the epidemic or challenge the stereotypes and misconceptions that have pervaded AIDS discourse thus far.

Many of the problematic conceptions surrounding women and AIDS were evident in a January 1988 article by the physician Robert E. Gould in *Cosmopolitan* magazine. Gould's article was designed to reassure *Cosmo*'s several million women readers about AIDS: "There is almost no danger," wrote Dr. Gould, a psychiatrist with no expertise in AIDS research or treatment, "of contracting AIDS through *ordinary sexual intercourse*"— which means, in his words, "penile penetration of a well-lubricated vagina—penetration that is not rough and does not cause lacerations" (p. 146). In addition to the article's sloppy language (failing to distinguish AIDS from HIV, unprotected from protected sex, an infected from an uninfected partner, and so on), it argued that a "healthy vagina" was protection enough against the virus. If it were not, he reasoned, the prevalence of AIDS in the U.S. heterosexual population would by now be extensive. To account for the existence of widespread HIV infection among heterosexual men and women in Central Africa, Gould offered two explanations: first, he asserted, homosexuality among African men is common but taboo and therefore not acknowledged to investigators; second, "many men in Africa take their women in a brutal way, so that some heterosexual activity regarded as normal by them would be closer to rape by our standards" (p. 146).

As chapter 2 above demonstrated, Gould's *Cosmo* article was not the first publication to make dubious claims about women and AIDS during the first decade of the epidemic, but it was certainly the most widely read. And it was the first to which women responded loudly, collectively, and politically. Women in the New York chapter of the activist organization ACT UP (AIDS Coalition to Unleash Power), formed the year before, read Gould's article and were appalled. They identified errors of fact, flawed assumptions, outdated statistics, and claims contradicted by their own knowledge and experience—above all, perhaps, their knowledge that women *were* infected with HIV and *were* dying of AIDS. To challenge Gould's misleading advice to women, they organized a protest at the offices of *Cosmo*'s New York publisher; asserting on picket signs, "The *Cosmo* girl CAN get AIDS," they distributed flyers that challenged Gould's claims, point by point, documented the impact of AIDS on women (e.g., AIDS in New York City is currently the leading cause of death among women age twenty-five to thirty-four), and urged the public to just "Say no to *Cosmo*" by boycotting the magazine.[1] This action had a number

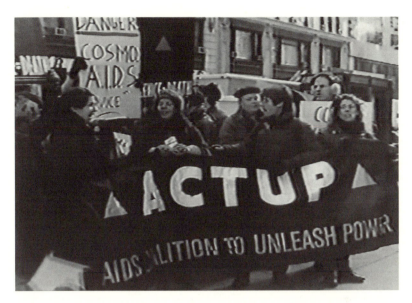

The decision by ACT UP *New York's Women's Caucus to protest* Cosmopolitan *magazine's facile reassurances to women about* AIDS *shifted the terrain of politics and possibilities in* AIDS *wars of representation. Documented in the video* Doctors, Liars, and Women *(8.1: Carlomusto and Maggenti 1988), the* Cosmo *action forcibly articulated a coherent narrative about women and* AIDS/HIV, *insisted that the failing patchwork of mainstream scenarios be abandoned, and challenged widespread medical and media complacency.*

of concrete outcomes: the women in ACT UP produced a documentary video called *Doctors, Liars, and Women: AIDS Activists Say No to Cosmo* (Carlomusto and Maggenti 1988), which recorded the debate as it continued in local and national media; they formed the ACT UP Women's Caucus, which organized subsequent actions; and they produced the book *Women, AIDS, and Activism* (ACT UP New York Women and AIDS Book Group 1992).[2]

The *Cosmo* action marked a significant step forward in understanding the realities of the AIDS epidemic for women and in challenging prevailing representations. In doing so, it came to terms with three important dimensions of the problem of identity. The first dimension involves classic philosophical questions of whether something is the same as or different from something else; the problem of identity, to repeat Stroll, entails trying to determine which features of the world account for its sameness, on the one hand, and for its diversity and change, on the other.[3] While the AIDS epidemic provides many examples, including technical questions about the nature and identity of HIV, an ongoing problem with regard to women and AIDS involves the identity of the AIDS epidemic itself. Questions of identity involving who is infected and how HIV is transmitted shape fundamental understandings of what AIDS *is*; in turn, these understandings have shaped the ways we identify and classify those whom HIV infects as well as its modes of transmission. In North America, the initial appearance of the epidemic among gay men, generating labels like *GRID* (Gay-Related Immune Deficiency) and *the gay plague*, encouraged physicians and scientists, in the face of seemingly disparate clinical symptoms, to perceive gayness as the common denominator underlying the condition of acquired immune deficiency. This history distorted the question of gender, encouraging women to feel immune. The question of whether AIDS is or is not "a gay disease" is still around, primarily because, in the United States, gay men continue to be affected in greatest total numbers statistically. Indeed, whole cultural narratives have been founded on what is essentially an accident of history. History is history, of course, and cannot be set aside because it might have been different. But neither does it fully dictate who has been infected or who will be in the future.[4]

Identity also encompasses personal identity, those features or properties that link each of us to other classes of people (groups, communities, populations) and distinguish us as unique individuals from other human beings. Recent work in critical and cultural theory suggests that gender is in many respects fluid, ambiguous, and fragmented, elements that are largely absent from the conceptions of gender that inform AIDS discourse, from medical journals to epidemiological surveillance reports to popular culture. Those accounts do contain ambiguities over identity: for example, the research literature sometimes collapses all sexually active unmarried women into a single category, a conflation that makes it impossible to figure out how sameness and difference might be meaningful (Cohen and Wofsy 1989).[5]

Finally, identity is relevant in a psychological or psychoanalytic sense— that is, as a process whereby we imaginatively identify with some aspect or attribute of another person, figure, or image. Such identification processes are assumed to shape our psychic and erotic lives as well as some sense of ourselves as part of a community, of a "we." In ordinary usage, the importance of identification is widely assumed: witness the transformative powers almost universally attributed to "media images" and "role models." But, as Harvey Milk said, "if media images were so powerful, I'd be heterosexual." How do representations influence our knowledge, self-perception, and objects of desire? In what ways do cultural stereotypes shape our fate?

With this brief introduction, I revisit the problematic representations of gender in AIDS discourse that I identified in chapter 2 above, here examining their 1990s incarnations. Returning to the *Cosmo* action and other feminist/lesbian/queer/AIDS activism, I then discuss intersections of identity, gender, and the cultural work of activism now and in the future. I conclude with some comments on the future of gender in/and the feminist movement.

Cosmo, *Identity, and Inscriptions of Gender*

Biological Identity: The Rugged Vagina Redux. Gould claimed that "there is almost no danger of contracting AIDS through *ordinary sexual intercourse.*" He goes on to define *ordinary sexual intercourse* as "penile penetration of a well-lubricated vagina—penetration that is not rough and does not cause lacerations (as it might in rape or violently macho thrusting or in the presence of severe vaginismus). Assuming that the genitals of both partners are healthy and intact—that there are no lesions or other openings due to infections—the virus, I contend, will not be transmitted during vaginal sex from an infected person to his or her partner" (Gould 1988, 146).

The fixed biological genderings that Gould evoked had, of course, appeared in scientific and medical journals as well as in magazines like *Cosmo.* Recall the rugged vagina/fragile urethra dichotomy described in chapter 1 above and the deeply divided debate in the mid-1980s and thereafter over whether it was possible for women to be infected with HIV and—especially—in turn to infect men through female-to-male sexual transmission of the virus. (For versions of this argument outside the United States, see chap. 7 above.)

One biological explanation was that a certain quantity of virus must be transmitted to cause infection; as one reporter put it, HIV infection "requires a jolt injected into the bloodstream, likely several jolts over time, such as would occur with infected needles or semen. In both cases, needle and penis are the instruments of contagion" (Fain 1985, 35). Obviously, male-to-female transmission better fulfills this projectile requirement for delivering viral jolts. Nevertheless, even when such a mechanism of infection was postulated and women were called "inefficient" and "incompetent" transmitters, the weakest link in the chain of HIV transmission, women could still get the blame. Like other populations of women found to have higher-than-average rates of HIV infection (sex workers, intravenous drug users, women of color, women from "Pattern II" countries), the prostitutes in Germany came to be characterized as "reservoirs," "vessels," "vectors," or "carriers" of infection. Presumably, the projectile penis became a sucking proboscis.[6]

Gould's basic claim depends on the equation of "ordinary sexual intercourse" with what is healthy and natural. In this, he closely echoed the argument made by the science writer John Langone, whose influential December 1985 article in *Discover* popularized the "vulnerable rectum"/ "rugged vagina" division; the vagina, he argued, "designed to withstand the trauma of intercourse as well as childbirth" (p. 41), was too tough for the virus to penetrate. Thus, the body's vulnerability to viral penetration is genderized, naturalized, and made to play out various versions of the "nature never intended" scenario: since nature never intended people to have anal intercourse, AIDS, as *Discover*'s cover blurb prophesied, "is— and is likely to remain—the fatal price one can pay for anal intercourse."[7] And elsewhere: AIDS is sexually transmissible "only in the sense that [it] can be transmitted by anal intercourse" (1985, 44). Langone also assumed, as Gould put it, that "the genitals of both partners are healthy and intact." Solicitous of the "fragile penis" (an ambiguous apparatus in all this talk about "homosexual" and "heterosexual" sex), Langone also argued that the vagina provides "armor" against viral invasion. The caption to the graphic illustration accompanying the article describes the vagina's lining as "composed of layers of plate-like squamous cells that resist rupture and infectious agents, presumably including the AIDS virus. Its tissue has fewer blood vessels and is usually naturally lubricated during intercourse" (Langone 1985, 41). Gould's three arguments for the safety of "ordinary sexual intercourse"—the vagina's tough mucous membrane, its lack of blood, and its natural lubrication—appear to have come straight from Langone's *Discover* article.[8] But Gould should have waited for the book. By the time *AIDS: The Facts* was published in 1988, Langone had rethought the vagina, presumably in the light of intervening evidence (see esp. pp. 82–108). Although he retained his basic argument that "a woman's genital anatomy seems to be in her favor insofar as AIDS is concerned," he now identified a number of conditions and "special circumstances" that may make a woman vulnerable to HIV:

> She is a "natural receptacle for large quantities of AIDS virus carried in semen."
> She menstruates.
> She may experience trauma during sex (e.g., a bruise of the vaginal wall).
> She may have "other diseases and conditions" that create lesions and "more potential host cells at the infection site."

She may have "any condition accompanied by vaginal bleeding, related or unrelated to menstruation—vaginitis, pelvic inflammatory disease, fibroid tumors, herpes, serious yeast infections, and even the stress associated with diabetes and ulcers—as well as by the use of IUDs and birth control pills, which have similar effects."
She may have anemia.
She ages.

If this does not cover the waterfront, he quotes the view that AIDS is "a mucous-membrane disease" and that the "vagina may be rugged, but it's not all that rugged" (Langone 1988, 95–96).

What are we to make of this? In evaluating these gendered accounts of the physical body, we need to ask what the stakes are. Implicit in claims of fixed biological difference is a conviction not only that AIDS is uniquely homosexual but that it represents a boundary transgression, a violation of natural difference. Yet an account of the vagina as "rugged . . . but not all that rugged" is fairly commonplace in the medical literature on sexually transmitted diseases in general or on toxic shock syndrome. There, the vagina is no longer so healthy and impervious to sordid pathogens; rather, it is shot through with cracks and lesions, punctures and sores. Langone's book is eloquent on the vagina's vulnerability: "If, for example, sex occurred during menstruation, the virus might invade her body through the blood; there are apparently times during the menstrual flow when the disintegrating blood vessels are open to microorganisms the same way a skin cut is. . . . Under the influence of oral contraceptives, and during pregnancy, the cellular lining of the uterine cervix, the narrow neck of the womb, may become fragile and crumble; blood vessels, which are often opened during intercourse, provide a pathway of entry similar to that resulting from rectal intercourse" (Langone 1988, 96).[9]

This final statement rewrites biological identity—and nature—in yet another way: having asserted the essential difference between the two objects (the vagina and the rectum), this argument accomplishes rhetorical repair work to show how they may appear to be "the same."

Epidemiological and Statistical Identity: Getting a Piece of the Pie Chart. Gould claimed that AIDS was virtually absent among U.S. heterosexuals. But what is the overlap between "heterosexuals" and "women"? And does it matter? As early as December 1981, women accounted for more than 3 percent of total reported AIDS cases in the United States. By early 1988, when the *Cosmo* article appeared, the Centers for Disease Control had reported 4,349 cases of AIDS in adult women, or 8 percent of the total adult cases. Of these cases in women, 1,251, or 29 percent, were attributed to heterosexual contact. This 1,251 total for heterosexual transmission represents 1,045 women who had "heterosexual contact with a person with AIDS or at risk for AIDS" and 206 women "without other identified risks who were born in countries in which heterosexual transmission is believed to play a major role although precise means of transmission have not yet been defined" (Rutherford and Werdegar 1989, 11). This same total of 1,251 cases among women attributed to heterosexual transmission constituted a bit more than half the total 2,285 cases attributed to heterosexual transmission; in turn, the total constituted 4 percent of total AIDS cases. The significance of this is that HIV was obviously being transmitted sexually to women, although, as we have seen, the role of gender in sexual transmission has been anything but clear.

For anyone not versed in epidemiology and statistics, the *Alice in Wonderland* quality of these numbers is frustrating. Meanwhile, the numbers themselves just keep getting worse. By 1991, women accounted for more than 11 percent of total cases; new AIDS cases in women were growing faster than those in men, with more than half the over 22,000 total cases reported in the previous two years. (This total included about 12,000 black women, 5,700 white women, 4,800 Latina women, 111 Asian women or Pacific Islanders, and 48 Native Americans; several hundred of these women were reported to be lesbian or bisexual.) By the early 1990s, it was estimated that 100,000–200,000 additional women were infected with HIV. Although the U.S. male-female ratio was conventionally given as 7 : 1—seven men with AIDS to one woman—this averaged figure was (and is) misleading: because such a ratio depends on the composition of the particular population being measured, it can vary according to sex and sexual orientation, geography, ethnic and social subculture, class, and so on. In some communities, men with AIDS may outnumber women by twenty or thirty to one; elsewhere, the ratio may approach one to one. It is perhaps more accurate to think of *the* AIDS epidemic in the United States as being constituted of multiple if intersecting local epidemics, each with its own dynamic.[10]

To make sense of statistics and "statistical identity," we need to think about how and why we collect statistics and to remember that they serve a number of functions. Obviously and ostensibly, they provide a critical scientific database for studying an outbreak of illness, define the scope and nature of the problem, and track change. To accomplish these functions, public health surveillance of illness and disease typically wants to know two things—who gets sick and how they get sick—thus yielding the classification of each case into a "risk group" and a "mode of exposure" (or, in the parlance of AIDS discourse, "who you are" and "what you do"). This also yields two broadly different analytic strategies: one seeks to learn why, within a given population, person A gets sick while person B does not; the other seeks to learn why population C has a higher incidence of sickness than population D. Whatever their purpose, statistical accounts are about aggregates and probabilities, whether for individuals or populations, risk groups or modes of exposure. They are not intended to convey absolute certainty about individual risk, encourage personal self-identification, or describe lived experience.

Women's statistical identity poses special problems because numerous features of AIDS surveillance reporting thwart our attempts to decipher what even the aggregate figures mean. Women *as women* are often not clearly identified in reports, whether of risk groups or modes of exposure, so data about them must be deduced from data in other categories. In the familiar pie charts that show percentages of AIDS cases represented by different groups, women were for many years invisible within official categories called "undetermined mode of exposure," "no identified risk" or—most ironically—"other." This poses great problems when, in the 1990s, we attempt to reconstruct the history of the gendered epidemic, for any such retrospective claim must take into account the uncertainties built into the catchall categories "undetermined" and "other" as well as the effects of periodic reclassifications, renaming of categories, and redefinitions of "AIDS" itself.

The belated acknowledgment of heterosexual transmission probably confuses as much as it solves the problem of women's invisibility. A pie chart in *Newsweek* (18 November 1991, 59) was headed "Who Has AIDS?" The 196,000 U.S. cases then reported were broken down into the following categories:

> homosexual/bisexual males;
> heterosexual intravenous drug users;
> male homosexual/bisexual intravenous drug users;
> heterosexuals;
> transfusions;
> hemophiliacs;
> undetermined.

Apart from the apparent mixing of "risk groups" with "modes of exposure" (thereby confusing "who you are" with "what you do"), this list contains few clues as to which of these identities might be gendered fe-

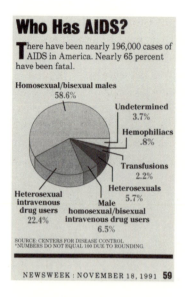

Who Has AIDS?

There have been nearly 196,000 cases of AIDS in America. Nearly 65 percent have been fatal.

Homosexual/bisexual males
58.6%

Undetermined
3.7%

Hemophiliacs
.8%

Transfusions
2.2%

Heterosexuals
5.7%

Heterosexual intravenous drug users
22.4%

Male homosexual/bisexual intravenous drug users
6.5%

SOURCE: CENTERS FOR DISEASE CONTROL
*NUMBERS DO NOT EQUAL 100 DUE TO ROUNDING.

NEWSWEEK : NOVEMBER 18, 1991 **59**

Although this pie chart (8.2: Newsweek, 18 November 1991, 59) is intended to show the growing diversification of populations with AIDS, its categories do little to highlight gender. In other words, if you were a woman who believed that AIDS/HIV was largely a "gay disease" or a "male disease," this gender-neutral chart would not surprise you or tell you anything you thought you didn't already know.

male. (Note the composite categories for males, which represent men reporting more than one mode of exposure.) Meanwhile, the CDC was classifying cases of AIDS among adult and adolescent females into the following "risk groups":

> intravenous drug users;
> sexual partners of intravenous drug users;
> sexual partners of homosexual or bisexual men;
> transfusion recipients;
> sexual partners of persons with hemophilia;
> heterosexuals born in Pattern II countries (countries where heterosexual transmission is endemic);
> mothers of pediatric AIDS patients.

Even though explicitly gendered female, the list does not necessarily translate into recognizable identities or even recognized groups of women. Rather, it is a list of grouped individuals who share certain characteristics—not necessarily self-identified—that allow *someone* to assign them to the same category. Again, they are artificial categories constructed for the purpose of *disease surveillance.* Now, there may be occasions when people with these characteristics would also form real-life groups or form a salient category in some other way. In a given town, for instance, some of the people classified as "intravenous drug users" might know each other and might congregate at some of the same places. But "sex partners of intravenous drug users" are less likely to constitute a real-life group: its members probably do not know each other; they may not even know that their partners use drugs. And who thinks of themselves as a "sex partner" anyhow? ("That was no sex partner, that was my wife"?) This point is eloquently made by Stephanie Kane and Theresa Mason (1992) in their ethnographic study of intravenous drug users and their sex partners; making a strong critique of the rigid emphasis on "risk groups" rather than "risk behaviors," they emphasize that, with regard to intravenous drug users, AIDS research and public health interventions take place "in a political climate increasingly unfavorable to the illegal behaviors that define the 'group' of drug injection users"; conversely, the risk-group category "sex partner" lacks correspondence with "any shared social scene and identity" (p. 201).[11]

Moreover, the *Newsweek* list reads like something out of Margaret Atwood's *The Handmaid's Tale*, in which each handmaid's name is determined by the powerful male to whose household she is assigned and whose semen she receives—thus, the handmaid attached to Fred's household becomes Offred (of Fred). The CDC reporting mode still reinforces the prevalent view that women's identities are not autonomous but established by the significant others to whom they are attached; in some cases, of course, this is precisely what we need to know, but it also shows how a way of thinking about women that erases them shows up in areas where surveillance is irrelevant. In one review article on psychological issues in AIDS, women were mentioned only under such headings as *pediatric AIDS* (Lehman and Russell 1986). A 4 March 1992 *New York Times* article described efforts to prevent transmission of the virus from mother to fetus, expressing little interest in the mother's fate. The sexual partners of people with hemophilia and blood disorders, for the most part women, have primarily been dependent for information on their male partners (the patients); yet, because these men may have determined not to let the disease interfere with their lives, they may exclude their partners from opportunities to gain medical information—including information about AIDS and HIV risks. A workshop organized in 1989 to address issues affecting "women in the hemophilia community" began the transformation of this official "risk group" into a lived identity and real community; the Women's Outreach Network of the National Hemophilia Foundation (WONN) is now a national organization with local chapters across the country (Broullon 1992).[12]

The exclusion of lesbians from surveillance reporting and research represents a different problem; here, a "real," lived identity has no official

recognition. Lesbians and bisexual women are not counted as a population at risk, nor is women's same-sex behavior listed as a potential mode
of HIV transmission. Despite questions that we can raise about how they
are identified and defined, the categories male-to-male, male-to-female,
and female-to-male sexual transmission *exist* as modes of exposure to
HIV; female-to-female sexual transmission does not. The few reports
(e.g., Calabrese and Gopalakrishna 1986; Marmor 1986; Sabatini et al.
1984; and Sanders et al. 1989) that document apparent woman-to-woman
sexual transmission of HIV identify cases to "traumatic" modes of sexual
activity—that is, in Gould's words, activity other than "ordinary sexual
intercourse." But these cases are so isolated as to be discounted; rather,
lesbians' generally low incidence of sexually transmitted diseases is used
to justify their exclusion. Clay Stephens (1988), however, suggests that
researchers' lack of interest in lesbians also reflects a common view that
sex between women is too infrequent, gentle, or boring to transmit a
virus. (It is worth recalling that, in the early days of the epidemic, some
leading scientists discounted the possibility that AIDS could be caused by
a sexually transmitted virus: gay men were mainly infected, they argued,
and how could a virus get from one man's body to another man's? What
orifice would it enter?)[13]

As I said in chapter 2 above, prostitutes are not an official "risk category"
in AIDS surveillance, yet they are a major group cited when "women"
are discussed. Nevertheless, ongoing studies suggest that prostitutes are
likely to be infected through sharing contaminated needles, not through
sexual activity; because they routinely use condoms, they do not constitute a significant source of HIV transmission. As Nancy Shaw and Lyn
Paleo reported in 1987 on the basis of their studies in the San Francisco Bay
Area, some prostitutes do get AIDS, but "neither the number of sexual
contacts nor the receipt of money for sex . . . seems to put women at higher
risk for getting AIDS" (1987, 144). At the same time, the *clients* of prostitutes are rarely mentioned as risks.[14]

Finally, as I noted briefly above, some researchers define any single
unmarried sexually active woman as a prostitute or establish no clear
definitions for "sex with multiple partners," "promiscuity," or "prostitution"; this makes it impossible to sort out the potentially salient issues of
risk and prevention that each term connotes. Some lump as one risk factor
"sexual contact with multiple partners, including prostitutes"; and some
health jurisdictions classify cases in this category as "heterosexual transmission," others as "no identifiable risk" (Cohen and Wofsy 1989; Gorna
1996, 265). Terminology is tricky in other ways as well. Researchers have
grown sensitive to terminology about gay men and people with AIDS, and

one now routinely finds relatively neutral references in the journal literature to "sexually active men" and "gay men with multiple sexual partners." But, in the absence of monitoring by women, old sexist stereotypes persist, and alongside the nonpejorative references to men one finds references to "promiscuous women." Similarly, studies of AIDS in Africa may contrast "men who migrate to the cities to look for work" with "women who come to the cities to be prostitutes"—as though being a sex worker is not work.

My discussion of biological identity and epidemiological/statistical identity has been somewhat extended to suggest the most pervasive ways that identities are officially represented and interpreted. Taken together, these authoritative discursive constructions shape a commentary not likely to enlighten women readers as they try to determine in what ways they are the same as or different from "women with AIDS." In the rest of this section, I will more briefly review problems in AIDS discourse that continue to discourage a clear conception of women's risk and the formation of an organized political response.

Heterosexual Identity: Can the Cosmo *Girl Get AIDS?* Reviewing statistics for "heterosexual AIDS victims," Gould suggested that, if HIV could easily be spread heterosexually, the heterosexual population would be much more widely infected. The United States has been virtually unique in its obsession with "heterosexual AIDS"; in France, where cases among men and women, straight and gay, were acknowledged from the beginning, AIDS was never a "gay disease." In the United States, terms like *heterosexual intercourse* and *heterosexual victims* were used ambiguously for years, often failing to distinguish persons infected through sexual contact with a person of the other sex (*heterosexual transmission*) from infected persons identified as heterosexuals. Since human beings live inconvenient lives, these are not the only confusions. When HIV-infected "heterosexual intravenous drug users" and their "sexual partners" both use drugs, HIV transmission is officially attributed to needle sharing, although in actuality we do not know the relative likelihood of HIV transmission via sexual contact versus shared needles. Where two factors are involved, the epidemiology becomes what Kane and Mason call a "logistical nightmare" (1992; see also Kane 1990; 1991; 1998). And the gender-neutral term *heterosexual* is sometimes used in gender-specific ways; paradoxically—or lopsidedly—although women are a necessary component of "heterosexual spread," they are not always included when the term *heterosexual* is used.[15]

Statistics have implicit functions as well that further complicate their role in the AIDS epidemic: in any given context, they may serve to justify budgets, provide evidence of competence or modernity, given an illusion of control, feed demographic computer models, justify in the name of protection mechanisms for increased surveillance, and create rhetorical dramas (see also chap. 3 above). When the noted sex researchers William Masters and Virginia Johnson claimed in their book *Crisis: Heterosexual Behavior in the Age of AIDS* (Masters et al. 1988) that "the AIDS virus is now running rampant in the heterosexual community," they certainly created a stir; in actuality, however, they meant a small middle-class sample that was not accurately tested. Michael Fumento's book *The Myth of Heterosexual AIDS* (1989) also makes a dramatic claim: that there is *no* scientific evidence of HIV or AIDS among heterosexual men and women. When Fumento claims that "heterosexual AIDS" is a myth (excoriating Masters and Johnson in the process), he too is defining *heterosexual* so that it exempts heterosexual people of color, heterosexuals who are too poor, sick, shoot drugs, or live in Africa (or Haiti, Miami, New Jersey, etc.). Infected non-U.S. women are assumed to have engaged in something other than "ordinary sexual intercourse" or other risky practices; infected U.S. women of color are assumed to be drug users; infected U.S. white women are assumed to be flukes. The bottom line: educated white middle-class heterosexual people with Cuisinarts do not get AIDS: the "myth" that they do, according to Fumento, is largely the creation of "the media" and what he calls "the homosexual lobby."[16]

Divisions between "us" and "them" are part of the history of responses to epidemics, of efforts to achieve control and reduce the mystery of infectious disease. Despite its ambiguity and meaninglessness, the term *the heterosexual population* serves, in *this* epidemic, as a mobile cultural marker that helps shore up the division. In his history of epidemiological thinking, Mervyn Susser (1973) reminds us that "risk groups" during epidemics were invented for a reason—originally, to tell the bourgeoisie when to leave town (both Defoe [(1722 1960] and Camus [(1947) 1948] recount the plague's movements, street by street, house by house, from the ports and periphery to the centers of commerce). The comedian Richard Pryor puts it differently: "An epidemic is when white folks get it." Deploying sexuality and gender as ideological barriers to protect the *Cosmo* girl from AIDS is predictable and, in itself, probably meaningless, yet it highlights the anxiety caused by gender at this historical moment. But to obsess over sexuality as an absolute and to embrace gender as a protective barrier obscure the multiple ways that people with HIV and AIDS may experience the disease as sexualized and gendered beings. This is apparent in the clinical effects of HIV.

Clinical Identity: Is HIV an "Equal Opportunity" Virus? A special AIDS issue of *Scientific American* in October 1988 included a schematic diagram (106) showing the effect of HIV on the human body. The male figure pictured is supposedly "generic," implying that gender has little effect on how HIV behaves. But, as women recount their experiences, it is clear that gender is relevant in several ways. On 6 June 1991, for example, the *Champaign-Urbana News-Gazette* published a story about a woman infected with HIV (Vaughn 1991). "Dee," as she is called in the story, was infected by her ex-husband, an intravenous drug user who had since died of AIDS. A former user of drugs and alcohol herself, she remembers sharing needles twice with her ex-husband but may also have been infected through sexual contact during a brief period of reconciliation in 1983; diagnosed with HIV in November 1987, she has three children who are not infected. She is asymptomatic, having had none of the symptoms or opportunistic infections that conventionally signal HIV infection or define AIDS. In Champaign-Urbana, where she moved from Chicago, she has found both medical and social support less adequate than in Chicago; she has stopped seeing her physician because he wanted her to keep taking AZT, which caused overwhelming anxiety and depression. She has now joined an HIV-positive women's group and finds this more helpful. Her main concern is her children; she wants to stay healthy because she is worried about their fate.

Dee's story is in many respects typical of the thousands of women in the United States infected with HIV who now encounter a clinical model of AIDS that was developed over the first decade of the epidemic on the basis of experience with men. For example, according to this model, she is asymptomatic; but she has been treated in recent years both for a salmonella infection and for cervical cancer, illnesses that may signal HIV in women. Although Dee sought testing because she knew she was at risk, women more typically learn that they have been at risk when they experience symptoms, seek care, and are tested and diagnosed. If they seek care, it is still common for physicians not to perceive women as candidates for HIV infection, even where AIDS is common. New Yorker Alison Gertz, who died in 1992 six years after she was diagnosed with AIDS, was not in any of the stereotypical risk groups when she got sick: "Ms. Gertz was none of the above. She was a strong, heterosexual woman, raised on Park Avenue, educated at private schools, aspiring to be an illustrator. Ms. Gertz seemed so unlikely to be infected with HIV, the virus that causes AIDS, that, when she became sick at the age of 22, doctors put her through three weeks of exhaustive tests for other illnesses before they diagnosed the disease" (Bennet 1992).[17] The lag between infection and diagnosis continues to mean that women live less average time after the diagnosis of AIDS than men, although much uncertainty surrounds the various differences in disease progression in different groups and individuals.[18] With early intervention now shown to improve both quantity and quality of life, this lag time is obviously worrisome for women. Early intervention has posed other clinical dilemmas. Studies suggesting the benefits for women of early treatment (AZT, e.g., seems to delay disease progression in a diversity of populations) do not always seem to have women in mind. Commenting in the *New England Journal of Medicine* on an account of HIV treatment of pregnant women, Cooper et al. note, "Ironically, the authors discuss therapeutic advances only as they pertain to children" (1992, 646). In a treatment update, *PI Perspective*, the fine newsletter from Project Inform, likewise reported the success of early drug intervention— for the fetus.

It has taken years for gender to acquire even potential theoretical or clinical significance. Since the diagnosis of AIDS can now be made in the presence of more than thirty distinct clinical conditions, an important question is whether the gender of the host influences the virus's behavior and its clinical manifestations—whether, that is, HIV infection and AIDS become different entities in women. As early as 1991, Kathryn Anastos and Carola Marte asked other questions as well:

> Fundamental questions about the progression of this disease in women have not been asked or answered. Is cervical cancer more common in HIV-infected women? How does HIV infection affect pregnancy and childbirth? Do the different hormones in women and men affect the course of HIV infection? Do women fall prey to different opportunistic infections than men do? Do women respond differently to treatment regimens established for male patients? Do women suffer different side effects and toxicities from AIDS medications? Do women survive a shorter time after the diagnosis of AIDS has been made? Are the causes of death in women different than in men? (192)

Dee also mentions her reaction to AZT and struggle over medication with her physician. Not only do women report different reactions to a range of AIDS drugs, but until recently they have been largely excluded from clinical trials of most experimental drugs; this exclusion limits both women's access to such drugs and our knowledge of those drugs' effects on female patients. While the exclusion policy is attributed to the thalidomide scandal of the 1950s, Wolfe and Long (1989) point to cultural stereotypes as well: "Women have historically been thought to be undesirable research subjects in clinical trials for non-reproductive oriented drugs [because] (a) women exhibit cyclical hormonal fluctuations which may influence the results of clinical trials; (b) the drug may only be good for men since men and women have hormonal differences; (c) women may become pregnant which results in the loss of a test 'subject' and puts the fetus at risk; (d) the disease may be different in women than in men" (pp. 49–50).[19]

Social service and support groups, established on the model of Gay Men's Health Crisis or Shanti Project, have been striving valiantly to identify and meet the needs of new and different clients. But, despite progress in some arenas, what has prevailed in clinical medicine is a generic patient with AIDS who is affected systemically by the action of the virus. Although "vaginal fluid" is assigned to the figure in the *Scientific American* illustration, this schematic human being, like policy governing how AIDS is defined, remains pretty unambiguously male. (For a rare exception to these weird schematic characters, see Aggleton et al. 1989, 14.)

Popular Images: Welcome Back to the World of AIDS. As its title suggests, *People* magazine's 14 March 1988 cover story "AIDS and the Single Woman" was a deliberate effort to follow up Gould's (1988) *Cosmo* claims. The cover suggests that a diversity of women may be at risk (characteristically, they are shown as individuals, not as part of a group). The opening two-page photograph shows a white urban heterosexual couple looking intently into each other's eyes; standing in what appears to be the center of a dark, rain-streaked intersection, they may be worrying about AIDS, but they should probably also be worrying about being hit by a car. Who are these two? Perhaps they are the yuppie couple documented in chapter 1 above who graced the 12 January 1987 cover of *U.S. News and World Report* and hailed us with the words, "AIDS: What You Need to Know, What You Should Do"; the story inside spelled it out: "Now the disease of *them* is the disease of *us*" (McAuliffe et al. 1987, 60). But, in *People*, the woman looks up at the man, who remains faceless. She is obviously the "single woman" of the title; is he "AIDS"? Should women beware? Based on a television survey of five hundred single women, the article cannot seem to decide. One woman, pictured lying in bed with her cat, is quoted as saying, "No one knows what the rules are, and everyone's scared. We talk more." Another says, "They can campaign all they want; they won't get me to buy a box of condoms." Another, pictured with her daughter, says, "Men lie 90 percent of the time. They're not going to tell you if they have AIDS." A guy says, "I wouldn't take a woman home from a singles bar for all the money in the world." And another: "I'm just looking for a woman I can spend the next 40 years with." The *People* article concludes approvingly, "That's one side effect that doesn't necessarily call out for a cure" (Dougherty 1988, 102–5).

In chapter 2 above, I recounted a popular urban legend circulating long before media reports of women with AIDS. The 1990s version goes something like this. In October 1991, the television newsmagazine "Prime Time Live" (ABC) broadcast a story about a woman in Dallas who called herself CJ and who, in a September letter to *Ebony*, had claimed to be deliberately infecting several men a week with HIV. The story of the "Angel of Death" or the "Black Widow" mushroomed into a full-blown media sensation via local, regional, and national talk shows and news coverage. "She says she has AIDS," Diane Sawyer told the "Prime Time Live" audience (accompanied by visuals of bar scenes and topless dancers and pounding disco music), "and she's bent on revenge. She says she's going to clubs and bars and sleeping with lots of men so that she won't be the only one to die. No one knows who she is, but she's the most talked about and most feared person in Dallas." Frantic calls to a black talk show host in Dallas following CJ's *Ebony* letter led to an on-air exchange between the host and a woman purporting to be CJ. Investigators then turned up other women claiming the honor, although all were revealed as imposters who had neither AIDS nor HIV infection. The media scholar Elizabeth Bird watched the CJ saga unfold, "convinced that no actual CJ would ever be found or arrested. The reason? I saw the story of CJ as undoubtedly an urban legend run wild—a product of oral folk tradition that, because of its cultural salience, had become transformed into 'news' " (Bird 1996, 45). Interested in how this happened and what it tells us about our understanding of "news," Bird reviewed not only the urban legend I noted in chapter 2 ("Welcome to the World of AIDS!"—reported by Fine [1987] and also, under the title of "AIDS Mary," by Brunvand [1992]) but also its U.S. permutations, its European, U.K., and Australian versions, its historical prototypes (e.g., a report in Defoe's 1722 *Journal of the Plague Year* and tales of GIs in Vietnam reported to be infected by prostitutes with an incurable venereal disease called "Black Rose"—cf. "Black Widow" in the CJ update), and its circulation on the Internet. Bird argues that the media took up the CJ story as news because news, like folklore, is also a culturally constructed "narrative that tells a story about things of importance or interest." "Most important in this context," she continues, "news reflects and reinforces particular cultural anxieties and concerns. It goes in waves; many scholars have demonstrated, for example, that waves of reporting about teenage suicide or child abuse do not necessarily reflect actual changes in the rates of these problems. Rather, they reflect waves of interest, and in turn feed the anxieties that have produced the interest in the first place" (Bird 1996, 47). Like the film *Fatal Attraction*, such legends are routinely read as morality tales about sexually active single women. Similarly, despite Magic Johnson's own admission of unprotected sex with multiple partners, the blame was immediately placed on the person (widely assumed to be a woman, although not by Michael Fumento) who infected him—a figure given a blurred reality on the cover of the *National Enquirer.*

Real women with HIV and AIDS have gradually begun to compete with and replace the phantasmatic creatures of these legends. In chapter 2 above, I discussed the 1987 film *Suzi's Story* (I. Gillespie 1987), which chronicled the life and death of a young Australian woman with AIDS. Other figures have had the force of revelation for many adolescents, including Pedro Zamora on "The Real World," the characters of Stone Cates and Robin Scorpio on "General Hospital," and sports figures Magic Johnson and Greg Luganis. Alison Gertz, a young white woman from New York City, spent her life after diagnosis in pilgrimages to high school auditoriums and college classrooms all over the country (a television movie with Molly Ringwald told her story—without, unfortunately, mentioning the word *condom*). The "African-American woman with AIDS" looked very different in a 1994 story in *Essence* in which Rae Lewis-Thornton described her diagnosis in 1986 and life with HIV since then: "I am the quintessential Buppie [black urban professional]. I'm young—32. Well-educated. Professional. Attractive. Smart. I've been drug- and alcohol-free all my life. I'm a Christian. I've never been promiscuous. Never had a one-night stand. And I am dying of AIDS" (Lewis-Thornton 1994, 63). Lewis-Thornton also makes her pilgrimages, estimating that she has talked to at least seventy thousand high school students about HIV prevention (a message that in her case emphasizes God, not condoms). As with Gertz, we can criticize many features of the "good girl" role model figure that Lewis-Thornton embodies, but she is giving her time and energy to education and, through her material presence, challenging the shadowy CJ stereotypes that previously dominated media accounts.

Cultural Identity and "Third World AIDS". Gould explained HIV transmission via heterosexual contact in Africa by positing cultural differences in sexual practices, an argument he was neither the first nor the last to make (see Gilman 1985; Packard and Epstein 1992; Bond et al. 1997; and chaps. 3 and 7 above). Statistics from Africa on apparent heterosexual transmission are repeatedly attributed to a variety of cultural practices of "the Other" (Gould's article, in fact, mentions a number of these): unadmitted homosexual or quasi-homosexual transmission, unadmitted drug use, the practice of anal intercourse as a method of birth control, the widespread use of unsterilized needles, a history of immune suppression and infectious disease, scarification, clitoridectomy, circumcision (its presence in females and absence in males), and violent, excessive, or exotic sexual practices. And, of course, prostitution. Erik Eckholm wrote in the *New York Times* that prostitution was "always an engine of sexually transmitted diseases," claiming it "has played a major role in African AIDS" (1990a). These are the kind of self-righteous Anglo-American morality tales that Simon Watney (1989) derides as "missionary positions." African women are marked as different from women in the United States; they, meanwhile, ask how they can possibly have the same disease as rich white men in the West. Like other stereotypes that have guided the interpretation of AIDS data, these supposed cultural differences have both practical and symbolic effect in establishing us/them divisions—for "them" as well as for "us."

Will the 1990s be different? The Eighth International AIDS Conference in Amsterdam declared that this would be "the Decade of the Woman" (Jonathan Mann quoted in L. Altman 1992), sounding ironically almost like an award with its echoes of the media celebration of the UN Decade for Women and its frenzy in the United States in 1991–92 over the "Year of the Woman." Meanwhile the *New York Times* announced that "AIDS Rich Held Twice as High in Women" (1994). A 1992 *Los Angeles Times Magazine* cover story attempted to emphasize gender without showcasing prostitution, promiscuity, or little-known sexual practices; the article tried instead to examine AIDS in terms of women's status and social powerlessness. The author quotes a psychologist at the University of Zimbabwe: "You cannot have a heterosexual AIDS epidemic in which women have power or close to equality" (Kraft 1992, 12). This is welcome in that it is what many longtime advocates of women have been calling for. Yet a peculiar semantic transformation is occurring here. The *Los Angeles Times Magazine* cover blurb, for instance, read: "AFRICA'S DEATH SENTENCE: Where Women are Powerless, AIDS Is Spreading Relentlessly from Husband to Wife, Mother to Child. And a Continent Is Dying." This line of argument casts women monolithically as victims, raising familiar theoretical and political problems. It also runs the risk of duplicating, under the cover of a more sophisticated and compassionate rendering, the approach formerly taken by white colonial governments toward the health problems of "natives"—that is, as Randall Packard and Paul Epstein (1992) have argued, it is the natives' fault. The *Los Angeles Times* article argues that the primary reason for the spread of AIDS in Africa is women's low status and subservience. Here, women's powerlessness, the *result* of oppression, becomes the *cause* of the spread of AIDS. In keeping with this reading, calls go up for "assertiveness training" to solve the problem.

Elizabeth Reid, consultant for the Australian Department of Community Services and Health, Canberra, called for an acknowledgment of women's "socialized passivity," particularly in developing societies. Pointing out many problems that make women especially vulnerable to HIV infection and the crucial role of women's organizations in educating communities and households about AIDS and in fighting rape and alcoholism in men, Reid goes on to argue that one positive outcome of the global epidemic may be that women are required "to take a more active role in social and interpersonal relations. . . . To survive uninfected, particularly from sexual or intravenous transmission, women must learn not only to be assertive but to choose or create relationships based on mutual concern and respect. This in itself should lead to an improvement in the quality of their relationships" (1988, 21).

The confounding of individual and socioeconomic vulnerability is common in "First World" contexts as well. While Canadian physician Catherine Hankins had argued for years that AIDS and HIV in women must be understood in the context of social inequality, media interpretations at the Montreal AIDS conference often rendered her position in terms of women's passivity. Mann and Tarantola (1996) provide a useful framework for assessing different kinds of vulnerability, while Farmer et al. (1996) offer a detailed, extensive critique of the substitution of individual responsibility for structural inequality in the social sciences literature on AIDS/HIV. At the same time, research findings make clear that "communication" and "assertiveness" are not merely neutral "strategies" that women can choose to employ but may themselves constitute sources of material risk. As summed up by Marcia Ann Gillespie (1991): "Depending on the degree of pressure to be submissive in sexual or social matters, the woman who tries to use the information to prevent infection may become the target of mockery, rejection, stigmatization, economic reprisal, violence, and death" (p. 16). Communication change must therefore parallel economic and legal change for women, along with AIDS 101 information, condom training, and consciousness raising for *men*.

Sexual Identity: Is the Cosmo *Girl Heterosexual?* The medical model of sexuality, with its tripartite division of sexual identity into homo, hetero, and bi, is familiar and used widely as a system of mutually exclusive classification. I have noted problems that this model creates in classifying and understanding data on HIV infection and in predicting the course of the epidemic. Conceptual problems are also created by a system of naming so commonplace as to be understood as natural, even when specific categories (like homosexuality) are judged "unnatural." An enormous body of research at this point makes clear that sex and sexuality are complicated, with no fixed or fully predictable correspondence between sexual desire, past practice, current practice, self-perceived identity, and official definition. How much more complex this becomes when cultural and linguistic differences are also present, and how futile to make facile generalizations about whole populations.

On the basis of his ethnographic work on AIDS and sexuality in Brazil, Richard Parker (1987) argued more than a decade ago that the ubiquitous homo/hetero/bi model is by no means universal and is indeed often seriously at odds with "the fluidity of sexual desire" in contemporary urban Brazil. While it has become familiar in recent years through the media, it remains largely part of a recent, elite discourse; an older, more deeply embedded classification system constructs both gender and sex in terms of a division between masculine *atividade* (activity) and feminine *passividade* (passivity). Traditional enough on the surface, the division is in fact not bound to commonsense notions of male and female. Two males engaged in anal intercourse are distinguished by who is the active masculine penetrator, who the passive feminine penetrated. Neither would necessarily perceive this activity as "homosexual," although the term would more likely be applied to the "penetratee." In contemporary urban Brazil and elsewhere, Parker argues, this is only the beginning of the complex permutations worked on the initial dichotomy (Parker 1987, 155). Similarly, Gill Shepherd's analysis of sexual options for both women and men in Mombasa, Kenya, shows an ongoing "interplay between heterosexual gender roles and homosexuality, in a society with marked sexual segregation in most contexts" (1987, 240). Among Shepherd's findings is that, between two men, being penetrated is not what labels a man *homosexual* but being paid for sex rather than paying (see also Herdt and Lindenbaum 1992; Patton 1997; Abramson 1992; Abramson and Herdt 1990).

The boundaries that separate conventional categories of sexual identity and gender role are further eroded by challenges to the very categories of *male* and *female* as a fixed dichotomy. AIDS discourse largely takes this binary division for granted, rarely articulating or, presumably, even examining which criteria are being treated as defining or essential. In fact, it has been notoriously difficult to fix the specific characteristics, qualities, or behaviors that define what is male while excluding what is female. Gina Kolata, investigating current gender testing protocols for Olympic athletes, reported that no single criterion is now considered ultimately reliable. "For all its dazzling discoveries about the genes that guide a human embryo along its path to maleness or femaleness," she concluded, "science, it appears, cannot provide a simple answer" (1992, 6). How about having a vagina or having a "real" vagina as opposed to a constructed one? Presumably espousing the view that birth sex is forever, a feminist publishing house prohibited a feminist researcher from using the pronoun *she* in reference to a male-to-female transsexual.[20] Meanwhile, in cities like New York and Miami, the term *gender community* is now sometimes used to encompass the various mix-and-match experiments and experiences of progressive urban humans, although birth sex gets its due through labels like *GGs* (genetic girls) and *RGs* (real girls). Quite apart from the problem, then, of whether the *Cosmo* girl can get AIDS are more fundamental questions of identity. Can we assume that the *Cosmo* girl is heterosexual? Can we assume that she is a girl? Do we know what we mean by either of these terms?

Education, Prevention, and Community: Who Are the "We"? These ambiguous reports and contradictory representations have made it difficult to conceptualize communities or cohorts of "women at risk" and have discouraged the formation, among women, of a collective female identity—a "we"—around the issue of AIDS. Virtually none encourage women to feel concerned about *themselves.* Thus, as I noted, most women find that they "have AIDS" and thus have been at risk only when they experience symptoms and are diagnosed; most men, in contrast, seek a diagnosis because they already know that they are at risk.[21] Official prevention campaigns have still failed to find appropriate forms of address for meaningful groups of women at risk, consistently to distinguish "risk groups" (*who*) from "risk behaviors" (*how*), to create a consistent set of representations, and to place issues of AIDS and HIV within larger social, cultural, and political contexts. Except for a small number of projects and organizations that targeted education and prevention for women (Project Aware, the San Francisco AIDS Foundation, and others), women essentially heard nothing in the media or from their government until 1988, when Koop's mailer was sent to U.S. households (see chap. 2 above).

Meanwhile, the first wave of euphemisms, like *exchange of body fluids*, was giving way to terms and concepts that AIDS researchers originally worked hard to clarify but that now, for official prevention purposes, are deliberately muddied. Hence, *promiscuity* is now used not unthinkingly but deliberately, precisely because it is pejorative; *the AIDS virus* is used precisely because it collapses the long period of HIV infection (whose length is uncertain and effects often invisible) with the specter and all the terrifying connotations of AIDS; *promiscuity* and *drug addiction* are labeled as intrinsically risky precisely to avoid the politically volatile burden of providing information about safer sex and cleaner needles. This package of terms has been well marketed. Surveys show that multiple partners and promiscuity per se are now associated in the public mind with an increased risk of HIV transmission and that monogamy is believed to decrease risk—whether or not the partner is infected or safer sex is practiced. At the same time, a research team found that not everyone had an adequate understanding of these terms: an adolescent woman in a focus group defined *monogamy* to mean sleeping with only one sexual partner at a time, not with only one sexual partner over a period of time. And a Planned Parenthood survey asked, "Are you presently sexually active?" a bread-and-butter question the organization thought it could count on. "No," wrote one young woman in response, "I just lie there."

Feminist Identity: What's Missing from This Picture? While the 1980s were unfolding, cases of AIDS and HIV infection among women were slowly but steadily increasing; some could be attributed to "heterosexual transmission," some could not; some obviously involved "women," some did not. Up until now in this essay, I have addressed some of the constructions within official AIDS and media discourse that discouraged attention to the issue of women and AIDS. But this is not to say that women and feminists were paying no attention to the epidemic. As I have documented elsewhere, authorities in public health and in AIDS programs concerned with women were convinced that the problem would grow worse and said so. Important articles appeared in both scientific and popular literature (see chap. 2 above). Nevertheless, established conceptions of women shaped a cycle of research, representation, and analysis and perpetuated a view of AIDS as a "man's disease." In the culture at large, stereotypes flourished and generated visions of women as impervious to infection or as uncontainable contaminators. So, despite efforts at clarification, the question of women and the AIDS/HIV epidemic remained a messy component of AIDS discourse that discouraged sustained focus on issues for women.

Unfortunately, feminists were not immune to the constructions of dominant AIDS discourses, which women's magazines and feminist journals tended to reproduce rather than challenge. As I argued in chapter 2 above, the centrist women's magazines did a better job on women and AIDS in the 1980s than many more leftist feminist publications. By the end of the 1980s, the centrist magazines had published at least one "what women should know about AIDS" article, but most either discounted AIDS's relevance for women or represented it rather narrowly as a personal health risk that the adoption of basic precautions could virtually eliminate. Perhaps most striking, and in sharp contrast to gay men's media, the feminist media generally failed to treat AIDS as a social issue, to call for solidarity with people with AIDS, or to show women in any kind of political relationship toward the epidemic, unless one can call *political* a kind of retrograde paroxysm that cast men as unclean sex-obsessed liars and *Cosmo* girls as their duped sluts (Treichler 1988a; Treichler and Warren 1998). Some feminists tended to be sympathetic to explanations of AIDS that directly implicated patriarchal practices (e.g., clitoridectomy). For others, AIDS appeared to provoke a nostalgic return to the sex wars of the 1970s and early 1980s. When lesbian activists began to raise questions about lesbians' potential risk, they were rebuked by other lesbians for "scapegoating lesbians," for implying that lesbians might have had sex with men, or for suggesting any similarity between the sexual practices of lesbians and those of gay men. Women who argued for solidarity with gay men were accused by some of their sisters (and, it cannot be denied, by some of their brothers as well) of being resentful wannabes trying to insert themselves into the AIDS crisis. Some journals argued that AIDS was the price that men had to pay for their aggressive sexual appetites. In one way or another, these visions of men and women, gay men and lesbians, were fairly widespread. For example, opening her mail to find an invitation to a lesbian craft fair, a friend of mine said, "There's the difference—put women together without men you get jewelry; put men together without women you get AIDS."

This subtext of the 1980s intensified in a November 1991 *Off Our Backs* article entitled "Does Lesbian Sex Transmit AIDS? GET REAL!" (Elliot 1991). The author, Beth Elliot, cited many of the arguments against lesbian transmission that I have reported here, arguing that lesbians' real priority should be to tell the public that "lesbian sex sure looks like safe sex." The claim of known cases of lesbian transmission "is an urban legend . . . like the story of the poodle in the microwave." Gay men foster the lie that lesbian sex is risky, charges Elliot, "because they want to keep women subservient." But "woman-identified, feminist lesbians can emerge from the silence to tell the truth about our lives and sexuality." As for lesbian "safer

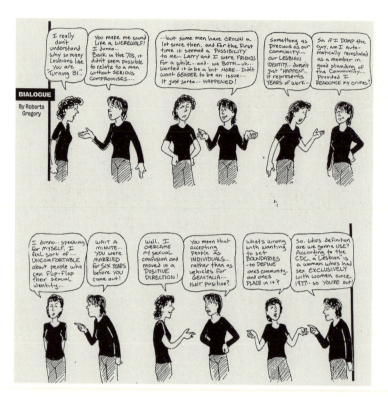

In the 1990s, AIDS discourse continues to diversify, often employing what John Greyson has called "strategic compromises" to challenge simple-minded formulas yet communicate effectively to a target audience. The tripartite division of human sexuality into homo, hetero, and bi, for example, reified in so much AIDS discourse, has been as confusing and inadequate for women as for men. Both the Roberta Gregory comic strip and the Advocate profile of Rebekka Armstrong (8.3: "Bialogue," Out/Look, Summer 1992, 6–7; 8.4: cover, Advocate, 6 September 1994) insist, in contrast, that sexual definitions and identities are not self-evident or universal. 4 Sisters Only unfolds into a comic strip about the risks and realities of heterosexual sex, scripted as a phone conversation in colloquial language between two adolescent African-American women (8.5: Urban League [U.S.]). The flip side summarizes facts, figures, and resources. "Julio y Marisol," appropriating a soap opera or photonovella format, was posted in serial installments in New York City subway cars, in English and Spanish (8.6: 1996, New York City Department of Health). Although conservatives protested the inevitable presence of sex and drugs, most New Yorkers were happy to read anything with a storyline. The Condom Comebacks wheel was designed for statewide California AIDS intervention programs in the early 1990s aimed at young women (8.7). Its novel presentation format is appeal-

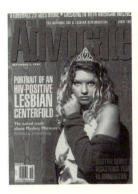

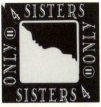

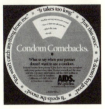

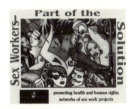

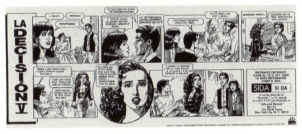

ing and adaptable for use in workshops and
other settings. No, it does not challenge fundamental structural inequalities, but it substitutes
concrete suggestions for the meaningless injunc-
tion to "use a condom" and sends a clear message to both men and women that their situation is not unique (and that a guy's excuse for
avoiding condoms is rarely original). By the 1998
World AIDS Conference in Geneva, sex workers
had formed a global network and were carrying
out a wide range of projects to promote health
and human rights (8.8). Finally, "Death Talks
about Life" is a safer sex booklet tipped into a
late run (1993) of Neil Gaiman's popular comic
Sandman (8.9); Death is a leading character in
Gaiman's pantheon and no doubt the figure
most likely to get the attention of the comic's
mainly straight male readership.

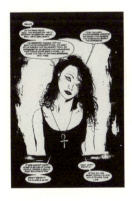

sex" precautions, Elliot is scornful: "Are all those dental dams keeping their mouths out of contact with their brains?" New York writer Monica Pearl responded, reiterating (as I have) that the absence of a *woman-to-woman* category precludes the gathering of accurate figures and that "the lesbian community is not a monolithic one: lesbians have children, have sex with men who shoot drugs, and get raped—all risks for HIV" (Pearl 1991). And some lesbians may use sex toys, practice S/M, have yeast infections, or do other things that compromise *Off Our Back*'s "thoughtless and dangerous" no-risk presumptions. "It's true that *being* a lesbian itself is not a risk. It's what we do that puts us at risk." Seven lesbians from Oklahoma responded that Pearl's letter made them ashamed. Sex toys, S/M, yeast infections—"We don't know about the women in New York, but here in Oklahoma, most of us have morals and observe cleanliness rules" (Seven Sisters 1992). They continue: "Perversion is what you're talking about, and if you're perverted enough to do those things, you probably have sexual intercourse with men also, and that puts you in a heterosexual category. Pure lesbian sex does not transmit AIDS. . . . Wake up and smell the coffee, baby!"

Although history suggests that there is no generic female purity and no generic female oppression, the idea that gender is magical and women are somehow immune to HIV is powerful, functioning in part to create an "us," a global sisterhood. Yet ultimately these notions of identity are incompatible. They make it difficult to preserve, within the women's movement, any reasonable working definition of *sisterhood* and *feminist identity*; nor do they help women make their way through the inconclusive data, conflicting media reports, and fragmented scientific constructions of AIDS discourse. In the end, women have remained confused about AIDS and HIV, and feminists have understandably resisted adding the epidemic to already overburdened agendas.[22]

Reinscribing Gender: The Cosmo *Action*

To sum up: for women, even in the late 1990s, AIDS's long-standing identity as a "gay disease" and a "man's disease" still places a burden on them to prove their own significance—as spokespersons, persons at risk, objects worthy of scientific and medical attention, and as agents of social justice and political change. But, for all the reasons I have noted, this has proved very difficult to do. The current state of affairs in the United States with respect to women and AIDS is that we lack knowledge, social policy, and cultural consensus—in part because we lack conceptual coherence about the role of gender in HIV transmission and about the impact of the AIDS epidemic on women, on families, and on society at large. The negative consequences are material and immediate: women encounter barriers to diagnosis and care, exclusion from treatment and social support programs, lack of information about sexuality and reproduction, lack of preventive technologies designed for women, and lack of resources and support services for women, children, and families. There are long-term consequences as well. As the 1990s end, questions about gender and identity are both theoretically important and politically pressing. Even as the AIDS crisis reveals the unreliability of everyday categories, those categories continue to be codified in policies and regulations for special classes of women, including sex workers, poor women, lesbians, women in Third World countries, intravenous drug users, inmates, and childbearing women at large. Lisa Bowleg (1992) argues that, where women in AIDS/HIV policy are not invisible (which is most of the time), they are conceptualized as "pollutants, criminals, and incubators." Nan Hunter's (1992) review of women and AIDS law details many problems, including existing criminal penalty laws for female sex workers and the legal vulnerabilities of many other women in many states. The AIDS epidemic fuels a conservative agenda for women—marriage, family, children—and amplifies already vocal calls for protection and surveillance. Should we doubt that this agenda is capacious and accommodating, the spectacle of Bill Clinton's impeachment identified all the demons in the "family values" pantheon: sex, queers, gay issues, minorities, godless Democrats, the cultural elites, public education, public funding for health, the 1960s, abortion, single mothers, working women, poor women, "radical feminists," Communists, and rock and roll. For women in many Third World countries, surveillance and repressive legislation are even more widespread, and less protection is available.[23]

In this larger context, the response of the ACT UP Women's Caucus to Gould's *Cosmo* article represents a significant step forward. The *Cosmo* action and the projects that it directly generated—the documentary *Doctors, Liars, and Women*, the *Women and AIDS Handbook*, and *Women, AIDS, and Activism*, its updated book version, and other activist interventions on behalf of women—demonstrate one model of feminist activism that accomplishes a certain kind of cultural work. In taking the *Cosmo* action as a turning point, I am of course not claiming it as the only authentic feminist response to the epidemic. Rather, I am using it to illustrate a general shift in our understanding of the multiple intersections between gender and the AIDS epidemic. Although to give a full account of other important developments and activist interventions by and about women would be another project, I will try to suggest their diversity.

As a model, the *Cosmo* action is uniquely useful because it was designed both to intervene and to demonstrate and document *how* to intervene. Moreover, it directly and self-consciously reinscribes gender by challenging the problematic representations of women and AIDS that had discouraged a collective feminist response; in particular, it addressed the three problematic dimensions of identity that I introduced at the outset: the identity of the epidemic itself, personal and collective identity, and the relation of identity to representation.

Redefining the Epidemic. In redefining the epidemic, the women in ACT UP began with the indisputable fact that *women have AIDS.* But their analysis did not turn simply on the question of whether women are or are not at risk or to what degree they are at risk. Rather, they defined the epidemic as a significant cultural and political crisis that threatens women's *and men's* lives and future well-being. They correctly saw the AIDS epidemic as a political and symbolic battleground that demands a widespread mobilization effort but also offers women an opportunity to gain power over their future. They resisted statistical conceptions of HIV and AIDS to the extent of refusing clearly to distinguish women who are *in*-fected from those who are *af*fected; while they continued to lobby for research that will generate more accurate figures, this general tactic provided some independence from the ongoing and changing calculation of which women are "at risk," revealing this for what, in some sense, it is: a scholastic exercise. At every point they challenged assertions of absolutes ("women can't get AIDS"). They also insisted on solidarity with gay men with AIDS while asserting the unique importance, at this point, of visibility for women.

The handbook on women and AIDS produced as a follow-up to the *Cosmo* action elaborated on this broad feminist framework, relating the AIDS epidemic to ongoing scientific, clinical, and social issues for women and showing its negative effect on civil rights, equality in the workplace, childbearing and reproductive freedom, and other areas. Now revised, expanded, and published by South End Press as *Women, AIDS, and Activism* (ACT UP New York Women and AIDS Book Group 1992), the book links the AIDS epidemic to long-standing struggles in women's health. Like other work, it argues that what happens with AIDS will influence what happens in women's health. Women's ability to obtain access to experimental drugs and other forms of treatment will influence future policy and practices with regard to other drugs—for example, women's access to experimental drugs and treatments for breast cancer. Thus, the AIDS epidemic was at last linked to long-standing struggles in women's health.

Although the word *activism* in the book's title unfortunately scares off some of the people (including health professionals and policymakers) who would find it most useful, *Women, AIDS, and Activism* has appeared to influence feminist perceptions of the epidemic. *Ms.* magazine, for example, dramatically changed its take on AIDS from the cavalier yet peppy coverage of the 1980s (see chap. 2 above). By 1991, AIDS had become a serious cover story: Explicitly influenced by *Women, AIDS, and Activism*, the January/February issue treated AIDS as a serious health concern for women and the epidemic as a social and political crisis.[24] Marcia Ann Gillespie's (1991) article, for example, addressed the epidemic as something beyond self-protective measures and something that women cannot solve alone. It highlighted women's connections to others and called attention to men's behavior toward women. Other publications also connected the fight for freedom in treatment to women's autonomy and their right to choice. These connections invoked not only broad philosophical and political questions but practical and strategic ones as well. The experience of AIDS treatment activists in smuggling illegal or unapproved drugs provided a model for access to drugs like RU-486 or breast cancer treatments. The epidemic also highlighted the many negative effects of sexually transmitted and vaginal infections, suggesting that AIDS initiatives could serve to reenergize basic reproductive research. The female condom, welcome in principle, is only a shard of what is possible. The feminist task is to reshape research priorities, encouraging research on a wide range of contraceptive and antidisease technologies for women, including anti-HIV spermicides that can be activated without a partner's cooperation or knowledge.[25]

Clarifying Personal and Collective Identities. The decision to protest the *Cosmo* article helped the women participants clarify more than the behavioral continuum of risk for women. It also clarified their own work within ACT UP. Before the action, as Maria Maggenti put it, "We were these lesbians and we would have these dyke dinners and we would sit around and try to figure out why we were involved with AIDS activism at all" (Carlomusto and Maggenti 1988). Maxine Wolfe (1992), another participant in the *Cosmo* action, put the same issue somewhat differently:

"How could a nice Jewish girl from Brooklyn, who once described herself as a bisexual, Trotskyist, anarchist, Reichian, lesbian-feminist, end up in an organization people continually describe as white, male, bourgeois (worse yet, upper middle class), single issue, not gay identified, arrogant, resource rich, and every other thing that people who describe themselves as 'progressive' don't like?" (p. 233). In carrying out the action, members of the women's caucus articulated their identity not only as friends and supporters of people with AIDS but as women, as feminists, and especially as lesbians. This is important, for, as Stoller (1995) writes, AIDS has affected lesbians in many different ways, often illuminating generational as well as political differences. In answering her own question, Wolfe writes: "I came to AIDS activism and to New York ACT UP out of a queer consciousness, a consciousness forced on me by the sexism and homophobia of the male-identified left in this country and by the homophobia of the women's movement. I came to ACT UP because of the inability of lesbians to organize around or even figure out what their issues were and because of the dead-end of the 'identity' politics of the early 1980s" (1992, 233). Through the *Cosmo* action, carried out in the name of ACT UP and women, the caucus successfully escaped rigid identity politics, a strategy akin to that outlined in Donna Haraway's "Manifesto for Cyborgs" (1985) and Kobena Mercer's (1992) notion of radical pluralism. By focusing on a single issue, the *Cosmo* article, the caucus brought together many different kinds of women and men to form a collective activist response that did not depend on across-the-board consensus on all other issues. Subsequent actions and related projects were similarly targeted and fostered links to other groups: gay men, Latinos, African Americans, health professionals, academics, drug education and treatment programs, drug users, sex workers, adolescents, lesbians, and straight women. Meanwhile, as Crimp and Rolston's *AIDS Demo Graphics* (1990) documents, many gay men committed to AIDS activism now began to participate in actions directed toward women's issues, acknowledging in some cases their debt to feminist and women's health organizing. While by no means always successful, women's coalition building has crossed national boundaries. High-profile actions at the 1989 International AIDS Conference in Montreal, for instance, included a protest against the scapegoating of prostitutes and a lesbian kiss-in (Block 1989, 10): sample signs read, respectively, "Whores are safer sex pros" and "Hi! Dykes get AIDS too." Also meeting at Montreal was the International Working Group on Women and AIDS, a loose network of women leaders from developing and industrialized countries that focused on ways to achieve equity for women. In these efforts to create international feminist networks around the issue of AIDS, generalizations proceeded by way of local knowledge, identities, and geographies. The women's group that composed the UN document on women and AIDS noted that many feminists think of the epidemic as a medical problem that should be solved by professionals; but, it was argued, AIDS is also facilitated by such nonmedical factors as women's economic dependence—broad social conditions that medicine cannot solve.

Keeping in mind the diverse material conditions in which women live, feminist AIDS initiatives potentially address another aspect of personal and collective identity: communication surrounding prevention and risk-reduction practices. Although transmission occurs as a result of practices, the function and meaning of those practices have evolved in the context of an individual's life and may be profoundly linked to identity. To think about changing one's practices may entail thinking as much about who one is as about what one does. These identities that we temporarily or partially inhabit are no less powerful for their instability and transience and are precisely what are needed to create a strong political voice for women. This statement incorporates a major insight of the feminist movement: we do not passively receive and internalize definitions and facts provided by authorities; rather, we talk about them with our friends, argue about how to interpret them, think about how they will apply to our everyday lives, and work out what is gained or lost by adopting new behavior and what that implies for our identity. In responding to information about HIV transmission, then, one problem for women has been that the "how to" questions of everyday life can rarely be discussed intelligently because authorized sources skip the details. This problem has been partially addressed by the publication of materials and guidelines for women.[26] But, as the guidelines themselves point out, women need to be able to talk about these issues in terms of their own lives; this requires establishing discussion networks and support groups, a project that depends on identifying existing groups of women or bringing interested women together: whether through face-to-face interaction, journals and newsletters, radio and television talk shows, or electronic networks.[27] Some things that women do may be illegal or stigmatized and not easily discussed with strangers or authorities. An important task, then, has been to find forms of address and identification that are as concrete as possible and circumvent the moral and semantic baggage already attached to the official AIDS lexicon.

In an insightful analysis of the burdens of this task, Robin Gorna (1996, 368) quotes a New York City lesbian:

I am bored with gay men. . . . And most of all I feel a nauseating boredom with AIDS, the virus that won't go away, the fight that I can't abandon, the spectacle of gay death that makes lesbian life seem so insignificant. Or maybe I'm not bored, maybe I am just tired of envy. . . . It is not a clean, honest envy but a guilty one, like the resentment a healthy child feels for a sick sibling who is getting all the attention.

Gorna comments as follows on the dilemma the epidemic poses:

For many queer women, AIDS reinforces the trauma of being raised as little girls who should not have needs, who should let the boys speak first. Just as women learn to acknowledge their own needs and desires, to speak up for themselves, to feel worthy and know that they matter, just at that moment the boys get something really awful. And so women are silenced again, letting go of their needs and feeling churlish for even daring to mind. Health has arisen as such a defining lesbian issue, because it seems like the only decent thing to do. How could queer women say that what really matters is being out as a mother, being out in the workplace, finding housing? These are all concerns which may be high priorities for queer women in their twenties and thirties—but it is hard to compare these with the high priority which queer men have in their twenties and thirties.

As Cindy Patton and Janis Kelly suggested in their groundbreaking *Making It: A Woman's Guide to Sex in the Age of AIDS* (1990), another possibility is to rethink eroticism. Or, as Lynne Segal put it, if sex is constructed, then it can be reconstructed: "We need to use our imaginations to explore the edges of safety, to redefine danger, to engage fantasy, to develop play in the arena of sex now marked by this epidemic" (1989, 145). Should such projects of reconstruction continue, it may indeed be the case that, as Gillespie suggests, historians will "look back and see the epidemic as a turning point in history" (1991, 16).

Eloquent and practical commentary from "anti-antiporn" survivors of the feminist sex wars includes an enlightening exchange between Gayle Rubin and Judith Butler in *Differences* (Rubin 1994a) on the malleability of erotic arrangements. Taking her position from feminist psychoanalytic theory, Butler suggests, rather pessimistically, that structures of desire are essentially fixed, intractable, despite the earlier feminist vision of sexual plasticity. Maybe not, Rubin replies; experimentation with the plasticity of desire is barely a generation old: our knowledge of sexual diversity in other cultures as well as our own suggests that there is considerable flexi-bility in our social and sexual arrangements, flexibility that we have only begun to explore. Inventive feminists like Pat Califia (1988, 1997) and Susie Bright (1995, 1997) likewise contribute to these dialogues of pos-sibility, while Lisa Jean Moore (1997) describes the myriad ways that sex workers are field-testing protective latex barriers, coming up with in-genious modifications and detailed feedback about real-world practices. Worthy of publication in *Consumer Reports* were their critiques of the "uniformly hated" female condom, one of the shockingly few devices developed after the advent of AIDS to prevent disease transmission. Sex workers told Moore that they were hard to use, awkward, clumsy, and unsightly and reflected hasty research and development and no consulta-tion with users. "I would love to have a good talking to whoever thought that shit up," said one woman Moore interviewed. "It is the most sexist archaic thing." Said another, "It looks like a colostomy bag." And, they added, not only does the female condom decrease feeling for the female user, but on top of everything else it is expensive: better to buy condoms at a quarter each than three female condoms at $8.95 (Moore 1997, 450–52).

Clarifying identities also entails contesting the stereotypes of "women with AIDS" in the larger culture, which sees women intravenous drug users as ignorant, unreliable, and incapable of caring for their infected babies, following a treatment program, or engaging in political action. Similarly, these projects challenge the criteria used to divide "women at risk" from "women in general." An important example is documented in *Doctors, Liars, and Women*; indeed, the video takes its title from this challenge. Shortly after the *Cosmo* article appeared, the women from ACT UP arranged to meet with Robert Gould and videotape their interview. They confronted the "healthy vagina" hypothesis, pointing out the extent of sexually transmitted diseases and other conditions that make it im-possible to separate women who are safe from those who are at risk. When they tell Gould that they themselves know women who have become in-fected through heterosexual intercourse, Gould replies that what women say does not necessarily mean that "it happened this way"; as a psychia-trist he knows that people lie, especially about practices like shooting drugs and having anal intercourse. Denise Ribble, a nurse and health coun-selor, responds forcefully: "I know many HIV positive women. They're not drug users, they're not the sexual partners of drug users, they're not prosti-tutes, and they're not liars." Ribble is in part responding to Gould on scientific grounds: many factors clearly influence the probability of trans-mission and hence suggest a continuum of risk where there are no absolute separations between *high risk, lower risk,* and *no risk.* Such a continuum is also made evident in Moore's analysis of safer sex practices among sex workers, with experimentation, negotiation of guidelines, and usage greatest in the "gray areas" of practices that are "possibly" or "probably" safe or unsafe. Like Ribble's challenge to Gould, other voices are demanding that women be made able to speak for themselves and be listened to. Both Judith Cohen, of Project AWARE in San Francisco, and June Osborne, dean of the School of Public Health at Michigan—both progressive forces in AIDS research and policymaking from early on in the epidemic—used their speaker slots at conferences not to present their own work or views but to speak for women not in positions to speak. Osborn jettisoned her own concluding keynote speech at an AIDS conference to read instead a manifesto of anger and frustration from women attending the conference who had been denied any forum for communication (reported by Corea 1992). Teare and English (1996) detail the areas of policy where crucial work is still needed on behalf of women, emphasizing the need not only to change official policy (such as the CDC's revised definition of AIDS to include conditions more likely to be present in women) but also to follow through at all levels to ensure that changes from above filter down systematically to the "real world of care delivery." Such initiatives are political in demanding a voice and visibility for women, in refusing to segregate "women at risk" from other possibilities for collective identity, and in striving explicitly to foster discussion among women across divisions of race, sex, class, and ethnicity. Yet, in this area where representation is so crucial, the examples that I have just given suggest how difficult representation is to achieve. Again, the *Cosmo* experience furnishes lessons.

Controlling Representations, Influencing Interpretation. For the women in ACT UP, several things came together during their interview with Gould. It confirmed their view that Gould was not well informed about the AIDS epidemic and that the *Cosmo* article was therefore irresponsible. That *Cosmo*'s publishers believed that they could publish such "advice" with impunity demonstrated the pressing need to place women's health care on the activist AIDS agenda. The *Cosmo* debate next entered high media mode. The day after the *Cosmo* action, Gould appeared as a panelist on "People Are Talking," a New York talk show hosted by Richard Bey on television station WOR in New York. An invited member of the audience was Chris Norwood, author of a 1987 book about women and AIDS and chair of the AIDS Committee of the National Women's Health Network. Roaming the audience with his microphone, Bey interrogated Norwood:

Richard Bey: Chris, is a woman at risk from heterosexual inter-
course?
Chris Norwood: Richard, she is specifically at risk from having panels
like this. Virtually all panelists on women and AIDS—
Bey: I asked you a question, Chris!
Norwood: —are men—
Bey: OK, thank you. [*Moving to other side of the audience.*] Any
questions over here?

Norwood then crossed to the dais and sat on the coffee table in front of
Gould. As Bey called for security guards, Norwood tried again to make her
point that women should speak for themselves and that misleading information "is dangerous to—" At this point, Bey interrupts, thrusting the
microphone at her:

Bey: Are you a medical doctor?
Norwood: —people's lives.
Bey: I can see you're a propagandist— Are you a medical doctor?
Norwood: I spent three years writing a book about AIDS—
Bey: Are you a medical doctor?

Bey broke off this exchange by turning to the studio and television audience: "One of the reasons we have hysteria in this country is that people
like this do not want the exchange of information."[28]

As director Jean Carlomusto points out in the video, the *Cosmo* action
was successful as long as the activists could remain in control; when they
lost control—on the WOR show, but especially in later shows that barred
them from the studio, and on *Nightline*, where activists had no representation at all (although Ted Koppel and Mathilde Krim effectively challenged Gould and *Cosmo*'s editor, Helen Gurley Brown)—they were at the
mercy of stereotypes and silencing. Like the growing body of independent
AIDS videos, *Doctors, Liars, and Women* graphically demonstrates why
the AIDS epidemic is a feminist issue: it shows the cultural silencing of
women, their exclusion from debates about their own fate, and their dependence on those who are more powerful to represent them. As Clay
Stephens writes of women and AIDS, "Most of the problems are not new;
they are simply viewed through another set of distorted lenses. AIDS is a
paradigm for the condition of women within our society" (1988, 387). Yet,
while it demonstrates this, the video of the *Cosmo* action—widely shown
and distributed—challenges this version of reality by reclaiming women's
right to represent themselves and tell their side of the story. Further pub-

lic actions detailed in the *Handbook*—from the Shea Stadium action directed at heterosexual men to lesbian kiss-ins directed at scientists and clinicians who believe that lesbians do not have physical or sexual relationships—similarly demonstrate this symbolic battleground. Such initiatives are supplemented by a growing body of productions from many sources—feminist and lesbian films and videos, photographs, posters, books and booklets, telenovellas, publications, comics, and cartoons—that offer many potential positions of identification and inscribe women in AIDS discourse in multiple ways.

Representation, Identity, and Power: Beyond Cosmo

This "war of representation," as Crimp and Rolston (1990) put it, does crucial cultural work with regard to AIDS, to activism, and to women. It moves beyond the intense gender politics of the 1980s in which—to oversimplify—the theory-practice split came to stand for a host of other divisions and differences among women: discourse-reality, male-female, white women–women of color, straight-gay, First World–Third World, technology-nature, academe-community, constructionist-foundationalist, pleasure-pain, and so on. Deconstruction, postmodernism, and other antifoundationalist (constructionist) frameworks offer numerous strategies for subverting binary and essentialist divisions, and, in many respects, I believe that they have been a godsend in the struggle against AIDS. It is also the case, however, that postmodern fragmentation and dispersion do sometimes deflect attention from realities that *should be* brutally (rather than strategically) essentialized. As Jody Berland (1992) argues, to embrace fragmentation uncritically runs the risk of duplicating the move to a market-driven consumerist model of human populations in which the fragmentation of conventional identities is a fine art. Political and intellectual action in the name of women is not inevitably incompatible with the postmodern vision embodied in some of ACT UP's tactics, provided that we acknowledge the difficulty of arriving at "truth" and concentrate instead on understanding the rules of discourse whereby truth in various universes is produced, sustained, deeply experienced, or contested. To take the most overexposed example, it is true that breast cancer is a pressing health issue for women. But it is also a rhetorical strategy, one that by the end of the 1980s had come to be the attack mode of choice against gay male activism. With its energy, knowledge, and uncompromising high style, ACT UP, in particular, attracted unprecedented media attention and public commentary; but it also drew the anger and resentment of other health lobbies. From public policy groups like the National Women's Health Network to conservative writers like Michael Fumento, breast cancer was used as evidence that AIDS research budgets and media coverage were draining resources needed by women. But this is a dead end. Women are also struggling over abortion, contraception, lung cancer, ovarian cancer, heart disease, osteoporosis, repetitive strain injury, infertility, developmental and physical disability, tuberculosis, infant mortality, teenage pregnancy, depression, schizophrenia, domestic violence, substance abuse, chronic fatigue syndrome, malnutrition, assault, and murder. These can be seen as threats to women's health as great as the AIDS epidemic or breast cancer. A turning point came in 1991 with the formation in New York of CAN ACT, the Cancer Patients' Action Alliance, WHAM, and other high-profile activist health groups: ACT UP had become a model for the 1990s and an ally instead of a competitor.[29] In the future, the pie itself, like the pie charts that I mentioned earlier, needs to be redrawn—and baked in bigger pans, not half baked by the Pentagon.

I said at the beginning of this chapter that an effective response to an epidemic (as to any widespread cultural crisis) depends on the existence of identities for whom that epidemic (or crisis) is meaningful—and stories in which those identities are taken up and animated. I have sought to show how identities and narratives about women and AIDS have not encouraged an effective response. Today, many challenges remain.

A July 1997 story in the *New York Times* on the "AIDS gender gap" demonstrates the unrivaled skill of major media outlets in recuperating stereotypes from stories that challenge them. Reporting that AIDS cases have for the first time leveled off for gay men, the *Times* story warns that cases among women continue to rise. "In a sense the AIDS gender gap reflects the history of women and AIDS, a history in which women have always lagged behind men." Just as women were faulted in the early 1980s for their role ("by virtue of their anatomy") as wet blankets at the spread-of-AIDS party (see chap. 1 above), they are described even now as "lagging behind men"—poor competitors in the AIDS marathon? AIDS first made its appearance among homosexual men, the *Times* then reminds us; in contrast to women, their head start means that they are now "reaping the benefits of early education and prevention efforts." There is nothing wrong with giving credit to the groups that pioneered safer sex and cleaner needles. But "reaping the benefits"? Of seventeen years of crushing burden and several hundred thousand deaths?

Even within the AIDS establishment and AIDS activism, there remains the need for voices to speak on behalf of women. A 1995 issue of the PWA newsletter *Newsline* on HIV and pregnancy makes clear that childbearing women with HIV still have few champions: "For people with AIDS/HIV, the right to privacy and self-determination have been of paramount importance. Many battles have been fought over these issues and some have been won. Most people with AIDS and those affected are strong advocates for the right to make personal choices about everything from treatment to disclosure. Yet when people with AIDS are also female and pregnant, the discourse around privacy and individual rights often takes a huge shift" (People with AIDS Coalition of New York 1995, 7).

In reviewing fifteen years of AIDS discourse on women and gender, what I find truly dizzying is the ease and simultaneity with which women can be both invisible and culpable, transparent instrumental carriers and reservoirs of contagion, dangerous and willful infectors and naive, irresponsible infectees. While there were occasions during the 1980s in which the entity *woman with AIDS* was fluid, complicated, and open to multiple meanings, the woman with AIDS produced by the major public discourses of the epidemic was largely nonnegotiable and the apparatus of production difficult to sabotage. That is, as I have been arguing, entrenched biological and social narratives about gender, scientists' stereotypes about particular kinds of women, and the established surveillance system were all highly overdetermined. The same can certainly be claimed for race and ethnicity. The long overdue 1993 recommendation that U.S. populations at high risk receive aggressive targeted interventions was set back years by media mishandling and public misinterpretation. (For background, see Wallace 1991; Wallace et al. 1994; National Minority AIDS Council 1991; Sobo 1993; and Leary 1993.)

Many promising initiatives and research projects continue, collectively, to challenge the nonsense. I have cited and discussed such work at many points throughout this book (e.g., Farmer et al. 1996; Stoller 1995; Moore 1997; Hammonds 1997; and Rubin 1994b). While not addressing AIDS/HIV in particular, Moore and Clarke's (1995) chronological review of medical representations of the clitoris is part of an ambitious research agenda designed to effect a major overhaul of institutionalized medical representations of genitalia. Intellectual projects of this kind complement the NIH initiative on women's health and other large-scale programs; they also provide a much-needed critical perspective on the positivist assumptions underlying conventional medical investigations (whether of male or female health). Sex worker organizations in Australia represent a stunning HIV/AIDS initiative. Now linked in a national network called the Scarlet Alliance, sex worker organizations have provided input for programming and policy as well as grounded sex information since almost the beginning of the epidemic (Perkins et al. 1994; Saunders 1997). That sex workers in the United States could play a comparable role in this country is demonstrated by Moore's (1997) interviews about safer sex technologies with practicing sex workers, whose knowledge of sexual diversity and genitalia and skill at linking devices to desires have been largely absent from heterosexual safer sex campaigns (not to mention the design of problematic inventions like the female condom). The basic research of the physiologist Richard Cone seeking to synthesize disease prevention and birth control likewise demonstrates the power of imaginative thinking about new technologies, even while institutional funding sources rigidly support research on contraception or disease prevention, but not both at once (see, e.g., Cone and Martin 1998). Charis Cussins's (1997) ethnographic research in infertility clinic settings confronts head-on the slippage between women's agency, identity, and "transparency." Given the unconventional technologies (e.g., in vitro fertilization) and social arrangements (e.g., gestational surrogacy) that routinely characterize reproduction in such settings, Cussins's goal was to see what resources participants used to construct and keep track of who "the mother" was, resources she calls "technologies of motherhood." She schematized this by developing a contrast between the "transparent" role of the woman (egg donor, gestational mother, or whomever) who was not to become "the mother" and the mother-to-be, whom she designated "opaque." As Cussins points out, the clients of infertility treatment programs tend to be carefully selected, with the result that, in her study, the "opaque mother" was almost always part of a heterosexual couple. She concludes that the negotiation of these categories—"the real mother" versus other designations—was extremely important but that "nature" and "biology" were not the governing determinants; rather, participants negotiated the categories on a case-by-case basis, drawing on the circumstances and resources of their particular social and biological configuration.

Sex work, too, is undergoing an overhaul. I have already contrasted the work of feminist researchers like Shaw and Paleo (1987) with the taken-for-granted assumptions of most "prostitute research." Another example is Akeroyd's (1997) decision to discuss HIV and prostitution in Africa within the context not of deviance but of occupational risk:

> There are few published studies which pay detailed attention to occupational and class issues in respect of women: attention has been directed primarily to "prostitutes" or "sex workers." "Downmarket"

prostitution, women serving a relatively poor clientele, has been emphasized . . . though it would be interesting to know how much power [women working in the small, expensive high-class prostitution sector] have in sexual exchanges compared with their poorer counterparts. The work of Schoepf and others, however, shows how misleading is the constant reiteration of the image of African women as prostitutes and barmaids created by epidemiological studies and the media. (p. 18)

Akeroyd goes on to show, further, that "prostitutes" are not always marginal and that many factors enter into women's choice of sex work over other options. She concludes that "generalized discussions of 'AIDS in Africa' may not be sufficiently sensitive to the differences in women's economic position and power within and between different countries and societies" (p. 19). Schoepf (1992b), similarly, insists that gendered activities and identities be placed within their larger socioeconomic context; only research "linking the macro-level political economy to micro-level ethnography" (p. 279) can illuminate the meaning, purpose, and (sometimes fatal) outcome of women's survival strategies.

As Rubin (1984, 1997) has written, there are continuous battles over definitions, evaluations, arrangements, privileges, and costs of sexual behavior. In defining the population of "sex workers" whom she interviewed about safer sex, Moore (1997) not only problematizes the notion of definition but also asks how and why the category "prostitute" has been created within social science research. What makes some women engaging in the exchange of sex for sustenance "prostitutes"—either self-defined or labeled by others—and others not? Moore herself bases the definition of *sex worker* for her own study on the following underlying assumptions: first, ideas and terms emerge out of specific historical, social, and discursive processes that label and create certain behaviors as deviant, a labeling that often facilitates some form of social control; second, social, institutional, and economic environments constrain and constitute what sex work can be; and, third, sex workers are not wholly determined by their labelers or by their environments: "Sex workers interact, deploy, resist, and manipulate their multiple identities and local environments" (p. 441).

Whither feminism? Along with cultural, postcolonial, and queer theory, AIDS activism extends insights in ways that help explain why, despite its enormous appeal and importance in building a movement, the notion of universal sisterhood has itself become impossible—and unnecessary—to sustain in the face of the very realities, diversities, and identities that feminism has brought to light. To bring the seemingly incompatible worlds of different feminisms and activisms together means refusing to make unappealing and, indeed, impossible choices: choices like whether to maintain that AIDS is a "man's disease" and keep it off the feminist agenda, thus ignoring its continuing toll of suffering and death on men and women, or to assert AIDS's urgency and primacy *for women* and thus divert resources from other urgent women's health problems. Instead, we must assert that AIDS is a premier symbolic battleground of our times where war will be waged incessantly, where language and reality will continually shape each other, where women's futures—all our futures—will in part be determined, and where the health-care system in its unacceptable entirety should be challenged and transformed for good. Informed by a feminist analysis that takes its historical and cultural context seriously and specifies its tasks carefully, the story of women and AIDS can be read as a dense narrative about women's health and American society; economic opportunity and political power; sexuality and safety; law and transgression; individual autonomy and reproductive freedom; the right to social services and health-care resources; the deformities of the American health-care system; alliances with others; and the significance of identity in everyday life.

The success of these efforts depends in part on their respect for such basic feminist tenets as the importance of self-definition and self-representation and the recognition that *women* is not a monolithic category even while it is inscribed as unitary in given discourses. What the role will be of the actual, historical feminist movement in these struggles remains a question.

9

How to Have Theory in an

Epidemic: The Evolution of

AIDS, Treatment, and Activism

I got the drug right here, it's called acyclovir,
And though it's used for herpes I have no fear.
Can do, can do, my Doc says the drug can do.
If she says the drug can do, can do, can do.
—Ron Goldberg, "Fugue for Drug Trials"

A remarkable development in the evolution of the AIDS epidemic has been the ongoing movement of AIDS activists to speed the testing and release of experimental drugs by the FDA, to participate in the design and implementation of clinical drug trials, and to have a voice in shaping the AIDS/HIV research agenda. The struggle over AIDS drug trials and treatments has required sophisticated technical information about the structure and functions of the FDA, the Department of Health and Human Services, and the NIH; about the process and economics of developing, evaluating, and releasing new drugs; about the conceptual and statistical grounds on which standards for clinical drug trials are based; about drugs themselves (where they come from and how they work); about viruses in general and the pathogenesis of HIV in particular; about how treatment interventions might act to bring about prevention, retardation, or cure; and, finally, about the nature and politics of basic and clinical biomedical research.

The epigraph to this chapter is the opening verse of "Fugue for Drug Trials," Ron Goldberg's adaptation of the famous curtain-raiser from *Guys and Dolls* in which each of three seasoned denizens of the New York racetrack, armed with statistics, insider tips, and the daily *Racing Form*, claims "I got the horse right here."[1] Performed by Goldberg and his colleagues in March 1989 after a successful demonstration by New York AIDS activists against Mayor Ed Koch and City Hall, "Fugue for Drug Trials" captures the Runyonesque combination of unquenchable optimism and bitter experience that characterized the first years of AIDS treatment activism. The horse-race analogy, echoed in the title of Arno and Feiden's (1992) study of AIDS drug development, *Against the Odds*, points to the enormously complex and often agonizing decisions about diagnosis, treatment, and the doctor-patient relationship that have had to be made daily—individually and collectively, personally and politically—by people living with HIV disease. And the lyrics suggest the degree of technical sophistication required in the age of AIDS, together with the element of ironic distancing, even of camp, that was regularly used to frame and contain technological overload. Disillusionment, death, and the intense pain of what Steven Epstein (1996) calls "clinical trials and tribulations" eventually took their toll on the high spirits and unity reflected in "Fugue for Drug Trials" and further complicated commitments to AIDS treatment activism. But it is this entire trajectory, however sobering and difficult, that offers a genuine model for the democratic engagement with science and medicine that the twenty-first century will demand of us.

This chapter explores the ongoing contributions of AIDS activism to the fight against AIDS/HIV and its enduring legacy to progressive political action more broadly. As the final cultural chronicle in this study, AIDS treatment activism demonstrates how theory may be used in an epidemic and, hence, gives this book its title. My discussion draws on published scholarship and media coverage, discussions and interviews with participants, field notes from meetings and conferences, reports and other documents from activist and advocacy groups, and resources from newsletters and websites. I first review the evolution of drug regulation in the United States and the intervention of AIDS activism in that process. I then look more closely at these interventions and the knowledge and resources that guided them. The early debate over the drug zidovudine (the antiviral drug also known as azidothymidine, or AZT) illuminates key theories and practices that served to shape AIDS research, treatment, and activism. On the one hand, this debate represents a set of overdetermined cultural narratives about scientific proof and practice (what Epstein [1996] calls, after Foucault, "regimes of credibility"), professional identity, the doctor-patient contract, the interaction of conflicting social priorities, and nature itself. Yet, on the other hand, it also suggests possibilities for rethinking and reconfiguring the processes of producing and interpreting knowledge. Like the cultural construction of HIV discussed in chapter 5 above, the AZT debate is of great contextual importance for more recent developments in HIV theory and treatment strategies, including the crucial research finding that, during its latency period, HIV is anything but latent; the "new era" of

AIDS/HIV treatment initiated with the development of protease inhibitors and sophisticated combinatory treatment regimens; and the structural inequalities, both material and conceptual, that the epidemic has so relentlessly exposed. AIDS treatment activism and the still more ambitious activist engagement with clinical and basic research offer an extraordinary demonstration of how to have theory in a crisis. Like medical technologies pioneered in wartime, they also offer a model applicable after the epidemic, a legacy for incisive engagement with biomedicine and the health-care system. But we are not in peacetime yet. So this chapter is also a chronicle of courage under fire: of people with AIDS fighting and dying in a war for which they will receive no medals. Like AIDS activism in particular and health-care activism in general, the debate about AZT is inevitably, in the late twentieth century, a debate about the uses and consequences of technology, biomedical theory, and human bodies in everyday life. Hence, it is a debate, with mortal stakes, about the evolution, value, and conditions of possibility for a radical and democratic technoculture.

The Industrial-Regulatory Loop

As the bearer of organic disease, the object of study made manifest, the body is denied its social and cultural embodiment and comes to stand for the disease itself. Hence research on the body becomes legitimated; the body becomes the object of research (a kind of walk-in, skin-encapsulated test tube) and people become the legitimate subjects of research.—Meurig Horton, "Bugs, Drugs, and Placebos"

In college, I had studied critical theory, where I had been struck by Michel Foucault's emphasis on two themes. First, that in political activism, it is necessary to master the language of your adversaries and use it to advance your own ends. This we did with medical jargon surrounding clinical trials, drug development, and FDA regulation. Second, the necessity to mobilize on a number of fronts and advance whenever a position gives way. We couldn't know in advance which front would give way. Once we had gained a strategic position, we needed to continue occupying it. The work, as we learned, goes on for years.—Mark Harrington, "Some Transitions in the History of AIDS Treatment Activism"

The public revelations of Nazi experimentation with human subjects during World War II led to the international adoption of the Nuremberg Code. Although the possibility of regulating human experimentation in the United States was discussed by the U.S. Public Health Service (PHS) during the immediate postwar period, medical scientists resisted regulations and guidelines on the grounds that the Nazi experiments were aberrations, carried out by deranged individuals. The regulation of medical research has evolved alongside the regulation of drugs. Public outcry over deaths from untested sulfa drugs forced the passage in 1938 of the Food, Drug, and Cosmetic Act, requiring companies to prove that their drugs were safe. The thalidomide tragedy led to the passage in 1962 of further amendments to the 1906 Pure Food and Drug Act, also known as the Kefauver-Harris amendments. For the first time, federal law explicitly imposed controls on human experimentation and directed doctors to inform patients when they were being given drugs experimentally. And, for the first time as well, as Arno and Feiden (1992, 30) put it, "the federal government demanded proof not only that a drug was safe but that it worked. And for the next twenty-five years the Kefauver amendments stood unchallenged."

This history of regulation has unfolded within a highly contested arena in which several powerful, value-laden narratives come into conflict: social and ethical concerns for individual rights, physicians' autonomy in determining treatment for their patients, the needs and principles of scientific investigation evolved by biomedical researchers, and the God-given right of U.S. capitalists to make money. The guidelines of the 1964 World Health Organization Declaration of Helsinki set out in less legalistic terms than the Nuremberg Code the broad ethical principles that should govern research with human subjects. Although the declaration was widely endorsed by medical organizations in the United States, strong objections to actual regulations persisted, and, not surprisingly, an NIH report that same year revealed no generally accepted codes of clinical research among medical scientists. In response, in 1966 the PHS issued Policy and Procedure Order 129, that agency's first set of guidelines on clinical research and training grants. Revised again in 1969 and in 1971, the guidelines challenged the widespread premise that the judgment and integrity of medical researchers provided sufficient protection of the rights and welfare of research subjects. New FDA regulations in 1971 mandated the review of experimental protocols and provisions for obtaining informed consent. Still, these regulations concerned procedural rather than ethical principles; moreover, they did not apply to the federal government's own research.

In 1972, however, the Associated Press broke the story of the Tuskegee syphilis study (Jones 1981). The American public learned that, since 1932, the PHS had been conducting research in the South on several hundred black men with syphilis, providing them neither information about their condition nor medical treatment. The PHS responded to the public storm—as it had responded to earlier private objections—by arguing that the goal of the research was to learn the natural history of untreated syphilis, that treatment would have compromised this goal, that the men would not have understood their condition or benefited from treatment, and that critics of the research did not understand science.

But this response was no longer good enough; indeed, it was no good at all. After Senator Edward M. Kennedy in 1973 conducted Senate hearings on human experimentation, an ad hoc panel was created to investigate the Tuskegee study. Loud and uniform public outrage persisted, and a class action suit was filed on behalf of the men with syphilis and their families. As a result, tougher controls for clinical research and protections for patients were finally put in place. The National Research Act of 1974 established the National Commission for the Protection of Human Subjects of Biomedical and Behavioral Research. Reflecting the growing cultural consensus that science should take social and ethical concerns into account, the commission was charged with identifying "the basic ethical principles that should underlie the conduct of biomedical and behavioral research" and developing guidelines to ensure that research be conducted in accordance with those principles. Such ethical principles, outlined in the final report of the President's Commission on Ethical Problems in Medicine and Biomedical and Behavioral Research (President's Commission 1983), include autonomy, beneficence, and justice.[2]

The FDA has thus evolved as a complicated repository of history, incorporating the products of liberal reform, biomedical achievement, and the free market. Charged with protecting the public from dangerous or useless drugs made available by inexpert clinicians or profit-seeking drug companies, the agency stands in an inevitably close relation to clinical medicine and pharmaceutical manufacturing as well as to biomedical research.

The FDA's process for overseeing the development of new drugs embodies this uniquely contradictory historical legacy (see Arno and Feiden 1992; Rothman 1991; Rothman and Edgar 1992; Grady 1995; and Epstein 1996). Studies of experimental drugs and therapies are called *clinical trials*, defined by Levine and Lebacqz (1979, 728) as "a class of research activities designed to develop generalizable knowledge about the safety and/or efficacy of either validated or nonvalidated practices." Thus designed to determine both safety and efficacy, clinical trials require that a drug be studied first in vitro (in a test tube), then in vivo (in living beings—animals and humans). A plan, or protocol, to study the drug in human beings is submitted by the drug's sponsor to the FDA; it must include results of earlier in vitro and animal testing and describe in detail how it plans to carry out the clinical (human) trial process. The FDA and its

Institutional Review Board (IRB) must approve the drug and the protocol before the drug can be released for experimental use on human beings; the IRB is specifically charged with protecting the rights of human subjects and ensuring that informed consent provisions are adequate. The research itself is carried out by the drug's sponsor; what the FDA and IRB see is the application for permission to proceed with the research that, with all its supporting documentation, may run to 100,000 pages.

Before AIDS, the routine at this stage was as follows. If the FDA decided that the drug and the protocol would not place subjects at unreasonable risk, the drug was given *investigational new drug* (IND) status, granting its sponsor the right to begin human testing. Phase I trials, typically lasting less than a year and involving only a small number of subjects, served to establish the drug's toxicity and the highest tolerable use (*maximum tolerated dose*). Phase II trials then tested the drug under highly controlled conditions in wider populations to determine efficacy (including *minimum effective dose*) and to provide more information on safety (toxicity and side effects). "Controlled" conditions seek to ensure that any demonstrated effectiveness can legitimately be attributed to the drug being tested: in a standard placebo study, one group is given the drug, and a control group is given an identical but innocuous medication; in a double-blind study, neither the experimenter nor the subject knows which is which. In an active control study, the control group receives existing treatment for the condition rather than a placebo. Phase III trials sought to confirm the drug's usefulness and obtain more detailed information about dose, duration, efficacy at various stages and in various populations, and rarer side effects. Throughout the clinical trial process, most drugs were tested primarily on white males. Approximately 25 percent of the drugs that entered clinical trials successfully completed Phase III trials, at which point the sponsor could file a *new drug application*. If approved, the drug could be placed on the market, where Phase IV studies were supposed to test its actual performance in the "real world." If the sponsors of the drug (including a vitamin or an herb) claimed unsupported therapeutic effects when they marketed it, or if the drug caused unforeseen problems, it could be recalled by the FDA at this stage.

Overall, through the mid-1980s, the drug approval process was laborious: eight years was the average time required for a drug to move from test-tube research to final market distribution. Two alternative regulatory options, however, were available. First, by filing an application for *compassionate use IND*, a physician could request permission from the drug's sponsor and the FDA to administer a drug to a patient who was seriously ill. Second, if, before controlled clinical trials were completed, tests appeared to demonstrate that a drug would not put patients at unreasonable risk, the drug sponsor could apply for *treatment IND* status to distribute the drug to patients with immediately life-threatening conditions; continuing research to establish efficacy accompanied the release for treatment. Neither option was as rational as it sounds: applications were time-consuming to produce and often rejected, and, even if an application was approved, typically the drug was made available only on a small scale.

The obvious problems inherent in this process were not helped by the intimate connection between federal regulations and corporate interests that protects the process itself from open scrutiny on the grounds of trade secrecy. Seeking to get more drugs tested and approved rapidly, AIDS advocates denounced both the secrecy and the glacial pace (e.g., the *Treatment and Data Handbook* [Bohne et al. 1989, 6] charged the FDA with "murderous lies and bureaucratic sloth"). They noted that the industrial-regulatory loop was also a revolving door: in the satiric video *Rockville Is Burning*, the character playing an FDA official advises AIDS advocates that, if they want information, "talk to Burroughs Wellcome—that's where I'm going when I leave this pissant job—that's where the *real* money is" (Huff 1989). Activists were by no means alone in their view. Other critics charged that the federal anti-AIDS effort was underfunded and understaffed (Presidential Commission 1988) and that the drug approval process was "politically contaminated" (quoted in Mahar 1989, 22). The medical ethicist Carole Levine described the clinical trials process as a system "designed to be cautious. It's designed to stop bad drugs—not to hurry up good drugs" (quoted in Zonona 1988).

As the debate broadened in the mid- to late 1980s, one proposed modification for AIDS drugs would have eliminated all restrictions on access for patients diagnosed with full-blown AIDS (Krim 1986, 1987). A second proposal took a laissez-faire approach and recommended that informed consent be the only determinant of access (Gieringer 1987). While the FDA adopted neither proposal outright, it did broaden and liberalize the category *treatment IND* (Young et al. 1988). Yet, under treatment IND, drug companies could charge for drugs, not only reversing the standard practice under conventional clinical trials of providing drugs free, but also lessening the incentive of drug companies to complete all stages of testing since they could begin to recover their costs before safety and efficacy had been fully established.

This history is studded with conflict and compromise. While the Tuskegee study clearly abused any reasonable definition of *experimental sub-*

ject, the format and regulations for clinical drug trials were developed precisely to determine safety and efficacy by stringent scientific criteria. Failure to apply such criteria was what led to the thalidomide tragedy as well as to widespread side effects in women used as subjects to develop oral contraceptives, the drug DES, and the IUD. It was, in fact, these abuses that spurred the formation of the women's health movement and eventually induced further regulation: in 1974, the Department of Health, Education, and Welfare developed guidelines to curb sterilization abuse, and, in 1978, the FDA gained statutory power to regulate medical devices. Yet, as Doris Haire's 1984 report to Congress for the National Women's Health Network makes clear, the regulatory process remains full of loopholes: FDA approval does not mean that the drug has been approved as safe for general use; safety has usually not been tested in nonmale populations, including the elderly, infants and children, pregnant women, and lactating mothers; no laws or regulations prohibit a doctor from prescribing or administering a nonapproved drug; the FDA often accepts manufacturers' safety data on faith, accepts unpublished data as evidence, may be influenced by economic pressures, does not evaluate drugs in combination, and shields safety research from public scrutiny.[3] During the 1970s, moreover, enthusiasm for tighter oversight waned as the entire health-care system began to shift from regulation toward a competitive market model. In the end, perhaps, regulation cannot fully resolve fundamental conflicts of interest between experimental science and patient care, between the need to obtain sound aggregate data and the duty to protect the rights of individual patients, between the duty to guard the public from unsafe or useless drugs and the need to make potentially useful drugs available rapidly, and between the willingness of afflicted people to risk anything and their special vulnerability to nonvalidated drugs and treatments (for a review of these issues with regard to AIDS therapies, see Freedman and McGill Boston Research Group [1989] and Grady [1995] as well as Eisenberg [1993]; Dixon [1990]; Amolis et al. [1993]; and Levine et al. [1991]).

The AIDS epidemic came to pass, then, in a health-care system fraught with unsolved problems and incompatible philosophical commitments. Add to this the conservative political appointments and budget cuts of the Reagan presidency, a slashed and demoralized staff at the FDA, bandwagon enthusiasm for deregulation, renewed faith in the invisible hand of natural market forces, and a growing awareness in Congress of AIDS as a sensitive political issue, and one better understands the terrain from which "AIDS drugs" so slowly and inconsistently emerged.

Yet, significantly, as Harrington's invocation of Foucault (quoted above)

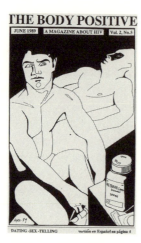

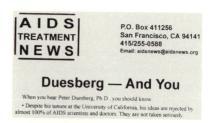

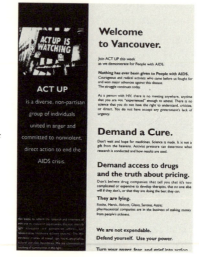

AIDS treatment activism has been hailed by many commentators, myself included, for its courage, politics, style, and media savvy. But a movement created to get "drugs into bodies" depends above all on the material experiences of hundreds of thousands of bodies and the record and interpretation of those experiences constituted in part by biomedical sci- ence. *But only in part: from the moment in 1981 that the* New York Native *decided to do its own investigative reporting on* AIDS, *biomedical reporting and interpretation have been closely and skeptically scrutinized and myriad publications established to amplify other voices. One cover of* The Body Positive *(9.1: vol. 2, no. 5, June 1989), for instance, shows* AZT *as a part of everyday reality for people with* AIDS, *looming large on the bedside table yet contemplated with clearly mixed emotions. To the man in the foreground, the* AZT *container may reveal a grim fact about his sexual partner—outing by prescription—but its presence also signals the profound changes in cultural values and practices that the epidemic has produced. Struggles surrounding* AZT *and other drugs and treatments have repeatedly served as a microcosm of broader struggles against* AIDS *(9.2:* ACT UP *flyer, June 1996) just as* AIDS *itself has proved a microcosm of larger social conditions. Aerosolized pentamidine, Compound Q,* AZT, ddI, *protease inhibitors: each has taught hard lessons about the conditions of production of scientific knowledge, the fitful and often contradictory accumulation of empirical data, the appeal of ostensible results, and the hardships of sustaining a mind-set of genuine equipoise. After more than a decade of relentless skepticism toward thousands and thousands of pages of data, some* AIDS *treatment activists decided that some propositions were more true than others and that it was time to say so (9.3: flyer distributed at a 1997 Duesberg lecture).*

recognizes, what are loopholes in one context may be footholds in another. Gaps in the FDA oversight that feminists and consumer advocates had long criticized also provided space for alternative approaches to AIDS drugs and treatment to take shape. By experimenting with combinations of legal, unregulated, and unapproved drugs and other potentially therapeutic substances, persons with AIDS and their advocates began to establish a body of personal testimony, anecdotal experience, and technological expertise sufficient to challenge the federal effort. I will come back to both positive and problematic sequelae to this challenge and to current developments in the politics of research and treatment. Here, I want to argue that treatment activists accomplished their earlier goals in three ways: (1) by providing drugs, treatments, and technical expertise through underground or alternative channels, (2) by working cooperatively with selected scientists, physicians, and drug manufacturers to explore new therapies and develop alternative strategies for testing and distributing new drugs and treatments; and (3) by publicly challenging the FDA and related scientific agencies to take charge of the epidemic.

First, as physicians and patients became increasingly convinced that treatment was an important variable in disease progression, guerrilla clinics and buyers' clubs formed to provide unapproved or illegal drugs and treatments (Arno and Feiden 1992). Such organizations as Project Inform in San Francisco and newsletters as *Treatment Issues, Body Positive, P.I. Perspective, Positively Healthy,* and *AIDS Treatment News* were founded to report and analyze the development of validated and nonvalidated therapies, scientific developments, and FDA action and inaction (see Callen 1987–88). Project Inform and the AIDS Coalition to Unleash Power (ACT UP) used the Freedom of Information Act to obtain documents pertaining to the FDA's approval of the drug AZT and proceeded to analyze flaws in the process and in the drug (see, e.g., Sonnabend 1989; Lauritsen 1989; and Erni 1994). Some medical researchers and clinicians, accordingly, recognized that people with AIDS were too well informed and technologically expert to submit passively to "controlled" clinical trials. Subjects enrolled in placebo trials, for example, would routinely take their samples to be privately analyzed; those on the "real" drug would then divide their supply with those on placebos. Others refused to enroll in clinical trials at all on the grounds that placebo studies for people with a deadly disease were unethical. Scientists familiar with these practices argued that, since PWAS were inevitably going to experiment with diverse treatment possibilities, scientists should find ways to study the effects systematically. (Arno and Feiden [1992] and Epstein [1996] describe these developments in detail.)

Second, in the absence of federal coordination and treatment guidelines, private physicians were prescribing drugs and treatments supported by their experience and that of their patients and colleagues. A notable discovery was the effectiveness of aggressive treatment of the symptoms and opportunistic infections associated with HIV infection; in particular, a regimen that included regular prophylaxis for *pneumocystis carinii* pneumonia (PCP)—the most common opportunistic infection in people with AIDS, which about 85 percent experience at some point in their illness—was found by many physicians to promote health and retard disease progression significantly (L. Altman 1988b). Yet, in the absence of official scientific and clinical recommendations, early intervention in general and specific treatment regimens in particular had limited the ability to save lives outside the cities where such forms of treatment were standard practice (Callen 1989a). By this point, important relationships had been formed among physicians, medical researchers, and patients over the question of AIDS treatments. Many of these physicians had large practices of AIDS patients and were frustrated, too. Further, many understood the drug approval process and could serve as informants and consultants. And their patients were ready to try new drugs, a fact of interest to pharmaceutical companies unable to get drugs tested. Congressional committees were exploring ways to facilitate these efforts. The desire to "fast-track" drugs also attracted supporters of deregulation and potential investors in AIDS drug development. These coalitions formed a potent lobby, generating proposals, as early as 1986, for community-based AIDS treatment research programs to speed the testing and release of safe drugs for treatment.[4]

Third, political activism directed at the existing system sought to modify most features of the FDA oversight process described above, activism documented by Crimp and Rolston (1990), among others. Congressional hearings were held in 1987 as a result of the agitation; as I noted above, the FDA subsequently approved *treatment IND* status for several AIDS drugs. By 1988, enough knowledge of the drug development and approval process had been amassed so that FDA commissioner Frank Young could be authoritatively challenged when in the summer of 1988 he stated that only two new drugs could be approved before 1991. Following a daylong protest by AIDS activists at the FDA in October 1988, which received extensive media coverage, the FDA relaxed some regulations; held discussions with AIDS advocates, community physicians, and others; and approved several AIDS drugs targeted by advocates. Notable among these was aerosolized pentamidine, a drug used in aerosol form to prevent and treat PCP; a lifesaving treatment for people who cannot tolerate more conventional

PCP drugs (including Bactrim, Dapsone, and injected pentamidine) and the target of sustained activism, the drug was at last given official sanction as an experimental drug (Torres 1989). At about the same time, standardized guidelines for treating PCP were released by the Centers for Disease Control (see CDC 1989).

In July 1988, the FDA reversed an earlier stand and approved the importation of unapproved AIDS drugs (although in small quantities and for personal use only [Boffey 1988c]). Activist protests, and the media coverage of them, influenced the makers of approved drugs to lower their costs. At the Fifth International Conference on AIDS in Montreal in June 1989, ACT UP presented its *National AIDS Treatment Research Agenda*, a comprehensive plan for AIDS treatment research. Extensive discussions of the agenda with FDA officials followed, focusing particularly on the need to expand access to clinical trials and better meet the ethical principles of autonomy, beneficence, and justice. Out of these discussions came more formal proposals to test promising new drugs through community-based research and make them accessible through parallel release programs (Harrington 1989, 1990). Federal and other funding was made available for such community-based treatment research in 1989. And, when Project Inform initiated unauthorized testing for trichosanthin (Compound Q) in 1989, the FDA advised against the trials but did not forbid them; when official trials were initiated, the FDA agreed to a protocol negotiated by Project Inform that would incorporate the patients from the underground trials (*Treatment Issues* 3 [15 May 1989]: 1–2).

This challenge to the federal regulatory process reflected a significant understanding of the health-care system; potentially, a broad range of policies for all drugs could be affected. AIDS treatment activism, including proposals for parallel release and community-based AIDS treatment research as well as continuing interest in a broad range of nonvalidated therapies, is tied to the AIDS movement's evaluation of technology and its determination to make technological resources available to people living with AIDS. This goal is in many ways incompatible with existing scientific and medical practice, with the current capabilities of an overburdened health-care system, and with the Left's long-standing distrust of technology. Also at stake, then, is the potential for the growth of a progressive democratic technoculture. By this, I mean that the strongest challenge to current conditions comes not from those who dismiss or denounce technology but rather from those who seek a more progressive, intelligent, and participatory deployment of science and scientific theory in everyday life.

Technology and Resistance

How was *AIDS Treatment News* financed? In 1986, there was no prospect of funding for this work, because of our lack of credentials, and because of the disinterest and hostility toward treatments in the AIDS community. "Beautiful death" ideas were strong in San Francisco, and treatment information was regarded as quackery, false hope which interfered with the process of accepting death.—John S. James, *AIDS Treatment News* (1989)

In the beginning, those people had a blanket disgust with us. And it was mutual. Scientists said all trials should be restricted, rigid and slow. The gay groups said we were killing people with red tape. When the smoke cleared we realized that much of their criticism was absolutely valid.—Anthony S. Fauci, *Washington Post* (1989)

People tell me, "You've lost your resistance." I say, "Not yet!"—Herbert Daniel, *Life before Death*

This first phase of AIDS treatment activism, which Mark Harrington later called "therapeutic utopianism" (1997), could be seen as a postmodern, post-Stonewall reworking of *Walden, Our Bodies Ourselves*, the *New England Journal of Medicine*, and *The Scarlet Pimpernel*. Its mix of strategies and sensibilities is evident in *Rockville Is Burning* (Huff 1989), a video-theater piece that takes the October 1988 AIDS action at the FDA as its starting point. The video opens with a Dan Rather–esque network anchor reporting the takeover and burning of the FDA by "AIDS terrorists," a "shadowy group that calls itself the New Center for Drugs and Biologics" and is described by inside sources as "extremely well informed and extremely dangerous." Then, during the commercial break ("When we come back: more on that puppy trapped in a well shaft in Texas"), three "terrorists"—two men and one woman—suddenly take over the broadcast studio in order to give their own account of AIDS treatment research. Using live "uplinks" from around the country to support their charges and illustrate their demands, they lay out a basic critique of the FDA's process (I return to this below). They conclude their broadcast with the following oration, which the three deliver sequentially:

> Two years ago most of us never would have conceived of marching in the streets, much less using flamethrowers or hijacking television sets. The truth is we never saw what was happening around us. We never saw beyond the facade. That is, until it hit home. Until we realized that the system was killing us and we started trying to figure out what was happening.
>
> Slowly we educated ourselves. We began to analyze the bureaucracy and the politics. We read stacks of tedious protocols and con-

tracts. We learned medical terminology and the tricks of the budget manipulators.

And slowly a pattern began to emerge. The very people with the firsthand knowledge of the epidemic were the last to be consulted. And while we were waiting for kind words and crumbs from the liberal managers of the epidemic we realized that they were simply links in the chain of command. It wasn't a question of saving lives or even of saving money—it was about power.

But when the first PWA chose to sit down and be dragged off in the middle of Wall Street, we started to take back some of that power.

This version of AIDS treatment activism, based largely on Huff's New York chapter of ACT UP, invokes several essential elements of the movement: a vision of the power structure that calls for unleashing the power and knowledge of resistant forces; expertise about technology and science, the politics of the federal bureaucracy, biomedical research, and economics; self-education; and the use of theatrical tactics, including civil disobedience, lawbreaking, infiltration, and seizing control of the media. To that repertoire, West Coast activists added the vital clearinghouse function so reliably pioneered by *AIDS Treatment News* and Project Inform. The mounting AIDS death toll was a permanent piece of scenery on the changing activist stage.

These strategies are not entirely recent.[5] Almost from the beginning of the AIDS epidemic in the United States, gay men had attempted, individually and collectively, to conceptualize scientific and clinical explanations of acquired immune deficiency, to articulate the meaning of the epidemic, and to decide for themselves what to do about it. The immediate historical context for this grassroots approach to the AIDS crisis included the antiauthoritarian legacy of post-Stonewall gay liberation; the successful struggle within the American Psychiatric Association by gay psychiatrists and gay rights groups in the early 1970s to remove *homosexuality* as an official category of mental disorder (Bayer 1981); the celebrated collaboration among physicians, research scientists, and the gay community in the clinical trials of a hepatitis B vaccine (Goodfield 1985); and the philosophy, knowledge, and tactics developed by the women's health movement. Within this context, education and prevention efforts began in the gay community even before there was general acknowledgment of a fatal epidemic disease. Randy Shilts (1987, 108) documented the élan with which Bobbi Campbell carried out his campaign as "the KS poster boy" in San Francisco's Castro District, Frances FitzGerald (1986) detailed the lengthy debates within the gay community about what to do, and Terry

Sutton's battle to change clinical trial rules was documented in *AIDS Treatment News* (see James 1991, 15–23).

While education efforts by health professionals advised abstention from "promiscuity" in general and specific "high-risk" sexual practices in particular, some gay men approached the crisis as a technical problem. The pamphlet *How to Have Sex in an Epidemic* (Callen and Berkowitz 1983) did not try to persuade gay men to abstain from sex or to relinquish the pursuit of sexual pleasure to atone for the excesses of the 1970s; instead, it provided an analysis that grew out of, rather than retreated from, the gay liberation movement. It analyzed the body (and specifically the gay male body) as an environment to be respected, technically manipulated, and cultivated to foster health rather than disease. For the authors of *How to Have Sex*, published before AIDS was officially linked to a transmissible viral agent, the epidemic was not a tale of either conservative morality or medical mortality but a crisis in which a unique body of knowledge would be needed. As Douglas Crimp (1988c) argues in "How to Have Promiscuity in an Epidemic," titled to celebrate the politics of AIDS activists, the sexual adventures of the 1970s should be seen as a key behavioral resource for inventing new, safer ways to have sex in an epidemic.[6]

Safer sex guidelines, soon taken up by health professionals and other constituencies at risk, are widely acknowledged to have affected both the scope and the public perception of the epidemic. Treatment, in comparison, seemed a will-o'-the-wisp in the light of the apparent reality that AIDS was "untreatable" and "incurable." On a local level, AIDS workers and PWAs sometimes discouraged the quest for treatments as a diversion of resources from human services and approved clinical management and sometimes, too, as a denial of death (for a fuller analysis, see Douglas and Pinsky 1989). A political effort for basic and treatment research at the federal level continued, producing appropriations from Congress in 1986 for scientific research and drug development.

At the same time, something else was happening at the grass roots. Although prevention was not a high-tech solution, it was nevertheless based on a body of technical knowledge and behavioral experience. By the mid-1980s, communication about living with AIDS through anecdotal reports and newsletters gradually put into circulation the news that more people seemed to be living longer. Some of the reported self-treatments relied on the established literature of holistic medicine and self-care; some testified to ways of clinically managing the opportunistic infections that were the main cause of suffering and death (I have mentioned prophylaxis to prevent and treat PCP); and some described drugs and treatments identified through original research, expert consultation, cross-cultural communication, and/or personal experimentation. These reports testified to the resourcefulness and determination of people who have decided that they will try anything, break any law, and do whatever is necessary to get the treatments they perceive to be needed. Underground networks were set up to provide drugs and treatment: the first guerrilla clinic was founded in San Diego in late 1985 (Geitner 1988); buyers' clubs also formed to obtain and distribute both gray market (unapproved) and black market (illegal) drugs, in some cases importing or smuggling drugs in bulk into the United States from Japan, Germany, Mexico, France, or wherever else they were available (Kolata 1988b; Greyson dir. 1989b; Arno et al. 1989; Arno and Feiden 1992; Epstein 1996).

An important catalyst for directing these efforts toward a systematic challenge of the industrial-regulatory loop was Larry Kramer's June 1987 speech to the annual Gay and Lesbian Town Meeting in Boston. I report this in some detail not because Kramer is a model of activism but because the speech exemplifies a vision of the federal AIDS effort that helped establish the direction and operating mode of ACT UP and articulated a general shift in emphasis among some activists from prevention to treatment. In this speech, Kramer, a writer and founder of Gay Men's Health Crisis in 1982 and ACT UP in 1987, tells the gay community that its successful efforts to get research funded have been for nothing because the system is not working.[7] In seven years, the only drug that has been produced is AZT, he says, which is highly toxic. Gay men must have a death wish, he says, to sit back and let themselves be killed, and he lists all the things they could be doing but aren't to make the federal system do its job.

Kramer's polemic is a brilliant call to activism and a stirringly cynical analysis of a government bureaucracy. To emphasize his main thesis, Kramer (1987, 37–39) dismantles, piece by piece, every institution in which his audience may still have faith:

> No one is in charge of this pandemic, either in this city or this state or this country. It is as simple as that. And certainly no one who is compassionate and understanding and knowledgeable and efficient is even anywhere near the top of those who are in charge. Almost every person connected with running the AIDS show everywhere is second-rate. I have never come across a bigger assortment of the second-rate in my life. And you have silently and trustingly put your lives in their hands. You—who are first-rate—are silent. And we are going to die for that silence.

The money appropriated by Congress to fight AIDS, says Kramer, is not being spent; for example, the NIH was given $47 million just to test new drugs, which it is not doing:

> When I found out about three months ago that $47 million was actually lying around not being used, when I knew personally that at least a dozen drugs and treatments just as promising as AZT, and in many cases much less toxic, were not being tested and were not legally available to us, I got in my car and drove down to Washington. I wanted to find out what was going on.

Kramer then tells his audience about each federal official in the AIDS chain of command. He says that Dr. C. Everett Koop, the U.S. surgeon general, is out of the loop—outspoken but powerless. He says that Dr. Otis Bowen, secretary of health and human services and the one official who reports directly to President Ronald Reagan, has still—after seven years—not said anything significant about the AIDS epidemic. He says that Dr. Robert Windom, Bowen's assistant, is exceptionally ill informed about AIDS and exceptionally dumb—"if his IQ were any lower," one aide told Kramer, "you'd have to water him." He says that Dr. Lowell Harmison, Windom's assistant, actually believes that gay people *intentionally* give blood to pollute the nation's blood supply. Kramer continues:

> Dr. Harmison reports to Dr. Windom, who reports to Dr. Bowen, who reports to the President. . . . I am here to tell you that I know more about AIDS than any of these four inhumane men, and that any one of you here who has AIDS or who tends to someone who has AIDS, or who reads all the newspapers and watches TV, knows more about AIDS than any of these four monsters. And they are the four fuckers who are in charge of AIDS for your government—the bureaucrats who have the ultimate control over your life.

Then he gets to the NIH, directed by Dr. James Wyngaarden, and to Dr. Anthony Fauci, director of the National Institute of Allergies and Infectious Diseases (NIAID) of the NIH,

> the single most important name in AIDS today . . . who has probably more effect on your future than anybody else in the world. . . . Dr. Fauci is an ambitious bureaucrat who is the recipient of all the buck passing and dumping-on from all of the above. He staggers, without complaint, under his heavy load. No loudmouth Dr. Koop he. . . . Dr. Fauci, of all the names in this article, is certainly not the enemy. Because he is not, and because I think he does care, I am even more

angry at him for what he is not doing—no matter what his excuses, and he has many. Instead of screaming and yelling for help as loud as he can, he tries to make do, to make nice, to negotiate quietly, to assuage. An ambitious bureaucrat doesn't make waves.

Yes, Dr. Fauci reports to Dr. Wyngaarden, who reports to Dr. Windom, who reports to Dr. Bowen, who reports to the President.

Kramer's house-that-Ron-built exposé of the federal AIDS effort confirmed in blunt language what official reports were saying more guardedly. It served as a bulletin from the front, and its content and anger also suggested a strategy for action. Between June 1987 and June 1989 ACT UP chapters formed in many U.S. cities with the aim to get "drugs into bodies" by whatever means possible. In July 1987, ACT UP New York staged a round-the-clock vigil at Memorial Sloan-Kettering Hospital in New York, a designated AIDS treatment evaluation unit (ATEU), one of nineteen centers across the country established by the NIH to test new AIDS drugs; with $1.2 million in funding, Sloan-Kettering had by July 1987 enrolled only thirty-one patients in drug trials. ACT UP's public protest and factual leafleting were appreciated by frustrated health care professionals; investigations in the wake of the vigil identified the many points at which the ATEU system was not working and initiated changes for improving it (Crimp and Rolston 1990). Calling for a "Manhattan Project" on AIDS, activists repeatedly used military metaphors to describe their situation. "Living with AIDS," said Vito Russo (1988, 65) at a rally at the Department of Health and Human Services in October 1988, "is living through a war which is happening only for those people who are in the trenches." "You cannot underestimate the therapeutic value of feeling like a soldier in the war against AIDS," said Dr. Nathaniel Pier (quoted in Zonona 1988). Invoking the grounds on which this war was being waged, Nancy Wechsler (1988) wrote of the 11 October 1988 action by twelve hundred demonstrators at the FDA that, "by the end of the nine-hour blockade, 176 of us had been arrested, and by current estimates, eighteen more Americans had died of AIDS."

If the fight for alternative AIDS treatments within PWA and HIV-infected networks underscored the self-empowerment and antiauthoritarian stance of AIDS activists, the organized challenge underscored a sophisticated understanding of the medical-industrial complex and how to turn its own tactics against it. "ACT UP! FIGHT BACK! FIGHT AIDS!" became ACT UP's working policy, a policy that paired extensive background research with an increasingly professional campaign to educate the media and, in turn, to influence public perception of the treatment crisis. According to Crimp and Rolston's documentary chronicle (1990), by the Fifth International AIDS Conference in Montreal in June 1989 ACT UP chapters had held successful actions at the Brooklyn Bridge, the Department of Health and Human Services, the FDA, Wall Street, the New York Stock Exchange, *Cosmopolitan* magazine, New York City Hall, Kowa Pharmaceuticals, the Democratic and Republican conventions, the Golden Gate Bridge, Rockefeller Center, the New York State capitol at Albany, University Hospital in Newark, New Jersey, Memorial Sloan-Kettering Hospital, the Los Angeles County Hospital, Shea Stadium, the Hall of Justice in Washington, D.C., and meetings of the Presidential AIDS Commission.

The goals of AIDS treatment activism were initially tailored quite precisely to the working procedures and principles of the FDA, outlined above. The *National AIDS Treatment Research Agenda* constructed by ACT UP (1989a) in consultation with many other groups and projects, called for changes in basic principles in the testing of AIDS drugs, proposed alternative models for clinical trials, and listed concrete research priorities (drugs and treatments).[8] The principles section of the document called for greater participation in the design and execution of clinical trials by people with AIDS and HIV and their advocates; rapid testing and distribution of all promising drugs; a search for drugs that fight the entire spectrum of HIV's clinical manifestations, not just flashy antiviral drugs; inclusion in clinical trials of women, people of color, children, and others traditionally excluded (including those found to be intolerant of AZT); the design of trials for the "real world" of health care in which treatment for infections is given but placebos are not; reasonable inclusion criteria; humane and compassionate evaluations of efficacy; and access to trials and promising treatments regardless of personal income. In addition, the agenda called for increasing funding of the entire drug research-and-development network and for the establishment of an international, up-to-date registry of clinical trials and treatments for HIV infection and related opportunistic infections. (Arno and Feiden [1992, 23] note, however, that, between 1982 and 1991, the FDA AIDS budget stayed virtually flat; in contrast, the NIH AIDS research budget increased from $5.5 to $87 million.)

At this point, several pioneering projects outside the federal establishment began attempting to institute some of these changes. Parallel-track programs would enable the testing of drugs on patients who had been excluded, for a variety of reasons, from conventional experimental trials (Harrington 1989). Community-based AIDS treatment research organizations, such as Project Inform in San Francisco and the Community Research Initiative (CRI) in New York City, began working directly with pharmaceutical companies to test drugs outside the rigidly controlled environment of major medical centers. Among other things, Project Inform organized underground trials of Compound Q, which for a time seemed to place the whole initiative in jeopardy (Kolata 1990; Epstein 1996). The CRI organized a number of trials, several sponsored by drug companies. The key trial, involving 225 patients, collected data that at last made possible the approval of aerosolized pentamidine (L. Altman 1988b; Torres 1989). Sixty physicians participated; the CRI's sponsorship guaranteed the speedy recruitment of research subjects. The CRI also launched quick studies to monitor the effects of unproved underground treatments used by many AIDS patients. "If people are taking it, that's almost reason enough to study it," said Tom Hannan. "If something works, great. If it is ineffective or harmful, we want to get the word out" (quoted in Zonona 1988).

Some academic researchers questioned the value of research data gathered by community physicians and charged that such programs would inevitably threaten the integrity of the clinical trials process and destroy the federal AIDS effort. Health care consumer advocates who had fiercely fought for tougher regulation agreed (Kolata 1988c). Yet scientific advisory committees of community-based AIDS research programs typically included representatives of academic medicine and basic science research. Both resistance and support reflected the growing ferment over the bureaucratic federal approval process as well as the urgently felt need to get more people with AIDS and HIV infection into clinical drug trials. Indeed, the federal government at last established a $6 million program to promote community-based AIDS treatment research throughout the country; a major goal was to enroll groups traditionally underrepresented in academic clinical research—HIV-infected women, minorities, drug users, children and infants, and those excluded from other trials for other reasons. Likewise, the American Foundation for AIDS Research announced that it would contribute resources to fund pilot programs. In part, the change was a pragmatic one: if a single "magic bullet" would not emerge to cure AIDS and its various manifestations and complications, the search would have to be made for a combination of agents to keep the virus inactive, to revitalize the immune system, and to treat the range of clinical problems that HIV can cause. Thus, dozens of drugs would have to be tested on tens of thousands of volunteer subjects. A serious impediment to this goal was the failure to enroll enough subjects in conventional controlled clinical trials. Breaking new scientific and ethical ground, these community-based programs sought to produce scientifically valid findings under more flexible conditions than conventional clinical trials and to reconcile the conflicting goals of scientific investigators and human experimental subjects.

The activist monologue that concludes *Rockville Is Burning* efficiently recapitulates the history and principles of AIDS treatment activism, including its commitments to civil disobedience, self-empowerment, and technological expertise ("Treatment: Understand it in order to demand it" [Douglas 1989, 2]). Like *Seize Control of the FDA* (Bordowitz and Carlomusto 1988), a documentary video of the FDA action, and *The Pink Pimpernel* (Greyson dir. 1989b), a romantic adventure about the smuggling of underground AIDS drugs, *Rockville Is Burning* manipulated conventional cultural narratives and representations to tell an alternate story. Finally, AIDS treatment activism did not depend on an us/them division in which the category *us* is good, pure, natural, and human while the category *them* is bad, profit seeking, contaminated, and cold-bloodedly technological. Rather, out of available resources it assembled a complex conception of the body and a multilayered strategy for rescuing it from disease and death. This conception was framed as provisional but nevertheless as a theory for everyday life that could be used to guide practical actions. Over the long term, experiments such as community research initiatives promise to make a unique contribution to the process of producing knowledge. The strength of their guiding theoretical frame lies not in a resistance to orthodox science but in strategic conceptions of "scientific truth" that leave room for action in the face of contradictions. This makes it possible to seek local, partial solutions and to give more attention to difference and diversity.

AZT on the Head of a Pin

I'm afraid that the AZT argument is a kind of magnet for people's anti-establishment feelings. Whereas that might be okay under a lot of circumstances, it's not okay when we're talking about life and death choices. This is a medical decision, not a political or philosophical one.—Martin Delaney, in Douglas 1989

Essential Oils are wrung—
The Attar from the Rose
Is not expressed by Suns—alone—
It is the gift of Screws—
—Emily Dickinson, "[Essential Oils are Wrung]"

The AIDS/HIV epidemic is, I have argued, cultural and linguistic. But it is also biological and medical and takes its continuing toll on real human bodies. Despite the energy, effectiveness, and uptopian moments of AIDS treatment activism, a democratic technoculture is not a pretty place. Deep divisions over theory, practice, and credibility mark the movement as much as its breakthroughs and coalitions. Armed with AIDS treatment activism as a model and the Internet as a vast new world of resources, we enter the "century of the life sciences" still burdened with uncertain knowledge, competing knowledges, and fragile bodies.[9] As AIDS treatment alternatives become available and yield failures as well as successes, tensions, disputes, and schisms are inevitable. I wish therefore to look closely at ongoing disagreements about zidovudine, or AZT. As consensus and routinization around treatment with zidovudine evolved, the divisions at the heart of treatment struggles tended to become less visible. The early AZT debate, then, helps illuminate questions of theory and practice that will continue to put AIDS and all treatment activism to difficult tests.

Manufactured by the Burroughs-Wellcome Corporation, zidovudine was for several years the only approved drug for the treatment of the spectrum of AIDS-associated problems. Derived from the sperm of herring, it had been tried as a cancer chemotherapy in the 1950s and abandoned as too toxic and expensive, then retrieved in the FDA's move to test drugs "off the shelf" for effectiveness against AIDS. As soon as benefits were claimed in corporate-sponsored Phase II trials in September 1986, the placebo trials were cut off, and the drug was distributed in limited quantities under a treatment IND until its full FDA approval in March 1987. In August 1989, the NIAID reported that AZT had been found to be beneficial in asymptomatic HIV-positive persons with fewer than five hundred T4 cells. According to the published study (Volberding et al. 1990), equal numbers of patients with T4 cell counts below and above five hundred were divided according to three conditions: placebo, five hundred milligrams of zidovudine daily, and fifteen hundred milligrams of zidovudine daily. Over the year in which the patients were followed, twice as many placebo patients developed AIDS or AIDS-related symptoms as those taking the drug; only 3 percent on the lower dose developed lowered counts of red and white blood cells, in contrast with 12 percent on the higher dose; and no statistical difference in efficacy was found between the higher and the lower dose, the latter being less toxic and cheaper. These findings appeared to offer a reasonable basis for optimism, and the FDA changed labeling instructions for prescribing to facilitate reimbursement by insurance or Medicaid. The price of the drug also changed over time. Because AZT was developed under the Orphan Drug Law, Burroughs-Wellcome had a seven-year monopoly (followed by a seventeen-year use patent). Protests over the cost of the drug ($8,000–$10,000 per year per patient) including pasting "AIDS Profiteer" stickers on Burroughs-Wellcome products in stores, draping a banner reading "SELL WELLCOME" above the floor of the New York Stock Exchange, and taking over an office at the company's headquarters. Although these activities, together with lobbying by a broad coalition of activists and legislators, forced Burroughs-Wellcome to lower the cost of the drug 20 percent, the company refused to share information on its production costs with congressional oversight committees (*Treatment Issues* 3 [30 October 1989]: 10).

Yet many were skeptical of the claimed benefits of AZT. Both physicians and patients in New York were perceived as uniquely recalcitrant in their resistance to AZT, with critics of the drug particularly opposing its use to prevent disease progression in asymptomatic HIV-infected people. They argued not only that the drug was toxic but that it might also destroy the very resources that the body needs to resist the destruction of the immune system. The report on AZT that led to its initial approval (Fischl et al. 1987a) was widely criticized, yet the drug's supporters argued that its potential benefits justified its release; although some subsequent studies appeared to confirm the positive results of zidovudine, at least over the short run (Friedland 1990), the negative results of the large European Concorde trial were depressing, calling into question the premises of treatment activism. By 1996, AZT was used routinely but no longer as a monotherapy.

Although the AZT controversy is gradually being resolved by what is perceived as the accumulation of scientific evidence and clinical experience, it was not the first such argument, nor will it be the last. Like other debates, it does not represent simply a local disagreement over "facts" and "truth"; it is also the distillation of deep-seated cultural discourses about how facts are produced and truth arrived at and about what values should shape this process. It is instructive, therefore, to examine these overdetermined cultural narratives in action at the second annual conference on AIDS/HIV treatment organized by the Columbia Gay Health Advocacy Project. Held at Columbia University on 19 November 1988, the conference was described in the program as designed "for the lay person on treatments and health maintenance strategies for people with AIDS, ARC, and asymptomatic HIV infection, featuring a distinguished panel of researchers, clinicians, and activists." Continuing updates on treatment information—found, for example, in the annual *Sanford Guide to HIV/AIDS Therapy* and AIDS treatment newsletters and Web sites—provide new data on the issues debated in the discussion that follows.

Panelists for the conference were told in advance to expect a well-informed and technically knowledgeable audience. On the morning of the conference, the organizer, Laura Pinsky, cautioned the audience that the day would be long and feelings would run high. Therefore: "We want to ask for a lot of cooperation in terms of not booing and hissing, which is going to take up time, alienate the panelists, and make it hard for us to invite people back next year (not to mention scaring the people from California)" (Douglas 1989, 1).

The opening speaker in the session on zidovudine was Craig Metroka, an M.D.-Ph.D. at St. Luke's/Roosevelt Hospital in New York and an editor of the *AIDS Targeted Information Newsletter.* Metroka first outlined the life cycle of HIV, noting six points in its replication process at which antiviral drugs can potentially intervene. AZT is one of a group of drugs called *nucleoside analogs* that interrupt replication fairly early on, binding with the virus's reverse transcriptase (its transcribing mechanism) and preventing it from copying its DNA into that of the host cell. Representing academic research tempered by clinical experience, Metroka is involved in the real world of AIDS treatment but is also equipped to analyze technical data in some detail. His presentation summarized what studies appeared to show as of November 1988. The results of the Phase II study showed improved short-term survival, reduced frequency and severity of opportunistic infections, and delayed progression to AIDS; it encouraged weight gain and improved overall functioning. Its toxicity was in some cases substantial, side effects including nausea, muscle ache, headache, fever, skin rash, and dementia. Because it interrupts cell replication, especially in bone marrow, it can severely deplete red and white blood cells, causing fatigue, shortness of breath, and severe anemia; after eight months, some patients experience severe leg pain (from muscle wasting).

Metroka then addressed the most controversial question: when to start AZT treatment. We know most about the severest cases, he argued; much less is known about asymptomatic seropositive patients. While a European study of three hundred patients had shown that the usefulness of AZT seems to decline after six months, the results of large studies are not expected until 1991 (but see Volderbing et al. [1990]—these studies were released early). High toxicity must be taken into account; thus, Metroka's bottom line as of November 1988 was to "use AZT only in those groups in which a survival benefit has been claimed, that is, in patients with fewer than 200 T4 cells" (Douglas 1989, 25). He makes exceptions for people whose T4 cell count is not so low if other clinical and laboratory findings suggest that their health is deteriorating. Metroka was conservative in wanting to see published scientific research before reaching conclusions about treatment yet more flexible than some biomedical scientists would be in his willingness to depart from strictly orthodox protocols. Accordingly, he provided PCP prophylaxis for patients with low T4 cell counts and argued for the discontinuation of placebo testing and the concurrent provision of helpful drugs.

Martin Delaney, founder of Project Inform in San Francisco and a central figure in negotiations between the FDA and the PWA community, then described the West Coast experience with AZT, which had been somewhat different. An early organizer of underground drug runs, Delaney operates according to fairly pragmatic rules and is loyal to a real-world constituency, not to a body of abstract biomedical principles. Speaking at the conference, he confirmed the negative side effects and agreed that the drug was overpriced, that Burroughs-Wellcome is "ripping us off," and that the drug produces serious toxicities. But, despite flaws in the original studies (Delaney was one of those who obtained the FDA data through the Freedom of Information Act), studies taken together now show, he believes, a clear pattern of usefulness and benefits that have not been duplicated by any other drug. Delaney commented as follows on coastal differences: "AZT use has not become as much of a religious debate on the West Coast as it has on the East Coast, for a variety of reasons. But I think it's important in entering this discussion to realize that AZT is not the enemy, and the people who disagree over AZT use are not the enemy. AIDS is the enemy, and we are all seeking to find solutions" (Douglas 1989, 25). Delaney then went on to outline new thinking about AZT. As treatment has matured, it has been used flexibly and carefully in particular treatment regimens rather than in a blanket, uniform fashion for everyone. AZT may be appropriate only for patients in whom viral replication is the main problem: "That's not East Coast opinion or West Coast opinion, but a simple fact of what is in the scientific literature." As for its use with asymptomatic people, West Coast logic is that, since AZT is most toxic with the sickest patients, it will be least toxic with asymptomatic people: "A lot of the problem with AZT is that we're using it at the wrong time with the wrong people." Delaney recommends early use: "The drug is *not* a poison. We do ourselves a disservice by starting from that premise or trying to prove it's a poison" (Douglas 1989, 26). Speaking for the AIDS community and arguing that people at least should be given options, Delaney values personal autonomy and individual experience.

Familiar with the script of AIDS debates, Delaney anticipated "East Coast" objections. Joseph Sonnabend, M.D., an academic researcher practicing as a private AIDS physician in New York and a pioneer of the Community Research Initiative there, at this point produced the argument that Delaney had been anticipating. Sonnabend contended that AZT *is* a "poison"; because it is not selective, it inhibits both "the replication of the virus *and* the replication of the host cell DNA. . . . It will effectively terminate chains of host DNA as well as viral DNA." In antiviral research, he observed, selectivity has traditionally been an important criterion: "For some reason in the case of HIV these principles have been abandoned." He repeated his continuing criticism that the AZT multicenter trials did not control for the quality and kind of medical care the patients received and reasserted his thesis that medical care is "the most important determinant of life and death in the short term. . . . This includes *pneumocystis* prophylaxis, but that's not the only thing" (Douglas 1989, 28; and see Sonnabend 1989). He noted that there were still no federal guidelines for overall AIDS patient management.

In Metroka, Delaney, and Sonnabend, we can identify a spectrum of views on AZT. On the basis of the rules of good scientific evidence, Metroka is ready to endorse AZT within the limits of the data. Sonnabend, often described as an independent thinker (not always a compliment in private medicine), bears the burden (no doubt at times a tiring one) of questioning the rules themselves—that is, what constitutes good scientific evidence. To do so, he must repeatedly speak his piece and get his resistance on the record. Delaney, a pragmatist with an agenda that calls for expanded options, predictably calls it counterproductive to harp on the problems of the original multicenter study—"a little like having study groups on the Council of Trent." As a representative of the activist community, Delaney signals his own credentials not by invoking science but by asserting that AZT is now endorsed by "people who hate Burroughs-Wellcome as much as I do—and there's no one who hates them more than I do" (Douglas 1989, 33).

Next to speak was Michael Lange, M.D., an associate professor at Columbia University College of Physicians and Surgeons, who contributed his own laundry list of AZT's problems. Like Sonnabend, Lange argued that the claims for the drug were not supported by good evidence and cited seven criticisms. Nor was Lange convinced that AZT has any antiviral effect or works in human beings at all. He noted that the truth about AZT is crucial to obtain, not only for the sake of patients in the United States, but because Third World countries were now discussing whether to invest in it at its unaffordable price. Not to be "strict with ourselves" here (in the First World) is to play "into the hands of the military-industrial complex at a tremendous cost" (Douglas 1989, 30).

At this point, Ronald Grossman, M.D., a private internist in New York, entered as peacemaker: "*Pace, pace* Joe, *pace* Michael. Despite all the disclaimers to the contrary, I've heard war words, and I think we need to avoid that desperately in this situation. . . . I am a clinician, not a researcher. I see real live patients who are achieving real live benefits from this drug—and plenty of them who get toxic effects, just as we see with every other drug we use in medicine." Grossman then related the apparent benefits of AZT to the familiar tripod model in which the three determinants of health care are (1) medical care, including the doctor-patient relationship, technology, and medications; (2) self-care, including diet, rest, and lifestyle; and (3) spirituality and positive thinking. "If we're offering hope with AZT," he concluded, "that strengthens the clinical benefit" (Douglas 1989, 30).

Michael Callen, an AIDS activist who had been diagnosed with AIDS in 1982, was a founder of the PWA Coalition, a writer and musician, and a patient of Joseph Sonnabend's. At the Columbia conference, he emphasized the difficulty of expressing skepticism in the context of AIDS theory. Despite his own attacks on AZT, Callen typically manages to construct a self-reflexive commentary that is always in some respects about the politics and purposes of speaking: "I realize," he said at the conference, alluding to his experiences speaking around the country, "that you can't breeze into a city or a group of people whose buzzers are going off all the time and say, cavalierly, as I have said, AZT is Drano in pill form, that it is poison." He says that he is often told to cool out, but he believes that the "rational" procedure is to look at both sides and decide. ("In prison, I've been told, if somebody with AIDS chooses not to take AZT, they're diagnosed as suffering from HIV dementia!") "In response to Dr. Grossman's curious point that AZT is hope," he added, "let's give people some non-toxic substances that are also offering hope" (Douglas 1989, 31).[10]

Neither Delaney nor Callen was a trained medical professional; nevertheless, both had extensive knowledge, a conceptual grasp of drug actions, and influence in their communities (Callen died in 1995). On AZT, they were on opposite sides, and at this point in the debate Delaney lost patience with Callen's skepticism and self-reflexivity: "This isn't an argument about how many angels can dance on the head of a pin. People's lives hang in the balance of this decision." The discussion then became heated. Lange demanded to be shown one good study on AZT. Delaney and Grossman responded that many good papers were presented at the Stockholm conference. Lange asserted that those papers also showed that AZT does nothing for the wasting syndrome that characterizes AIDS in Africa and is therefore probably *not* an antiviral drug. Delaney retorted that *of course* AZT is an antiviral: "I can't find many people outside this room or outside of this table who suggest that that's the case" (Douglas 1989, 33). Laura

Pinsky, the moderator, intervened at this point by asking Metroka, as coeditor of a treatment newsletter, to sum up AZT's efficacy. "Reviewing the literature," Metroka responded, "I would say that AZT has efficacy, while the drug is clearly not for everyone." Pinsky then commented that the conference organizers deliberately set up this panel to reflect differing opinions but that the audience should know that Sonnabend, Lange, and Callen were very much in the minority. Someone from the audience shouted, "That doesn't mean they're wrong!"

Donald Kotler, M.D., associate professor of clinical medicine at St. Luke's/Roosevelt, suggested that AZT can be viewed as a "negative co-factor" in disease development, just as the existence of other viruses or infections is a "positive co-factor": "I think we've all fallen into the trap of believing that a prospective randomized placebo-controlled double-blind trial is the ultimate arbiter of truth. In point of fact, it's not. . . . I would think that as a physician there is perhaps a better truth, and the better truth is one's own experience. My experience is that in some people AZT really has worked very well, and in some people it has not. . . . [He provides two examples.] I feel looking at both those experiences that the personal experience to me is irrefutable. The FDA does not see it, but the FDA doesn't see my patients, they look at report forms" (Douglas 1989, 36). Kotler's position here is almost classically distinct from Metroka's; whereas Metroka relies on published controlled aggregate data to certify—and guard against—less formal perceptions and reports of success, Kotler trusts to the empirical lessons of observed clinical experience. The bottom line of this "better truth" is not necessarily that AZT is always good but that only the physician and patient can determine whether, for individual patients, AZT "really has worked." Direct clinical observation and individual experience are taken as unique sources of knowledge.

These perspectives roughly represent the universe of discussion regarding zidovudine at the 1988 Columbia conference.[11] But the same issues, tensions, and perspectives have surrounded subsequent developments: the apparent confirmation through U.S. clinical trials (e.g., Volberding et al. 1990) that AZT does confer benefits and the acceptance of surrogate markers (raised CD4 counts and, later, lowered viral loads) as grounds for evaluating effectiveness; debate over the precise point of intervention (what, in a forceful 1990 New England Journal editorial on early intervention, Gerald Friedland called "the golden movement") as well as the optimum drug regimen; growing tension among AIDS activists over the wisdom of the "drugs into bodies" agenda but profound disagreement over how it should be altered; the last unified ACT UP demand for better drugs and treatment research, a mass action at the NIH in May 1990; over-simplified press coverage that threatened community-based drug trials (Kolata 1989, 1990; "Don't Blame Drug Program for AIDS Deaths" 1990); the FDA's adoption in 1992 of *accelerated approval*, a new procedure for releasing promising drugs; the adoption of aerosolized pentamidine as the standard of care for PCP; the departure from ACT UP New York of leading treatment activists in January 1992 to form TAG, a treatment and action group committed to a longer haul and closer working relations with "the enemy" (i.e., the biomedical establishment); the creation by President Bill Clinton of the Office of AIDS Research at the NIH, designed to oversee and coordinate AIDS research; news from the Concorde trial, a larger, longer-term clinical trial of AZT in Europe (which researchers refused to terminate early), that AZT's benefits were short-lived, apparently conferring no sustained improvement and no overall prolongation of life; the despair of the 1993 and 1994 International AIDS conferences, where the Concorde results coincided with news that other promising drugs had also flunked their trials; basic scientific discoveries about the pathogenesis of HIV (Levy 1993), including the key 1995 finding that, from the moment it enters the body, HIV is in constant struggle with the immune system; the reiteration of hope and a proposal for new direction by John S. James, Martin Delaney, and other longtime treatment activists; the development of successful new treatments for opportunistic infections; the considerable promise of yet a new generation of drugs culminating, at the 1996 Vancouver International AIDS Conference, in widespread optimism for the first time in years; renewed leadership in primary care by the AMA (1996); and release in 1997 of four U.S. government documents formally outlining a new standard of care for HIV disease (James 1997).[12] Over this same period, the cumulative number of AIDS cases in the United States passed half a million: "a relentless tide of death" (Harrington 1997, 280).

Accompanying these developments was Peter Duesberg's continuing campaign to discredit HIV theory and to call on the population of the HIV positive to refuse drug treatment, including protease inhibitors; this increased tension between Duesberg's supporters and the majority of AIDS organizations and treatment activists. A Duesberg lecture in the Bay Area, promoted by some local AIDS groups, provoked a collective, public response. A consensus letter, addressed to the National Academy of Sciences and signed by a long list of AIDS organizations, expressed concern that Duesberg's views would have negative health consequences. *Aids Treatment News* distributed flyers outside Duesberg's lecture headed "Duesberg—and You." "When you hear Peter Duesberg, Ph.D.," the flyer began, "you should know [that] despite his tenure at the University of California, his ideas are rejected by almost 100% of AIDS scientists and doctors. They are not taken seriously" (James 1997, 7).

Important lessons for the present and future are therefore offered by the narrative themes and competing regimes of credibility on display at the 1988 Columbia conference. One central subtext is power. Callen and Delaney demonstrate a significant feature of AIDS activism: the refusal of patients to be patients and the corollary determination of research subjects to be speaking subjects. It is said of Western medicine that the patient comes to the physician's office with an illness but leaves with a disease. Disease is thus taken to represent the medical model and illness the patient's subjective experience; the primary-care physician plays a crucial role in mediating between individual subjective experience (illness) and the objective system of biomedical science (disease). But, here, we also see an insistence that patients' interests must, in some contexts, be treated as distinct from the interests of physicians. This insistence recalls anthropologist Michael Taussig's (1980) argument that the clinician's attempt to understand the patient's cultural construction of illness—the "native's point of view"—does not adequately recognize the institutional power structures that traverse the clinical experience. Despite the physician's desire to identify with the patient, "there will be irreconcilable conflicts of interest and these will be 'negotiated' by those who hold the upper hand, albeit in terms of a language and a practice which denies such manipulation and the existence of unequal control." The issue, Taussig argues, is not "the cultural construction of clinical reality" but the "clinical construction of culture" (1980, 12; for related discussion, see Clarke [1994], Odets [1995, 1996]; and Boyd [1992]).

A second underlying narrative concerns technology, equity, and who determines their distribution. Lange's invocation of responsibilities toward the Third World is one place where this surfaces explicitly. But, as Paul Douglas and Laura Pinsky (1989) have argued, concerns about equity implicitly shape domestic AIDS debates as well. The resistance to early intervention in New York, they suggest, in part reflected the sorry state of health-care delivery and social support services. It is not responsible, some activists and clinicians believe, to advocate early intervention—whether early use of AZT, PCP prophylaxis, good nutrition, or combination therapies—when such treatment cannot be obtained by most HIV-infected people. When Friedland (1990) emphasized the obvious medical benefits of early use AZT, he also acknowledged the staggering economic and policy implications of adopting early intervention strategies (see also

Arno et al. 1989). In the 1990s, although U.S. media coverage of AIDS remains remarkably noninternational, our relationship and responsibility to people with AIDS in less-developed countries have become increasingly controversial. A prominent dispute in the *New England Journal of Medicine* (Angell 1997) brought many of these issues into public view: Martin (1997) produced a briefing book on the controversy for the ACAS, the Association of Concerned African Scholars; related ethical and economic questions are raised by Garrett (1992), Bond et al. (1997), L. Altman (1995), Connors and McGrath (1997), Farmer et al. (1996), "AIDS Epidemic, Late to Arrive" (1996), and Mann and Tarantola (1996).

Appeals to established scientific fact function to support positions already held. At one extreme are officials and scientists upholding the value of strict clinical trial protocols, at the other AIDS activists who likewise support their views by referring (as Delaney does) to the "simple fact of what is in the scientific literature." As Karl Mannheim long ago argued in *Ideology and Utopia* ([1936] 1985), out of prolonged social debates arise steadfast defenders and passionate challengers of the status quo who are equally skilled at constructing different interpretations about the "facts" of the world to support their cause. To dispute these "facts" becomes increasingly difficult over time because the gradual acceptance of one interpretation tends also to naturalize the processes and assumptions through which it was arrived at. At the same time, as observers of scientific practice have argued, once "facts" are widely accepted, they become synonymous with reality and truth and in some sense render the quest for truth irrelevant or uninteresting (Fleck [1935] 1979; Knorr-Cetina 1981; Latour and Woolgar [1979] 1986; Fujimura and Chou 1994; Epstein 1996).

Latour and Woolgar ([1979] 1986) go further, however, when they suggest that the authority to define reality is reinforced by an intersection of interests; *reality*, indeed, may be defined as that set of statements that has become too costly to give up. This takes us to the heart of the impatience that "practical" people often express toward "theory"—Delaney's charge, for instance, that to continue to criticize the early AZT data is "like holding study groups on the Council of Trent" or that "this isn't an argument about how many angels can dance on the head of a pin." This is always a dismissive comment, designed to characterize the opponent's argument as scholastic when "people's lives hang in the balance of this decision." But it is also an enactment of power that asserts that "reality"—the set of statements too costly to give up—is now taken as settled and is no longer vulnerable to questions of abstract theory.[13]

Beyond Vancouver 1996: The Crisis Is Not Over

I'm wanting something new
Say, have you got a clue
where I can get a hold of some
Compound Q?
Compound Q—Antabuse—Acyclovir:
I got the drug—right—here!
—Ron Goldberg, "Fugue for Drug Trials"

As a person with HIV, there is no meeting anywhere, anytime that you are not "experienced" enough to attend. There is no science that you do not have the right to understand, criticize, or direct. You do not have to accept any government's lack of urgency. . . . Science is made. It is not a gift from the heavens.—"Welcome to Vancouver," ACT UP flyer, Eleventh International Conference on AIDS, 1996

There was a lot of euphoria, but there was also a wistfulness about crossing over. From then on we were sort of inside/outside, and not just outside; and [we] sort of lost innocence. I knew that we would never be so pure and fervent in our belief that we were right, because we were actually going to be engaged and, therefore, be more responsible for some of the things that actually happened.—Mark Harrington

In October 1988, when activists stormed the FDA, two people with AIDS in the United States were dying every hour. By May 1990, when activists targeted the NIH, the ACT UP poster claimed ONE AIDS DEATH EVERY 12 MINUTES. As we approach the third decade of the epidemic and the relation of AIDS prevention to treatment to research grows more intense and fraught with controversy and responsibility, how to have theory in an epidemic becomes an even more crucial question. Like AZT, Compound Q, and aerosolized pentamidine, protease inhibitors and AIDS cocktail therapies hold out, for a brief time, the promise of a magical cure for HIV— a cure that AIDS scientific theory had long declared impossible and that was at odds with the provisional, partial vision of science and truth that I have been attributing to the first phases of AIDS activism. This makes the horse-racing metaphor underlying "Fugue for Drug Trials" all the more appropriate, for, as both the history of science and the *Racing Form* testify, magical things sometimes happen, and no movement can or should fully arm itself against hope or fully repress the desire that the unfulfillable will be fulfilled. A significant requirement for effective AIDS intervention is informed democratic involvement in the production and deployment of research and treatment. Involvement in both the agenda-setting and the procedural practices of biomedical science seeks to guarantee that long shots as well as favorites, proletarians as well as blue bloods, will all have their chance to run.

Although resistance to AZT has faded as newer therapies have superseded or supplemented it, its story retains symbolic importance—and pedagogical value, too, as other new and controversial drugs and treatments and technologies arrive that must be understood and evaluated. In one form or another, divisive debates and seemingly irreconcilable positions about research and treatment are here to stay. Indeed, informed activism about the politics and practice of knowledge is a requirement if we are genuinely to face the "permanent crisis" that constitutes the U.S. health-care system.[14] But, in a society with great wealth and profound structural inequities, informed activism must also preserve some degree of fluidity— and therefore of permanent crisis—about its own goals and strategies. Although what seem to be mutually exclusive discourses and world visions offer many points of contact, coalition, and negotiation, their differences cannot be transcended by commonsense assertions about what is true, natural, human, or "best" or by the eventual emergence of apparently consensual truths about AIDS, HIV, treatment, and other once controversial questions. Apparent resolutions in such a crisis can be neither stable nor permanent because they are always, to some degree, conjunctural.

Yet, as Meurig Horton (1989, 171) argues, innovative structures like community-based AIDS treatment research programs offer "a social and theoretical space where the possibilities of research and treatment can be thought differently." Like the debates that generated them, such programs furnish lessons about the rules, conventions, and values that anchor the production of knowledge and determine how "truth" in any given context will be decided. This will be useful as the struggle broadens, as it eventually must, to challenge the health-care system itself. It is also clear that contradictory evidence and widely divergent interpretations exist, although these are not always neatly correlated with particular professional systems (Abbott 1988). As I have argued throughout this book, we draw on diverse cultural resources to make sense of a complex and devastating crisis. The AIDS epidemic and the clinical reality of HIV infection and AIDS are intrinsically complicated and can be simplified only for specific strategic purposes. What is incontrovertible is that the volatile interactions entailed by these broadly inclusive debates—in both the short and the long term—will have consequences not only for people with HIV infection but for the culture as a whole. For they involve significant renegotiations of the geography of cultural struggle—of sources of biomedical expertise, relationships between doctor and patient, relations of the general citizenry to science and to government bureaucracies, and debates about the role and ownership of the body. Not only are the basic definitions and self-images of many constituencies at stake but also the institutional and cultural structures and the concrete material resources that shape their relations to each other and their relative empowerment and effectivity within the culture as a whole.

Like that for the right to experience pleasure, the struggle for the right to preserve health is founded on a political and theoretical analysis of the body—how it works, what it experiences, and how it exists and is valued in society. Community-based treatment research does not make treatment decisions easier, but it enables them to take place in a context radically different from what was available a decade ago. And it provides a way of engaging, as a lived reality, with the question of how many angels can dance on the head of a pin. This is what theory in an epidemic requires; it is one way to begin to put one's body where one's head is (or vice versa), to show courage when too many people have already died, and to try to come to terms with what Donna Haraway (1989a, 32) calls "the problematic multiplicities of postmodern selves." The activist struggle against the AIDS epidemic has required intense vigilance, ongoing self-education, continually revised strategies and alignments, and the gradual acceptance of the reality that certainty may often be temporary and contextual. This struggle can be seen as a narrative about the evolution of a radically democratic technoculture and about whose rules, in this democracy, we are to live by. But changing the rules, or whose rules they are, will not make the world easier, more stable, or less postmodern.

Earlier, I described Bob Huff's 1989 video *Rockville Is Burning*, which laid out the activist agenda to get "drugs into bodies." Only such an agenda—presented unequivocally and pursued relentlessly—had any hope of success. The truth as ACT UP dramatized it was a powerful narrative, worthy of challenging the soothing story of scientific method and progress that it sought to disrupt. But it was not, could not have been, free from dogma. Activists had to learn to appeal to—indeed to generate and to believe—facts, statistics, experiences, conclusions, and scientific arguments supporting their own positions. Even at its most strategic, their argument, in part, had to be, We are the ones who are dying, and we are the ones whose knowledge and experience must dictate what is to be done. Eventually, the treatment activists who moved closer to the site of scientific production also, almost inevitably, moved closer to the positivist criteria for evaluating truth that they had earlier questioned or satirized, thereby accepting one set of rules over others.[15]

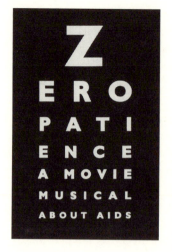

Early in Greyson's musical Zero Patience (1993), the character of Sir Richard Burton performs an ode to empirical science: "A culture of certainty," he sings, "will wipe out every doubt." By the end of the film, virtually every apparent certainty has been called into question, including some of the most treasured certainties of AIDS treatment activism (9.4). The character of George, losing his sight from CMV, is also losing his patience with treatment orthodoxies, no matter whose they are. But even as his poignant refrain asserts this condition of radical uncertainty—"I know I know I know I know that I don't know"—Greyson's story of the stories of the epidemic never forgets what we do know: that a narrative can be powerfully persuasive, that a democratic technoculture must find ways to acknowledge the power of competing narratives, and that, for all the power of narrative, this epidemic leaves hundreds of thousands of people dead.

John Greyson's 1993 feature-length musical *Zero Patience* takes up the story of the epidemic and treatment activism a little further down the road. Envisioning a democratic technoculture better equipped to acknowledge the persuasive power of competing narratives, *Zero Patience*, performing its own unique cultural work, is ultimately a dense critique of arrogance and taken-for-granted certainties, no matter whose they are.

In *Zero Patience*, Greyson tells the story of the stories of the epidemic, condensing into one hundred minutes most of the staple narratives and counternarratives of the 1980s and giving them his own matchless spin. At the center is the figure of Patient Zero, the French-Canadian flight attendant Gaetan Dugas, whose story Randy Shilts told, or mistold, with such relish and repugnance in *And the Band Played On* (1987). As Douglas Crimp says, Shilts's account was not about a human being but about an obligatory agent of contagion, the Typhoid Mary that every epidemic requires ("The Man Who Brought Us AIDS," trumpeted the publicity for *Band*). "The real problem with Patient Zero," writes Crimp, "is that he already existed as a phobic fantasy in the minds of Shilts' readers before

Shilts ever wrote the story" (Crimp 1997, 645). In contrast, in Greyson's musical, Zero anchors his own story and inspires many more. The lyrical opening number, in which several delicious young men gathered at a swimming pool sing, dive, and perform Busby Berkley–style synchronized swimming, sketches the life stories of gay men in the AIDS epidemic ("We were boys who loved our bodies") and asks for continued storytelling on their behalf—as though such stories, like Scheherazade's in *The Arabian Nights*, could save their lives. Counterposed to Zero is Sir Richard Burton, legendary Victorian sexologist and dashing translator of *The Arabian Nights*, himself still miraculously alive and employed to keep others alive, in a way, through his position as chief taxidermist at the Toronto Museum of Natural History. Burton wishes to tell Zero's story yet again, making it the jewel in the crown of his "Hall of Contagion" exhibit at the museum ("It will create a King Tut–like sensation when it opens," he assures his superior). Where Zero's swimming pool anthem is silhouetted against a radiant sky, Burton's ode to empirical science— "Culture of Certainty"—is delivered against a back projection of scientific slides, a familiar kaleidoscope of clichéd AIDS images.[16]

As the musical unfolds, these stories and other codes and conventions of AIDS narratives are self-consciously framed, contrasted, and denaturalized: repeatedly called "tales," "stories," and "histories," they are used and manipulated to furnish data for grant proposals, fed to the media, distorted by the media, juxtaposed to other stories, told differently by different people, espoused and repudiated, hammed up, camped up, acted out, politicized, ridiculed, idealized, and discredited. In this sense, they represent competing regimes of credibility (Epstein 1996, 355), placed in visible collision.

"For Shilts," writes Crimp (1997, 648), "history is the story of what actually happened. For Greyson, history is what we make by telling a story." This is a musical about theory in an epidemic: it asks us to think about how knowledge is produced, about how we come to accept truths about AIDS, about the contingent status of what we know, and about the beneficiaries of competing accounts. By the end, Burton himself has fallen in love with Zero; they have screwed in one of Burton's own dioramas (not to mention a hot tub); in an intimate duet of assholes, they have pondered some of AIDS's persistent philosophical preoccupations ("An asshole's just an asshole," sings Zero. "Your rectum ain't a grave"); the stuffed creatures in the Hall of Contagion (Typhoid Mary, the African green monkey, etc.) have come alive as sexual beings to speak (and sing and dance) for themselves; "Mis HIV" has appeared to Zero under the microscope to "tell the story of the virus" and outsing her competitors ("Weep for me, Scheherazade"); and Zero's story has been turned every which way. "A culture of certainty," sang Burton at the outset, "will wipe out every doubt"; "a culture of certainty will put us back on top." By the end of the film, virtually every self-contained "story" has been called into question, including the certainties of AIDS activism: "I know I know I know that I don't know" is an underlying musical refrain near the end. Finally, *Zero Patience* is the story of people with AIDS yet simultaneously an array of many stories always already still needing to be told.

Epilogue

Given the complexities and historical significance of the AIDS epidemic that this book has attempted to chronicle, I cannot bring myself to call this final section a *conclusion.* Indeed, in the face of an epidemic that continues to continue, the word is arrogant and untrue. "The end of AIDS" is loudly trumpeted, but statistics at home and abroad tell us otherwise. Every revision of the bibliography of this book, for that matter, has kept death alive for me as authors whose work has deeply affected my own keep dying. An epidemic, like a war, marks us for decades. Even so, these chronicles of AIDS offer several lessons about language and culture that may usefully be summarized here.

By the end of the 1980s the AIDS epidemic had been invested with an abundance of meanings and metaphors. Scientists, physicians, and public health authorities argued repeatedly that AIDS represented "an epidemic of infectious disease and nothing more." This uncompromisingly medical argument had been developed over the course of the twentieth century as medicine and public health wrenched themselves free of moral understandings of disease, and its value and power for the AIDS epidemic must not be minimized. Continually eluding such containment efforts, however, the AIDS epidemic has produced a parallel epidemic of meanings, definitions, and attributions. This semantic and cultural epidemic—what I have come to call an *epidemic of signification*—has been the subject of this book.

The sheer volume and wild diversity of AIDS's rapidly multiplying meanings underscore the strength of this semantic epidemic. The following examples represent only some of the efforts in the epidemic's first decade to articulate "what AIDS is":

1. An irreversible, largely untreatable, and ultimately fatal infectious disease.

2. A disease of the "4-H Club": homosexuals, heroin users, hemophiliacs, and Haitians.
3. A modern plague and the most urgent and complex public health problem facing the world today.
4. A minor or possibly even nonexistent health problem, sensationalized by the media for its own titillation and profit.
5. The price paid for homosexuality, anal intercourse, and/or "the homosexual lifestyle."
6. The crucible in which the field of immunology will be tested.
7. A sign that the end of the world is at hand.
8. The product of government research labs developing "Andromeda strain"–type mutant viruses for chemical and biological warfare.
9. An extraterrestrial conspiracy to weaken the human immune system and make the earth more vulnerable to alien invasion.
10. A massive human tragedy demanding charity, compassion, and care for the afflicted individuals.

Like other cultural events that are mysterious, life threatening, and indefinitely extended over space and time, the AIDS epidemic compels us to try to make sense of it—hence its enormous power to generate meanings. Yet we need to push past this commonsense conclusion and ask more precise questions about the conditions under which meanings proliferate. What are the key cultural and structural characteristics that promote the generation of meanings? What are the processes and mechanisms through which individual meanings originate? Whose discourses speak through particular understandings of the AIDS epidemic? Whose are obscured? And what are we to make of them?

The documented record of the AIDS epidemic, constituting a rich corpus for the exploration of these questions, provides several instructive lessons about the workings of language in culture. As even this partial inventory suggests, language, culture, authority, and evidence—and undoubtedly other factors—interact in the production of meaning.

Moreover, the term AIDS has come to be linked to a series of preexisting worldviews, institutional discourses, material realities, and cultural phenomena—which in turn represent a range of positions and interests, draw on multiple resources and strategies, originate from different places within the culture, and point toward different strategies for treatment and control. Although "AIDS" is new, it is already peopled.

Third, although it is commonplace to speak of "our society" and "our culture," these myriad perspectives on AIDS—what I am loosely calling *meanings*—do not testify to a monolithic zeitgeist or historical moment. Rather, they suggest that generalizations about "the culture" should be made with great caution: *the culture* produces a diversity of meanings. Only a careful examination and analysis can identify where these meanings come from, who they represent, to what degree they are disseminated, what cultural and intellectual work they accomplish, and what ends they serve.

Fourth, the multiple meanings attributed to AIDS in the United States attest to the individuality and creativity that can exist within a complex democracy and even be preserved in print. At the same time, these meanings do not enjoy perfectly equal status in the marketplace of ideas. For much of the 1980s, the notion of AIDS as an irreversible, communicable, largely untreatable, and usually fatal viral disease (the first example cited above) represented a widely accepted view among scientists, physicians, and other opinion leaders, not to mention people with AIDS themselves. Disseminated through public health institutions, the biomedical and the general media, and the arts, this view of AIDS constituted the media's boilerplate on the epidemic—that is, the authoritative, consensus view that could be taken for granted as a starting point for commentary—and dominated research, prevention, and treatment efforts long after counterevidence had begun to emerge. An important goal of people with AIDS and their advocates from at least the mid-1980s was to challenge each element of mainstream AIDS orthodoxy, but to do so required concentration and unrelenting efforts to refute claims of rampant contagion, develop strategies to reduce transmission, demand and document experimental treatments, and publicize evidence of long-term survival.

Fifth, as contexts change, so do the ways that meanings function. That is, meanings do different things in different times and places. Broad in scope and deeply entrenched in history is the tenth meaning listed above, a liberal humanist view of AIDS as a terrible human tragedy that demands care and compassion. In the United States and elsewhere in the world, in both secular and religious societies, perhaps no single view of the epidemic has done more important cultural work: the call for compassion and caring has served important social ends, asking citizens to rise above prejudice, discrimination, and fear and help the suffering. At the same time, no other single view is so overarchingly irrefutable, so unreflectingly embraceable, or so glibly deployable in short-circuiting discussions of structural inequalities, politics, and economic needs. Thus, this meaning, too, AIDS activists came to believe they must challenge—and they did so by mapping onto this "human tragedy" the repeated failure of social, biomedical, and political institutions to carry out their traditional responsibilities in times of epidemics and comparable disasters. Hence, this inventory enables us to compare precisely how "the massive human tragedy" of Western humanism was strategically rewritten to produce an activist account and encourage collective, political action. In this rendering, AIDS is "a massive human tragedy compounded and prolonged by prejudice, ignorance, structural inequalities, and gross political negligence" (see, e.g., Crimp 1992; Düttman 1996).

Sixth, some meanings live their lives in public; others do not. Gradual shifts in the *dominant meaning of AIDS* (roughly synonymous here with *mainstream media boilerplate*) took place very much in the public eye: the annual international AIDS conferences, for instance, regularly producing revised consensus views, were consistently covered by major media outlets. Other meanings on the list, in contrast, were systematically excluded from such arenas. The view that AIDS is a sign that the world is ending, for example, has a different and more specialized domain; despite its revelatory intensity for believers as well as the Christian Right's efficiently orchestrated influence on U.S. responses to the epidemic, an apocalyptic formulation of AIDS's ultimate meaning has not supplanted the secular boilerplate. Similarly, despite the zest and ingenuity with which so-called conspiracy theories (like entries 8 and 9 above) have been embraced by individuals and groups around the world, the numerous scenarios of HIV and AIDS as products of clandestine chemical and biological warfare or extraterrestrial activity are not among the AIDS 101 official building blocks (although they are certainly linked to AIDS in popular culture). Nor does a view of AIDS as a media concoction rate much air time on "World News Tonight with Peter Jennings," for the agenda-setting processes of major media outlets largely filter out ideas that depart too extravagantly from the dominant view. Nevertheless, of course, these "minor" or "minority" meanings may enter implicitly or explicitly into specialized or local debates about AIDS and, indeed, into debates about issues other than the AIDS epidemic itself—debates, for example, about borders, tariffs, and immigration policies, about the value of a "global marketplace," about the costs and scope of health care, about the value of government research, about attitudes that churches should adopt toward sex and drugs, and so on. (Moreover, we need not stray very far from "World News Tonight"— "Tony Brown's Journal," e.g., on PBS—to find "alternative" views given serious air time.)

Finally, the coexistence of dominant meanings with corollary and alternative meanings confronts us with the problem of truth, a prominent theme in AIDS discourse, and how truth can most legitimately be found. Battles over "the truth about AIDS" are sometimes little more than phatic rituals that, on the one hand, invoke "truth" in scare quotes to mark it as a deluded legacy of the Enlightenment or, on the other hand, invoke Truth, with a capital *T*, to trivialize problems of representation or politics by appealing to an underlying, stable, external "real" that dictates what truth is, whether we transcribe it right or not. Contests over the nature and formulation of truth, in turn, invoke other debates over verification of evidence, nature, scientific investigation, delusion, cultural perspective, and appropriate context. Tracking the meanings of AIDS over the years helps us formulate the professional, disciplinary, moral, political, or philosophical rules by which such battles are fought. But it also enables us to track the emergence and maintenance of more fragile, contingent, and provisional kinds of truth: scientific hypotheses to be explored, perhaps, or predictions of phenomena that are subtle and undramatic, or ideas that provide useful resources or perform important cultural work for particular communities at particular times, or truth provisionally understood or accepted in particular contexts, or truth that is understood as multifaceted and complicated.

As AIDS moves through time and through more and more communities, its narratives and explanations move with it, to recur, like urban legends, in new places, with locally inflected players and plot twists. Tracking the main themes of the meanings listed above through time and space could produce an extensive inventory of assertions of "what AIDS is," and I have identified and discussed many of these in the course of this book. For the moment, a further inventory will illustrate the ease with which these pronouncements travel, incorporate or revise new information, and adapt to diverse social and political formations:

11. A creation of the state to legitimize widespread surveillance over people's lives and regulation of their social and sexual practices.
12. A creation of biomedical scientists and the CDC to generate funding for their activities.
13. An imperialist plot to destroy the Third World.
14. A fascist plot to destroy homosexuals.
15. A CIA plot to destroy subversives.
16. A KGB plot to destroy capitalists.
17. A capitalist plot to create new markets for pharmaceutical products.
18. A scientific experiment on human beings (gay men) that will not jeopardize women's reproductive capacities.

19. A scientific experiment on human beings (people of color, women in the Third World) that will deliberately jeopardize their reproductive capacities.
20. A plague stored in King Tut's tomb and unleashed when the Tut exhibit toured the United States in 1976.

Again, this inventory offers several lessons. First, meanings that have been repeatedly discredited by the historical record and appear to retain little authority or demonstrable effect on policy do not simply stop existing. Steadfastly, and no doubt appropriately excluded from official U.S. AIDS 101 packages (which have typically held, e.g., that HIV is "an equal opportunity virus"), the notion of epidemic disease as a plague on particular kinds of people moves so easily across time and space that its very mobility is worthy of investigation. Narratives that posit some mythic "cause" or "origin" of epidemic disease were readily resurrected in the case of AIDS, even, in some cases, claimed to have tracked HIV's travel route backward from San Francisco to New York to Haiti and, finally, to "darkest Africa" (i.e., central Africa). Although some of these scenarios simply fulfill predictable patterns of blame, others more concretely reproduce the geographic origin stories of syphilis, plague, and other past epidemics.

Second, however, it is important to explore what specific cultural work these differing accounts accomplish and what material outcomes they might entail. In the 1988 congressional hearings on AIDS in Africa, for example, some experts characterized AIDS in Africa as "a new disease," others as merely one of many chronic diseases endemic to many regions of Africa. The seemingly commonsense question of whether AIDS is *new* in fact represents loaded terminology with significant economic and political stakes. In terms of economic development and foreign aid, the question involves routine and long-standing budget politics: if AIDS is "new," it can be argued that new money should be appropriated to address it; if it is "not new," its funding can legitimately be cannibalized from such existing programs as population control or maternal and child health. At the same time, the issue of AIDS's "newness" to the African subcontinent is central to continuing debates about whether HIV originated in Africa—an origin largely taken for granted by experts in the United States (one of whom suggested, at a conference in the mid-1980s, that AIDS could be taken as "Africa's revenge for the slave trade"). More fully debated outside the United States (in Europe, the United Kingdom, and, not surprisingly, many African countries), the origin of HIV and AIDS remains a question of great scientific interest and connects to other important questions: Is HIV the true cause of AIDS? Indeed, is "AIDS" a new phenomenon anywhere, that is, a new human condition caused by a new virus, or is it a widening and dramatic manifestation of growing immune system depression? And what kind of evidence should be sought and credited in exploring such questions?

Third, boundaries among popular culture, science, policy, and media are fairly permeable, each offering discursive archives—linguistic or semantic reservoirs—that furnish resources (and perhaps legitimacy) to the others. Popular culture borrows elements from science, while science borrows narratives and images from popular culture. Long after fears that HIV was a readily transmitted Andromeda-type virus gave way to accounts of less aggressive transmission, the killer virus remains alive and well in a powerful cultural imaginary—a space from which it is periodically resurrected for medical thrillers like *Outbreak* and *The Burning Zone* or documentaries like *The Hot Zone* and *The Coming Plague* and as a staple story in even the lowliest local media outlets (Ebola, flesh-eating bacteria, mad cow, etc.).

Fourth, many items on this second list seem far-fetched in the extreme, unsupported by any shred of scientific evidence or even common sense. In contrast, many items in my earlier inventory (e.g., 1, 2, 3, 5, 6, 10) include meanings that scientific authorities on AIDS/HIV have embraced at some point in the epidemic's development, pointing in support to a body of established scientific evidence. Yet scholars in the sociology of science argue that appeals to established scientific fact often function to support positions already held. At the same time, once established, scientific fact becomes increasingly difficult to dispute, for the gradual acceptance of one interpretation, one way of seeing the world, tends to naturalize the processes and assumptions through which it *was* established. As observers of scientific practice have argued, established facts become synonymous with reality and truth and in some sense render the continuing quest for truth irrelevant or uninteresting. The sociologists of science Bruno Latour and Steve Woolgar go further, however, when they suggest that the authority to define reality is reinforced by an intersection of interests, including material interests: "reality," they suggest, may in fact be defined as that set of statements that has become too costly to give up (Latour and Woolgar [1979] 1986). In examining these lists of ideas about AIDS, we should not be too eager to divide them mechanically into those that are correct and those that are not, those that represent sound scientific thinking and those that represent ignorance, stupidity, or paranoia.

There are circumstances in which such a division may be appropriate and necessary (I have mentioned public health brochures—not a perfect example, but one that will work for the moment). But, if we are seeking to chronicle the cultural life of the AIDS epidemic and understand how people have come to think about it, other observations are more interesting. Like science, many of these accounts try to make sense of AIDS by building on known facts. Take item 20, for instance—the notion that AIDS is caused by a virus released when King Tut's tomb was unsealed and unleashed on the populace when the Tut exhibit toured the United States in 1976. This account acknowledges that AIDS seemed to be new, possibly caused by some hitherto-unknown pathogen; that it first appeared in the late 1970s in major U.S. cities; and that several years might elapse between exposure and symptomatic disease. In suggesting that the opening of King Tut's tomb unleashed an ancient killer virus, the theory rather ingeniously draws on the fact that archaeologists who have entered sealed sites actually have contracted and indeed died from strange pathogens. That the Tut exhibit toured the United States in 1976 explains why the disease began showing up when it did. That it primarily afflicted homosexual men is less directly addressed: perhaps an assumption that urban gay men are well educated and therefore active museum goers played a role. Interestingly, these early AIDS theories never really die. Like urban legends with footnotes, they disappear only to rise again. Hence, in a communication to *Emerging Infectious Diseases*, Richard J. Ablin (1996) argues that ancient Egyptian papyrus texts may document the existence of HIV in the time of the pharaohs.[1]

Finally, meanings that can be loosely grouped as "conspiracy theories" warrant special attention. The list above is a tiny sampling of those cited in this book and of the vast heterogeneous corpus of accounts that exist elsewhere—their only unifying element the notion of a collusion among allied parties (often "shadowy forces") carried out in secret. Conspiracy theories help us understand what is important to people and offer lessons about why, at some level, all meanings matter. Whether the theory holds that information about AIDS is tightly controlled by an "AIDS Mafia" (an elastic category that now and then encompasses the queen of England, the pope, and Larry Kramer but more commonly features a medical and scientific elite), or an international depopulation strategy coordinated by the World Health Organization and the United Nations, or a creation of our very own "alphabet agencies" (DOD, CIA, FBI, NAS, NCI, NASA, and so on) to rule the new world order, or "Africa's revenge for the slave trade," or a way to strengthen the gene pool on Altair 7, conspiracy theories are part of the larger "epidemic of signification" that the AIDS epidemic has generated—an epidemic that must be examined and interrogated, not eradicated.

Clearly, some meanings attributed to the AIDS epidemic may reflect odd visions of the world, some apparently incompatible with the values and practices of orthodox science. Or are they? When all is said and done, few of these accounts, no matter how apparently iconoclastic, are, in the end, fundamentally incompatible with the pervasive germ theory world-view that has dominated twentieth-century life sciences. Indeed, it is striking how often these accounts—even the most tortuous conspiracy theories charging "science" with corruption, fraud, hypocrisy, and fail-ure—adopt the rhetorical apparatus of empirical scientific research: statis-tics, findings, citations, counterevidence, graphic documentation, histori-cal records, first-person testimonials, and reports of observed results.

We can point out that documenting a scenario in print does not make it so. But who are the "we," and to whom are we pointing this out? And what do we expect to accomplish? A scenario that casts "the media" or "the government" as complicit in duping the public about AIDS will not be dislodged by network news reporting or a lecture from the U.S. surgeon general. Evidence, facts, the assertion of authority: none of these will function to discredit an alternative account of truth. Indeed, as the soci-ologist John Gagnon has deftly put it, the difference between a conspiracy theory and a scientific theory is that a scientific theory has holes in it.

Finally, these inventories of meanings help us understand processes of linguistic mediation—processes, to borrow Allan Brandt's phrase, through which language enables biology and culture to meet. They help us under-stand the role of authority in the creation and maintenance of cultural capital—why, to put it somewhat differently, some meanings languish in a long-forgotten letter to the editor while others become official definitions with considerable power to shape our realities and our lives. Identifying and exploring this diversity of meanings do not tell us what the "truth" about AIDS and HIV is. But they do help us understand the rules, as I have put it throughout this book, by which truth in a given context, commu-nity, or culture is generated, accepted, or rejected.

The emergence and fate of the term AIDS over the past two decades offer a dramatic case study of a novel word and concept, just as the proliferation of meanings cited above suggests that linguistic theory and cultural the-ory have much to contribute to the analysis of the epidemic. At the same time that "AIDS" is new, however, it is always already occupied, peopled with discourse that predated it and establishing precedents for language not yet invented. The proclamations since 1996 that "AIDS is over" or that "the cure" has been found must likewise be read from within this discursive trajectory.

The evolution of the AIDS epidemic, and with it the scientific entity HIV, has occurred in a historical era when language has achieved great prominence. The language of the AIDS epidemic enables us to see language in the process of being created, modified, institutionalized, and put to use. Because we can date the beginning of the epidemic's official written record fairly precisely (i.e., with the publication of the 5 June 1981 issue of the *Morbidity and Mortality Weekly Report*), AIDS offers us a unique opportunity for investigating language at work in the culture. Many of the struggles over naming, definition, and lexicon illustrate what the philosopher Hilary Putnam (1975) calls the "division of linguistic labor" and what the historian of science Donna Haraway (1979, 1991a) calls "contests for meaning." The dissension and debate over the naming of "the AIDS virus" (HTLV-III, LAV, ARV, HIV) provide an example of such a contest for meaning—for "the struggle to construct reality." Each such cultural chronicle involves an effort to understand and evaluate a range of complicated scientific assumptions and practices, the reliability of clinical diagnosis and case definition, contradictory interpretations of serologic data and test results, highly technical genetic comparisons among different viral strains, and the various clinical manifestations of what we have come to call *AIDS*. These debates also raise questions about their own origins—that is, about the social and historical contexts in which scientific data are produced, interpreted, and put to use; about the discourses that further or complicate that mission; and about seemingly straightforward and commonsense understandings of identity, language, representation, and cultural practice.

Historians helped greatly in this task. Early on in the epidemic, those charged with managing it desperately searched history for applicable lessons. Commenting on the early 1980s, the medical historians Elizabeth Fee and Daniel Fox (1992b) wrote that "most accounts presented AIDS as a radical break from the historical trends of the twentieth century, at least in the industrialized nations: a sudden, unexpected, and disastrous return to a vanished world of epidemic disease. Epidemic disease belonged to history, a history that most had comfortably forgotten. But faced with the new threat of AIDS, people felt a need to reach back into history to discover how previous epidemics had been handled: how had societies dealt with plague, cholera, and polio?" (pp. 1–2). Accordingly, Fee and Fox titled their first edited collection of essays, published in 1988, *AIDS: The Bur-*

dens of History. By the early 1990s, however, Fee and Fox could title their second collection *AIDS: The Making of a Chronic Disease* (1992a). "The patterns of research, services, and financing of care in the 1990s," they wrote, suggest that "we are dealing not with a brief, time-limited epidemic but with a long, slow process more analogous to cancer than to cholera" (1992b, 4, 5). This transition from a concept of AIDS as a classic epidemic of acute infectious disease to that of AIDS as a chronic, potentially manageable disease represents one of the pervasive, influential, yet still contested shifts in meaning in the course of the 1980s and 1990s, one debated through personal observation and testimony, epidemiology, laboratory studies, clinical trials, and actuarial statistics.

Other histories will further illuminate this shift and the trajectory of the future (e.g., Berridge 1996; Bayer 1997). In this book, I have documented many efforts to subvert a series of conventional Western responses to fatal disease: grand modernist narratives of aesthetic transcendence, humanist celebrations of art and other eternal verities, and visions of AIDS as a tragic inevitability that must be faced, accepted, and learned from. Subversion cleared space for anger, politics, aggressive treatment and social service initiatives, safer sex campaigns, grassroots organizing and other collective actions, marches, media interventions, lawsuits, and a range of other responses. As Douglas Crimp (1989) warned, militancy must not preempt mourning. But subversion of the "beautiful death" tradition made possible experimentation and activism in memorializing activities as well. Faced with higher mortality rates than wartime and no offers of aid from Arlington National Cemetery, communities with AIDS had to pioneer new ways of burying their dead. Thus grew a diverse array of rituals, from memorial performances, commemorative videos, and underground musicals to graphic novels, rock albums, and political funerals—and, of course, the AIDS quilt, a dazzling and monumental legacy. But, for those who did not want to be remembered as "another faggot on that fucking quilt," still more alternatives evolved. In *Diseased Pariah News*, the zine-like creation of PWAs in the Bay Area, deadpan black humor and the absence of sentiment are the order of the day. When one of the magazine's founding editors died, his send-off was a funeral pyre of blazing teddy bears, photographed for *DPN*'s next cover. For others who might desire this form of solace, the editors included instructions for getting teddy bears to burn really well.

Death is not the only sacred cultural site invaded by AIDS. In January 1991, ACT UP briefly took over the "CBS Evening News with Dan Rather" and was able to shout "Fight AIDS, Not Arabs!" before the show's pro-

Eb; H; Blo; L.38 (13,4)   L 38

(13,3)   Blo 189

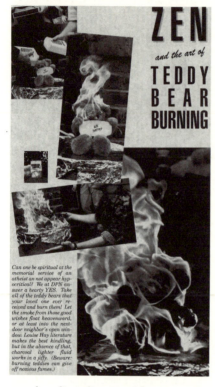

ZEN

and the art of

TEDDY
BEAR
BURNING

Can one be spiritual at the
memorial service of an
atheist an not appear hyp-
ocritical? We at DPN an-
swer a hearty YES. Take
all of the teddy bears that
your loved one ever re-
ceived and burn them! Let
the smoke from those good
wishes float heavenward,
or at least into the next-
door neighbor's open win-
dow. Louise Hay literature
makes the best kindling,
but in the absence of that,
charcoal lighter fluid
works in a jiffy. (Beware:
burning teddies can give
off noxious fumes.)

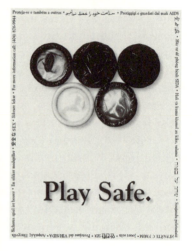

Play Safe.

Continuing chronicles of AIDS
and HIV: E1: translations of Papyrus
texts from ancient Egyptian literature are said to suggest that HIV
may have existed in the time of the
pharaohs (Ablin 1996); E2: Diseased
Pariah News (no. 3 [1991]: 10) hon-
ors a founding editor; E3: Olympic condom rings, 1996 International Olympics,
Atlanta (color Xerox, 8 x 11 inches).

ducers cut to a commercial. I have elsewhere noted the safe sex demonstration in Shea Stadium directed toward straight men, the insertion of an
AIDS critique called the *New York Crimes* into newsstands around New
York City, wrapped around its lookalike, the real *New York Times*, and so
on. At the 1996 Olympics in Atlanta, the five gold rings symbolizing the
International Games were commandeered for a safer sex message. Posters
adorned with five multicolored interlocking condoms were widely pasted
up on the walls of the Olympic Village before they were torn down by
officials for contaminating both the spirit of the games and a copyrighted
symbol.

I have argued in this book that linguistic constructions and cultural stereotypes are pervasive and play a powerful role in shaping our understandings and perceptions—among them the meanings attributed to the AIDS epidemic, HIV, and a whole constellation of surrounding issues. That linguistic constructions of the world shape our understandings of natural phenomena, from molecular structures to epidemics of infectious disease, is not good or bad; it is a condition of human life. In this book, I have tried to ask more interesting questions about language. How do particular verbal constructions (*the genetic code, the immune system, the AIDS epidemic*) develop and flourish, taking hold in cultural discourse so profoundly that they come to seem obvious even as they cloak their alternatives? What are the relations and material entailments between such a construction (e.g., the *genetic code*), the constellation of metaphors it has generated (transcription, writing, reading, errors, translation), and the material practices and performances through which these discursive realities are enacted? How, precisely, do linguistic, social, and cultural constructions shape research investigations or treatment interventions, how do they interact with the phenomena that we call *data, facts*, and even *experience*, and how, in a given historical context as well as in the intellectual and emotional existence of institutions, communities, and individuals, do they come to perform unique cultural work? The AIDS epidemic has furnished many case studies for exploring these questions, even as it reminds us that the practices that we call *science* have evolved in part as a series of safeguards against the seductive power of culture, society, language, and individual consciousness to perceive and define reality in ways that are scientifically or aesthetically appealing, politically or personally palatable.

I have several times cited Latour and Woolgar's proposition that reality is that set of statements that has become too costly to give up. Like "reality" in this sense, a "definition" is a set of statements with authority putting up the collateral. Where meanings are relatively democratic and individual and, under many circumstances, can simply be left to the individual minds in which they exist, a definition is a phenomenon of the public sphere that purports to signify what *is*. It is a meaning that has donned a public face, has been transformed into policy, and is often serving a policing function. But definitions are not simply neutral labels for things in the world; rather, like constructions of "reality," they represent the outcome of struggle. A number of factors contribute to the process by which a given meaning may be transformed—or fails to be transformed—into an official definition. These include the historical moment at which a given definition is put forward, its cultural and social origins, the strength of its institutional backing, its harmony with existing scientific and medical models, its linguistic and aesthetic appeal, its ideological associations, its economic consequences, its implications for existing policy, and its material entailments.

This general model challenges conventional wisdom about what definitions do, the primacy and superiority of scientific and medical accounts of reality, the privileged status given scientific facts, and the taken-for-granted nature of scientific discovery. Conventional media gatekeeping serves a useful public health function in filtering out some of the more extravagant, even "crazy" ideas about the AIDS epidemic. Yet a more inclusive view of what people think AIDS means enables us to study more precisely how meanings—some meanings—become official definitions while others do not. These meanings raise interesting questions about the function of cultural authority and cultural institutions in anchoring our understandings of a cultural crisis as well as about the reasoning, evidence, interests, and social positioning that such attributions represent. At the same time, although my argument intersects with what is sometimes called the *constructionist* tradition in analytic philosophy and semantics and with a body of research in the philosophy and sociology of science, I have not argued that AIDS and HIV are ultimately in the mind or that "everything is discourse."

Culture is not merely an overlay on the "real world" of nature and science; it is not a tidy domain of social life that is—to return to the importance of syntactic constructions—unilaterally "affected by" the AIDS epidemic. Nature and culture, reality and language, are interactive; they constitute each other. What this does not mean, however, is that nature and reality are fixed, certain, and unyielding while culture and language—"the social"—are up for grabs, purely arbitrary, or accidental. It is on this point that researchers in cultural studies (and some strains of thought within philosophy, anthropology, sociology, and history) are emphatic—the social is as much the reality we inherit as a river or a body or a virus and often even more intractable. Hence, meaning is held in place by social as well as natural reality.

These cultural chronicles of the AIDS epidemic help us know the ways in which we have come to understand AIDS, its interaction with culture and language, the intellectual debates and political initiatives that it has engendered, and its symbolic function as a staging ground for both ideological and material struggles. Like other linguistic constructions, *AIDS* and *HIV* are not simply labels, provided us by science and scientific naming practices, that we attach to precise entities in the real world. They are also, in and of themselves, material things with a life of their own—in journal articles and medical records, in scientific and biomedical discourse, in conversations and dreams, in art and museums, in newspapers and books, in dictionaries and computer databases. They exist in material spaces, that is, quite distinct from but as real as those inhabited by the entities to which they are presumed to "refer." Certainly, the story of the AIDS epidemic, its nature and future, takes place in cells, bodies, test tubes, hospitals, laboratories, bodily fluids, and death. But it also takes place in language and discourse, where *AIDS*, the word, is constructed, where it becomes a story, where it is rendered intelligible, and where it is acted upon. Language itself is "real" and "material," a concrete vehicle that lays a trail of its existence in documents, policies, conversations, and other sites and routes of cultural circulation. We cannot, therefore, look "through" language, as though it were a plate glass window, to see what AIDS really is. I have tried here to look at the window itself, where language, like a series of special effects, constructs what we come to think we know about AIDS. *AIDS*, a material sign, a set of sounds, four letters on a page, animates our thinking; it produces convictions and meanings; it generates plans, policies, terror, rage, grant proposals, research and clinical interventions, cultural practices, cultural artifacts, computer searches, voluminous media attention, and a proliferation of specialized discourses. Ultimately, the activities and ideas that we organize around the sign *AIDS*—including the chronicles that we write—have the power to change the fate of the epidemic that, as I write this, in the United States alone has killed more than half a million people and will kill still more. It is in these chronicles that the histories of the AIDS epidemic will be preserved and its lessons offered. Will we heed these lessons or, like Camus's fictional citizens of Oran, calmly deny, "in the teeth of the evidence, that we had ever known a crazy world in which men were killed off like flies"? ([1947] 1948, 268). These are the crucial cultural chronicles that remain to be written. And there is still time, for those of us fortunate to have it, to read, more closely and carefully, the chronicles we are in.

Notes

1 AIDS, Homophobia, and Biomedical Discourse

An early version of this essay was presented in New York in December 1986 at the annual meeting of the Modern Language Association. For publication history, see Treichler (1988b). I have left the 1988 text substantially unchanged in the present book.

1. Discussing the validity of their interpretation of everyday life in a science laboratory, Latour and Woolgar claim, similarly, that the "value and status of any text (construction, fact, claim, story, this account) depend on more than its supposedly 'inherent' qualities. . . . [T]he degree of accuracy (or fiction) of an account depends on what is subsequently made of the story, not on the story itself" ([1979] 1986, 284).

2. The term *signification*, derived from the linguistic work of Ferdinand de Saussure ([1916] 1986), calls attention to the way in which a language (or any other "signifying system") organizes rather than labels experience (or the world). Linking signifiers (phonetic segments or, more loosely, words) and signifieds (concepts, meanings) in ways that come to seem "natural" to us, language creates the illusion of "transparency," as though we could look through it to "facts" and "realities" that are unproblematic. Many scientists and physicians, even those sensitive to the complexities of AIDS, believe that "the facts" (or "science" or "reason") will resolve contradiction and supplant speculation; they express impatience with social interpretations that they perceive as superfluous or incorrect. Even Leibowitch writes that, with the discovery of the virus, AIDS loses its "metaphysical resonances" and becomes "now no more than one infectious disease among many" (1985, xiv). The position of this essay is that signification processes are not the handmaidens of "the facts"; rather, "the facts" themselves arise out of the signifying practices of biomedical discourse.

3. These conceptualizations of AIDS come chiefly from printed sources (journals, news stories, letters to the editor, tracts) published in the first five years of the epidemic. Many are common and discussed in the course of this essay; the more idiosyncratic readings of AIDS (e.g., as a force destroying the Boy Scouts) are cited to suggest the dramatic symbol-inducing power of this illness as well as the continuing lack of social consensus about its meaning. Sources for the more idiosyncratic views are as follows: (2) Senator Jesse Helms; (6) Gallo's introduction to Leibowitch (1985, xvi–xvii); (8) gay rights activist on Channel 5 television broadcast, Cincinnati, 18 October 1985 (compare the French joke that the French acronym for AIDS, SIDA,

stands for Syndrome Imaginaire pour Decourager les Amoureux [Nordland et al. 1986, 47]); (9) Langone's (1985) characterization of the popular view; (10) GRIA (1982) (and see Pally 1985); (12) Lee (1985); (13) Langone (1985), citing a story in a Kenyan newspaper; (14) a *National Inquirer* story cited by Becher (1983); (15) Rechy (1983); (16) the Soviet view, cited by Lieberson (1986, 45); (17) Gathorne-Hardy (1986); (18) cited by Check (1985, 28); (19) Toby Johnson (1983, 24) ("Perhaps AIDS is just the first of a whole new class of diseases resulting from the tremendous changes human technology has wrought in the earth's ecology"); (20) example of AIDS "humor" cited by Black (1986); (23) acronym cited by Van Gelder and Brandt (1986, 89); (24) Goldstein (1983); (25) Black (1986), citing one view of plagues; (31) cited by Pally (1985); (37) Gallo (1987). In the epilogue, I revisit, update, and discuss the implications of the multiple meanings that have attached to AIDS.

4. Sontag (1978) argues that the confusion of illness and metaphor damages people who are ill, and certainly with AIDS there is ample evidence for this argument. Arguing that "the metaphor essentially creates the framework for the individual's experience of the disease" (p. 18), Tancredi and Volkow (1986), e.g., cite studies indicating that many people with AIDS experience a variety of psychological difficulties as a result of its symbolic (as opposed to its prognostic) message. But metaphor cannot simply be mandated away. Goldstein (1983) writes: "Since we are so vulnerable to the erotic potential of metaphor, how can we hope to be less susceptible when illness intersects with sex and death?" Sontag argues that, once the cause and cure of a disease are known, it ceases to be the kind of mystery that generates metaphors. But her view that biomedical discourse has a special claim on the representation of reality implies as well that the entities that it identifies and describes are themselves free from social construction (metaphor). As Durham and Williams (1986) insist, however, despite the origins of the AIDS crisis in the domain of microbiology, the "greatest obstacles to establishing a cure for AIDS and a rational, humane approach to its ravages do not flow from the organic qualities of the [virus]."

5. Brandt summarizes the ways that AIDS thus far recapitulates the social history of other sexually transmitted diseases: the pervasive fear of contagion; concerns about casual transmission; the stigmatization of victims; the conflict between the protection of public health and the protection of civil liberties; increasing professional control over definition and management; and the search for a "magic bullet" (1987, 199). Despite the supposed sexual revolution, Brandt writes, we continue through these social constructions "to define the sexually transmitted diseases as uniquely sinful." This definition is inaccurate but pervasive: and as long as disease is equated with sin "there can be no magic bullet" (p. 202).

6. Allan Sollinger, Ph.D., Department of Immunology, University of Cincinnati Medical Center, speaking as an expert guest on a local television documentary, Cincinnati, October 1985. By this time, a number of leading authorities on AIDS had come to believe that scientists had to begin communicating to the public with greater clarity and certainty. The Centers for Disease Control issued a "definitive statement" in October 1985 that AIDS *cannot* be spread by casual contact. Dr. Mathilde Krim, director of the American Foundation for AIDS Research, discussed transmission with emphatic clarity on the "MacNeil/Lehrer News Hour" (4 September 1985): "AIDS is contagious strictly through the transmission of a virus which passes from one person to another during sexual intercourse or with contaminated blood. It is not contagious *at all* through casual interaction with people, in normal social

conditions such as living in a household with a patient or meeting patients on the bus or in the work place or in school" (Krim 1985b). Interestingly, as Merritt's (1986) comprehensive review makes clear, constitutional precedents for addressing public health problems give broad latitude to the state; strong scientific "evidence" is essentially not required as a basis for interventions.

7. Visual representations of AIDS are not the subject of this essay, yet it is worth noting that they have been a source of continuing controversy. In Watney and Gupta's (1986) textual and visual "dossier" on the rhetoric of AIDS, one writer calls the magnified electron micrograph of the HTLV-III virus "the spectre of the decade." The cover of *Time* (12 August 1985) also treats a photograph of the virus as proof of its reality; "magnified 135,000 times," the virus is pictured "destroying T-cell." (See McGrath's [1984] analysis of the cultural and political role of medical photography in naturalizing the biomedical model.) Some members of the San Francisco gay community complained early that public health warnings used euphemistic language ("avoid exchange of bodily fluids") and, through innocuous pictures, subverted the message that AIDS was a deadly and physically ravaging disease (FitzGerald 1986, 52; see also Gilman 1988a). On other aspects of the media coverage of AIDS, see Becher (1983), O'Dair (1983), Schwartz (1984), Check (1985), and Black (1986). Controversies over graphics were not limited to popular journals: a photograph published in *Science* purporting to be an isolated strain of Gallo's AIDS virus figured in the international dispute over its discovery (Gallo et al. 1986; Norman 1986).

8. See, e.g., *Newsweek*, 3 November 1986, 66–67, and 24 November 1986, 30–47; Eckholm (1986a) in the *New York Times*; McAuliffe et al. (1987) and Zuckerman (1987) in *U.S. News and World Report*; Leishman (1987; and see 1986) in the *Atlantic*; and "Science and the Citizen" (1987) in *Scientific American*.

9. The Second International Conference on AIDS, held in Paris in June 1986, revealed no major scientific breakthroughs (Barnes 1986, 282); rather, answers to several crucial questions were clarified or strengthened. Check notes that, as health and science reporting on AIDS has evolved, "articles about the spread of AIDS to the so-called general public do not have to be pegged to any specific new data" (1985, 31). Some of the sources useful in grasping the evolution of the epidemic are *Abstracts* 1985 through the present (the abstracts of papers given at the regular International AIDS conferences); American Medical Association 1987; *AIDS: Epidemiological and Clinical Studies* 1987 and 1989; *AIDS Medical Glossary* 1995; and such journals as *AIDS Treatment News* (see James 1989a, 1991, 1994). See also Lawrence Altman's coverage in the *New York Times* beginning with Altman (1981), and Kulstad (1986, 1988).

10. The Paris conference was one of several fact-pooling and consensus-building events in 1986 that influenced new readings of existing evidence. Also influential were the *U.S. Surgeon General's Report on Acquired Immune Deficiency Syndrome* (U.S. Surgeon General 1986), which advocated comprehensive sex education in the schools; an investigation by the Institute of Medicine and National Academy of Sciences (1986), which emphasized the dangers of heterosexual transmission; and a World Health Organization conference, which concluded that AIDS must now be considered a pandemic of catastrophic proportions. (An epidemic disease is prevalent in a specific community, geographic area, or population at a particular time, usually originating elsewhere; a pandemic disease is present over the whole of a country, a continent, a world). I describe these reports at greater length in chap. 2 below.

11. Black: "I realized . . . that any account of AIDS was not just a medical story and not just a story about the gay community, but also a story about the straight community's reaction to the disease. More than that: it's a story about how the straight community has used and is using AIDS as a mask for its feelings about gayness. It is a story about the ramifications of a metaphor" (1986, 30). AIDS is typically characterized as a "story," but whose? For AIDS as a story of scientific progress, see Relman (1985, 1), Nichols (1986, 1989), Gallo (1987, 1988, 1991), and Lieberson (1983). But, for Lynch (1982), Goldstein (1983), Kramer (1983), Gunn (1985), Ault (1986), D. Altman (1986), FitzGerald (1986), the San Francisco *A.I.D.S. Show* (Artists Involved with Death and Survival) (Adair and Epstein 1986), and others, AIDS is the story of crisis and heroism in the gay community. In the tabloids, AIDS has become the story of Rock Hudson ("ROCK IS DEAD," ran the headline in the *London Sun* on 3 October 1985, "THE HUNK WHO LIVED A LIE"), Liberace, and other individuals. A documentary film about the Fabian Bridges case, a young man with AIDS in Houston, is called *Fabian's Story*. For Mains, AIDS interrupts the adventure story of leather sex, a "unique and valuable cultural excursion" (1985, 178). And, in Thom Gunn's (1985) poem "Lament," AIDS is a story of change and the death of friends. The stories we tell help us determine what our own place in the story is to be. FitzGerald writes that the "new mythology" about AIDS in the San Francisco gay community—that many gay men are changing their lives for the better—was "an antidote to the notion that AIDS was a punishment—a notion that . . . lay so deep as to be unavailable to reason. And it helped people act against the threat of AIDS" (1986, 62). But, for Mohr, this new mythology—in which the loving relationship replaces anonymous sex—is a dangerous one: "The relation typically is asked to bear more than is reasonable. The burden on the simple dyad is further weighed down by the myth, both romantic and religious, that one finds one's completion in a single other. White knights and messiahs never come in clusters" (1986, 56).

12. Articulate voices had taken issue with the CDC position from the beginning, warning against the public health consequences of treating AIDS as a "gay disease" and separating "those at risk" from the so-called general population. See, e.g., comments by Gary MacDonald, executive director of an AIDS action organization in Washington: "I think the moment may have arrived to desexualize this disease. AIDS is *not* a 'gay disease,' despite its epidemiology. . . . AIDS is not transmitted because of who you *are*, but because of what you *do*. . . . By concentrating on gay and bisexual men, people are able to ignore the fact that this disease has been present in what has charmingly come to be called 'the general population' *from the beginning*. It was not spread from one of the other groups. It was *there*" ("AIDS: What Is to Be Done?" 1985, 43).

One can extrapolate from Bleier's observation that questions shape answers (1986, 4) and suggest that the question, Why are all AIDS victims sexually active homosexual males? might more appropriately have been, *Are* all AIDS victims sexually active homosexual males? It is widely believed (not without evidence) that federal funding for AIDS research was long in coming because its chief victims were gay or otherwise socially undesirable. Black describes a researcher who made jokes about *fagocytes* (phagocytes), cells designed "to kill off fags" (1986, 81–82). Secretary of Health and Human Services Margaret Heckler was only one of many officials who expressed concern not about existing AIDS patients but about AIDS's potential to spread to the "community at large" (with the result that Heckler was called "the Secretary of Health and Heterosexual Services" by some activists in Gay Men's Health Crisis in New York [see "AIDS: What Is to Be Done?" 1985, 51]).

There is evidence that the "gay disease" myth interferes with diagnosis and treatment. Many believe that AIDS may be underdetected and underreported in part because people outside the "classic" high-risk groups are often not asked the right questions (physicians typically take longer to diagnose AIDS in women, e.g.). Health professionals and AIDS counselors sometimes avoid the word *gay* because, for many people, this implies an identity or a lifestyle; even *bisexual* may mean a lifestyle. Although *homosexually active* is officially defined as including even a single same-sex sexual contact over the past five years, many who have had such contact do not identify themselves as homosexual and therefore as being at risk for AIDS. Nancy Shaw (1985, 1986) suggests that, for women as well, the homosexual/heterosexual dichotomy confuses diagnosis and treatment as well as the perception of risk. Murray (1985), Patton (1985a), and Pally (1985) all argue that AIDS is a "women's issue" and should receive more attention in feminist publications (and see COYOTE 1985; Switzer 1986; and Zones 1986). The persistence and consequences of the perception that AIDS is a disease of gay men and IV drug users are documented in a number of recent publications, notably Leishman (1987) and "Science and the Citizen" 1987. CDC interviews with members of two heterosexual singles clubs in Minneapolis documented that, as of late 1986, this already-infected population had made virtually no modifications in its sexual practices (CDC 1986b). DiClemente et al. (1986) found that many adolescents in San Francisco, a city where public health information about AIDS has been widely disseminated, were not well informed about the seriousness of the disease, its causes, or preventive measures.

13. Minson (1981) and Weeks (1985) analyze the evolution of homosexuality as a coherent identity. Bayer (1981) and Bayer and Spitzer (1982) document the intense and acrimonious "contests for meaning" during the American Psychiatric Association's 1970s debates over the official classification of homosexuality.

14. On the reclassification in 1986 of the CDC's 571 previously "unexplained cases," see Nichols (1986) and Associated Press (1986b). Formerly classified as *none of the above* (i.e., outside the known high-risk categories), some of these cases were reclassified as heterosexually transmitted.

15. Even after consensus in 1984 that AIDS was caused by a virus, there continued to be conflicting views on transmission and different explanations for the epidemiological finding that AIDS and HIV infection in the United States were appearing predominantly in gay males. One view holds that this is essentially an artifact ("simple mathematics") created because the virus (for whatever reason) infected gay men first and gay men tend to have sex with each other. The second is that biomedical/physiological factors make gay men and/or the "passive receiver" more easily infected. A third view is that the virus can be transmitted to anyone but that certain cofactors encourage the development of infection and/or clinical symptoms. For more information, see Cahill (1983), Gong and Rudnick (1986), Krim (1985a, 4), Leibowitch (1985, 72–73), and Leishman (1987). Many scientists suggest that, whatever sex the partners may be, infection, as Fain (1985) put it, "requires a jolt injected into the bloodstream, likely several jolts over time, such as would occur with infected needles or semen. In both cases, needle and penis are the instruments of

contagion." Since women have no penises, they are "inefficient" transmitters. For more detailed discussion, see Bolognone and Johnson (1986) and Treichler (1988a) and chaps. 2 and 8 below.

16. Brandt (1987) and Walkowitz (1983) review the long-standing equation of prostitutes with disease and the conceptual separation of infected prostitutes (and other voluntarily sexually active women) from "innocent victims" (see also Douglas [1975] 1982; Eckholm 1985; COYOTE 1985; Shaw 1986, 1988; and Shaw and Paleo 1987).

17. Discussions of AIDS and heterosexual transmission in Africa include Patton (1985b), Osborn (1986), Marx (1986b), Lieberson (1986), Hosken (1986), Feldman (1987), L. Altman (1985b), Treichler (1988a), and "New Human Retroviruses" (1986). See also chap. 3 below.

18. Congressman William Dannemeyer, October 1985, during a debate in the Massachusetts Legislature on a homosexual rights bill (quoted by Langone 1985, 29).

19. In the gay community, the first reaction to AIDS was disbelief. FitzGerald quotes a gay physician in San Francisco: "A disease that killed only gay white men? It seemed unbelievable. I used to teach epidemiology, and I had never heard of a disease that selective. I thought, They are making this up. It can't be true. Or if there is such a disease it must be the work of some government agency—the F.B.I. or the C.I.A.—trying to kill us all" (1986, 54). In the San Francisco *A.I.D.S. Show* (Adair and Epstein 1986), one man is said to have learned of his diagnosis and at once wired the CIA: "I HAVE AIDS. DO YOU HAVE AN ANTIDOTE?"

20. For an example of the view that, although the virus is the sine qua non for AIDS, the syndrome actually *develops* "chiefly in those whose immune systems are already weak or defective," see Lieberson (1986, 43). For broader discussion of public health issues in relation to scientific uncertainties and questions of civil liberties, see Bayer (1985), Silverman and Silverman (1985), and Matthews and Neslund (1987).

21. L. Altman (1985a) and Black (1986) discuss changes in scientific terminology as a result of gays' objections; *sexually promiscuous* generally shifted, e.g., to *sexually active* or *contact with multiple sex partners*. A new classification system for AIDS and AIDS-related symptoms (presented and agreed on at the Second International AIDS Conference in Paris, June 1986) is based on the diverse clinical manifestations of the syndrome and its documented natural history without using presumptive terminology like *pre-AIDS*. Jan Zita Grover's (1986) useful review of *Mobilizing against AIDS* (Nichols 1986) points out a number of problematic terms and assumptions that occur repeatedly in Nichols's book and other scientific writing on AIDS: (1) the term *AIDS victim* presupposes helplessness (the term *person with AIDS* or *PWA* was created to avoid this), prevention and cure are linked to a conservative agenda of "individual responsibility," sex with multiple partners and/or strangers is equated with promiscuity, and "safe" sexual practices are conflated with the cultural practice of monogamy; (2) "caregivers" are differentiated from "victims," scientific/medical expertise from other kinds of knowledge, and "those at risk" from "the rest of us"; and (3) existing inequities in the health-care system are noted but not challenged. Dobrow (1986) notes the dramatic and commercial appeal of the common "cultural images" in popular press scenarios of AIDS.

22. The *Journal of the American Medical Association* study is quoted by Langone to support the "vulnerable anus" hypothesis: "It is not unlikely that these prostitutes had multiple partners during a very short period of time, and performed no more

than perfunctory external cleansing between customers" (Langone 1985, 49). But reports from prostitutes in many countries, summarized in the June 1985 *World Wide Whores' News*, indicate familiarity with AIDS as well as concern with obtaining better protection from infection and better health care (see also COYOTE 1985).

23. Some scientists outside the federal health-care network charge that this "AIDS Mafia" dictates a party line on AIDS. Joseph Sonnabend, M.D., e.g., former scientific director of the AIDS Medical Foundation, founded the *Journal of AIDS Research* to print scientific articles that he believed were being suppressed because they argued for a multifactorial cause rather than a single virus. For discussion, see Black (1986, 112–18).

24. The scientific account of retroviruses goes something like this. A virus (from Latin *virus*, "poison") cannot reproduce outside living cells: it enters another organism's "host" cell and uses that cell's biochemical machinery to replicate itself. These replicant virus particles then infect other cells; this process is repeated until either the infection is brought under control by the host's immune system or the infection overwhelms and kills or debilitates the host, making it susceptible to other infections (as HIV does). Alternatively, virus and host may reach a state of equilibrium in which both coexist for years. The virus's initial entry into the host cell may cause initial symptoms of viral infections. Certain viruses can remain inactive, or latent, inside the host cell for long periods without causing problems; they can remain integrated with the cell's DNA (genetic material) until triggered to replicate (typically when the organism is compromised by old age, immunosuppressive drug therapy, or infection by another virus or bacteria); at this point, the DNA is transcribed into RNA, which in turn becomes protein.

A retrovirus replicates "backward," transferring genetic information from viral RNA into DNA, the opposite of previously known viral actions. The retrovirus carries RNA (instead of DNA) as its genetic material along with a unique enzyme, reverse transcriptase (from which the name *retro* comes); this uses the RNA as a template to generate (transcribe) a DNA copy. This viral DNA inserts itself among the cell's own chromosomes; thus positioned to function as a "new gene" for the infected host, it can immediately start producing viral RNAs (new viruses) or remain latent until activated. In the case of HIV, the latency period can be as long as fourteen years (as of this writing), followed by a very sudden explosion of replication activity that may directly kill the host's cell—chiefly the T4 lymphocyte, a white blood cell that regulates the body's immune response. The rapid depletion of T4 cells, characteristic of AIDS, leaves the human host vulnerable to many infections that a normal immune system would repel. The HTLV isolated by Gallo in 1980 was the first identified retrovirus associated with a human disease (see Osborn 1986, 47).

25. Koch's postulates, developed by bacteriologist Robert Koch, require that, in order to establish a specific virus as the "cause" of AIDS, the virus would have to be present in all cases of the disease; antibodies to the virus must be shown to develop in consistent temporal relation to the development of AIDS; and transmission of the same virus to a previously uninfected animal or human must be demonstrated with subsequent development of the disease and reisolation of the infective agent. With AIDS, a lethal disease, this last requirement cannot be tested on humans, but a demonstration that the virus could be used to produce an effective vaccine would

more or less fulfill this requirement. (See Marx 1984, 151; and Feorino et al. [1983] 1986, 216.) As questions about AIDS's causation and the role of HIV became "the debate that would not die" (Epstein 1996), Koch's postulates were repeatedly invoked, revised, and reconstructed. Fujimura and Chou (1994) review the history of Koch's postulates, detailing the ways in which they have been adapted or reinterpreted to accommodate new knowledge and technologies: The shift of interest from bacteria to viruses, e.g., required serious reformulation of the criteria by which a given pathogen could be considered to cause a given disease; by the 1990s, many epidemiologists and bench scientists had already shifted to a more flexible model of disease causation.

26. For a fuller analysis of the theory and politics of these origin and alibi stories, see Patton (1985b), Fettner and Check (1985), Weeks (1985), D. Altman (1986), Chirimuuta and Chirimuuta ([1987] 1989), and Grmek (1990). The consensus developing in the mid-1980s was reinforced by the recommendation that the virus be called HIV, but stability was again threatened by the French patent suit. J. Feldman (1992) traces the Gallo-Montagnier phase of the dispute, examining the intertextual relations produced by published texts and other documents. The controversy was kept alive by John Crewdson's (1989) lengthy investigative report in the *Chicago Tribune*, although Crewdson focused more on the scientific process and laboratory practices that had produced HIV (a.k.a. HTLV-III, LAV, ARV, etc.) than on AIDS's retroviral etiology.

27. Hence Leibowitch likens the effort to identify the AIDS virus as a "medico-biological Interpol" on the trail of an international "criminal" charged with "breaking and entering" and asks, "Who is HTLV?" (1985, 41–42, 48). Describing the mechanism of AIDS transmission at the congressional AIDS hearing in 1983, Mervyn B. Silverman testified in comparable language that "many believe that this virus does not act alone" (U.S. House 1984, 125). In an article on a related finding in immunological research, Van (1986) refers to cells called "free radicals" who serve as the body's "terrorists." A *Consumer Reports* (1986) article entitled "AIDS: Deadly but Hard to Catch" inadvertently invokes the structural ambiguity of "catching" the virus (who is the catcher, who the catchee?). The policing metaphor (and the connection between *policy* and *police* has not gone unnoticed) carries over to efforts to control the spread of the virus. Lieberson (1986, 47) reports that some gay clubs have created "fluid patrol officers" who try to ensure that no "unsafe sex" takes place. Mohr (1986) argues that, like recommendations for celibacy, such attempts to promote "safe" sexual behavior seem "remote from reality and quite oblivious to the cussedness of sex and culture" (p. 51). Further, Mohr argues, "though in midcrisis it is politically injudicious to say so, safe-sex is poor sex" (p. 52); as an epigram for his essay, he quotes a former gay "reprobate," now reformed: "Who wants to suck a dick with a rubber on it?"

28. For discussion and analysis of the growing competition in AIDS research as the funding increased, see D. Altman (1986), Black (1986), Patton (1985b), Panem (1985), Schwartz (1984), Office of Technology Assessment (1985), "AIDS: Public Health and Civil Liberties" (1986), and Shilts (1987). For an account of the case of the French physician Willy Rozenbaum, see Raeburn (1986).

29. Despite whatever criticisms biomedical scientists may have about AIDS research, an ideology of heroism, progress, and faith in ultimate scientific conquest pervades dis-

cussions. Examples include Frederickson (1983), Francis (1983), Choi (1986), American Medical Association Council on Scientific Affairs ([1983] 1987), Landesman et al. (1985), Relman (1985), Sande (1986), and Gallo (1987). Sonnabend (1985) critiques the assumptions of a heroic stance, while Leibowitch (1985) is distinctive in his irony and political self-consciousness about the nature of the scientific enterprise.

30. As of December 1986, 10 million people were estimated to carry the virus worldwide; at least a quarter of these people are expected to develop AIDS within the next five years and many more to develop illnesses ranging from mildly disabling to lethal. By the end of 1986, almost 30,000 people in the United States had been diagnosed with AIDS, and half of them had already died. The number of diagnosed cases is expected to reach 270,000 by the end of 1991, with a cumulative death toll of 179,000. There will be a heavy financial toll. With repeated hospitalizations, a person with AIDS may have medical costs of $500,000. The cases of AIDS diagnosed in 1986 alone will eventually cost the nation $2.25 billion in health-care costs and $7 billion in lost lifetime earnings. Its expenses are seventy-five times what we are currently spending on it. (Costs vary greatly from city to city: the CDC estimated in 1986 that each case would average $147,000; the U.S. army estimated that a case could cost as much as $500,000 to treat; but, in San Francisco, use of nonphysician caretakers, home care, and nursing home services can bring the cost of a comparable case down to $42,000. For discussion of the politics of AIDS funding, see U.S. House [1984], Patton [1985b], D. Altman [1986], and Tuller [1987]. The Institute of Medicine/National Academy of Sciences report [1986] judges recent federal allocations to be "greatly improved" but still "woefully inadequate" and calls for spending $2 billion per year by 1990 for education and the development of drugs and vaccines. For predictions based on the current distribution of HIV antibodies, see American Medical Association Council on Scientific Affairs ([1983] 1987), CDC (1986c), Johnson and Vieira (1986), Redfield et al. (1985, 1986), and Winkelstein et al. (1987).

   In revising this book, I have left the foregoing summary of statistical estimates as it was originally written in 1988. Although in other places I have updated or qualified estimates made at particular times, this summary warrants comment as it stands. First, virtually every prediction made in the first five years of the epidemic regularly produced—as though it were a physical law—an "equal and opposite" prediction in the other direction. In other words, every prediction of thousands and millions of AIDS cases would be debunked, belittled, or shown to be impossible. Second, many questions raised at this point had no solid answers—cost estimates, e.g., fluctuated widely, in part because so many factors could influence the macro- and microtrajectories of the epidemic. Third, like others untrained in epidemiology (academics and nonacademics), it took me awhile to learn to interpret statistical claims and distinguish solid sources from the Panglosses and Pandoras making counterclaims. Fourth, statistical projections and their periodic revision came to have immense rhetorical and political power, and any upward or downward revision became a reliable predictor of ideological warfare. In my view, then and now, the worst-case scenarios should in every instance have been taken seriously until we knew enough to rule them out absolutely. In the face of uncertainty, prudence and foresight surely should have dictated that we prepare for the worst and hope for the best. If such terrible predictions did not come to pass, we could, simply, be glad—and be credited for furthering changes in knowledge and practices. Instead, any downward revision of statistics brought gloating cries of "Gotcha!" from the debunkers: As though liberal politicians and "special interests" had purposely inflated the figures and been found out. And as though half a million AIDS cases was a trivial total since more had at some point been predicted. Fifth, at the time this essay was originally written, few people, I think, actually believed that the monstrous figures predicted would ever be so close to the truth. We simply did not believe that an epidemic of infectious disease could, in the late twentieth-century United States, last so long and kill so many.

31. The concept of *saturation* did not last long in public AIDS discourse. For one thing, it presented the picture of a population as a passive mass, absorbing virus to capacity until the virus overflows and moves on to a new population. The instrumental image is troublesome but also inaccurate, for it suggests that a given population is homogenous, has uniform "absorbency," and takes no steps to reduce or prevent infection (and that the rest of the world stands by while the saturated population dies off). More useful, perhaps, is a concept of circles or networks of sexual/social contact, where the density of viral prevalence better predicts the infectability of the uninfected without assuming discrete, self-contained populations. Still, in later proposals for drug and vaccine testing, comparable concepts were evoked: the desire for a "virgin population," for instance.

32. Although Lieberson insists that a "heterosexual pandemic (comparable to Africa's) has not occurred in the United States" and criticizes those who suggest that it is going to (1986, 44), current data based on tests for HIV among 1986 army recruits (nongay non–drug using, so far as researchers could determine) argue for increasing heterosexual transmission (Redfield et al. 1986). For discussion and analysis, see L. Altman (1985a), D. Altman (1986), Marx (1986a), Osborn (1986), Patton (1985b), Hosken (1986), and Feldman (1987). See also Potterat et al. (1987). It has been suggested that malnutrition plays an important role in the rapid spread of AIDS in Africa. Worldwide, malnutrition is common associated with acquired immune deficiency, while poverty is the factor most consistently associated with disease in general.

33. We must even, perhaps, identify with the virus, an extraordinarily successful structure that has been comfortably making the acquaintance of living organisms for many more millions of years than we have. A virus that enters the human bloodstream and circulates through the body may ultimately negotiate with the host some mutually livable equilibrium. The relation may be a close one: it is difficult to separate the effects of the virus from those of the body's defenses; and any poison intended for the guest may kill the host as well. Any given species, including human beings, may sometimes prove to be an inhospitable, even unnatural host. To speak teleologically for a moment, it is obvious that to kill the host is not in the microorganism's best interests; this sometimes happens, however, when a virus adapted to a nonhuman host shifts, through some untoward turn of events, to the human body. Although, from our perspective, HIV is indeed virulent, killing quickly, in fact the long latency between infection and the appearance of clinical damage provides plenty of time—often years—for the virus to replicate and infect a new host. For the time being, we are sufficiently hospitable for this virus to live off us relatively "successfully"; if mutation occurs, our relation to the virus could evolve into something relatively benign or mutually disastrous.

34. This interview, conducted by Philip Horvitz in Berkeley in 1985 (and scrutinized, it's said, like the Watergate transcripts to find out what Foucault knew and when he knew it), concludes as Foucault enters the BART station: "Good luck," he tells Horvitz. "And don't be scared!" The interview is titled "Don't Cry for Me, Academia."

35. Although Check writes that "it sometimes appears that the only risk group that hasn't raised a ruckus is the IV drug users, who are not organized" (1985, 28), a few commentators are beginning to draw attention to this critical problem: Barrett (1985), Joseph (1986), Byron (1985), Shaw and Paleo (1987), and Clines (1987). Finally, aware that many drug addicts were avoiding information centers as well as medical authorities, the Gay Men's Health Crisis in New York took responsibility for going to shooting galleries, clinics, and drug treatment centers to provide AIDS education and training to drug users, who in turn could work with other drug users. (For an update, see Friedman et al. [1992].)

2 The Burdens of History

I first addressed the topic of women and AIDS in "AIDS, Gender, and Biomedical Discourse: Current Contests for Meaning," an essay I presented in various versions during 1987 and 1988 and published in *The Burdens of History*, a collection of essays about AIDS and history edited by Elizabeth Fee and Daniel Fox (see Treichler 1988a). Because "Current Contests for Meaning" overlaps significantly with "An Epidemic of Signification," the first chapter of this book, I have not included it in *How to Have Theory*. The present chapter 2, "The Burdens of History," which borrows its title from the Fee and Fox book, addresses the same issues and time period (roughly 1981–88), but it draws retrospectively from the firmer data and more comprehensive media studies that now exist, and it functions more as a "lessons from the 1980s" piece than as the contemporary critique and intervention that "Current Contests" was intended to be. Having said that, I should add that the earlier critique is still accurate and that few of the lessons of the 1980s have been heeded.

1. Second-wave U.S. feminism's analysis of women in medicine and science was formative for the women's health movement. One milestone of this analysis can be read from the successive editions of *Our Bodies Ourselves*, from its newsprint incarnation in the late 1960s to the substantial trade press twenty-fifth anniversary edition, which dominates its market niche (Boston Women's Health Book Collective 1994). The influential *Complaints and Disorders* (Ehrenreich and English 1973) was one of the first attempts to place women's health in a quasi-scholarly historical context. The large body of research and commentary produced over the last two or three decades cannot be easily summarized; here, I draw primarily on studies concerned with discourse and representation—i.e., concerned with the historically specific processes through which gendered biological entities are constructed. I also emphasize studies concerned with pathological and contaminated constructions of the female body. Important contributions include Gallagher and Laqueur (1987), Suleiman (1986), Irigaray (1985), Barker-Benfield (1976), Smith-Rosenberg (1985) (esp. her chapter "The Hysterical Woman"), Jacobus et al. (1990), Jordanova (1980, 1987, 1989), MacCormack and Strathern (1980), Laqueur (1990), Schiebinger (1993), Oudshoorn (1994, 1996), Buci-Glucksmann (1987), Walkowitz (1983), Martin

(1987), Bleier (1986), Ryan and Gordon (1994), Rapp (1988), Fausto-Sterling (1993), Scheper-Hughes (1994), and Terry and Urla (1995). Moore and Clarke (1995) offer a dense tour through this body of scholarship, and Eckman (1996) analyzes the trajectory of the women's health movement from the mid-1960s to the mid-1990s in the light of contemporary theoretical and feminist scholarship. (Eckman [1998] examines current initiatives in the light of that trajectory.)

2. Elsewhere (Treichler 1988a), I use Colin Douglas's 1975 novel *The Intern's Tale* to analyze duplicity as a significant feature of women's bodies. Set in a teaching hospital in Edinburgh, the novel savages virtually every aspect of modern academic medicine—including its rampant and unreflective sexism. But the end of the book betrays its satiric impulses when two of the interns, Campbell and his friend Mac, hospitalized with potentially fatal hepatitis B, deduce that the source of their infection is Maggie, an unmarried nurse who is well known to sleep around. The interns' realization suddenly transforms Maggie from a readily compliant sexual object into an unruly agent of disease, actively spreading hepatitis to her sexual partners—who include many of the hospital's medical staff. As they compare notes, the interns find that she has lied to them, passing off as a routine female complaint ("she said something about just finishing a period") the symptoms of serious pathology ("always dripping"). Her lie could succeed, of course, only because both interns were ready to attribute the signs of pathology to the expected vicissitudes of the female menstrual cycle. (Laqueur [1987, 31–32] and Martin [1987, 35] cite the vivid language of Walter Heape, a nineteenth-century antifeminist, antisuffrage zoologist at Cambridge, to suggest how extreme male views of menstruation could become. In menstruation, writes Heape in the late nineteenth century, the entire epithelium is torn away, "leaving behind a ragged wreck of tissue, torn glands, ruptured vessels, jagged edges of stroma, and masses of blood corpuscles, which it would seem hardly possible to heal satisfactorily without the aid of surgical treatment." Heape was the first to use the term *estrus*, a neologism from Latin for *gadfly*, to mean "frenzy, rut, heat." As Laqueur notes, Heape did represent an extreme, but Martin observes that the 1977 edition of a widely used textbook of medical physiology disrupts its characteristically "emotionally subdued prose" to inform the reader that, "to quote an old saying, 'menstruation is the uterus crying for lack of a baby.' " For a careful comparative review of the treatment of the clitoris and the rest of the "female apparatus" in anatomy textbooks from 1900 to the early 1990s, see Moore and Clarke [1995]; the authors also describe related projects.)

Like women elsewhere in *The Intern's Tale* (another woman tricks Campbell into thinking that she is a virgin, while a third woman's apparent indigestion turns out to be appendicitis), Maggie is not what she seems. From the perspective of the interns, she has tricked them into the potentially fatal risk of having intercourse "bareback," as they put it, without protective contraception. Even as Maggie's sexuality infects them with the possibility of their own mortality, they express no concern about hers. Their dialogue echoes the book's treatment of Maggie as a casually passive sexual object, twisting suddenly only with the revelation that she is the deeply duplicitous perpetrator of a crime against them. Not only that, in mimicking a menstrual period she plays a traditional female card, allaying the male fear of pregnancy and the one reason left to wear a condom. Her dupes are the interns, boys whose only crime was to be boys. The narrative's language also links the carrier or source of the disease with the disease itself, suggesting, indeed, that Maggie, not a virus, causes hepatitis: she who is infected is simultaneously both infectious (a state or condition) and infecting (an active agent of disease).

Duplicity and disguise as feminine characteristics figure elsewhere in medical discourse. Poovey (1987) cites a variety of ways in which women and their bodies are judged to be duplicitous, including the view of hysteria as mimicry, the "periodicity" of the menstrual cycle as creating inherent "instability," and the invisibility and mysteriousness of the origins of many "women's illnesses"; the female body, wrote one physician, "mocks the reality of truth," and another wrote of hysterics that "these patients are veritable actresses" whose lives are "one perpetual falsehood." (The long-standing equation of women's bodies with acting is echoed many years later in filmmaker Lizzie Borden's comment on *Working Girls*, her 1987 release about prostitutes: "Men's bodies are exposed and therefore vulnerable, whereas women have this ability to conceal. On some level, women have always dealt with theater" [quoted in Dieckmann 1987, 33].)

Duplicity and changeability have special implications in relation to the symptomatology of venereal diseases—especially syphilis, the "Great Imitator," with its diverse array of symptoms; "if you know syphilis," it used to be said, "you know medicine." Writes Ludvik Fleck ([1935] 1979, 12), "Syphilis is an extremely pleomorphic disease of many aspects. We read in many treatises that it is a 'proteoform' disease, since with its many forms, it reminds one of 'Proteus or Chameleon.'... There was hardly any disease or symptom that was not attributed to syphilis." In her detailed examination of the immune system, Waldby (1996) shows how stereotypical gendered binaries structure AIDS discourse and its regulatory technologies. Crucial features in this process are feminine formlessness, permeability, and receptivity.

3. Gilman (1995, 141) reproduces this poster in his review of AIDS education posters internationally. Note the text's uneasy form of pronominal address (who is supposed to get tested?) and reliance on "getting tested" to resolve the question of the woman's unknown HIV status. For further description of AIDS education campaigns and their imagery, see Carter and Watney (1989), Watney (1987c, 1987d, 1988), Watney and Gupta (1986), Berer with Ray (1993), Sabatier (1988), Berridge (1996), Berridge and Strong (1992, 1993), Grover (1988b, 1989a, 1989b), Ostrow (1987a, 1987b, 1987d), Aggleton and Homans (1988), and Aggleton et al. (1989, 1990, 1992, 1993). Scholarship on the evolving use of images in medicine and health education includes Treichler et al. (1998), Cartwright (1995), Fyfe and Law (1988), Kember (1991), Martin (1987, 1994), McGrath (1984, 1990), Reagan (1996), and Tagg (1988).

4. In analyzing the social history of venereal disease in the United States, of which these posters are a part, Brandt (1987) notes that gender entered these discourses (and their associated visual images) through the contrasting figures of the innocent wife and the "fallen" woman and that real-life women were essentially forced to be one or the other. As Poovey (1988) argues, characterizations of women and women's bodies as diseased or pathological may not be explicit. Gilman (1985) shows how implicit cultural narratives about women's bodies (and black bodies) pervade scientific and medical texts. Martin's *Woman in the Body* (1987) identifies linguistic devices (metaphors, e.g.) in nineteenth- and twentieth-century medical texts used to describe human sexuality and reproduction; Martin's meticulous comparison of passages about women with comparable passages about men demonstrates the

ways in which female functions are conceptualized negatively. Within this vision, menopause is viewed as a breakdown in "production" or, in more recent texts, as a breakdown of "authority" and efficient communication—a management problem. Male functions, in contrast, remain heroic and full of energy. Martin's manipulation of the texts demonstrates how the same passages could be rewritten (but rarely are) to reverse the traditional conceptualizations. (Examples of gendered stereotypes in immunology texts assembled by Haraway [1991b], Martin [1994], and Waldby [1996] will astound even hardened veterans of the feminist language wars.)

Similar textual manipulation was used by Ruth Herschberger in her classic study *Adam's Rib* ([1948] 1970), a book that deserves to be better known within feminist scholarship on gender and science. Her hilarious rendering of chimpanzee studies demonstrated that a traditional—supposedly "objective"—account of male and female biological development seems so natural to us that its patriarchal foundations are revealed only when a "matriarchal account" is created and placed beside it (pp. 75–82). In one of the first close feminist readings of technical prose, Hilary Allen (1984) draws on the language and logic of British court decisions to reveal their implicit assumption that women are always already pathological (thus "premenstrual tension" is essentially a permanent—and potentially disqualifying—condition).

Poovey (1987) pursues the position of the prostitute in nineteenth-century literature not as a contrast to the virtuous married woman but as a disruption of the virtue/vice binary. Because of her relative economic independence, right to own property, and sexual freedom, Poovey argues, the prostitute challenged conventional social divisions; vast quantities of discourse were required in the effort to restore the fixed dichotomy between pure and fallen women. See also Bell (1987), Corbin (1987), Gilman (1985), Colwell (1998), and Walkowitz (1983). Such studies identify many contradictions in approaches to women, sex, and VD. Connelly (1984) argues that early twentieth-century education, conceptualization, and views on the regulation of venereal disease were curiously inconsistent. On the one hand, the antiprostitution crusade and call for premarital testing for both women and men clearly assumed that both women and men could transmit disease; yet this assumption was contradicted by the widespread view that men are always the authors of these social crimes, women always their victims. Connelly observes that "to insist that women could not spread venereal disease simply because they were women embodied an attitude that, even by 1915, was becoming increasingly absurd" (p. 202).

5. Silence is another theme that locates AIDS historically within the discursive universe of venereal disease. The Victorian "conspiracy of silence" surrounding VD referred both to broad conventions of silence about sexual matters in polite society and to a specifically "medical secret": the collusion of "physicians and male patients, either husbands or prospective husbands, which resulted in unsuspecting women being infected with venereal disease" (Connelly 1984, 202). Poovey (1987) discusses at length the role of silence in the nineteenth-century medical debates about the use of chloroform during childbirth, specifically, the value of the "quiet and unresisting body" for the physician. Above all, Poovey argues, "the silenced female body can be made the vehicle for any medical man's assumptions and practices because its very silence opens a space in which meanings can proliferate" (p. 152); she describes this as the "metaphorical promiscuity of the female body" (p. 153). Warren (1996) explores three kinds of silence: the silencing of the powerless

by the powerful, the silence of the powerless because they are not heard (not audible), and the silence that the powerful impose on themselves so as to fix the conditions of possibility about what can and cannot be said. Although she focuses on the silence of the medical establishment on the topic of the sexual abuse of patients by physicians, the "conspiracy of silence" on the subject of venereal disease is a parallel example. See also Limmer (1988).

6. The individual and the social body have often been articulated together in the context of disease, not just in such broad theoretical propositions as social Darwinism but also in vividly medicalized language and detailed technical analogies. To take just one example, the images of diseased blood, body fluid, and other liquids so prominent in the discourses surrounding sexually transmitted diseases mesh almost seamlessly with descriptions of buildings, cities, nations, and societies to argue that "bad blood" functions like a polluted stream, an overwhelming tide, or blocked sewers to contaminate the larger body through which it flows. (Fleck [(1935) 1979], Jones [1981], and Brandt [1987] discuss "bad blood" in syphilis; Jones explores the special significance of blood and "bad blood" for African-American communities.) The discursive processes that articulate the body to the social order may operate in both directions, taking the larger body to stand in for or govern the individual human body. Hence, Turner (1984, 2–3), e.g., argues not only that disorders of the body, especially women's bodies, are often treated as disorders of society but also that order is restored through macro regulatory systems designed to control women's bodies (see also pp. 115–76 and 204–26). Turner renews and elaborates his argument in his foreword to Petersen and Bunton (1997), a collection of essays and case studies anchored in Foucauldian theory that explores bidirectional material effects of body-society links in health and medicine.

These articulations have taken on great urgency in the AIDS epidemic, prodding investigators to examine more closely what discursive links actually do. Some studies attempt to assess the actual power of the literal analogies inscribed through such authoritative media as medical illustration (Martin 1994; Haraway 1991b). Others examine how particular images and metaphors function to shore up particular interests.

Dangerous Bedfellows (1996) and Rubin (1994b, 1997), e.g., add a cogent specificity to broad analogies between body and society, examining how certain bodies and their practices come to be read as dangerous to the "general population" and how such readings may further particular economic and political interests. Rubin's historical study of San Francisco's leather community investigates the effect of the AIDS epidemic on rhetoric, community identity, and specific sexual practices as well as their representation in the gay and general Bay Area media. The Dangerous Bedfellows volume uses New York City's 1994 "public sex" crackdown as its case study, showing that new data on rising HIV rates among younger gay men fueled a movement to step up, "under the sign of HIV/AIDS," a regime of intensified surveillance, regulation, and closure of sex-related businesses and clubs. During an epidemic disease, it is no surprise to find public health and moral arguments articulated together in calls (both liberal and conservative) for the identification, targeting, and removal of supposed sources of contamination. In both San Francisco and New York, however, these AIDS-cleansing initiatives also created matchless development opportunities in the cleansed neighborhoods.

Catherine Waldby's *AIDS and the Body Politic* (1996) systematically examines analogies employed by biomedicine to establish normative standards of health, arguing that any biomedical representation of disease can be read as a technical description of bodily pathology, as a guide for distinguishing the normal from the pathological, and as "an immanent narrative of social order" (p. 51). Complementing the work of Foucault, Haraway, Martin, Brandt, and Sontag, among others, Waldby pursues in greater detail the implications of analogies between bodies, social systems, and the figuring of the immunocompetent body as a military nation-state. Especially in her discussion of "the primal scene of immunology" and its bio-military metaphors, she demonstrates in detail how "the militarized immune system" shapes "what HIV infection is understood to *be*" and simultaneously sets up "binaries of sexual difference in association with contagion and abjection" (p. 53). She argues not only that the fundamental immunological binary of self-other is sexualized and gendered to equate "self" with heterosexual masculinity but also that this binary in turn constructs the entire apparatus of the epidemic. Not only is the individual body read as a nation-state, but the nation-state (society) is read as a body, and, in AIDS, this body—the "general population" that public health measures are designed to protect—"includes men but not women, and heterosexual men, but not gay and bisexual men" (p. 86). As part of this package, she writes, the "heterosexual masculine body . . . must suppress its capacities for passivity and anal and oral receptivity, capacities which are then projected onto the bodies of women and gay men. In other words, the permeability of the heterosexual male body is suppressed in dominant forms of cultural representation" (p. 14).

7. This booklet, located in the U.S. Public Health Service archive in the National Library of Medicine and reproduced in Gilman (1995), was part of a larger Australian public health campaign targeting women. The first of industrialized nations to develop a broadly based public health campaign against AIDS, Australia developed flashy posters and public service announcements for television for its Grim Reaper series. In the signature television spot, the Grim Reaper relentlessly knocks down bowling pins representing different kinds of people. The last to go are a blonde middle-class mother embracing her small middle-class child. As in the United States, the campaign was criticized for highlighting the danger to extremely low-risk groups at the expense of those who more urgently needed the information (and, predictably, for seeming to suggest that bowling could cause AIDS). Parmar (1987) includes the bowling clip and discussion of it. Waldby (1996) describes the Australian campaign in detail and its varied strategies for appealing to women.

8. For the convenience of the reader, citations of *MMWR* articles will be given in the text. Full citations for all *MMWR* articles used in the book are alphabetized in the bibliography under "Centers for Disease Control."

9. Shilts (1987, 171) describes the coining of the acronym *AIDS*, an event also dramatized in the 1992 HBO version of *And the Band Played On.* The Discovery Channel documentary *A Time of AIDS* includes an interview with the official who actually proposed the change. Oppenheimer (1988) draws attention to the power of epidemiology during the first few years of the epidemic in naming both GRID and AIDS. Black (1986, 60) comments that the CDC task force director James Curran called the new names "reasonably descriptive without being pejorative," but, Black adds, "names have power." Indeed, charged with naming "the AIDS virus," the International Committee on the Taxonomy of Viruses had to make a number of decisions

along these lines, among them whether to incorporate the term *AIDS* into the virus's official name. An argument against doing so was that the term *AIDS* would place further stress and stigma on patients found to be infected. The counterargument was that any term would, before long, acquire whatever stigma continued to exist; according to the committee chair, Harold Varmus, the committee came to refer to this as "the evanescence of euphemism" (1989, p. 6). (I might note that Francine Frank and I argue similarly that "politically incorrect" language must be frankly faced and analyzed; it cannot simply be decreed away. Although many social mechanisms exist for holding meanings in place—giving a virus its "official name," e.g.—language is not a single obedient system, standing still and awaiting our command; on the contrary, linguistic processes also exist that enable stigmatized or objectionable features of particular terms to migrate with surprising efficiency to their newly cleansed alternatives [see Frank and Treichler 1997].)

In the end, *AIDS* was left out of the name *HIV*. The name *HIV* specifies the pathological/clinical effect of the virus (immune deficiency) rather than (as *HTLV* or *LAV* does) the type of cell it attacks. The terms *HIV infection* or *HIV disease* have come to be used as a generic name to signify the entire spectrum of possibilities (from asymptomatic infection to full-blown AIDS). Brown (1986) objects to the name *HIV* as being "conciliatory" but too nonspecific because all microbes associated with AIDS are immunosuppressive. Duesberg (1987) argues that HIV is at most a precipitating agent in AIDS. According to Epstein (1996), Duesberg told John Lauritsen of the *New York Native* that many respected scientists agreed with him in private but were afraid to do so in public. On the meaning trajectory, see Juengst and Koenig (1989).

10. Steve Rabin, who for the agency Ogilvie and Mather directed the ARTA campaign for several years, objected to the collapsed categories, scathingly pointing out that "war-MIPP-sa" was not likely to speak to the assortment of "risk groups" that it was supposed to represent (personal communication). Despite the negative close readings to which it was subjected by various constituencies, *Understanding AIDS* (U.S. Surgeon General 1988) was judged by several researchers to have successfully accomplished its major objectives (see, e.g., Gerbert and Maguire 1989; and Macro Systems 1990). Veeder's (1994) enlightening rhetorical analysis of the booklet incorporates information from the numerous successive drafts to which it was subjected.

11. Just the text of the journal itself? Annotations, elaborations, or retrospective interpretations of the CDC's models and predictions (such as, e.g., Anderson and May 1988; Anderson et al. 1988; May et al. 1988; Fumento 1989; King 1993, 1997; and Mann and Tarantola 1996)? Behind-the-scenes narration ("the highly sexual lifestyle of the early victims was beginning to persuade Jaffe . . . that a sexually transmitted bug might be behind the unexplained cancers and pneumonia" [Shilts 1987, 86])? Interviews with CDC officials (e.g., Curran 1988)? During the heterosexual panic of 1986–87, e.g., Harold Jaffe repeatedly told reporters that the agency did indeed acknowledge the threat of heterosexual transmission but believed that "the virus is more likely to spread gradually over a period of years, rather than explosively, into the heterosexual population" (quoted in L. Altman 1987b). What is to count as AIDS? Usages of the actual term *AIDS*? Instances from the late 1970s and early 1980s, written before the term *AIDS* existed, of cases of Kaposi's sarcoma, *pneumocystis* pneumonia, and other diseases and conditions retroactively incorporated into the official definition of acquired immune dysfunction? What

about much older cases of immune dysfunction unearthed from medical journals and clinical records?

These questions are critical to any analysis of discourse but carried out differently by different researchers. For discussion of the relation of discursive universes to processes of definition and diagnosis, see Epstein (1996), Hopkins (1990), Treichler (1989b), and Johnson (1996). The question of how AIDS is defined by the CDC, the agency responsible for surveillance, exemplifies the nontransparent nature of language in relation to reality: as knowledge of the "reality" of AIDS increases, redefinition is regularly called for; but a new definition reorganizes the scope of phenomena under surveillance. The CDC's revised classification systems for AIDS cases are regularly reported in the *MMWR*.

12. Feminist theorists will not miss the irony of a surveillance scheme in which women show up as *none of the above* or *other*. The extensive feminist literature on Woman as Other includes de Beauvoir (1953), Benstock (1987), Irigaray (1985), Woolf (1929), Nelson (1985), Culler (1982, 43–64), Moi (1985), Belsey (1980), and Wolf (1992).

"Otherness" and "othering," however, appear to be a permanent feature of epidemic disease. Brandt (1987) cites "otherness" in the history of venereal diseases, which are always said to originate in other races, other places, other classes; among the poor, among immigrants; among aliens (see also Walkowitz 1983). During the Black Death of the fourteenth century, Jews were accused of "poisoning the wells" and were massacred. In the fifteenth and sixteenth centuries, the Spanish called syphilis "the Portuguese disease," the Portuguese called it "the Moroccan disease" (Ladislav Zgusta, personal communication). According to Jamie Feldman (1988), in France, where AIDS was at first called "the Moroccan plague," French researchers and clinicians had little difficulty incorporating Africans with AIDS into the French/ European population of people with AIDS, while American gay men seemed to remain for some time the Other (see also Feldman 1993). In central African countries struck by AIDS, the epidemic was in each case claimed to have originated in one of the other countries. In Japan, the Other figured in efforts to safeguard the national blood supply and divided Japanese from non-Japanese (foreign—including homosexuals, who were, ipso facto, non-Japanese). Because Japan carefully screened out "foreign" blood from blood sources given to Japanese people, the Japanese government claimed transfusion-related AIDS cases to be nonexistent. For a different account, see Dearing (1992). On parallels between Japanese government policy on blood transfusions and other forms of transmission, see Treat (1994). Albert (1986a, 1986b) reviews accounts of the general process through which communities create distinctions between the normal and the deviant; he uses this division to discuss media accounts of AIDS.

Waldby argues that epidemiology's later shift away from "risk groups," designed to reduce the consequences of othering and stigmatization, could not overcome the logic that considers the bodies of risk group members "to form contagious circuits within the body politic." A shift to the seemingly neutral categories *modes of transmission* and *sources of infection* in fact does nothing to disrupt the process of metonymic displacement that sustains a phallocentric public health apparatus (see Waldby 1996, esp. 101–11).

The epidemiological case studies in Bond et al. (1997), carried out primarily by social epidemiologists and sociologists in various settings in Africa and the Caribbean, identify numerous ways in which ostensibly transparent disciplinary measures contribute to establishing and maintaining "us/them" divisions within societies already "othered" by the postindustrial world.

13. Indeed, as many sources indicate, the CDC's official reports were produced out of often-conflicting voices (see Chase 1986; Clark et al. 1986; Shilts 1987; Fettner and Check 1985; Connor and Kingman 1989; and Corea 1992; and cf. Johnson 1996).

14. Childbearing has been a historical concern in epidemic disease. Reviewing the "primitive epidemiological data" available, Ell (1986, 151) writes that the 1531 plague in Venice "spared no one," killing about one-third of the total population. Among the 93,661 mortalities in Venice and the surrounding area were 11,486 pregnant women, "a catastrophic blow to the reproductive capacity of the city. Yet, this inclination toward pregnant women is quite in keeping with the fact that pregnancy acts as a nonspecific immune-suppressant." Barbara Tuchman (1978, 92–125) provides a dramatic account of the Black Death, tracing the social and economic consequences of curtailed reproduction over subsequent decades (consequences borne out by modern demography).

But demography is only one reason that epidemics highlight reproduction. More fundamentally, a vast body of discourse on conception, childbirth, and mothering already freezes women in a series of permissible and forbidden tableaux (for background, see Treichler 1990a; Hartouni 1997; and Cussins 1997). When vertical transmission emerged as a source of HIV infection, these tableaux came to life. The first studies of HIV prevalence in babies in New York State in December 1987 revealed that one of ninety babies tested was infected and one of sixty in New York City. As Corea (1992, 121) tells us, "Dr. Helen Rodriguez-Trias was one of many health officials and professionals shocked by the results. . . . Horrendous, Rodriguez thought. . . . What was also stunning to Rodriguez was that the obvious conclusion from this study didn't hit people: 'Hey, these are infected *women!*'" Infection in women did not galvanize the public health establishment or the media until they could perceive "women-and-children as a package deal" (p. 46). Until this point, women concerned about their vulnerability to HIV infection, requesting the antibody test, or reporting symptoms to their physicians were dismissed as hypochondriacs, tested for other things, or given mental health referrals. Those who did test positive found as little help in the literature as the clinicians and researchers concerned about women; indeed, what they found were the stereotypes, biases, misinformation, and bizarre theories that I have reported here. Corea uses the metaphor of a "funhouse mirror" to describe the distortions produced by science about women. Some women look in the mirror and see themselves reflected as crazy, irrational, hysterical, maternal. Other women see nothing: "What they feel, what they experience—none of it is reflected in the funhouse mirror" (p. 266). While to my mind the mirror analogy is as problematic as the notion that language is a transparent vehicle for content (Lacan aside, what on earth would an "undistorted reflection" look like?), the funhouse mirror image does capture one striking feature of scientific AIDS publications and pronouncements about women and gender: designed for the funhouse, the mirrors do their work in a closed environment, all facing each other to reflect, re-create, and endlessly distort whatever images enter their world. Not only is "reality" produced through a series of coconstructions; no "reality check" from another perspective is available.

15. Kinsella's (1989) profile of Kramer notes that the reputation he established with *Women in Love* was somewhat eroded by his publication of *Faggots*. Arno and Feiden's admirable 1992 book *Against the Odds* indexes *Women in Love* but also includes genuine index entries under *women*. To be fair, Shilts's index does not have an entry for *homosexuals* or *gay men* either (although there are various sub-entries under *gay*, and certainly both terms are used extensively throughout the book). The listing for *intravenous drug users* is extensive. Now, of course, I'll have to put *Women in Love* in this index, too.

16. In her masterly study of San Francisco leather communities, Gayle Rubin contrasts these stereotypes with the actual diversity of activities and preferences of the community's members in everyday life and emphasizes the range of meanings that various practices may hold for different subcultures and individuals. While in the early 1980s it was widely believed that, of all U.S. male homosexual populations, "the leather community" was at highest risk for HIV infection—an assumption held by some insiders as well as those outside the community and certainly fueled by Randy Shilts's reporting (culminating in *And the Band Played On* [1987])—Rubin argues that little empirical research actually bears on this precise question (see Rubin 1994b, 1997; Bolton 1992; and Waldby 1996; as well as Ostrow 1987a, 1990).

17. Researchers seem to have made their classificatory decisions without consulting any lesbians and to have remained in a cultural vacuum throughout the 1980s; this is in sharp contrast to decisions made about gay men, who demanded that they be consulted and to some degree were able to shape terminology, classifications, and methodology. Stoller (1995) describes the complicated intersection of lesbians and AIDS, analyzing the meaning of AIDS for lesbians and lesbian communities of different geographic locations, political commitments, and generations, and tracing the evolution of many 1980s lesbian AIDS activists into the queers and queer theorists of the 1990s. Her discussion suggests how illuminating such contributions might have been to conventional AIDS epidemiology. Stoller, of course, carried out crucial research on AIDS and women for the San Francisco AIDS Foundation, furnishing us with some of the earliest empirical work on women (including lesbians, prostitutes, and many other kinds of "women") and, along with the statistics, a more intelligent conceptual framework and nuanced vocabulary. Her thoughtful analysis reduces the scientific dithering of the 1980s about gentle sex vs. SM to nonsense. (I think, however, that the "gentle sex" stereotype may help explain a radio talk show comment I heard a couple of years ago. The topic was a controversial lesbian retreat then being planned for the Virginia countryside, and a woman, a future neighbor if the deal went through, called in to air her grievances. "I don't care about them being lesbians," she said, "but they're *feminists*.")

18. See, e.g., the pie chart in "AIDS: Science, Ethics, Policy" (1986, 2), which includes women within the category *other*—which at this point meant unknown, no known risk factor, or a risk factor that could not be established. Poggi (1987) satirized the ubiquitous AIDS pie charts in her attack on the leftist publication *In These Times*'s uninformed endorsement of mandatory HIV testing.

19. Corea's (1992) narrative, a kind of Shiltsian behind-the-scenes story of women and AIDS, highlights the "network" of U.S. clinicians and health researchers that she interviewed. Like Shilts, Corea is less interested in genuine ambiguities of data and how different constituencies make sense of them than in telling a morality tale of

good and evil. Specifically, her goal is to show that "male supremacy provides the wings on which the human immunodeficiency virus flies around the world" (p. 87). Others, including myself, would undoubtedly reconstruct this narrative differently. As recounted by Corea—unquestionably a compelling version of events—the major participants would include, although not be limited to, Judith Cohen, Constance Wolfsy, Anke Ehrhardt, Margaret Fischl, Janet Mitchell, Nancy Klimas, Zena Stein, Dooley Worth, Alexandra Levine, Vickie Mays, and Joyce Wallace.

20. On the mucous membrane, see Martin and Cone (1998), Moore and Clarke (1995), Merson (1993), Mann and Tarantola (1996), and Royce et al. (1997).

21. See the acknowledgment note to this chapter.

22. On sexism in language about AIDS, see Treichler (1988b), Grover (1988a, 1988b, 1992), Watney (1994), and Treichler et al. (1998). Other examples of linguistic slippage involve the terms "heterosexual AIDS," "heterosexual population," "through heterosexual contact," and "heterosexual partners." Another confusion is between "sexual contact" and "casual contact": "casual contact" is always assumed to be in complementary distribution to "sexual contact," thereby leaving a space for ambiguity in cases of "casual sexual contact." In non-U.S. discourses, greater specificity has produced terms like "casual nonsexual contact" and even "sexual contact without penetration."

In epidemiological parlance, the frequent reference to women as the "reservoir" in which HIV can be "harbored" calls to mind not only a whole catalog of liquid and landscape metaphors for women's bodies but also the more familiar insect and rodent "reservoirs" for diseases like plague. When a study of urban prostitutes in central Africa calls them a "major reservoir of AIDS virus" and heterosexual African males "vectors of infection," human bodies are literally implicated by a piece of technical shorthand, by the careless linguistic migration of language from a technical discourse to a more general one.

Watching the HBO movie version of Shilts's *And the Band Played On* (toward which, as I say in chap. 4 below, I am generally favorable), I was struck by scenes that casually and inadvertently reproduced the sexism of the whole epidemic. The following exchange is from a scene in the early 1980s in which members of James Curran's CDC task force on AIDS are trying to get a grip on their data:

Curran: OK, What do we think? What do we know? What can we prove? Only gays?

Male staff member: Think but can't prove.

Curran: Only males?

Male staff member: Think but can't prove.

Mary Guinan: Semen depositors. It's in the semen. Unless there's something specifically unusual about this disease, it shouldn't matter what orifice the semen is deposited in, whether it's in the anus or in the vagina. Which could mean women will be getting it also.

Curran: That's a good point—you should focus on that.

So much for women and AIDS. Although, as I relate in this chapter, in "real life" Mary Guinan did go on to coauthor the first major epidemiological paper on the subject, this is virtually the last we hear about women in the movie.

23. Media studies include Shilts (1987), Colby and Cook (1991, 1992), Buxton (1992), Check (1985), Fettner and Check (1985), Dearing (1992), Dearing and Rogers (1988),

Juhasz (1995), Kinsella (1989), McAllister (1989), Kaiser Family Foundation (1996), Kitzinger and Miller (1991), Nelkin (1984, 1985, 1987b), Schwartz (1984), Treichler and Warren (1998), Watney (1987c), Norton and Hughey (1990), Alwood (1996), A. Baker (1986), R. Baker (1994), and Albert (1986b). Albert (1986a) and Becher (1983) discuss media treatment across a range of publications; Becher's examples show that early AIDS stories on male physicians and researchers fastidiously pictured them at home with their wives, kids, and pets. Dobrow (1986) notes the dramatic and commercial appeal of the common "cultural images" in popular press scenarios of AIDS. A theoretical analysis of media accounts in relation to questions of identity and desire is offered by Simon Watney (1987c, 1994). Continued monitoring of AIDS coverage was provided by Geoffrey Stokes in his *Village Voice* column "Press Clips" (e.g., 11 October 1985, 3, 10); O'Dair (1983), Alter (1985), Winsten (1985), and Watney and Gupta (1986) cover some of the earlier media treatments. Nelkin (1985) discusses the so-called Ingelfinger rule of the *New England Journal of Medicine*, which prohibited release of findings prior to publication; Relman (1985), then the *Journal*'s editor, discusses suspension of the Ingelfinger rule and other changes in editorial policy designed to speed up publication of AIDS-related research (see also L. Altman 1988c; and D. Altman 1992).

24. I am not proposing these precise questions, of course, but recommending a shift in framework and approach to emphasize the production and deployment of knowledge rather than "knowledge" as a bag of bricks. A small but growing body of research moves in this direction: see, e.g., McAllister (1989), Buxton (1992), Reeves and Campbell (1994), Kitzinger and Miller (1991), Epstein (1996), and Williams and Mathery (1995). Likewise, a small number of reporters on science and medicine try to place knowledge within the context of its production: certainly, Crewdson's (1989) investigation for the *Chicago Tribune* qualifies as a model, even if the two years the paper's editor gave him for background research—rare these days—enraged the *Tribune*'s board of directors. Discussing the role of gender in media coverage of women's health and biology, Bertin and Beck (1996) note that general cultural perceptions of social dislocation and change increase the appeal of biological frames and explanations. See also Balsamo and Treichler (1990), Barrett and Phillips (1992), Cayleff (1989), and Sacks (1996).

25. Other work includes Patton (1985a), Patton and Kelly ([1987] 1990), Richardson (1987), Grover (1986), Pally (1985), and Shaw (1985, 1986). See also Byron (1985), Bowleg (1992), Califia (1988), Bristow et al. (1987), and Ardill and O'Sullivan (1987). Gay press coverage includes Mass (1982, 1990, [1983] 1997), Ortleb (1982, 1987, 1997), Bronski (1987). For more systematic treatment of AIDS coverage in alternative media outlets, see McAllister (1989), Kinsella (1989), Cohen (1993), Epstein (1996), and Alwood (1996).

26. Interviewed about the event and photographed for various media, the women explained their objections to Clause 28 and its restrictions on the free flow of potentially lifesaving information. AIDS activism was crucial for lesbians, they commented, adding that such activities were more useful and worthwhile than "spending a night at the disco." Interestingly, one publication captioned their photograph with this phrase: "Better than a night at the disco." Out of context, the remark was likely to be interpreted to mean something closer to "More fun than a night at the disco."

27. For more on programs and projects developed during the 1980s and 1990s in the

United Kingdom, see Aggleton et al. (1989, 1990, 1992, 1993), Berridge and Strong (1993), Watney (1994), Connor and Kingman (1989), King (1993), Gorna (1996, 1997), Oppenheimer and Reckitt (1997), and O'Sullivan and Thomson ([1992] 1996). On Australia, see Bray and Chapman (1991), D. Altman (1986, 1988, 1992, 1994), Gander (1993), Waldby (1996), and Saunders (1997). On the United States, see ACT UP New York Women and AIDS Book Group (1992), Adam and Sears (1996), Farmer et al. (1996), Corea (1992), Essoglou (1995), Meyer (1995), Kramer (1989a), ACT UP (1989a, 1989b, and 1990), and ACT UP et al. ([1989] 1997). The GPA is now UNAIDS (see Piot 1996).

3   AIDS and HIV Infection in the Third World

1. For an excellent discussion of the vexing terms *First World, Second World*, and *Third World*, see Pletsch (1981). Pletsch argues that the notion of the Third World is bogus; indeed, he writes that, except for the political categories *left* and *right*, "the scheme of three worlds is perhaps the most primitive system of classification in our social scientific discourse" (p. 566). I agree with Pletsch that, as a framework for investigation, this classification system yields studies in which non-Western civilizations—i.e., the Second and Third Worlds—are "almost pure fantasies" (p. 566). Because it is these fantasies that I am attempting to chronicle, I deliberately use the First World/Third World terminology in this essay along with such alternative signifiers as *colonial, postcolonial, industrialized, developing*, and *poor*. (See also Farmer et al. 1996; and Mann and Tarantola 1996.)

2. Homi Bhabha (1983) and Chandra Mohanty (1984), among others, argue that colonial discourse defines the colonized in such a way that increased surveillance over them is made necessary, for their own good.

3. For discussion of arrival scenes, see Pratt (1986, 35–45). The Clifford and Marcus collection *Writing Culture* (1986) offers an extended reflection on relations between anthropology, ethnography, and travel writing. See also Wolf (1992).

4. Conspiracy theories of AIDS are reviewed by Lederer (1988), Bearden (1988), Rense (1996), Gilbert (1996), and Bratich (1997). Clumeck (1989) and Konetey-Ahulu (1988), in contrast, identify and counter the main myths and misinformation held in the West *about* AIDS in Africa. The function of conspiracy theories in postcolonial settings is discussed by Farmer (1990) and Gottlieb (1990) and explored at length by White (1993), who offers several methodological pointers about the collection and interpretation of such accounts. First World conspiracy theories make their own use of "Third World AIDS," sometimes rhetorically to invoke the universality of the victims of transnational elites, sometimes instrumentally to provide verisimilitude for narratives of power, greed, and evil. For examples, see Douglass ([1987] 1996), Keith (1993), Null with Golobic (1987), and Shenton (1990). See also Herek and Capitanio (1994) and M. Novick (1995).

5. A parallel shift took place in representations of gay men in the United States, as illness and death transformed a threatening and alien community into a vulnerable one, worthy of achieving a redemptive ending (see Pratt 1986, 44–50). Working against redemption is the ethnographic paradox that the Other becomes worldly wise through contact with "modern civilization"—often in the guise of ethnographers themselves. In Selzer's encounter, the fact that he pays the prostitutes to talk to him parallels the further irony of ethnographic research in which the privileged

investigator enters into a commodity exchange with the native informant—an exchange that, as Pratt puts it, turns the "anthropologist preserver-of-the-culture" into the "interventionist corrupter-of-the-culture." Wolf (1992) explores these questions at length.

6. See also the photographs in Nordland et al. (1986) and Pierce (1986). Images of AIDS in Brazilian magazines like *Veja*, first brought to my attention by Elisabeth Santos, are further analyzed in Seijo-Maldonado and Horak (1991). The "truth" of these images cannot be decided by appeals to realism or statistics about the number of ambulances in Brazil, although such information may be relevant to interpretation. We also need to know the story's context, its aim, and the conventions of the medium and genre in which it is told. Linkages among photographs, captions, and text that seem natural to us do not occur only in Third World context, of course. A story on AIDS in the Canadian journal *Macleans* (24 August 1987), e.g., includes a photograph of pedestrians on a crowded Toronto city street; shot from behind so that the pedestrians are moving away from the camera, the photograph appears to illustrate the caption: "Toronto sidewalk traffic: Growing fear of AIDS virus spreads to general public" (p. 31). We have learned from years of reading news stories that such a photograph is not literally picturing pedestrians fleeing from the virus.

7. In his 1990 book *Slim*, Hooper provides an illuminating account of the circumstances under which the photographs were taken and considerable insight into the production and circulation of images produced by professional photojournalists. Hooper's discussion is in turn used by Matthew Little (1994) to argue that textual analyses of images like the photograph of Florence are enriched and tempered by "on-the-ground" perspectives, like Hooper's. Little tracks the circulation of Florence's images in more detail than I have here. For other cultural critiques of First World media representations of AIDS/HIV in Africa and in the less-developed world more generally and debates about the grounds for such critique, see Sabatier (1988), Patton (1990), Watney (1989, 1994), Kitzinger and Miller (1991), Hooper (1990), Karnik (1998; forthcoming), McGee (1996) and Seijo-Moldonado and Horak (1991).

8. Renée Sabatier quotes a Nigerian prostitute named Juliet as follows: "Although white clients generally pay better than their African counterparts, I will never go to bed with a white man unless he wears a condom. As far as I am concerned, AIDS is a white man's disease" (Sabatier 1988, 96). Similarly, a letter to the editor of the Kenyan *Weekly Review* inverted the Western argument for gender-neutral transmission (it happens in Africa) to argue that heterosexual contact is an unlikely source of AIDS in Africa: "it seems illogical to assume that a method that doesn't work in the U.S. should be the main route in Africa" (Rowell, 1986).

9. Jean William Pape, a leading AIDS researcher in Haiti and one of the physicians Selzer consulted, expresses disenchantment with the Western press for consistently ignoring "the efforts of the Haitian people to fight, with almost no resources, the most devastating disease of this century." He told the Panos Institute: "I have given over 60 interviews to American and other reporters about AIDS in Haiti. It is very time-consuming and exhausting, and takes energy I would like to put into my work. Of all those interviews there are only one or two that recorded what I said, and the context in which I said it, accurately. The others often painted a picture of AIDS in Haiti that was unrecognizable to me" (quoted in Sabatier 1988, 90; see also Johnson and Pape 1989; and Farmer et al. 1996). (I do not know whether Pape found Selzer's report objectionable.) But negative reactions to Western media reports do not neces-

sarily disrupt cycles of representation. Some African governments, e.g., angry at what they believed to be inflations of AIDS statistics or simply wishing to deflect attention from the AIDS problem, prohibited AIDS researchers and physicians from giving interviews to the Western press. "One result of such attempts at control," said James Brooke, West Africa correspondent for the *New York Times*, in an interview with the Panos Institute in November 1987, "has been to force foreign reporters to rely more heavily on foreign researchers working in those countries, making it more difficult than before to convey an authentically African point of view" (quoted in Sabatier 1988, 95). See also Brooke (1988a, 1988b), Kinsella (1989). In chap. 7 below, I discuss a series in the *New York Times* entitled "A Continent's Agony," which ran from 16 to 19 September 1990.

10. Here, discussing the word *experience* in *Keywords* ([1976] 1983, 126–29), Williams refers to his earlier analysis in *The Country and the City* (1973, 215–32) of experience and statistical analysis as different ways of producing knowledge.

11. See, e.g., the testimony of Bradshaw Langmaid, Bureau of Science and Technology, USAID, on funding criteria for AIDS aid to African countries (U.S. House 1988).

12. Most studies depend on some degree of cooperation between the First and the Third Worlds and are thus influenced by the scientific and political commitments of given agencies and their ability to find common grounds of inquiry as well as resources. Scarce resources have created wide variation in scientific research in Africa; yet much more research goes on than stereotypes about Africa would suggest. Needless to say, views on cooperation with Western scientists are also highly variable, reflecting in some respects the ideological commitments of the state as a whole. On the distinction between the many long-term collaborative projects that predate AIDS and what African commentators call "parachute research" or "tourist research," in which foreign researchers drop in "to collect blood samples, data or clinical observations, and just as quickly [take] off again, to write up their findings for a (Western) scientific journal," see Sabatier (1988, 108–9).

13. For recent updates and detailed discussion of the methods used to make statistical measures of and predictions about AIDS/HIV, see Mann and Tarantola (1996)—who also lay out the theoretical foundation for shifting from the old WHO Pattern I, II, and III classifications to a much more sophisticated system that groups nations and regions by geographic and cultural affinities and takes into account resources, religion, infrastructure, and the like. The appendix to their book, rare among AIDS publications, lays out the procedures used to arrive at quantitative outcomes, noting sources of uncertainty. Monthly statistical updates are available from the Pan-American Health Organization in Washington, D.C., WHO's regional health office for the Americas. Although the worldwide estimate of HIV infection at the end of the 1980s was often given in the press as 5–10 million, official estimates were somewhat lower: 6–8 million was the estimate given at the Sixth International Conference on AIDS in San Francisco by Michael Merson, Mann's replacement as head of WHO's Global AIDS Program (De Wolk 1990, A1, A4). Merson (1993) estimated 14 million infected. By the 1996 International Conference on AIDS in Vancouver, estimated worldwide cases totaled 21.8 million (L. Altman 1996a).

Many countries produce their own version of "Patient Zero," and these sometimes reflect patterns of geopolitical conflict. The former Soviet Union reported its first official "indigenous" death from AIDS in September 1988—a pregnant Leningrad prostitute named Olga Gaeevskaya ("Epidemiologists Were Incensed" 1988, A2).

Previous cases were attributed to sexual contact with Westerners. Japan resisted the possibility of "indigenous AIDS" for many years, but a Patient Zero emerged eventually. Treat (1994) describes the months-long saga in the Japanese media during 1987 of "Miss A," a Japanese woman found to have AIDS and reportedly the first case to involve a Japanese citizen who had never traveled abroad; before long, it emerged that she had had "sexual contact" and possibly "cohabited" with "a foreigner." According to a report in the *London Independent* (14 February 1987), Miss A was a Japanese prostitute in Kobe who, it was concluded, had acquired AIDS from sexual contact with a foreigner; a Japanese newspaper was quoted: "Her death was the result of an infatuation with Europe." Sabatier notes that "in the red light district of Tokyo warnings signs suddenly appeared: '*Gaijin* [foreigners] off limits'" (1988, 114), and Treat (1994) reports their appearance in the neighborhoods where foreign students and faculty could afford to live. (See also Dearing 1992.) Corea (1992) relates the cases of two female Patient Zero figures in the United States. A case in Edmonton in 1988 enabled the press to create a female Canadian Patient Zero. A comparably high-profile 1989 case in Australia involved an HIV-positive sex worker known as Charlene; she was incarcerated in a psychiatric hospital in Sydney under the Public Health Act for allegedly having unprotected sex with clients—at their request (Waldby 1996, 153; see also Lupton 1994). In the previous chapter, I noted the "Welcome to the World of AIDS" urban legend; in chapter 8 below, we will encounter this legend resurrected for the 1990s. Another "outbreak" of HIV infection (the headline says "AIDS") occurred among twenty-seven babies and five of their mothers in a hospital in Elista, capital of a region along the Caspian Sea. Transmission scenarios abounded; in the end, authorities blamed unsterilized needles for the babies' infection and suggested that the mothers' infection was contracted through breast-feeding the infected babies (Burns 1989). In retrospect, this incident seems almost to be a prototype for the AIDS reports that would pour out of Eastern Europe and the former Soviet Union after its breakup. Where earlier stories had tended to report cold war AIDS conspiracy charges or contrast official denials of homosexuality in the Soviet Union with visits to gay bars, journalists "after the fall," with new access to the former "Second World" (WHO's Pattern III AIDS), now seemed to produce transmission narratives featuring (like this report of infants infected by a single contaminated hospital syringe) chaos, systemic breakdown, and the devastation produced by decades of centralized control (the "AIDS orphans" in Romania, e.g.).

14. For assessments of the nature and effect of AIDS in Third World countries in the 1980s, see UNESCO (1986), U.S. House (1988), WHO (1988a, 1988b, 1988c), Panos Institute (1986), Altman (1985c), Netter (1987), Roberts (1987), Sabatier (1988), Patton (1985b), Miller and Rockwell (1988), Anderson et al. (1988), Biggar (1988), Bygbjerg (1983), Copson (1987), Hawkins (1988), Hunt (1988), Institute of Medicine and National Academy of Sciences (1986, 1988), Krieger (1987), Over et al. (1988), Prewitt (1988), Perlez (1988a), Venter (1988), Waite (1988), and Watson (1987). Jonathan Mann, former director of the Global AIDS Program, advocated aggressive, activist strategies to achieve global cooperation (Mann et al. 1988a, 32). Mann's departure from WHO interrupted the momentum of program and policy development at a critical stage in the epidemic. Mann and Tarantola (1996), Farmer et al. (1996), and Bond et al. (1997) point to many relevant sources and resources. Brooke (1993), Buckley (1997), Piot (1996), and *UNAIDS Report* (1998) update the global epidemic.

15. My discussion of language in chap. 2 above identified several problems with the

term *prostitutes* as used in the AIDS literature, problems that are more fully amplified in the work of sex workers themselves. Two scholarly collections provide an interesting contrast on this point. Bond et al. (1997), a collection of epidemiological and ethnographic studies of AIDS/HIV in Africa and the Caribbean, addresses many problems of terminology and definition and sees such problems as integral to research design. Plant, editor of a collection titled *AIDS, Drugs, and Prostitution*, acknowledges only that prostitutes are called by many different names, many of them pejorative: "For the purposes of this book prostitution may be defined as the provision of sexual services in exchange for some form of payment such as money, drink, drugs, or other consumer goods" (Plant 1990, xiv). See also Kreiss et al. (1986), the first major "prostitute study" to be published in a leading medical journal.

16. For an overview of problems associated with diagnosis and testing, see Gunn et al. (1988), Sher et al. (1987), Wendler (1986), and WHO and CDC (1988). See also the essays in Koch-Weser and Vanderschmidt (1988), especially Konotey-Ahulu (1988). Existing studies on Africa are summarized by Clumeck (1989), Hilts (1988), and Torrey et al. (1988). On the clinical manifestations of AIDS in Haiti, see Johnson and Pape (1989). A detailed treatment of "the African data" (blood samples, etc.) is provided in Grmek (1990).

17. An influential anthropological source for rumors about exotic behaviors has been Hrdy (1987). The rumors preserve bits and pieces of anthropological research studies without their larger cultural context. A detailed critique of many studies can be found in Chirimuuta and Chirimuuta (1989), who also suggest that "underreporting" is no more a problem than "overdiagnosing." See also Chirimuuta et al. (1987), Haq (1988), Torrey et al. (1988), and other papers in Miller and Rockwell (1988). A general critique of studies of AIDS in Africa is provided by Cerullo and Hammonds (1988) and Krieger (1987). An attempt to place AIDS statistics within a broader political and economic perspective is presented in Barker and Turshen (1986). An elaborate web of speculation about Haiti can be found in Moore and LeBaron (1986). The historical debate over "the Haitian origin of syphilis," of course, goes back centuries, a debate noted by Paul Farmer (1990) in his critique of Moore and LeBaron. Farmer and colleagues (1996) review much of this literature in detail.

18. For differing interpretations of the situation in Cuba, see Wade (1989) and Goldstein (1989). Fee (1988) talked with Cuba's minister of health about AIDS and other health issues. Scheper-Hughes (1992, 1994) argues that Cuba's approach has been successful in many respects and represents no more than a traditional public health approach (quarantine the infected). On the basis of her fieldwork on AIDS among poor communities in Brazil, she expresses considerable exasperation with U.S. AIDS activists for their condemnation of Cuba. Only First World leftists, she implies, can afford to embrace individual civil liberties as an absolute right, sacrificing conventional approaches.

19. Although these dichotomies are primarily social, the differentiation among types of AIDS and strains of HIV is also a scientific and clinical question (see Clumeck 1989; and Grmek 1990).

20. Hilts (1988, 12) notes the incredulity that greeted the appearance of AIDS in Africa. He quotes a pulmonary specialist in Uganda who first saw AIDS there in 1983: "It looked like the new American disease. But none of us could believe it." (Compare the comments quoted in n. 8 above.) But, before too long, AIDS began to be blamed on the loose morals of African people—always those in other countries, classes, or

ethnic groups. Thus, an editorial in the *Kenya Times* ([Nairobi], 26 May 1987) blamed Uganda for lax sexual behavior, noting that "nature has its own law of retribution." See the discussion in Sabatier (1988, 105). In contrast, see Browning (1988), who says that most descriptions of U.S. subcultures involved in AIDS make them sound "as strange as those of Bantu twig gatherers" (p. 70).

21. Schoepf et al. (1988) observed (as USAID, apparently, did not) that condoms "which hurt their wearer or break during normal use may limit the effectiveness of AIDS prevention efforts." See also Schoepf (1991, 1992a, 1992b), Hooper (1990), and Treichler (1996).

22. I have greatly oversimplified Parker's intricate representation of Brazilian sexuality, which, as he emphasizes, is not the mere overlay of a Western ethnographer but permeates language, slang, informal discussion, and ongoing open debate about sexuality as an essential aspect of cultural identity and "Brazilianness." The penetrator/recipient and other distinctions that construct masculinity/femininity between same-sex partners occur elsewhere, including the United States. For an illuminating review of recent research on "same-gender sexual behaviors" in several cultural settings, see Turner et al. (1989) as well as Bolton (1991). For an analysis of sexuality from a different perspective, but one potentially helpful in articulating women's concerns, see the conclusions and recommendations "adopted by the group of experts" at a UNESCO conference in Madrid, 12–21 March 1986 (UNESCO 1986; see also Carrier (1995) and Merson (1993). In chap. 7 below and elsewhere in this book, I return to permutations of gender, including recent work in the fields of cultural anthropology, postcolonial studies, and queer theory.

23. Ratafia and Scott (1987) make clear the size and diversity of the "AIDS market" for the development of clinical products. In the 1990s, this market has become more sophisticated and more selective; as hot button ethical questions about vaccine testing and treatment have become topics of intense public debate, even less scrutiny is given everyday market development.

24. See Kolata (1988a), the "AIDS Monitor" column in the *New Scientist* (18 February 1988), and Perlez (1988b). Perlez, reporting vaccine discussions at a conference in Tanzania on AIDS and Africa, writes: "In Africa, unlike the United States, the virus is most commonly spread through heterosexual contact. Officials believe that, despite warnings to use condoms and avoid multiple partners, further spread of the virus is inevitable. . . . Because of behavioral changes brought about by extensive education about AIDS, the spread of the infection among gay men in the United States has slowed. Thus, there would be few new infections in a study group, whether or not its members took the vaccine, the scientists said. The scientists said they regarded intravenous drug users, a group that continues to have a high incidence of AIDS in the United States, as unreliable for the necessary follow-up that is needed for a study group" (p. B5). According to Perlez, a WHO committee developing ethical guidelines for vaccine testing said that the decision to go ahead should be made by three groups: scientists developing the vaccine, scientists knowledgeable about vaccine development but with no academic or commercial stakes in it, and "government officials and their scientific advisers from the population where the vaccine is to be tried." No representatives of the population to be tested were mentioned. For more recent developments, see chap. 7 below.

25. I know of no comprehensive description and analysis of the names given to AIDS

and HIV internationally and interculturally, but it would be of great interest. Of equal interest and even greater policy significance would be the debates in various nations over the official naming and defining of AIDS and HIV and the circumstances and implications of differing positions. Feldman (1995) discusses a number of reasons why French and U.S. AIDS physicians have developed different practices of naming, defining, referring to, and charting the dimensions and course of HIV infection. Not the least of these reasons are the national health care systems in the two countries and their vastly different arrangements for covering the costs of care.

4 Seduced and Terrorized

This chapter began as a presentation at SIDART, a conference on art and culture held in conjunction with the Fifth International Conference on AIDS in Montreal (June 1989), and was revised and updated twice for publication (Treichler 1992b). Although I would probably write this whole essay differently today, I have left my original argument more or less intact and added commentary on the 1990s.

1. The green snake phenomenon was described to me by Leland C. Clark Jr., professor emeritus of pediatrics and director of neurophysiology, University of Cincinnati College of Medicine.

2. Selected readings of television and media coverage of the AIDS epidemic include Alcorn (1989), D. Altman (1986), Crimp (1988a, 1988c), Grover (1988c, 1989a, 1989b), Herzlich and Pierret (1989), Kinsella (1989), Landers (1988), Hughey, Norton, and Sullivan (1986), Norton and Hughey (1990), Norton et al. (1990), Packer and Kauffman (1990), Shilts (1987), Sturken (1997), Tagg (1988), Treichler (1988a, 1988b), and Watney (1987c). See also Gitlin (1986) and Friedman et al. (1986). Several papers on television were presented at "AIDS: Communication Challenges," a day-long conference held in conjunction with the annual meeting of the International Communication Association, San Francisco, 27 May 1989.

3. The value of such control becomes especially clear when it is absent—as it was, e.g., on a November 1986 segment of "Wall Street Week" during which a guest expert was asked by a visiting panelist to recommend stocks that might go up as a result of the AIDS epidemic or on a 1989 segment of the conservative Washington talk show "Tony Brown's Journal" (21 May 1989) during which several AIDS conspiracy theorists presented their views to a largely black audience with virtually no challenge or contradiction. Eva Lee Snead, e.g., listed as "Dr." and author of *Win! against Herpes and AIDS*, argued that "AIDS is a figment of the media," that the "HTLV virus" was deliberately used to contaminate Zairean gamma globulin, and that the World Health Organization was behind it. She was supported by a young black man in the audience who feverishly documented places in the *Congressional Record* where this could all be verified. He also supplied the motive, about which Dr. Snead was murky: to obtain the natural resources of central Africa by killing off the black population there and in the United States. At this point, the largely black audience burst into applause. In the entire half hour, reservations were expressed only twice: a representative from WHO forcefully but briefly took issue with Dr. Snead's theory, and a young black woman in the audience said, "I do AIDS education, and what you're saying in this room would set me back ten years; I'd like to know what credentials, what business you have saying what you're saying?" Both were ignored.

The program ended with a Lyndon LaRouche follower (white) rising from the audience to commend the entire event and attempt to fill the audience in on the role of the Trilateral Commission. Important theoretical questions can be asked about why conspiracy theories are so appealing and in precisely what ways (and on what grounds) they are to be distinguished from scientific theories.

4. "The AIDS Quarterly," to which Greyson refers, greatly improved in its later installments and broadened to become "The Health Quarterly." At the time of Greyson's comments, the single independent feature aired by PBS was *The A.I.D.S. Show* (Adair and Epstein 1986). Since then, additional independent videos have been aired.

5. Many of the alternative films and videos to which I refer here are compiled on *Video against AIDS*, a set of three tapes curated by John Greyson and Bill Horrigan (1990). Likewise, many are described more fully in Carlomusto (1992), Saalfield (1992), Grover (1989a), Boffin and Gupta (1990), and Juhasz (1995). Interesting *AIDS* videos for health professionals have been produced by Norman Baxley (e.g., 1991, 1994).

6. As actor Tom Hulce said in his presentation at SIDART (June 1989), what shocked audiences at Larry Kramer's play *The Normal Heart* was not "the medical details about AIDS—the seizures, the lesions, etc.—they're used to medical stuff. What shocked them was seeing two men kissing." Concern about job discrimination in Hollywood was addressed on "Saturday Night Live" in 1986; linking AIDS panic to McCarthy-era blacklisting, a sketch showed a gay male actor worried about being "pinklisted" and trying to establish his heterosexual credentials by swaggering into a bar, flirting with the waitress, and talking about the Dallas Cowboys. Ironically, Aidan Quinn told "TV Guide" that, since his performance in *An Early Frost*, he has received more scripts calling for him to play "more normal, human guys" instead of the narrowly typecast rebel hunks he played before. For a more detailed discussion of *An Early Frost*, *Our Sons*, and other made-for-television movies, see chap. 6 below.

7. *Fabian's Story*, widely criticized as unethical, nonrepresentative, and exploitative, shows a black male prostitute who continues to have unsafe sex even after his diagnosis: Martha Gever (1988) pointed out that, in contrast, a positive film about a man with AIDS, *Chuck Solomon: Coming of Age*, by Mark Huestis and Wendy Dallas (1986), was turned down by PBS (although shown by Channel Four in Britain). The figure of "Patient Zero," the Canadian flight attendant represented as a kind of Typhoid Mary character by Shilts (1987), is discussed in Crimp (1988c). Buxton (1991) uses the "Midnight Caller" episode as a detailed case study of production processes in broadcast television, showing that considerable negotiation among different groups brought about significant changes in the script (see also Gerard 1988). See also chaps. 6 and 9 below.

8. In the chapter on AIDS in his memoirs, former Surgeon General C. Everett Koop (1991) details his ferocious battles with the Reagan White House over AIDS policy; describing pressure to tone down his hard-hitting AIDS report (U.S. Surgeon General 1986) before releasing it, Koop says that, in the end, they wanted him to delete the word *condom*. Koop refused (although he makes clear that, as a Christian and a conservative, he was not especially thrilled to be dubbed "the king of condoms"). In my essay "How to Use a Condom" (Treichler 1996), I discuss condoms and television at length.

9. On Reagan's surgery, see Bob Huff's amazing 1987 video *The Asshole Is a Tense*

Hole. The evolution of explicit usage is discussed by Colby (1989), Kinsella (1989), and Packer and Kauffman (1990). Generally, *penis* and *anal intercourse* have been considered to be the most sensitive words, and, even now, some stations do not permit them. Interestingly, in the first years of AIDS coverage, the only phrase prohibited by the relatively liberal National Public Radio was "full-blown AIDS," which they perceived to be sexually suggestive. Michael Callen commented that "one distressing presumption that runs through this asshole coverage is that anal intercourse and male homosexuality are synonymous. When will someone point out that heterosexuals can *and do* engage in anal intercourse?" (1988, 218).

10. As Schoepf et al. (1988) point out, discussing their experiences working with women in Zaire, the country's deepening poverty presents added difficulties for condom use: for many women, only the provision of new income-generating activities would provide real alternatives to multiple-partner sex. Elsewhere, Schoepf describes an experimental condom education program based on cooperation with traditional tribal elders (1992a).

11. Screenings of activists' and artists' videos at the Montreal conference were very popular; after the conference, with little additional publicity, many orders for *Video against AIDS* (see n. 5 above) came in to Video Data Bank and V/Tape from community health organizations and health educators—precisely the viewers conventionally believed to require "straight" materials.

12. Analyzing the Gulf War and its televised spectacle, Elaine Scarry observes that Americans' intense obsession with the war's daily chronicle on CNN was widely interpreted to signify a level of interest and involvement wholly appropriate to the citizens of a participatory democracy in the information age. Yet, argues Scarry, the mesmerizing images of the Gulf were really offered U.S. citizens *in place of* genuine participation in deliberations about U.S. involvement. It may have looked like deliberation, it may even have felt like deliberation, but what it really represented, in Scarry's view, was "a mimesis of deliberation." This is, of course, a serious concern.

5 AIDS, HIV, and the Cultural Construction of Reality

1. In addition to the conference program, sources for examples of discourse at the conference include texts of lectures, press kits, press releases, published newspaper and journal articles, and the author's notes from press conferences and press briefings. For Morisset's introduction, see *Abstracts* (1989).

2. In the 1970s, the sociologist Pauline Bart designed a T-shirt with the statement "Everything is data" on the front, "But data isn't everything" on the back. In other words, everything is potentially material for an analysis based on cultural construction, but this enterprise by no means exhausts the world or one's ways of being in it. To hold on to a point of perfect equipoise between what we say to the world and what it says back to us is perhaps the major intellectual challenge of working in the domain of cultural investigation.

3. Kroeber and Kluckhohn (1952) trace the two ideologically contradictory meanings that the term *Kulture* acquired in Germany as both in league with and resistant to *Zivilisation*: the first meaning was international and progressive and involved the desire to go forward toward democracy; the second was introverted and romantic and represented a fight for Germany's unique cultural heritage (and the wish to go

backward toward "nature"). We do not know which meaning would have won out because the word was deleted from German dictionaries until after 1848, by which point its radical connotations had been forgotten.

4. The social and cultural construction of reality, as I am interested in it here, is, of course, addressed in the work of Dilthey, Weber, Merton, Benedict, Sapir, Firth, Halliday, Whorf, and Putnam as well as Weber, Schutz, Ricoeur, Mead, Freud, and Giddens. And see Hill (1988), Ortony (1979), Sperber (1985), and Wuthnow et al. (1984). Kroeber and Kluckhohn's review is a definitive starting point for any discussion of culture. They invoke the old realist/idealist divide—what Ortony (1979), updating the terminology, calls "the realist/constructionist divide"—only to reject it: "We are not too sure we can properly classify ourselves as cultural realists, idealists, or nominalists" (Kroeber and Kluckhohn 1952, 190). Bourdieu also insists on a radical attention to practice, leading him to the notion of the *habitus*—a term designed to move beyond "the common conception of habit as a mechanical assembly or performed programme" and instead emphasize a specific intersection in time and space (Bourdieu [1972] 1977, 218 n. 47). By emphasizing the situatedness of practice, its unique possibilities within a network of constraints, Bourdieu can envision a system that transcends conventional dichotomies.

   The sociology of science and science studies take up these questions in detail, rigorously employing several methods to construct a nonrealist account of scientific discovery and truth. Interviews, ethnography, and discourse analysis are among the strategies used to develop detailed case studies of specific scientific developments and controversies. See, e.g., Barnes and Bloor (1982), Fujimura and Chou (1994), Pickering (1995), and Epstein (1996). Veldink's (1989) dissection of the "honeybee language controversy" is less well known but highly relevant to AIDS and HIV debates. Adrian Wenner, one of the principals in that controversy, co-authored a more philosophical explanatory framework, based in part on Latour's work, to account for scientific controversies and allegiances (Wenner and Wells 1990).

5. Given their radical and uncompromising version of construction, Latour and Woolgar no doubt took some pleasure in reporting, in a note to the 1986 (second) edition, that, when the book was originally published, they were forced to remove such disclaimers to certainty as "*all* texts are stories" and "the reader can never know for sure"; the publishers (Sage) said that they were not in the habit of publishing anything that "proclaimed its own worthlessness" (p. 284). Latour and Woolgar also note their decision to drop the term *social* from the book's original subtitle (*The Social Construction of Scientific Facts*): "By demonstrating its pervasive applicability, the social study of science has rendered 'social' devoid of any meaning. Although this was our original intention, it was not clear until now that we could simply ditch the term" (p. 281).

6. Perhaps because physicians worked so systematically to establish medicine as a science equipped to define reality—anywhere, anytime—their resistance to constructionism is considerable. Indeed, *resistance* is perhaps the wrong word, for it implies a perceived and articulated challenge. It is more accurate to see medicine as an ideological system that works tirelessly and smoothly, in Berger and Luckman's sense, to keep its reality coherent, a reality that cannot by definition be challenged. Hence, when anthropology and ethnography encounter medicine as a signifying system, they come into contact with a deeply entrenched realism. Nevertheless, a

view of medical reality as constructed does now figure in the work of some medical sociologists, historians, linguists, literary critics, and anthropologists. (Again, of course, a point that I pursue in chap. 9 below, the practices that constitute and confirm a given vision of the world in everyday life—and clinical medicine—are not carried out within an explicit framework of radical provisionality and indeterminacy; indeed, I dread the day my primary care physician first refers to my medical record [or my body] as a text, moreover a text to be deconstructed.) Writings in medical anthropology particularly germane here include Caplan (1987), Gaines (1987), Gaines and Hahn (1985), Marcus and Fischer (1986), Marshall and Bennett (1990), Payer (1988), Holland and Quinn (1987), Rapp (1988), Scheper-Hughes and Lock (1986), Schneider (1980), Sperber (1985) and Wright and Treacher (1982). On anthropology and AIDS, see Farmer and Kleinman (1989), Parker (1987, 1991), and Bolton's comprehensive bibliography (1991). See also Brieger (1980).

While some anthropologists would place themselves on one side or the other, others suggest that the division grows out of the way the world is. Dorothy Holland and Naomi Quinn write, e.g., "Undeniably, a great deal of order exists in the natural world we experience. However, much of the order we perceive in the world is there only because we put it there. That we impose such order is even more apparent when we consider the social world, in which institutions such as marriage, deeds such as lying, and customs such as dating happen at all because the members of a society permit them to be. D'Andrade contrasts such culturally constructed things with the cultural categories for objects such as stone, tree, and hand, which exist whether or not we invent labels for them. An entity such as marriage, on the other hand, is created by 'the social agreement that something counts as that condition' and exists only by virtue of adherence to the rules that constitute it" (1987, 3).

Atwood Gaines (1987) summarizes with great confidence the assumptions of a constructionist position in medical anthropology: medical knowledge is seen as problematic, not given; medical knowledge is not distinct from social knowledge; diseases are not naturally existing entities; the study of medicine and its development must include the study of external social forces. But, in the absence of the detailed cultural context and meticulously circumscribed ground rules established by studies like Knorr-Cetina's, an uneasiness with a constructionist model of biomedical phenomena sometimes emerges. The introduction to Gaines and Hahn, e.g., includes the statement: "The editors note here a difference between them which also divides anthropologists more widely; in the determination of human affairs, Hahn gives more weight to an external 'real' 'physical' world while Gaines emphasizes particular cultural constructions of reality as sources and guides of human action" (1985, 5).

7. Recent ethnographic research on sexuality and sexual identity could be said similarly to challenge epidemiology's narration of the real (see Caplan 1987; Herdt 1981; Kane and Mason 1992; Leonard 1990; Lindenbaum 1984; and Parker 1987, 1991). Gill Shepherd (1987) describes sexual relationships in Mombasa, Kenya, where "same-sex" behavior indubitably occurs but differs in cultural meaning according to sex, social rank, and age; because same-sex relationships are constituted within this dense network of social and symbolic relationships, they are said not to exist in virtually all nonscholarly literature on "homosexuality" in Africa (see also Bolton 1991; Dean 1993; and Duberman 1997).

8. Press briefing reports are based on my field notes.
9. The Montreal conference provides other examples as well. A second understanding of culture at Montreal was reflected in public health and social science papers. In the tradition of Virchow, Sigerist, and Dubos, these accounts emphasize the broad social conditions that encourage and sustain epidemics of infectious disease in various cultures—conditions ranging from poverty, malnutrition, endemic disease, population shifts, and inadequate health care to discrimination, capitalism, colonialism, environmental toxins, cultural and linguistic barriers to communication, government inaction, drug use, and problems of postcolonial development. Here, information about social conditions and cultural practice is crucial to defining the epidemic and developing strategies for addressing it; the 1989 conference was enhanced in this respect by the participation of people of color from developing countries (scientists, policymakers, media representatives, and people with AIDS). As the correspondent for the magazine *West Africa* commented, the Montreal conference was a landmark for Third World people ("Symptoms of Global Malady" 1989).

Another understanding emerged in the events explicitly labeled *cultural*: educational dramas and dances designed for rural villages in the Caribbean and central Africa, exhibits of historical and contemporary art on infectious and venereal disease, and panels of writers, television producers, artists, activists, and academics featured in SIDART (a series of panels, exhibits, films, and other cultural events organized in conjunction with the conference). Here, *culture*—designating, on the one hand, the actual objects and artifacts resulting from cultural production and, on the other, the intellectual apparatus of symbolic production and meaning (signification, cultural difference, cultural production, interpretation, and representation)—addressed what Brazilian writer Herbert Daniel (1989) called "the staging of the epidemic"; notions of cultural construction were explicit elements of debate.
10. No doubt in part this is because the Canadian press has a tradition of deflating U.S. puffery. Press coverage relevant to the Montreal conference includes Charles (1989), Crewdson (1989), Dunn (1989), Kuitenbrouwer (1989), Picard (1989), Regush (1989a, 1989b), and Treichler (1992b). For a similar critique of U.S. arrogance, see Konotey-Ahulu (1988). See also "AIDS Victims Live Longer" (1989).
11. Questions at these briefings were sometimes passed forward in writing. In this case, the questioner was writer and activist Michael Callen, one of Joseph Sonnabend's AIDS patients and a participant at Sonnabend's press briefing the day before. In asking his question orally, Callen noted that the written version had been torn up rather than read out. (Thus, gatekeeping can take place even when no gates are visible.) When a couple of quasi-technical follow-up questions failed to elicit any concession from Gallo that other factors might be involved, Callen started to turn away; but Gallo stopped him, saying with some sarcasm, "Wait a minute, wait a minute—I probably know as much about this as you." He then proceeded to talk at length, concluding: "I don't control who gets funded. If it meets peer review, it gets funded. If you or Duesberg or Sonnabend wants to work on something other than HIV, be my guest."
12. The often-amorphous conditions and diverse injuries caused by the stress of repetitive motion are considered a legitimate occupational disease category in Australia but not in the United States. It has been persuasively argued by Andrew Hopkins

(1990) that in part this is because the Australians early settled on a single term—*repetitive strain injury* (or *RSI*)—that was conceptually meaningful in terms of its causes; in contrast, the United States has confused the picture with a plethora of terms, including the narrowly medicalized *carpal tunnel syndrome* and the broader but vaguer *cumulative trauma syndrome*, a term few would readily associate with work-related problems. What is at stake, Hopkins argues, is individual vs. social (and corporate) responsibility—and hence accountability and cost of care. Within Australia's national health care system, the incentive is to identify socially produced disease as early as possible and determine how to prevent it. As the United States shifts from private coverage to managed care, one would expect a growing acknowledgment of socially produced disease, yet no doubt some version of individual risk and culpability will remain dominant in discourse.

13. Quote from author's interview with Sonnabend, Montreal, 7 June 1989.

14. This is in transition; in abstracts of papers given at Montreal and San Francisco, one finds both military and coding metaphors. On the development of coding and language as the metaphors underlying molecular biology, see Woese (1967). On the evolution of representations in twentieth-century medical textbooks, see Haraway (1989a). On metaphor, see Brandt (1988a), Geertz (1973), Lakoff and Johnson (1980), Martin (1988), McGrath (1990), Miller (1989), Ortony (1979), Sontag (1989), Sturken (1997), Varmus (1989), Vedder (1996), Verghese (1994), Waldby (1996), Watney (1989), Williamson (1989), and Zuger (1995).

Consider the ways, as described by Crewdson (1989), that the Pasteur group and the Gallo group approached the problem of identifying "the AIDS virus." From the beginning, Gallo believed that AIDS was caused by a leukemia retrovirus like the two HTLV viruses his laboratory had already isolated. The discovery process was, therefore, shaped by this conception: when he introduced infected cells from AIDS patients into cell cultures, he expected them to replicate as a cancer virus like HTLV would; instead, the cultures died. As a metaphor, the tenor of Gallo's conception was that AIDS was caused by a human retrovirus; the vehicle for him was the HTLV leukemia model. The French, meanwhile, began with no such preconception: the tenor was identical, but the vehicle was not nearly so narrow. Accordingly, they explored different ways to keep the cell culture alive, discovering before long that the virus killed cells rather than causing them to replicate; because the French scientists kept adding fresh cells, the cultures did not die.

For a detailed analysis of the Gallo-Montagnier dispute and its status as a continuing narrative, see Feldman (1992). More recently, the Gallo-Montagnier-Duesberg dispute is analyzed in Fujimura and Chou (1994) and Epstein (1996).

6   AIDS Narratives on Television

1. Made for NBC "Monday Night at the Movies," *An Early Frost* was directed by John Erman and produced by Perry Lafferty, with story by Sherman Yellin, teleplay by Daniel Lipman and Ron Cowen, music by John Kander, and photography by Woody Omens. The movie stars Gena Rowlands as Kay, Ben Gazzara as Nick, Aidan Quinn as Michael, and Sylvia Sidney as Bea, with D. W. Moffett as Peter, John Glover as Victor, Sydney Walsh as Susan, and Terry O'Quinn as Dr. Redding.

2. On the basis of a study of two weeks of television programming in November 1985,

Joseph Turow and Lisa Coe (1985) conclude that the treatment of illness on television merely exaggerates a general characteristic of television's program formats in presenting a straightforward, short-term, single-perspective take on a problem. They call representations "textured" when they present multiple points of view and multiple discussions of the illness by different characters and show the illness itself as multifaceted—e.g., with both acute and chronic and sometimes uncertain aspects. Overall, only 5 percent of television patients in their sample had textured medical problems; soap operas and movies were most likely to represent textured representations. Turow and Coe point out a number of further ways in which the dimensions and representations of illness are influenced by program formats and constraints. For example, while the unusual or taboo illness can be treated in the expanded time offered by the television-movie format—and provides a focal point for the network's promotional efforts—chronic illness lends itself particularly well to the continuing story lines of soap operas (and hospital sets are cheap and good for low-budget productions).

The important difference between a straightforward, single-perspective treatment of AIDS and a more complex, multifaceted reporting is explored in a number of contexts: e.g., nightly television news coverage in the United States (Colby and Cook 1991), reporting in three newspapers between 1983 and 1985 (McAllister 1989), and media coverage of AIDS in Africa (Kitzinger and Miller 1991). On the made-for-TV movie, see Schulz (1990).

3. Depicting the "homosexual community" on television is problematic in that it involves showing homosexuals not as single stereotypes or abstractions but as social beings—i.e., as gay men and lesbians in the process of "being" (living their lives as) gay men and lesbians. Karpf (1988) and Watney (1987c) discuss media treatment of AIDS as a classic example of a "moral panic" generated by the gay equals sex equals death connections (but Watney 1994 questions the utility of the concept). Shilts (1987), Kinsella (1989), and Colby (1989) discuss the reasons that AIDS is deemed hard to cover and hard to show visually. Howard Rosenberg's review in the Los Angeles Times praised An Early Frost as "a wise, honest and tender drama" that had somehow, surprisingly, remained resistant to the more typical media treatment of AIDS—which tended to be, in Rosenberg's words, "exploitive," "opportunistic," "sensational," and "obsessive" (1985, 1). "Yet even as the decade drew to a close," writes Rodney Buxton (1991, 37), "AIDS remained a topic that television drama could only address with some difficulty." The networks' reluctance to accept ads and PSAS on condoms is discussed from an advertising perspective by Christopher (1986, 1987). Simon (1991) addresses the Fox network's decision to begin accepting such advertising. Christen (1989) discusses television's overall impact on the course of the epidemic.

4. Independent videos include such documentaries as *Doctors, Liars, and Women, Born in Africa, Absolutely Positive,* and *The Los Altos Story*—the first shown on "Living with AIDS" (New York cable television), the second and third on PBS ("The AIDS Quarterly" and "P.O.V.," respectively), and the fourth on Fox; alternative and independent videos that self-consciously manipulate existing narrative genres, such as *Ojos Que No Ven, Rockville Is Burning,* and *The Pink Pimpernel;* and experimental videos that deliberately depart from conventional narrative structure, such as *Tongues Untied* (also shown on "P.O.V.," with much controversy), *Chuck Solomon: Coming of Age,* and *Danny.* Although broadcast only in the San Francisco

Bay Area, *Paul Wynne's Journal* received national attention (Rosenberg 1990b). Taken together, these represent a range of network, cable, and independent video productions whose target audiences range from prime-time mainstream or public television viewers to the markets of local cable outlets and specialized and alternative audiences—or a mixture of all the above. A sampling is available on the six-hour compilation *Video against AIDS*. For further discussion, see Chris (1989), Crimp (1988b), Gever (1988), Grover (1989a), Landers (1988), Lerner (1991), Saalfield (1992, 1995), and Saalfield and Navarro (1991). On AIDS cinema, see Hoctel (1990), Lew (1991), and Russo (1987). Juhasz (1995) explores the unique role in the AIDS epidemic of what she classifies as "indigenous media"—film and video that is local, personal, and "speaks from the inside" (i.e., is by and about those to whom it is addressed). Lorraine Kenny's (1989) interview with the Testing the Limits Collective includes a useful discussion of conventional narrative techniques deliberately adopted by video artists for certain kinds of AIDS projects.

5. As Mim Udovitch (1991, 50) writes, progress on prime-time network television is always relative; thus, reviewing the 1991–92 blossoming of "single girl sitcoms" with their various unconventional pregnancies and other revelations, she can write, "I reluctantly applaud these unclosetings, compromised by the wishy-washy fairy-godmothering of their scripts as they may be." In this spirit, we can acknowledge that television does AIDS 101 rather well. Research regularly presented at the International Conferences on AIDS finds that television is the main source of AIDS information for virtually all populations surveyed, including, in the United States, urban intravenous drug users (Liza Solomon et al., abstract FD 851, *Abstracts* 1990, 2:294), sexual partners of intravenous drug users (Les Pappas et al., abstract SC 750, *Abstracts* 1990, 3:276), and randomly selected respondents in the Southwest, including black and Hispanic residents (Christine Galavotti et al., abstract WEP 58, *Abstracts* 1989, 869). Outside the United States, populations studied include intravenous drug users in Montreal and Toronto (Janine Jason et al., abstract FD 852, *Abstracts* 1990, 2:295; urban residents of Kinshasa, Zaire (M. Kyungu et al., abstract FD 846, *Abstracts* 1990, 2:293), teenagers in Copenhagen (Bjarne Rasmussen et al., abstract SC 727, *Abstracts* 1990, 3:270), the "general population" of France (Mitchell Cohen et al., abstract FD 847, *Abstracts* 1990, 2:293); and hospital patients in Delhi (A. B. Hiramani and Neelam Sharma, abstract E647, *Abstracts* 1989, 910). Significantly, only one study surveyed gay men and bisexuals, reproducing an apparently pervasive inability to count these citizens among the "audience" envisioned for television.

6. In addition to prime-time dramas like *An Early Frost* and *Our Sons*, there are also docudramas like *Rock Hudson, Born in Africa*, and *The Ryan White Story*, scientific documentaries on series programs like "Nova," and AIDS episodes on drama and comedy series like "Roseanne," "Trapper John, M.D.," "Thirtysomething," and "L.A. Law." AIDS episodes on "Midnight Caller" and "Miami Vice" are analyzed in depth by Buxton (1991) and Braddlee (1989), respectively. O'Connor (1991b) discusses the controversial aspects of these shows. O'Connor (1991c) discusses what he calls "straight AIDS" on such shows as "DeGrassi High," "A Different World," and "First Love, Fatal Love." AIDS has also been featured on daytime dramas, network and cable comedy shows, and talk shows (including the appearance of basketball superstar Magic Johnson on the "Arsenio Hall Show" (7 November 1991), just after he announced that he had tested positive for HIV). In chapter 4 above, I

note some of these programs, including the well-crafted AIDS story line on the soap opera "General Hospital" in 1995–96. Buxton (1992) analyzes AIDS in the context of several of these broadcast formats and describes in detail several specific examples; he also lists production information about all AIDS made-for-TV movies as of that date.

7. A number of critics keep track of television's "flip-flops" on AIDS. Collins (1991) observes that, on the positive side, "In the Shadow of Love: A Teen AIDS Story" aired 18 September 1991 on PBS and (in an unusual cooperative arrangement) on ABC as an "Afterschool Special" the next day; ABC also scheduled an eight-episode AIDS story line on "Life Goes On." Yet, during the same period, the PBS series "P.O.V." showed Peter Adair's "daring" *Absolutely Positive* (1991) yet decided that the documentary *Stop the Church* (Hilferty 1991) "went too far" and pulled it. Weinstein (1990a, 1990b) documents NBC's repeated postponements of the "Steven Burdick" episode on the excellent medical series "Lifestories," the account of a television news anchor who learns that he is HIV positive; the network finally ran the episode many weeks after it was originally scheduled. Contradictory stances on sex are chronicled by Berry (1991), Du Brow (1991), Farber (1991), Kogan (1991), and O'Connor (1991a). Many critics (e.g., Rosenberg 1990a) considered ABC's *Red, Hot, and Blue*, broadcast on 1 December 1990 (World AIDS Day), a superlative example of AIDS-related programming.

8. Turow (1990b) provides a relevant historical account of the influences of outside institutions on early medical dramas on television, specifically, the relation between the Los Angeles County Medical Association and the American Medical Association and the programs "Medic," "Dr. Kildare," and "Ben Casey." Buxton (1991) analyzes the effect of diverse interest groups on a controversial AIDS episode of "Midnight Caller." Hill and Beaver (1991) provide an overview of the relation between advocacy groups and advertisers in television programming. See also Alcorn (1989), Associated Press (1991), and Turow (1990a, 1990b).

9. After a feverish bidding war while it was on the best-seller list, *And the Band Played On* languished "in development" as various studios tried and failed to get the project off the ground. Rights were finally purchased by Home Box Office and developed—again, not without difficulty—into a largely successful 1991 television movie. On mass media gatekeeping processes (including shortsightedness, ambivalence, conflict of interests, and so on) affecting AIDS, sexuality, and homosexuality, see Buxton (1992), Colby and Cook (1991), Dearing and Rogers (1988), Du Brow (1991), Elm (1989), Foltz (1985), Graham (1989a, 1989b), Grossberg et al. (1992), Harmetz (1987a, 1987b), Hoctel (1990), Hulce (1989), Kenny (1989), Klusaček and Morrison (1992), Leahy (1986), Lippe (1987), Litwin (1990), Miller (1989), Nelkin (1987b), O'Connor (1991a), Pastore (1993), Planned Parenthood of America (1986), Rogers (1989), Russo (1987), Saalfield and Navarro (1991), Strnad (1990), and Sturken (1997).

10. *The Return of Ben Casey*, a made-for-TV movie broadcast in February 1988, played on the contrast between the heroic tradition of medical dramas and the faster and grittier approach of such ensemble shows as "St. Elsewhere" and "ER." Vince Edwards returned to reprise his role as the arrogant, brilliant, macho male neurosurgeon of the 1961–66 series; arriving at County General, his old hospital, he finds problems everywhere and takes it on himself to solve them—just like old times. But

this is the late 1980s; the rules of the game (and the television show) have changed: Casey finds himself hauled up before the hospital administration for carrying inappropriate credentials, using unorthodox procedures, and committing a host of other offenses. Meanwhile, the new generation of house staff treats him less like a legend than like a neanderthal, and one of the women physicians has to try to fill him in on twenty years of feminism. Had the movie more consistently played with these ironic and self-conscious narrative conventions, it might well have fostered an interesting series. Instead, it was a hodgepodge that ultimately depended on an old cliché—Ben Casey *cares*—to resolve and transcend the myriad problems of contemporary medicine the show so graphically presented. For a perspective on the old and new Ben Casey, see Stanley (1988) and Atkinson (1988). For an overview of changes in the representation of physicians over time, see Malmsheimer (1988) and Turow (1990b).

11. For further critical perspectives on traditional American medicine and disease narratives, see Kalisch and Kalisch (1985), Turow and Coe (1985), Poirier and Borgenicht (1991), Karpf (1988), and Turow (1990b). Baker (1994), Murphy and Poirier (1992), and Pastore (1993) trace AIDS/HIV through many forms of narrative.

12. Research in feminism and film theory usefully explores the function of identification in television narratives—and suggests that it is variable and diverse, entailing multiple transactions between what are ostensibly masculine and feminine positions. See, e.g., Deming (1988), Doane (1986), Flitterman-Lewis (1988), Kaplan (1983), Lipsitz (1988), Mann and Spigel (1988), Rodowick (1982), and Penley (1989). With respect to AIDS, Buxton (1991) examines the ways in which the various interested parties negotiated the controversy over the "Midnight Caller" "As It Happened . . ." episode; Buxton argues that the final script's lack of closure opens up, if somewhat inadequately, its potential meanings in ways not typical of prime-time series dramas. Braddlee (1989) looks similarly at how "God's Work," a 1989 episode of the series "Miami Vice," is "at odds with itself over the issue of sexuality and AIDS." While, Braddlee argues, the overt narrative presents the central gay character in a positive way, the show's production codes present his relationship as incomplete, his sexuality as a prison, and solitude, ultimately, as the price of virtue. Baker (1994) discusses the handling of AIDS/HIV across different television and video genres, noting ways in which distinct conventions and audiences influence which aspects of the epidemic are emphasized or played down.

13. Miller (1990) calls this seemingly straightforward structure of narratives "by no means innocent." In somewhat more detail, his three elements include (i) an initial situation, change or reversal, and a revelation; (ii) the use of personification or some other mechanism for bringing issues "to life" through the positions of a protagonist, an antagonist, and a witness who learns; and (iii) a formal textual pattern that repeats key elements or nuclear figures—a trope, a system of tropes, or a complex word. For this last category, Miller draws on Empson's (1967) notion of a complex word, with some modification. He suggests also that, like fictional accounts, scientific and historical accounts have narrative structures that give order to phenomena, but the formal constraints and referential restraints are different—primarily in the way that science and history purport to be constrained by reality and claim to represent events as they "really happened" or nature as it "really is." Analysts like Poovey (1991), Latour and Woolgar ([1979] 1986), and Knorr-Cetina (1981) challenge

the position that fictional discourse can readily be separated from scientific or historical discourse by either formal or referential criteria. Recent work in narrative theory asks questions about the appeal of narrative structure, the role of form and representation in creating narrative pleasure, the relation of fictional narratives to "real life" and of narrative texts to each other (intertextuality), the construction of narrative meaning through form, character, and language, the purposes of narrative, and the function of narrative discourse as a staging ground for cultural struggles taking place elsewhere. As Miller notes, recent decades have generated a "swarming diversity of narrative theories" (1990, 67). There is not space in this essay to enter this swarm, but interested readers may consult Miller. See also Murphy and Poirier (1992), Sharf and Freimuth (1993), Stein (1990), Sturken (1997), and Wolf (1992).

14. In comparison, *Roe v Wade*, the made-for-TV movie about the Supreme Court's decision to legalize abortion, went through seventeen rewrites before it was broadcast on 15 May 1989 (Elm 1989). Like the abortion-related "Cagney and Lacey" episode originally broadcast in competition with *An Early Frost*, *Roe v Wade* drew much fiercer objections from conservative groups than any AIDS programs to date. At least one network affiliate pulled the "Cagney and Lacey" episode in response to objections by antichoice organizations, calling it too one sided; prolife boycott threats, likewise, caused numerous sponsors to withdraw their support from *Roe v. Wade*. Rick Du Brow (1991) comments, "One person's boundary on good taste is another person's censorship. But the question of where to draw the line has never been more difficult than it is at present." He quotes producer Steven Bochco: "The networks are all in a panic. When you cut through the bull, it's all money." See also Berry (1991), Farber (1991), Harmetz (1987a, 1987b), Kogan (1991) and Strnad (1990).

15. According to Turow (1990a), sponsors did not regularly intervene directly in week-by-week programming but sometimes established policies or ground rules; e.g., sponsors of the "Dr. Kildare" series included a cigarette company that prohibited use of the word *cancer* and Bayer, which prohibited episodes showing overdose or death from aspirin. Hill and Beaver (1991) find that, although a number of companies today have developed policies or guidelines for programming and advertising on television, most have none and appear to anticipate problems in no systematic way. They conclude that a decade of deregulation has on the whole exacerbated rather than decreased such tension. Buxton's 1991 study shows that the "Midnight Caller" controversy took executives and scriptwriters by surprise in part because no policy existed for anticipating problems (see also Associated Press 1988a; and Buxton 1992).

16. A number of critics have used the example of Peter and the cup to show irrational fears of contamination. Yet is it not a bit harsh to ask that Peter immediately adjust to living with an infectious disease when even experienced health professionals take a bit of time to let their knowledge overcome their initial fear of contagion and to learn what is safe and what is not? And need the shot necessarily signify that Peter is contributing to the isolation that develops around the person with AIDS? Could it not also signify that he does not yet realize that he may be infected himself, or that it is important to avoid further exposure, or that AIDS changes an entire household? What if he had started to throw the coffee out, then paused, then taken a drink? It seems to me that this would also have been ambiguous, even interpreted as a "death wish" or something similar. In Schulman's novel *People in Trouble* (1991,

200–201), when this issue has become clearly coded within AIDS discourse, two women encounter an acquaintance who is afraid that he is HIV positive. Afterward, one woman asks the other, "Why did you drink out of his [juice] carton when he might have AIDS?" "It's a rite of passage," says the other. "People who may be HIV positive inevitably offer you a drink out of their glass. It's a test of loyalty to see if you're prejudiced or not, to see if you are informed enough to know that you can't get it that way." In *Our Sons*, James and Donald are both familiar with this code.

17. The boundary between fiction and science breaks down at the same point that it is being reinforced. The physician, encapsulated in his two scenes, provides the core of scientific certainties that the audience is intended to receive. But the core is eroded from within by the doctor's factual admission that science is "not sure of very much." In chaps. 5 above and 9 below, I discuss Knorr-Cetina (1981), Latour and Woolgar ([1979] 1986), Fleck ([1939] 1975), Armstrong (1983), Epstein (1996), and others on the need to qualify and define statements with other statements vs. shorthand strategies that enable some statements to be treated as "facts."

18. The question of post-AIDS kissing in films has dramatically blurred the lines between the movies and real life, with a number of actors concerned about contracting HIV from on-screen kissing. The health professionals who viewed the premiere of *An Early Frost* emphasized that kissing was very unlikely to transmit HIV; but, in any case, as one commented, "I always thought actors and actresses could act. Isn't there a way to fake it?" (quoted in Steinbrook 1985, 9). Buxton (1992) provides a behind-the-scenes account of the conflicting views about the grandmother's kiss: ultimately, James Curran, the head of the Centers for Disease Control's AIDS Program, was called in as the final arbiter, successfully arguing that the kiss was pedagogically important to include. As the actor Tom Hulce (1989) has observed, the representation of homosexuality is far more shocking to American audiences than the representation of gory medical details, to which they are well acclimated (see chap. 4 above). These crossover fears recall Vito Russo's anecdote: "When the concerned mother of one young man up for a role in Arthur J. Bressan's *Abuse* asked the director if playing the part would make her son gay, he replied, 'No, and if he plays Hamlet he won't inherit Denmark, either.'" (1987, 302). D. W. Moffett, who played Peter in *An Early Frost*, said in interviews that he agreed with the decision to omit "kissy-poo" behavior because it would turn viewers off. The prospect of same-sex kissing may also, for an actor, embody career concerns (discomfort if he is straight, fear of exposure or rumor—or discomfort—if he is gay). But, as Buxton's (1992, 384) interviews about the film indicate, its writers had very deliberately written in visual signals of physical affection between the two men and were unhappy when the scenes were edited out to satisfy Broadcast Standards and Practices. Originally, too, the writers intended to show Michael and Peter within a larger community of gay men: scenes showed them eating in a restaurant, discussing AIDS, and drawing support and information about the epidemic. Not only was this element jettisoned, but the final version goes so far as to show their friends canceling dinner plans once Michael's illness is known.

19. In *Ground Zero* (1988), Andrew Holleran writes that his protagonist is, "while homosexual, . . . a completely conventional person at the same time." Jan Grover (1988c) comments on this homogenization: "In American terms, that translates most vividly into his inability to turn sorrow into constructive anger and collective

action. Because he cannot envision a collective response to AIDS, Holleran remains stranded in his own loss—impotent, because 'writing could not produce a cure.' Because he cannot arrive at an individual solution to It (the plague, the epidemic), he despairs, turns inward: '[O]ne stops reading the stories finally, turns off the TV when the topic is introduced'" (pp. 24–34). See also Landers (1988), Juhasz (1995), Roof (1996), and Watney (1994).

20. *Our Sons* was directed by John Erman (who also directed *An Early Frost*), produced by Phil Kleinbart, coproduced by Micki Dickoff, and written by William Hanley. Executive producers included Carla Singer, Robert Greenwald, and William Hanley; the movie was edited by Robert Florio, designed by James Hulsey, and photographed by Tony Imi. The cast includes Ann-Margret as Luanne Barnes, Željko Ivanek as Donald Barnes, Julie Andrews as Audrey Grant, Hugh Grant as James Grant, and Tony Roberts as Audrey's friend Harry.

21. The metaphor of *an early frost*, central to the movie's universalizing trope, arises literally in the context of gardening when Bea holds up a rose and says to Kay, "They're so beautiful this year: I hope an early frost won't nip them in the bud." Although an early frost kills not just one beautiful flower but a whole season of them, the collective potential of the metaphor is left untapped. The title and linguistic core of *Our Sons* is taken from an exchange between Luanne and Audrey:
    Luanne: How'd you get used to it? That you had a son who was one of them?
    Audrey: My son is not "one of them." Your son is not "one of them." Our sons are two of us.

22. Answering machines have multiple functions in these films. Often they work to contrast "normal life" with a new reality or crisis (with the prerecorded message representing the earlier time of stability); in *Our Sons*, James and Donald's prerecorded message as well as Audrey's incoming call are set against the immediate crisis of Donald's health. As Timothy Murphy has suggested to me, Michael's phone arrangements in *An Early Frost* guard his gay existence against discovery; when Michael's mother calls and Peter picks up the phone, he violates the routine: technology, in other words, has for Michael been part of the closet. In other AIDS narratives, machines function to signal that the person is still alive. Sarah Schulman writes (1991, 92): "I just can't imagine another one of those times when you call up an old friend and get that damn tape announcing that his number has been disconnected."

23. Reviewing the small eddies of feminist programming amid the 1991–92 mainstream, Mim Udovitch (1991, 50) writes, "The most obvious advance represented by the new . . . shows is that it is now permissible to hire three actresses for the same project without it being an absolute necessity that one be a redhead, one a blond, and one a brunette." Of course, Luanne in *Our Sons* turns out to be wearing a blonde wig—the sedate head of chestnut hair underneath functions to suggest that the two women are not so different as they appear.

24. Aidan Quinn, playing Michael, initially objected to this decision, but he changed his mind as he talked to people with AIDS and their advocates and learned that many people do not look sick and go about their lives for years. Some of the debates about visually representing the physical status of people with AIDS are discussed by Douglas Crimp (1992, 117–33) and by several authors in Crimp (1988b).

25. In chap. 9 below, I discuss the evolution of AIDS treatment and AIDS treatment

activism, including the resistance by physicians and patients as well as the general public to the possibility that AIDS can be managed as other chronic diseases are managed. For more on this debate, see Epstein (1996).

26. Good studies of "real" audiences that also take cultural texts seriously would help determine the range and significance of differing interpretations of AIDS texts. Most current research, involving content analysis, attitude surveys, focus groups, or textual analysis, cannot really accomplish this (see several essays in Grossberg et al. 1992). An exception is Kitzinger and Miller's (1991) effort to identify and interpret the diverse audience understandings of media accounts of "African AIDS." A model is Reeves and Campbell's (1994) deconstruction of media coverage of the war on drugs.

27. Richard Meyer analyzes the shock expressed by those who had to rethink their conceptions of Rock Hudson when they learned that he had AIDS: "Because he has been revealed as homosexual through the spectacle of illness, Hudson is said to betray the projective fantasies of his heterosexual spectator, here a female one" (1989, 279). On the representation of specific kinds of bodies and the screen, see also Saalfield and Navarro (1991). Television critic Walter Goodman (1991) predicted that, in contrast to the Rock Hudson story, which the networks approached with great anxiety (see Lippe 1987; and Litwin 1990), the case of young, blonde, and bitter Kimberly Bergalis would be "the story TV can't resist." But the Kaiser Family Foundation study (1996) provides evidence that it was resisted. What is irresistible is Magic Johnson's story; his announcement in November 1991 that he was HIV positive touched off a new explosion of media construction and projective desire. How the facts of all these stories and their media constructions unfold over time will bear watching.

7   AIDS, Africa, and Cultural Theory

1. The *New York Times* series "A Continent's Agony," 16–19 September 1990, consists of Eckholm with Tierney (1990), Eckholm (1990a, 1990b), and Tierney (1990a, 1990b). The first article ran on the front page above the fold of the Sunday edition, and the subsequent articles all began prominently on p. 1 and received substantial space. This opening series initiated continuing periodic reports.

2. Media coverage of AIDS in Africa in the 1990s is discussed in Garrett (1992), Little (1994), Karnik (in press), Farmer et al. (1996), McGee (1996), and Mann and Tarantola (1996).

3. This and other examples are cited and discussed by Watney (1989). Similar claims of identity between "Africans" and "homosexual men in the West" appear in such publications as the *Journal of the American Medical Association*. See also Konetey-Ahulu (1988), Treichler (1989a, 1991a), Waite (1988), and chap. 3 above.

4. One source for the recycling of these obsessions in AIDS research may have been Hrdy (1987). An especially notorious example is Gould (1988), who writes that HIV can be transmitted heterosexually in Africa because "men take their women in a brutal way that would be more like rape by our standards" (see chap. 8 below).

5. In his opening lecture, Kakoma noted that "homosexuality is not even translatable in my language, nor is there a term for anal intercourse—so we have had to improvise." On Gottlieb's point regarding research on homosexuality in Africa, see Gill

Shepherd's (1987) ethnography of sexual practices in Mombasa as well as Patton (1990) and White (1990, 1993).

6. In this case, the researcher, a University of Illinois at Urbana-Champaign faculty member, was effectively silenced. I was not convinced that those mounting the protest—including some longtime compadres of mine on the left—knew enough about the AIDS epidemic or AIDS in Africa to discount the researcher's potential contributions. Nor was I persuaded that rumored "CIA sponsorship" should have deprived us, the conference goers, of the right to judge the merit of the work for ourselves. A better argument would be that no AIDS research should be classified. If the *New England Journal of Medicine* can adapt its procedures to the AIDS crisis, so can the U.S. government.

7. The International Women's Working Group on the AIDS Epidemic, linking women's AIDS issues to women's experiences worldwide as second-class citizens, is only one example of political analysis concerned primarily with Third World settings. Media coverage of First World politics was also flawed. Peter Jennings's coverage of the opening ceremony on ABC's "World News Tonight," e.g., emphasized the split between scientists and activists; thus, a scientist shown wearing a red armband was misleadingly represented as resisting conference politics—when in fact the red armband *was* a protest against INS policy as well as a symbol of solidarity with the international AIDS community. Jennings talked about "activists—all of them American," without saying that activists from other countries were absent because they had boycotted the conference. From visual footage of Peter Staley leading his anti-Bush chant the story immediately cut to what seemed to be a reverse shot showing the seated audience clapping in a desultory way; actually, at that point, the whole audience was on its feet chanting with Staley. Wachter (1991), a major conference organizer, gives a stirring account of the solidarity march in which scientists and People with AIDS/activists joined together. See also Cohen (1993), Gamson (1995), and Epstein (1996).

8. I return to this issue later. In 1990, when I spoke with Dr. Okware, the testing problem was largely hypothetical. Now, in the late 1990s, the logistics, science, and ethics of clinical trials in central Africa are more widely debated. But, as far as I can tell, the participants in the debate still appear to be government officials, scientists, policymakers, private-sector sponsors, and First World pundit-ethicists.

9. Many of the Wenner-Gren Symposium papers are available in Herdt and Lindenbaum (1992). The Wenner-Gren Symposia, a topic too broad for adequate consideration here, used to be held in a castle in the Alps (Donna Haraway's [1989b] fascinating history of the Wenner-Gren is supplemented by knowledgeable staff and participants at conferences in the form of lore, legends, and gossip). The hotel where we met in Estes Park was Stephen King's inspiration for *The Shining*, so a degree of gothic castle atmosphere was preserved.

The explosion, at a panel on AIDS research at the 1992 meeting of the American Anthropology Association in San Francisco, involved academic priorities and credibility: First, what can/should anthropology contribute to the fight against AIDS? Second, who has the knowledge and experience to address the question? At issue was the composition of the "panel of experts," senior anthropologists who were eminently qualified to speak about anthropology but perceived by those in or near the trenches as having no expertise about AIDS. Many of those attending the standing-room-only session wore T-shirts reading "These natives can speak for themselves"

(Coughlin 1992). Nancy Scheper-Hughes (1994), one of the panel organizers, provides another perspective on the event. See also Fujimura and Chou (1994), Connors and McGrath (1997), and Farmer et al. (1996).

10. The controversy over HIV drug testing in Africa erupted as I was completing this manuscript; although I cannot do it justice here, I do offer many resources for making sense of the issues. Another excellent resource, compiled by William Martin for the Association of Concerned Africa Scholars, is a briefing packet of key background essays, journal articles, and media reports on the controversy (Martin 1997).

11. The commentary is adapted from a letter from Colin Garrett accompanying a packet of AIDS education posters and brochures. Looking over these materials, Stacie Colwell observed that the CAR AIDS creature resembles a bat figure called Popo Bao found in Zanzibari media and employed politically in a particularly vicious political campaign in the mid-1990s. More information would be welcome.

8 *Beyond* Cosmo

A very preliminary version of this material was presented at the Inside/Out Lesbian and Gay Studies Conference at Yale in 1989. Since then, as pieces of it have been presented and published in various places, it has accumulated intellectual debts that citations can only begin to acknowledge. I do, however, want to thank the members of the ACT UP New York Women's Caucus, whose work was so important and contributed to my own in so many ways.

1. AIDS is now considered a leading killer of women aged fifteen to forty-four in many American cities. Unless otherwise indicated, statistics are based on the monthly *HIV/AIDS Surveillance* reports published by the Centers for Disease Control in Atlanta.

2. *Doctors, Liars, and Women* first aired on the weekly GMHC series "Living with AIDS" on New York cable television and has been shown widely in public screenings of AIDS videos. It is available in the compilation *Video against AIDS*, curated by John Greyson and Bill Horrigan (1990). *Women, AIDS, and Activism* (ACT UP New York Women and AIDS Book Group 1992) is available in both English and Spanish. *The ACT UP Women's Caucus Women and AIDS Handbook*, a 1989 photocopied version edited by Maria Maggenti, preceded the book.

3. The concept *identity* is a vast topic in philosophy, psychoanalysis, and other fields, and I cannot do it justice here. I wish to use it as a general conceptual framework that embraces the three dimensions that I have noted, not as a technical problem to be rigorously wrestled with. For more extensive discussion, see Laplanche and Pontalis (1973), Penelhum (1967), Watney (1992), and Weeks (1987). Questions of identification and/or media representations in AIDS discourse are addressed in Albert (1986b), Baker (1986), Chris (1992), Campbell (1995), Gorna (1997), Grover (1997), Grossman (1996), Danzig (1992), Sturken (1997), Watney (1987c), and several essays in Crimp (1988a, 1997) and Grover (1989a).

4. As a working task force on women and AIDS put it, the conception of AIDS as a gay disease "lulled many women into a false sense of security"—worldwide, not only in North America (United Nations Economic and Social Council 1989, 9). For citations of serious scholarly, political, or theoretical work on women and AIDS/HIV published in the 1980s, see chap. 2 above. Work in the 1990s includes Ingram et al. (1997), Blasius and Phelan (1997), Butler (1990, 1993, 1994), K. King (1992), Gray et

al. (1994), Haraway (1989b, 1991a, 1991b, 1996), Rubin (1994a), Hollibaugh ([1993] 1997), Stoller (1995), Duberman (1997), Califia (1988, 1997), Bright (1997), Kane (1993, 1994), Broullon (1992), Odets (1996), Gorna (1996), Schneider and Stoller (1995), Huber and Schneider (1992), Roth and Fuller (1998), Roth and Hogan (1998), O'Sullivan and Thomson ([1992] 1996), Hammonds (1997), Hanawa (1996), Treat (1994), Friedman et al. (1992), and Levine and Siegel (1992).

5. Useful feminist discussions of gender and identity include Adams (1989), Haraway (1985), Parmar (1989), Segal (1987), K. King (1992), E. King (1993), Fausto-Sterling (1993), Gray et al. (1994), Duggan and Hunter (1995), Hammonds (1997), and Detloff (1997).

6. Warning women to guard their "moist, vulnerable mucous membranes" and other "vulnerable entrance ports for the virus," sex therapist Helen Singer Kaplan presented a vivid scenario for viral transmission during penile-vaginal intercourse: "The man's infected pre-ejaculatory secretions, the little drop of clear fluid that sometimes comes out of the tip of the man's penis when he is aroused but before he ejaculates, as well as his seminal fluid, are squirted into the woman's vulnerable wet vagina and can infect her." But the penile proboscis places men in danger, too: "If the woman has the virus, her infected vaginal lubrications pour over the open moist entrance to the man's urethra (the small opening at the tip of the penis where the urine and semen emerge) and he can become infected through that route" (Kaplan 1987, 78, 79).

7. Lisa Duggan, among others, has observed that sexual injuries are more likely than nonsexual ones to be attributed to "unnatural" practices. Toxic shock syndrome provoked decrees that nature intended the rugged vagina for penises and babies but not for tampons; AIDS likewise is used to argue that nature never intended the vulnerable rectum for sexual pleasure (see also Bersani 1988 and Fausto-Sterling 1993). But a broken ankle does not prove that nature never intended people to use rollerblades. In much of the conservative writing on AIDS, one sees an obsession with "natural" receptacles, orifices, and bodily functions. In *My Program against AIDS* (1987), Lyndon LaRouche writes: "AIDS demonstrates afresh . . . that if society promotes the violation of the principles of our bodies' design, that society shall suffer in some way or another for this obscenity" (p. 6); whether blood transfusions violate "the principles of our bodies' design" is not addressed.

8. Gould added that "the secretions of a healthy vagina are very inhospitable to the AIDS virus" (1988), presumably alluding to the vagina's PH, whose acidity has virus-killing and sperm-killing properties. Once HIV was isolated in vaginal secretions, it was decreed that the vagina's acidity could be neutralized by the alkaline bath it gets from semen or by other STDs, infections, and various other conditions. (Royce et al. [1997] review all these issues.)

9. The language of this passage recalls Emily Martin's (1987) charge that medical rhetoric casts women's reproductive systems as factories, with menstruation as a monthly failure in production and menopause the sign of a crumbling, obsolete physical plant (see also Moore and Clark 1995).

10. At the point in the epidemic that I am discussing here, the CDC's data (through 15 August 1992) already showed women as the fastest-growing segment of new AIDS cases and AIDS as one of the five leading causes of death among women aged fifteen to forty-four. Discussions of data on women at this earlier point include M. A. Gillespie (1991), Hunter (1992), and Corea (1992). AIDS statistics for women in the

United States as of October 1997 have worsened. Despite a drop for the first time since the beginning of the epidemic in new AIDS cases and number of AIDS deaths per reporting period, incidence among women did not drop. Reasons are still unclear, although differential access to the latest drug therapies is presumed to be one factor (L. Altman 1997; *AIDS Treatment News* 1995–98).

11. Another example: after several babies in Los Angeles were diagnosed with AIDS in the early 1980s, their mothers—"mothers of pediatric AIDS patients"—were able to be traced and contacted through hospital and blood bank records. (This example shows the ambiguity of this category, however, because these particular babies were premature and received transfusions; they were infected through the blood supply, not through their mothers, who were mainly not HIV-infected themselves.)

12. The companion Men's Advocacy Network of the National Hemophilia Foundation (MANN) had its first meeting in 1991. The two networks organize joint activities as well. For a comprehensive discussion of women in the hemophilia community, see Mason et al. (1988). My thanks also to John Gagnon and Paul Wilson for sharing their knowledge with me. A detailed description of educational workshops for partners and caretakers of men with hemophilia can be found in Roth and Fuller (1998).

13. Nancy Solomon (1991) quotes Dr. Charles Schable at the CDC in the late 1980s: "Lesbians don't have much sex" (p. 50). On researchers' understanding of homosexuality in the early 1980s, see Panem (1985).

14. Discussion of sex workers and AIDS can be found in Alexander (1996), Leonard and Thistlethwaite (1992), Lupton (1994), Gorna (1996), and Gander (1993). See also COYOTE (1985), Leigh (1988), Leigh's video *Safe Sex Slut* (1987), and Delacoste and Alexander (1987). Historical attacks on sex workers during epidemics of sexually transmitted disease are recounted by Brandt (1987).

15. Patton (1990) argues that, when concern is expressed for "heterosexuals," the community at issue is "straight men." Kane and Mason (1992) indicate that the "intravenous drug users" enrolled in the multicenter NIDA studies are male by definition and that their "sex partners" are presumed to be female. Studying the incidence of HIV infection in women is sometimes justified because it provides an index to infection in the "heterosexual community" as a whole (e.g., Guinan and Hardy 1987). So, while the category *women* is almost always assumed to mean *heterosexual*, the category *heterosexual* is not always assumed to include women. For a general discussion of social variables in epidemiology, see Ross and Mirowsky (1980).

16. Actually, Fumento's argument is not that individual white middle-class heterosexual people *cannot* acquire or transmit HIV through heterosexual activity; he acknowledges that they can. Rather, he argues that an *epidemic* will never occur exclusively among heterosexuals because of heterosexual transmission. While widely assumed to be talking about individual risk of HIV infection, he is in fact talking about incidence in a large population. For detailed (and fairer) discussion of the parameters affecting transmission and the difficulties of accurately predicting the epidemic's future, see Anderson and May (1988a, 1988b) and U.S. General Accounting Office (1989). In Treichler (1990b) I discuss Fumento's book in more detail.

17. Addressing the International Working Group on Women and AIDS at the Fifth International AIDS Conference, Montreal, June 1989, Cindy Patton (1989) summarized several cases in which women were misdiagnosed, although she cited one instance in which this mind-set was used to advantage: when a Boston woman was told by a

social worker that she would have to give up her children because she was suspected of having AIDS, she ridiculed the charge—"Don't you know women can't get AIDS?" Three women talking at the Second Annual Conference on Women and HIV in Los Angeles (14 Nov. 1993) described the circumstances of learning that they were HIV positive. The white woman said she had visited eleven physicians before being tested, the Latina woman seven, and the African-American woman five. For further discussion of medical issues that affect women, see Hunter (1992), Gorna (1996), Teare and English (1996), O'Sullivan and Thomson ([1992] 1996), and Roth and Fuller (1998).

18. Some studies suggest that the quality and timeliness of clinical care are crucial factors in prolonging life (see, e.g., Anastos and Marte [1989] 1991; and Lemp et al. 1992). But other studies suggest that we do not yet know the causes of differential disease progression: factors may include the quality of health care, ease of access, the effects of HIV on different people, the specific clinical conditions that develop, the changing virulence of the virus over time and place, or something else. Nor do we know why some women are infected at a significantly higher rate than others (Byron 1991; Royce et al. 1997).

19. Evolving policies on women and clinical trials are traced by Wolfe and Long (1989), Associated Press (1992b), Epstein (1996), Dickersin and Schnaper (1996), Teare and English (1996), and treatment newsletters.

20. The researcher reported this at a conference. In our book on language and gender, Francine W. Frank and I (1997) discuss the linguistic problems that arise from efforts to map pronominal gender onto biological sex. See also Kessler (1996).

21. Reports from the Eighth International AIDS Conference in July 1992 indicated that, for the first time, men as well as women were experiencing symptoms before seeking a diagnosis (see the discussion in the *AIDS Weekly*, 3 August 1992). The implication is that HIV is increasingly affecting men who are unaware of their potential for exposure to HIV and the symptoms of infection.

22. For perspectives on the "lesbian question," see Appleman and Kahn (1989), Ardill and O'Sullivan (1989), Bristow et al. (1987), Byron (1991), O'Sullivan and Thomson ([1992] 1996), Hammonds (1987, 1997), Juhasz (1995), Meredith (1992), Parmar (1987), Rieder and Ruppelt (1988), and Gorna (1996).

23. The conservative agenda for women is addressed by, among others, Eisenstein (1989), Hunter (1992), Kolder et al. (1987), Irwin and Jordan (1987), Petchesky (1987), Faludi (1991), Schneider and Stoller (1995), Roth and Fuller (1998), and Treichler et al. (1998), and MacNeil (1997).

24. This issue on AIDS reflected the "new" *Ms.*—ad free and reportedly more feminist. It is certainly true that so much space devoted to AIDS in the "old" *Ms.* would have been unlikely.

25. Researcher Zena Stein, professor of public health and epidemiology at Columbia University, discussed women and AIDS at the Congressional Biomedical Research Caucus, Women's Health Issues hearing, 29 July 1991 (covered on C-Span). Focusing her presentation on the search for an effective barrier method for HIV (specifically, for a barrier contraceptive or spermicide that will actually work), she emphasized how many fundamental biological questions we cannot yet answer. A panel of women at the Eighth International AIDS Conference in Amsterdam similarly identified an array of issues raised by the realities of women and AIDS. Although the

Associated Press story was headlined, "Health Officials Say Women Need Safe Sex Training to Avoid AIDS," the panel also urged pharmaceutical companies to develop creams and jellies to prevent HIV transmission (Associated Press 1992a). For further discussion, see Corea (1992).

26. Such efforts are visible in pamphlets and other educational materials prepared by community agencies like the New York Women and AIDS Resource Network (WARN), Project AWARE, the Martin-Lyons Clinic, the San Francisco AIDS Foundation, and Gay Men's Health Crisis. Other examples can be found in Catherine Saalfield's inventory of AIDS videos by and about women and Denise Ribble's assessment of risk, both in *Women, AIDS, and Activism* (ACT UP New York Women and AIDS Book Group 1992). For further discussion of safer sex videos for women, see Juhasz (1995). The student handbook of the Concordia University Students' Association (1991) is another fine example of creative intervention.

27. This task is brilliantly set forth in *DiAna's Hair Ego: AIDS Info Up Front* (1989), a video directed by Ellen Spiro in which DiAna, proprietor of a hair salon in South Carolina, describes how she took up the cause of AIDS by making her salon a virtual condom/AIDS theme park and providing a place where people could talk. There are also "tupperware parties" in which women talk about safe sex. Parked in front of my television set as I worked through the final editing of this manuscript, I happened to catch a "Sally Jessie Raphael" (ABC) show about safer sex (29 October 1997). The featured guests included Luis, a sexually active thirteen-year-old who, the caption said, "won't use condoms during sex," and Luis's mother, who said she was fed up with his irresponsibility. For an hour the issue was vociferously aired, complete with footage filmed "during the break" in which various audience members told Luis in no uncertain terms to "keep that little thing in your pants until you learn what to do with it." "For God's sake," fumed one man, "it takes two seconds to put on a condom: it's no big deal!" The audience burst into applause.

28. The video itself is edited here to dramatize this exchange: Bey's interruption and query "Are you a medical doctor?" are repeated several times. For critical analysis of selected videos about AIDS made from within communities of women and people of color, see Saalfield (1992), Saalfield and Navarro (1991), Juhasz (1995), and Sturken (1997).

29. On the politics of breast cancer and lobbying for research and treatment, see Solomon (1991), Flood (1992), and Batt (1994). For a powerful account of the experience of chronic fatigue syndrome sufferers, see Johnson (1996). On endometriosis activism and advocacy, see Shohat (1998) and Sanmiguel (1999). On bodies, see Caspar and Moore (1995). On disease and race, see Hammonds (1993, 1994).

9   How to Have Theory in an Epidemic

1. Sung to the tune of "Fugue for Tinhorns" from the musical *Guys and Dolls*, music and lyrics by Frank Loesser, new lyrics by Ron Goldberg © 1989. Performed at the ACT UP talent show, New York, 30 March 1989. Used with permission. AIDS treatment activism has been discussed and documented by participants, media commentators, scholars, and assorted pundits. The fine journal *AIDS Treatment News*, edited by John S. James and periodically compiled in published collections (James 1989a, 1991, 1994), provides detailed annotations of the events sketched in this

chapter. See also Bishop (1987, 1991), Kingston (1990), and Gross (1987a, 1992). The publications of other activist treatment groups likewise provide an ongoing commentary and critique. David Rothman's work (Rothman 1987, 1991; Rothman and Edgar 1992; Edgar and Rothman 1990) places AIDS drug development in a historical context. Peter Arno and Karyn Feiden (1992) chronicle the politics of AIDS drug development, with great attention to the interplay among the various institutional constituencies involved. Complementary studies include Nussbaum (1990), Kwitny (1992), and Cohen (1993). The analysis most closely concerned with the production, interpretation, and deployment of knowledge—my fundamental question in this chapter—is Steven Epstein's *Impure Science* (1996), a meticulously researched exploration of two related arenas of the epidemic: causation theory (my subject in chap. 5 above) and treatment activism.

2. In 1997, some twenty-five years after the Tuskegee study ended, President Bill Clinton officially apologized to the survivors and their families. On the relation of AIDS treatment activism to prior ethical doctrine on clinical research, see Bohne et al. (1989) as well as Dixon (1990), Harrington (1990, 1997), Grady (1995), and Douglas and Pinsky (1989, 1996). Horton (1989) describes the clash that occurred when medical researchers organizing clinical trials of AZT in England refused to share detailed information with their very well-informed potential clientele. Watney's "Perspectives on Treatment" (in Watney 1994, 194–96) compares medical issues and activism in the United States and the United Kingdom. Oppenheimer and Reckitt (1997) include several reflective essays on treatment. On comparative practice styles of AIDS research and clinical medicine in the United States and France, see Feldman (1995).

3. In September 1990, the U.S. Congress mandated that all NIH research on human subjects include women as well as men. Anne Eckman (1998) reviews this mandate in a broader discussion of the NIH women's health initiative and other evidence of the new visibility of women's health research. On AIDS/HIV, women, and drug treatments, see Associated Press (1992b), Banzhaf (1992), Clarke (1994), and Denenberg (1992). On participation in clinical trials, see *Deciding to Enter an AIDS/HIV Trial* (1989), Schneider and Stoller (1995), Roth and Fuller (1998), Farmer et al. (1996), and Mann and Tarantola (1996). On the relation between AIDS treatment activism and activism surrounding other diseases, see Batt (1994), Johnson (1996), Dickersin and Schnaper (1996), and Treichler et al. (1998).

4. From the beginning, these coalitions were not unproblematic (Kolata 1988b; Cohen 1993; Minkowitz [1990] 1997; Nussbaum 1990) and have fragmented a number of activist and advocacy organizations (Cohen 1993; Epstein 1996). The unvarnished profit motive came as a shock to many liberals and activists; a faster approval process "translates into lower research costs and quicker profits" for pharmaceutical companies, a Biochem founder tells Toughill (1989): "That's why Biochem chose to research AIDS drugs." Similarly, according to the cover story in *Business* by Franklin et al. (1987), the problem with vaccines is their poor profit margin—they are needed only once. Yet, because Wall Street continues to debate whether the epidemic has "topped out" and how to separate "hype from hope" about AIDS drugs (Mahar 1989), its analysts are motivated to look closely and skeptically at scientific data, media coverage, and other forms of conventional wisdom (see "AIDS and 1962" 1988; McGrath and Sutcliffe 1987; Franklin et al. 1987; Ricklefs 1988; Glaser

1988; and Mahar 1989). While AIDS activists are willing to use the profit motive to their advantage, they do not trust it (any more than they trust the media with whom they have learned to work so effectively). *Rockville Is Burning* (Huff 1989) satirizes Wall Street's pleasure with the "cocktail approach" to AIDS treatments in which a whole range of products will be tried. In the 1990s, HIV and AIDS continue to generate new drugs, technologies, and practices, including more than 1,500 patents ("Market-place" 1996). The pharmaceutical industry also increased its contributions and subsidies on behalf of AIDS, and among the benefactors were academic organizations, conferences, and activist initiatives. Martin Delaney of Project Inform, John S. James of *AIDS Treatment News*, various members of treatment and data committees, and others are among those attacked for their apparent coziness with the industry—and with leading figures in the federal science establishment as well (see Wachter 1991; Epstein 1996; Cohen 1996; and Mannion 1997).

5. Self-care is an old American tradition ("Each man his own doctor" ran a nineteenth-century aphorism) that has gained new ground since the civil rights, women's liberation, and consumer movements of the 1960s and 1970s. Peer support groups have also exploded during this period, some modeled on the twelve-step program of Alcoholics Anonymous, others adopting different formats and goals. Self-help and self-treatment have been perhaps most fully developed within the women's health movement, and it is to books like *Our Bodies Ourselves* (Boston Women's Health Book Collective 1994) that some AIDS treatment activists acknowledge their greatest debt. At the same time, women AIDS activists may identify with the movement more as gay or queer people than as feminists, whom they perceive as less than helpful in the AIDS crisis (see ACT UP New York Women and AIDS Book Group 1992). On the women's movement, gay men and lesbians, and queer activism in relation to AIDS, see also Norsigian (1996), Stoller (1995), Gorna (1996), Hollibaugh ([1993] 1997); and Gamson (1996) as well as commentary from diverse perspectives in Schneider and Stoller (1995), Levine et al. (1997), Duberman (1997), and others. Information about and useful distinctions among self-help, validated, nonvalidated, and unorthodox therapies are given in Cassileth and Brown (1988), Freedman and McGill Boston Research Group (1989), and Eisenberg et al. (1993), the very influential study of unconventional medicine. Gamson (1989) and Epstein (1996) both identify features that make AIDS activism distinct as a social movement.

6. For a capsulized version of this history, see Harrington (1997), as well as Scott (1997), who argues that official histories of the epidemic erase the contributions of activists. Accounts that chronicle activist work include Dixon (1990), Arno and Feiden (1992), Wachter (1991), Cohen (1993), and Epstein (1996).

7. Kramer later left ACT UP. His 1987 speech reflects his long-standing view that the federal effort against AIDS is unspeakably inadequate, a view that he consistently articulated in vividly aggressive prose. As early as 1982, e.g., he wrote that "studies are constantly announced and undertaken by people who have only the vaguest notions of how we live" (in Kramer 1989a, 26). This quote served as an epigraph to ACT UP's (1989a) *National AIDS Research Treatment Agenda*. In 1990, he depicted pro-AZT researchers pumping "AZT down the throats of AIDS patients like they were Strassbourg geese being fattened up for the kill." Tensions between official and activist perspectives on the AIDS drug approval process are addressed in Arno and Feiden (1992), Bishop (1987), Boffey (1988a, 1988b, 1988c, 1988d), Burkett (1995),

Chase (1988b), Douglas and Pinsky (1989), Geitner (1988), Goldstein and Massa (1989), Gross (1987a), James (1989a, 1989b, 1989c, 1991, 1994, 1997), Kingston (1990), Kramer (1989a, 1989b), Leary (1988), Rothman (1987), and Epstein (1996). Erni (1994) explores tensions and fantasies in AIDS discourse around the vision of "a cure." Treatment and cure are also a central focus of Robert Wachter's account of his experience as an organizer of the 1990 International Conference on AIDS in San Francisco, which, he writes, represented "a microcosm of the clash of forces over the most volatile issue of the epidemic" (1991, 209). See also Bordowitz (1993).

8. The agenda lists twelve principles for a new AIDS drug–testing system; proposes new models and suggestions for speeding Phase I safety trials, pilot efficacy trials, new treatment protocols, and postmarketing surveillance; sets priorities for clinical research into several dozen specific AIDS drugs; and highlights "five drugs we need now" and "seven treatments we want tested faster." The final section on AIDS drug disasters list nine drugs whose development has been delayed, mismanaged, neglected, or prevented. While this document is directed toward the FDA system, complementary publications address decision making for individuals; see, e.g., ACT UP's *Deciding to Enter an AIDS/HIV Drug Trial* (1989) and the excellent educational video *Work Your Body* (Bordowitz and Carlomusto 1988), produced for the Gay Men's Health Crisis Living with AIDS series (see also Bordowitz and Carlomusto 1989). For a more detailed analysis of the problems for women and drug trials, see ACT UP New York Women and AIDS Book Group (1992). For a discussion of why some people resist treatment and some organizations do not emphasize alternatives, see Douglas and Pinsky (1989). ACT UP also has an Alternative and Holistic Treatment Subcommittee, but this is not my focus here. Also not my focus here, but of considerable interest, is the development of drugs and treatments in other countries. For an outline, if a contentious one, of the controversy surrounding the drug Kemron, developed in Kenya, see Burkett (1995, chap. 6). Trials of Kemron in the United States were discontinued in 1997.

9. In the Dickinson epigraph, "the gift of Screws" signifies the mechanical press that is used to extract fragrant oils from flower petals. In the summer of 1989, I was telling a young man in Illinois the saga of trichosanthin, an AIDS drug popularly known as Compound Q, a highly purified form of a protein derived from the root of *Trichosanthes kirilowii*, a Chinese cucumber (see McGrath et al. 1989). I said that, in vitro, the drug seemed to be relatively selective, killing HIV-infected cells but no uninfected cells; still being tested in both approved and underground trials, Compound Q had nonetheless been hailed in the media as the latest cure for AIDS. He was delighted with this story. "Wouldn't you know the cure for AIDS would be a cucumber—something natural," he said, "and not some horrible toxic chemical." Born a cucumber perhaps, trichosanthin the drug is "the gift of Screws"—of laboratory operations and biochemical manipulations and capital investment and human effort. Moreover, initial tests in vivo reveal it to have highly potent, complex effects on HIV-infected people, with numerous side effects. Its further development will depend on technology, and even then it will not likely be a "cure." Dickinson's poem, then, can be read as a statement about the natural as almost always already technological. On Compound Q, see Second Laboratory (1976), Goldstein and Massa (1989), Kingston (1990), *Treatment Issues* (3 [30 October 1989]: 9), Arno and Feiden (1992), Epstein (1996), and Kolata (1990). Paul Reed's (1991) *The Q Journal* is an

extraordinary first-person account of his encounters with the joys, ambiguities, and dogmas of experimental AIDS treatments.

10. An interesting set of discourses converged around the question of whether AZT was a "poison." A technical discourse may define a poison simply in terms of its effects on cells and DNA replication. That many antiviral drugs have a broad effect on cellular replication is one of their generic difficulties. But the charge of "poison" is also part of a readily available cultural narrative about the poisoning of the body, the environment, the earth; about the poisoning of the natural by the technological. The British treatment journal *Positively Healthy* (see Marshall 1989) makes a sustained critique of AZT and other potent medications on the grounds that they poison the body with the same kind of systemic toxins that poison the earth. What is needed is to rebuild the body through intensive work with nutritive substances, not further destroy its fragile structures. Nevertheless, the journal provides detailed and timely treatment information and from this highly engaged position contests the terrain of AIDS discourse in technical analytic terms.

This is quite different from the position of someone like Larry Kramer, who condemned AZT as poison not because it was not "natural" but because it was not doing the high-powered biomedical nuking job that needed doing. *Positively Healthy's* position is also quite different from, say, some New Age articulations of "the natural." A collection of "channeled teachings" on AIDS encourages the use of natural healing processes, inner guidance, and internal "chemical inducers" to boost the immune system (Spirit Speaks 1987). But its discourse is generic and out of touch with the details of AIDS research and treatment. Despite repeated charges of traditional medicine's misconceptions, in the end the book represents AIDS as something that happens on the "Earth plane"—indeed, *needs* to happen there, whatever that means—and is of no concern: "Those within the Spirit dimension will not interfere in *any way* with the Earth plane" (p. 168). At the same time, although condoms, drugs, and vaccines are represented as ultimately illusory and hollow, they are nonetheless recommended by the spirits, who also counsel individuals not to hassle doctors with the truth, which the doctors will not understand. One lesson of AIDS activism is that a challenge to any given version of "truth" must be anchored in a coherent counternarrative. Yet, in the case of channeling, an entire alternative referential apparatus is constructed to no earthly avail. Its theories and therapies refuse an orthodox biomedical worldview in favor of an alternate universe that has no observable consequences and places virtually no burden on institutions such as the FDA, existing as they do only on the "Earth plane." (See also Darril 1987; Kaiser 1993).

Contrast this with the oppositional and contentious universe of AIDS treatment activism, which, whatever its internal disagreements, regularly produces an ambitious agenda for established institutions. Sparked by Eisenberg et al. (1993) as well as the drive under managed care to develop cost-effective treatment regimens, U.S. health care in the 1990s reflects a dissolution of the strict boundary between "conventional" and "unconventional" treatments—these latter coming to be grouped under the rubric of complementary and alternative medicine, or CAM (see, e.g., Hanna 1997).

11. On 18 August 1989, the *New York Times* reported that findings of a thirty-two-center study indicated that AZT would help "AIDS cases with virus but no symp-

toms" (Hilts 1989a, 1), making it half as likely for those receiving the drug to develop symptoms. Secretary for Health and Human Services Louis Sullivan announced the findings in Washington, D.C.: "Today we are witnessing a turning point in the battle to change AIDS from a fatal disease to a treatable one." Fauci said that the findings made it important for people to get themselves tested. Samuel Broder, confirming what claimed to be the study's definitive nature, stated in the article that the issue regarding asymptomatics "has now been resolved" (p. 12). A growing body of studies contributed to the debate—see *Abstracts* (1990, 1991, 1992, 1993, 1994, 1996, 1998).

But other scientists and AIDS groups emphasized that the *Times* story was little more than a reprint of Burroughs-Wellcome's press release and urged caution until published data were available. And, on 16 October 1989, this full-page ad appeared in the *New York Times*:

BEFORE YOU

TAKE AZT AGAIN,

READ THE

November

ISSUE OF SPIN.

In that issue of *Spin*, Celia Farber's regular "AIDS: Words from the Front" column, titled "Sins of Omission: The AZT Scandal," reviewed loopholes in the approval process for AZT and quoted a number of dissident scientists. Peter Duesberg, for example, told Farber (1989, 117), that asymptomatic seropositive people who take AZT "are running into the gas chamber." In another postconference judgment, in a continuing series for the *New York Native* on AZT as "poison by prescription," John Lauritsen (1989, 117) negatively reviewed the Columbia conference: "On the whole it was a flop." He described Metroka's talk as "almost inhuman in its glibness" and called Delaney's talk "a hard-sell pitch for AZT." Lauritsen, in a sense, has a role in the script, too—that of the revealer of the conspiracy. He describes being harassed at the conference; denials are taken as confirming evidence (see also Gilbert 1996; and Lauritsen 1987, 1997). The compelling nature of the *Native*'s theories was evident in its fierce defenders. Yet one of my friends was finally given a formal prescription by his therapist not to read it; the therapist promised that, if any major developments occurred, he would communicate them. Many others would doubtless credit the *Native* with keeping them alive through this terrifying period. This is yet one more example of the hazardous path among sources that people must learn to weave for themselves.

AZT, as a monotherapy, is no longer the treatment of choice, but it is useful for many purposes when combined with other classes of drugs. The annual *Sanford Guides* provide typical tables of indications, combinations, and interaction effects for creating the "AIDS cocktails" of the 1990s. As the authors of the *Guide* point out, it is crucial that more physicians acquire the pharmaceutical sophistication to provide good treatment now that it is available. (As Kitahata et al. [1996] and L. Altman [1996b] report, doctors' experience with HIV patients has now been shown to affect survival significantly.)

12. On the 1996 International Conference on AIDS in Vancouver and ongoing developments, see *Abstracts* (1996, 1998), L. Altman (1996a, 1996c, 1996d, 1996e, 1996f, 1996g), Dunlap (1996), and the ongoing discussions and advisories in Project In-

form's *P.I. Perspective, Beta, AIDS Treatment News* and *AIDS Clinical Care,* and countless websites.

13. Steven Epstein's *Impure Science* (1996) provides a careful and illuminating account of AIDS treatment activism and its reorientation toward influencing basic research in the early 1990s, including the emergence of protease inhibitors and combinatory drug regimens. Emphasizing the interaction of experts and laypeople in the production of biomedical knowledge, Epstein suggests "directions for the development of a more comprehensive inquiry into the politics of knowledge in modern Western societies" (p. 5). Epstein's analysis is particularly welcome on the subject of what he calls "clinical trials and tribulations," including those surrounding the Concorde trial and its aftermath; carefully and evenhandedly deconstructing the accomplishments of conventional and activist approaches to research and treatment, he continues to uphold the theoretical and practical value of "impure science." Work from other perspectives on scientific practice includes Aboulker and Swart (1993), King (1997), Harrington (1997), Balsamo (1996), Geison (1995), and Pickering (1995).

14. I am indebted to my colleague Diane Gottheil for illuminating, through the Medical Humanities and Social Sciences Program seminar series that she designed and directed at the University of Illinois College of Medicine in Urbana-Champaign, the notion of health care in America as a "permanent crisis."

15. Epstein notes the apparent inconsistency of this move with the more provisional and antiauthoritarian operating procedure of treatment activism in prior years. Yet we must assume that intimacy with positivist science also means intimacy with the process by which scientific facts are constructed and the often circumstantial and probabilistic evidence on which such constructions are based. As Epstein suggests, perhaps activists will now be positioned to better articulate this provisional construction process to their fellow activists and to the public. Indeed, in Harrington's view, quoted above, activists' move toward "the inside" of the scientific establishment meant that "we would never be so pure and fervent in our belief that we were right" (quoted in Epstein 1996, 233).

16. Both Patient Zero and *Zero Patience* figure in John Whittier Treat's compelling account of his 1988–89 sabbatical in Japan at the height of that country's AIDS panic over "foreigners," especially those from "Homo Heaven" (the United States). In Japan researching a book on the literature of the Holocaust (subsequently published as *Ground Zero*), Treat writes: "I come from a long line of homosexual professors of Japanese literature. I perch on the upper branches of a special family tree where roots go deep" (1994, 655). Thinking of past and present Japanese loves and lovers, he feels linked to a distinguished history that includes, among others, Sir Richard Burton; in AIDS-phobic Japan, however, he now imagines himself identified by the Japanese health authorities and the media as the foreigner who brought AIDS to Japan. In this context, he describes seeing *Zero Patience* some years later in London, "where Burton's work and that of others on older branches of the tree fill the British Museum with booty that spills the secrets of their private desires as well as the Crown's imperial demands." For many gay men, he reflects, as he watches Greyson's musical, "Burton cannot be more than some nutty Brit who measured penises; and for the clueless heterosexual watching this movie, Dugas is just some queen with a funny accent. But for me, when I watch the film's two leading men screw on screen, I see the two parts of me at once, both the white man with a burden and the

wide-grinned Huck Finn of a boy in a new place. No difference, yet nothing the same—the bizarre and beautiful spectacle of an indivisible embrace" (Treat 1994, 655).

Epilogue

1. Ablin (1996) refers to an earlier publication of his data (Ablin et al. 1985); possibly this provided the source for the original tabloid story linking AIDS to King Tut. In suggesting that many of these theories of AIDS's origin seem generically parallel to urban legends, I might observe that the apparatus of scholarly documentation (such as it is, in some cases) takes the place of the anecdotal chain of evidence that grounds urban legends ("This happened to the friend of my sister's roommate").

Bibliography

Abbott, Andrew. 1988. *The System of Professions: An Essay on the Division of Expert Labor.* Chicago: University of Chicago Press.

Ablin, Richard J. 1996. "AIDS: Déjà Vu in Ancient Egypt?" Letter, *Emerging Infectious Diseases* 2, no. 2 (April–June): 155.

Ablin, Richard J., R. S. Immerman, and M. J. Gonder. 1985. "AIDS: A Disease of Ancient Egypt?" *New York State Journal of Medicine* 85: 200–201.

Aboulker, Jean Pierre, and Ann Marie Swart. 1993. "Preliminary Analysis of the Concorde Trial." Letter, *Lancet* 341: 889–90.

Abramson, Paul R. 1992. "Sex, Lies, and Ethnography." In *The Time of AIDS: Social Analysis, Theory, and Method,* ed. Gilbert Herdt and Shirley Lindenbaum. Newbury Park, Calif.: Sage.

Abramson, Paul R., and Gilbert Herdt. 1990. "The Assessment of Sexual Practices Related to the Transmission of AIDS: A Global Perspective." *Journal of Sex Research* 27: 215–32.

Abramson, Paul, and Steven D. Pinkerton, eds. 1993. *Sexual Nature/Sexual Culture.* Chicago: University of Chicago Press.

Abramson, Paul, and Steven D. Pinkerton. 1995. *With Pleasure: Thoughts on the Nature of Human Sexuality.* New York and Oxford: Oxford University Press.

Abstracts. 1985. First International Conference on AIDS, 15–17 April, Atlanta.

Abstracts. 1986. Second International Conference on AIDS, 23–25 June, Paris.

Abstracts. 1987. Third International Conference on AIDS, 1–5 June, Washington, D.C.

Abstracts. 1988. Fourth International Conference on AIDS, 12–16 June, Stockholm.

Abstracts. 1989. Fifth International Conference on AIDS, 4–9 June, Montreal.

Abstracts. 1990. Sixth International Conference on AIDS, 20–24 June, San Francisco.

Abstracts. 1991. Seventh International Conference on AIDS, 16–21 June, Florence.

Abstracts. 1992. Eighth International Conference on AIDS, 19–24 July, Amsterdam.

Abstracts. 1993. Ninth International Conference on AIDS, 6–11 June, Berlin.

Abstracts. 1994. Tenth International Conference on AIDS, 7–12 August, Yokahama.

Abstracts. 1996. Eleventh International Conference on AIDS, 7–12 July, Vancouver.

Abstracts. 1998. Twelfth World AIDS Conference, 28 June–3 July, Geneva.

ACT UP. 1989a. *A National AIDS Treatment Research Agenda.* New York: ACT UP.

ACT UP. 1989b. *Treatment and Data Handbook.* See Bohne et al. (1989).

ACT UP. 1990. *A Critique of the AIDS Clinical Trials Group.* New York: ACT UP.

ACT UP. 1996. "Welcome to Vancouver." Flyer distributed at the Eleventh International Conference on AIDS, Vancouver.

ACT UP et al. [1989] 1997. "Stop the Church." In *We Are Everywhere: A Historical Sourcebook of Gay and Lesbian Politics*, ed. M. Blasius and S. Phelan. New York: Routledge.

ACT UP New York Women and AIDS Book Group. 1992. *Women, AIDS, and Activism.* Boston: South End.

Adair, Peter, producer. 1991. *Absolutely Positive.* San Francisco: Adair Films. Film, 90 minutes.

Adair, Peter, and Rob Epstein, producers. 1986. *The A.I.D.S. Show—Artists Involved with Death and Survival.* San Francisco: Direct Cinema Ltd.

Adam, Barry D., and Alan Sears. 1996. *Experiencing HIV: Personal, Family, and Work Relationships.* New York: Columbia University Press.

Adams, Mary Louise. 1989. "There's No Place Like Home: On the Place of Identity in Feminist Politics." *Feminist Review* 31 (Spring): 22–33.

Aggleton, Peter, Graham Hart, and Peter Davies, eds. 1989. *AIDS: Social Representations, Social Practices.* New York: Falmer.

Aggleton, Peter, and Hilary Homans, eds. 1988. *Social Aspects of AIDS.* New York: Falmer.

Aggleton, Peter, et al., eds. 1989. *AIDS: Scientific and Social Issues: A Resource for Health Educators.* Edinburgh: Churchill Livingstone.

Aggleton, Peter, et al., eds. 1990. *AIDS: Individual, Cultural, and Policy Dimensions.* New York: Falmer.

Aggleton, Peter, et al., eds. 1992. *AIDS: Rights, Risk, and Reason.* New York: Falmer.

Aggleton, Peter, et al., eds. 1993. *AIDS: The Second Decade.* New York: Falmer.

"AIDS: A Public Inquiry." 1986. *Frontline.* 25 March. New York: PBS.

"AIDS and Africa: Facing the Facts." 1988. Special issue, *Africa Report*, vol. 33, no. 6 (November–December).

AIDS and the Arts. 1987. "MacNeil/Lehrer News Hour." 27 July. New York: PBS.

"AIDS and 1962." 1988. Editorial, *Wall Street Journal*, 14 July, 24.

AIDS and the Third World: The Impact on Development. See U.S. House (1988).

"AIDS Campaigns, The." 1987–89. "Ideas." Multipart radio series, prod. Coleman Jones. Montreal: Canadian Broadcasting Company Enterprises/Radio Canada.

"AIDS Carrier's Baby Free from Virus, Government Confirms." 1987. *Japan Times*, 19 April, 2.

AIDS: Chapter One. 1984. "NOVA." Boston: WGBH/PBS.

"AIDS: Déjà Vu in Ancient Egypt?" See Ablin (1996).

"AIDS Epidemic, Late to Arrive, Now Explodes in Populous Asia." 1996. *New York Times*, 21 January, 1.

AIDS: Epidemiological and Clinical Studies, Vol. 1. 1987. Waltham, Mass.: Massachusetts Medical Society. Reprints from the *New England Journal of Medicine*.

AIDS: Epidemiological and Clinical Studies, Vol. 2. 1989. Waltham, Mass.: NEJM Books. Reprints from the *New England Journal of Medicine*.

"AIDS: Global and Regional Perspectives on Assessment, Risk Reduction, and Prevention." 1996. American Medical Association and Henry J. Kaiser Family Foundation, executive summary of media briefing, Eleventh International Conference on AIDS, 6 July, Vancouver.

AIDS Medical Glossary. 1995. Baltimore: AIDS Research Information Center (ARIC).

"AIDS Monitor." 1988. Column, *New Scientist*, 18 February, 36.

AIDS Prevention and Control. 1988. See WHO (1988a).

"AIDS: Public Health and Civil Liberties." 1986. Special supplement, *Hastings Center Report*, vol. 16, no. 6 (December).

"AIDS Risk Held Twice as High in Women." 1994. *New York Times*, 1 November, B-11.

"AIDS: Science, Ethics, Policy." 1986. Forum, *Issues in Science and Technology* 2, no. 2: 39–73.

"AIDS: Syndrome of an Imperialist Era." See GRIA (1982).

"AIDS Victims Live Longer, U.S. Doctor Says." 1989. *Montreal Gazette*, 12 June, 1.

"AIDS: What Is to Be Done?" 1985. Forum, *Harpers*, October, 39–52.

"AIDS: What Women Must Know Now!" 1985. *Good Housekeeping*. November, 245–6.

Akeroyd, Anne V. 1997. "Sociocultural Aspects of AIDS in Africa: Occupational and Gender Issues." In *AIDS in Africa and the Caribbean*, ed. George C. Bond et al. Boulder, Colo.: Westview.

Albert, Edward. 1986a. "Acquired Immune Deficiency Syndrome: The Victim and the Press." *Studies in Communication* 3: 135–58.

Albert, Edward. 1986b. "Illness and Deviance: The Response of the Press to AIDS." In *The Social Dimensions of AIDS: Method and Theory*, ed. Douglas A. Feldman and Thomas M. Johnson. New York: Praeger.

Alcorn, Keith. 1989. "AIDS in the Public Sphere: How a Broadcasting System in Crisis Dealt with an Epidemic." In *Taking Liberties: AIDS and Cultural Politics*, ed. Erica Carter and Simon Watney. London: Serpent's Tail.

Alexander, Priscilla. 1996. "Bathhouses and Brothels: Symbolic Sites in Discourse and Practice." *Policing Public Sex*, ed. Dangerous Bedfellows. Boston: South End.

Allen, Hillary. 1984. "At the Mercy of Her Hormones: Premenstrual Tension and the Law." *m/f* 9: 19–43.

Alonso, Ana Maria, and Maria Teresa Koreck. 1989. "Silences: 'Hispanics,' AIDS, and Sexual Practices." *Differences* 1 (Winter) 101–24.

Alter, Jonathan. 1985. "Sins of Omission." *Newsweek*, 23 September, 25.

Altman, Dennis. 1986. *AIDS in the Mind of America.* New York: Doubleday.

Altman, Dennis. 1988. "Legitimation through Disaster: AIDS and the Gay Movement." *AIDS: The Burdens of History*, ed. Elizabeth Fee and Daniel M. Fox. Berkeley and Los Angeles: University of California Press.

Altman, Dennis. 1992. "AIDS and the Reconceptualization of Homosexuality." In *A Leap in the Dark: AIDS, Art, and Contemporary Cultures*, ed. Allan Klusaček and Ken Morrison. Montreal: Véhicule/Artexte.

Altman, Dennis. 1994. *Power and Community: Organizational and Cultural Responses to AIDS.* London: Taylor and Francis.

Altman, Lawrence K. 1981. "Rare Cancer Seen in 41 Homosexuals." *New York Times*, 3 July, 20.

Altman, Lawrence K. 1985a. "Heterosexuals and AIDS: New Data Examined." *New York Times*, 22 January, 19–20.

Altman, Lawrence K. 1985b. "Linking AIDS to Africa Provokes Bitter Debate." *New York Times*, 21 November, 1, 8.

Altman, Lawrence K. 1985c. "New Support from Africa as WHO Plans Effort on AIDS." *New York Times*, 22 December, 1, 11.

Altman, Lawrence K. 1986. "Study Says AIDS in Haiti Spreads Mainly by Heterosexual Activity." *New York Times*, 29 June, A-1.

Altman, Lawrence K. 1987a. "AIDS Virus Always Fatal?" *New York Times*, 8 September, 15–16.

Altman, Lawrence K. 1987b. "Anxiety Allayed on Heterosexual AIDS." *New York Times*, 5 June, 11.

Altman, Lawrence K. 1987c. "Study Examines Prostitutes and AIDS Virus Infection." *New York Times*, 27 March, A-14.

Altman, Lawrence K. 1988a. "AIDS Reported Rising in Thai Drug Users." *New York Times*, 19 April, 26.

Altman, Lawrence K. 1988b. "Inhaled Drug Is Found to Benefit against Pneumonia in AIDS Cases." *New York Times*, 15 June, A-21.

Altman, Lawrence K. 1988c. "Medical Guardians: Does *New England Journal* Exercise Undue Power on Information Flow?" *New York Times*, 28 January, 1.

Altman, Lawrence K. 1989. "Who's Stricken and How: AIDS Pattern Is Shifting." *New York Times*, 5 February, A-1, 28.

Altman, Lawrence K. 1992. "Researchers Report Much Grimmer AIDS Outlook." *New York Times*, 4 June, A-1.

Altman, Lawrence K. 1995. "Vitamin A Deficiency Tied to AIDS Virus in Newborns." *New York Times*, 3 February , A-9.

Altman, Lawrence K. 1996a. "AIDS Meeting: Signs of Hope, and Obstacles." *New York Times*, 7 July, A-1, A-8.

Altman, Lawrence K. 1996b. "AIDS Survival Linked to Doctors' Experience." *New York Times*, 1 February, A-11.

Altman, Lawrence K. 1996c. "At AIDS Meeting, Experts Find an Uneasy Mix of Hope and Fear." *New York Times*, 9 July, C-5.

Altman, Lawrence K. 1996d. "Discussing Possible AIDS Cure Raises Hope, Anger, and Question: What Exactly Is Meant by 'Cure'?" *New York Times*, 8 July, A-3.

Altman, Lawrence K. 1996e. "India Suddenly Leads in HIV, AIDS Meeting Is Told." *New York Times*, 8 July, A-3.

Altman, Lawrence K. 1996f. "Landmark Studies Change Outlook of AIDS Treatment." *New York Times*, 14 July, A-14.

Altman, Lawrence K. 1996g. "Scientists Display Substantial Gains in AIDS Treatment." *New York Times*, 12 July, A-1.

Altman, Lawrence K. 1997. "AIDS Deaths Drop 19% in U.S., Continuing a Heartening Trend." *New York Times*, 15 July, A-1.

Alwood, Edward. 1996. *Straight News: Gays, Lesbians, and the News Media*. New York: Columbia University Press.

American Medical Association. 1987. *AIDS: From the Beginning*, ed. Helen M. Cole and George D. Lundberg. Chicago: American Medical Association.

American Medical Association. 1996. *Guidelines for Primary Care Physicians on HIV/ AIDS*. Chicago: American Medical Association.

American Medical Association Council on Scientific Affairs. [1983] 1987. "The Acquired Immunodeficiency Syndrome: Commentary." In *AIDS: From the Beginning*, ed. Helen M. Cole and George D. Lundberg. Chicago: American Medical Association. Originally published in the *Journal of the American Medical Association* 252, no. 15 (19 October 1983): 2037–43.

Amolis, Steven, et al. 1993. "Unconventional Medicine: Correspondence." *New England Journal of Medicine* 329, no. 16: 1200–1204.

Anagnost, Ann S. 1988. "Magical Practice, Birth Policy, and Women's Health in Post-Mao China." Paper presented at a colloquium of the Unit for Criticism and Interpretive Theory, 7 December, University of Illinois at Urbana-Champaign.

Anastos, Kathryn, and Carola Marte. [1989] 1991. "Women—the Missing Persons in the AIDS Epidemic." In *The AIDS Reader: Social, Political, and Ethical Issues*, ed. Nancy McKenzie. New York: New American Library.

Anderson, D. J., and E. J. Yunis. 1983. " 'Trojan Horse' Leukocytes in AIDS." *New England Journal of Medicine* 309: 984–85.

Anderson, Roy M., and Robert M. May. 1988a. "Epidemiological Parameters of HIV Transmission." *Nature* 353: 514–19.

Anderson, Roy M., Robert M. May, and A. R. McLean. 1988b. "Possible Demographic Consequences of AIDS in Developing Countries." *Nature* 332: 228–34.

Andrews, Edmund L. 1989. "Equations Patented; Some See a Danger." *New York Times*, 15 February, D-1.

Angell, Marcia. 1997. "The Ethics of Clinical Research in the Third World." Editorial, *New England Journal of Medicine* 337, no. 12 (18 September): 847–49.

Anonimo (Anonymous). 1992. "No Puedo Confiar en Nadie" (I can't trust anyone). In *Women, AIDS, and Activism*, ed. ACT UP New York Women and AIDS Book Group. Boston: South End.

Appleman, Rose, and Linda Kahn. 1988. "Women and AIDS." *Radical America* 21, no. 2 (March–April): 3.

Appleman, Rose, and Linda Kahn. 1989. "Lesbians Face AIDS on Several Fronts." *New Directions for Women* (May–June): 12.

Ardill, Susan, and Sue O'Sullivan. 1987. "AIDS and Women: Building a Feminist Framework." *Spare Rib* 178 (May): 40–43.

Ardill, Susan, and Sue O'Sullivan. 1989. "Sex in the Summer of '88." *Feminist Review* 31 (Spring): 126–34.

Armstrong, David. 1983. *Political Economy of the Body: Medical Knowledge in Britain in the Twentieth Century*. Cambridge: Cambridge University Press.

Arno, Peter S., and Karyn L. Feiden. 1992. *Against the Odds: The Story of AIDS Drug Development, Politics, and Profits*. New York: Harper Collins.

Arno, Peter S., et al. 1989. "Economic and Policy Implications of Early Intervention in HIV Disease." *Journal of the American Medical Association* 262: 1493–98.

Associated Press. 1985. "AIDS Funding Boost Requested: Increase Would Bring $200 Million to Bear on the Disease." *Daily Illini*, 27 September, 7.

Associated Press. 1986a. "Doctors: Case Shows AIDS Can Spread Heterosexually." *Champaign-Urbana News-Gazette*, 10 April, A-7.

Associated Press. 1986b. "571 AIDS Cases Tied to Heterosexual Causes." *Champaign-Urbana News-Gazette*, 12 December, A-7.

Associated Press. 1988a. "Protestors Halt 'Midnight' AIDS Episode." *New York Daily News*, 28 October, 12.

Associated Press. 1988b. "U.S. Scores Low in Geography Test." *Champaign-Urbana News-Gazette*, 17 July, B-10.

Associated Press. 1991. "AIDS Activists Disrupt Start of Television News Shows." *Daily Illini*, 23 January, 4.

Associated Press. 1992a. "Health Officials Say Women Need Safe Sex Training to Avoid AIDS." *Champaign-Urbana News-Gazette*, 22 July, D-1.

Associated Press. 1992b. "New Medicines for Women Tested." *Champaign-Urbana News-Gazette*, 7 August, "etc!," 6.

Associated Press. 1997. "School District Scraps Girl's Science Project on Condoms." *Los Angeles Times*, 1 April, 7.

Atkinson, Terry. 1988. " 'Return of Ben Casey' Pilot for Possible Series Revival." *Los Angeles Times*, 1 March, sec. 6, p. 10.

Atwood, Margaret. 1986. *The Handmaid's Tale*. Boston: Houghton Mifflin.

Ault, Steve. 1986. "AIDS: The Facts of Life." *Guardian*, 26 March, 1, 8.

Avery, Caryl S. 1988a. "Flirting with AIDS." *Self*, July, 80.

Avery, Caryl S. 1988b. "Women and AIDS: How Real Is the Danger?" *Self*, June, 146–49.

Baker, Andrea J. 1986. "The Portrayal of AIDS in the Media: An Analysis of Articles in *The New York Times*." In *The Social Dimensions of AIDS: Method and Theory*, ed. Douglas A. Feldman and Thomas M. Johnson. New York: Praeger.

Baker, Rob. 1994. *The Art of AIDS: From Stigma to Conscience*. New York: Continuum.

Balsamo, Anne. 1996. *Technologies of the Gendered Body: Reading Cyborg Women*. Durham, N.C.: Duke University Press.

Balsamo, Anne, and Paula A. Treichler. 1990. "Feminist Cultural Studies: Questions for the 1990s." *Women and Language* 13, no. 1: 3–6.

Banzhaf, Marion. 1992. "Race, Women and AIDS." In *Women, AIDS, and Activism*, ed. ACT UP New York Women and AIDS Book Group. Boston: South End.

Barker, Carol, and Meredeth Turshen. 1986. "Briefings: AIDS in Africa." *Review of African Political Economy* 27, no. 105 (January–March): 51–54.

Barker-Benfield, G. J. 1976. *The Horrors of the Half-Known Life: Male Attitudes toward Women and Sexuality in Nineteenth Century America*. New York: Harper and Row.

Barnes, Barry, and David Bloor. 1982. "Relativism, Rationalism and the Sociology of Knowledge." In *Rationality and Relativism*, ed. Martin Hollis and Steven Lukes. Cambridge: MIT Press.

Barnes, Deborah M. 1986. "AIDS Research in New Phase." *Science*, 18 July, 282–83.

Barnes, Edward, and Anne Hollister. 1985. "AIDS: The New Victims." *Life*, July, 12–19.

Barré-Sinoussi, Françoise, et al. 1983. "Isolation of a T-Lymphotropic Retrovirus from a Patient at Risk for Acquired Immune Deficiency Syndrome." *Science*, 20 May, 868–71.

Barret, K. 1983. "AIDS: What It Does to a Family." *Ladies Home Journal*, November, 98.

Barrett, Michèle, and Anne Phillips, eds. 1992. *Destabilizing Theory: Contemporary Feminist Debates*. Stanford, Calif.: Stanford University Press.

Barrett, Wayne. 1985. "Straight Shooters: AIDS Targets another Lifestyle." *Village Voice*, 5 November, 14–18.

Bateson, Mary Catherine, and Richard Goldsby. 1988. *Thinking AIDS: The Social Response to the Biological Threat*. Reading, Mass.: Addison-Wesley.

Batt, Sharon. 1994. *Patient No More: The Politics of Breast Cancer*. Charlottetown, P.E.I.: Gynergy.

Baxley, Norman, producer. 1991. *Physicians and AIDS: The Ethical Response*. Urbana, Ill.: Baxley Media Group. Video.

Baxley, Norman, producer. 1994. *The Berlin International Conference on AIDS*. Urbana, Ill.: Baxley Media Group. Video.

Bayer, Ronald. 1981. *Homosexuality and American Psychiatry: The Politics of Diagnosis*. New York: Basic.

Bayer, Ronald. 1985. "AIDS and the Gay Community: Between the Specter and the Promise of Medicine." *Social Research* 52, no. 3 (Autumn): 581–606.

Bayer, Ronald. 1986. "AIDS: The Public Context of an Epidemic." Supplement, *Milbank Quarterly* 64, no. S1: 168–82.

Bayer, Ronald. 1997. "An Oral History of AIDS: Doctors in the First Decade of the Epidemic." Paper given at the symposium "The Culture of AIDS," Humanities Series Colloquium, 5 March, Johns Hopkins Univesity.

Bayer, Ronald, and Robert L. Spitzer. 1982. "Edited Correspondence on the Status of Homosexuality in DSM-III." *Journal of the History of the Behavioral Sciences* 18: 32–52.

Bayles, Martha. 1992. "The Testament of Philly Lutaaya." *Wall Street Journal*, 2 April, 11.

Bearden, T. E. 1988. *AIDS: Biological Warfare*. Greenville: Tesla.

Becher, Brian. 1983. "AIDS and the Media: A Case Study of How the Press Influences Public Opinion." University of Illinois College of Medicine, Urbana-Champaign. Photocopied manuscript in the author's collection.

Bell, Laurie, ed. 1987. *Good Girls/Bad Girls: Feminists and Sex Trade Workers Face to Face*. Seattle: Seal; Toronto: Women's Press.

Belsey, Catherine. 1980. *Critical Practice*. New York: Methuen.

Bennet, James. 1992. "Friends Remember Alison Gertz's Fight against AIDS." *Champaign-Urbana News-Gazette*, 10 August, A-11.

Benoit, Patricia, producer. 1989. *Se Met Ko*. New York: Haitian Women's Program. 16mm film, video.

Benstock, Shari, ed. 1987. *Feminist Issues in Literary Scholarship*. Bloomington: Indiana University Press.

Berer, Marge, with Sunanda Ray. 1993. *Women and AIDS/HIV: An International Resource Book*. London: Harper Collins.

Berger, Peter L., and Thomas Luckman. 1967. *The Social Construction of Reality: A Treatise in the Sociology of Knowledge*. New York: Doubleday, Anchor.

Berland, Jody. 1992. "Angels Dancing: Cultural Technologies and the Production of Space." In *Cultural Studies*, ed. Lawrence Grossberg, Cary Nelson, and Paula A. Treichler. New York: Routledge.

Berridge, Virginia. 1996. *AIDS in the U.K.: The Making of Policy, 1981–1994*. Oxford: Oxford University Press.

Berridge, Virginia, and Philip Strong. 1992. "AIDS Policies in the United Kingdom: A Preliminary Analysis." In *AIDS: The Making of a Chronic Disease*, ed. Elizabeth Fee and Daniel M. Fox. Berkeley and Los Angeles: University of California Press.

Berridge, Virginia, and Philip Strong, eds. 1993. *AIDS and Contemporary History*. Cambridge: Cambridge University Press.

Berry, Jon. 1991. "Think Bland." *Adweek's Marketing Week*, 11 November, 22–24.

Bersani, Leo. 1988. "Is the Rectum a Grave?" *AIDS: Cultural Analysis, Cultural Activism*, ed. Douglas Crimp. Cambridge: MIT Press.

Bertin, Joan E., and Laurie R. Beck. 1996. "Of Headlines and Hypotheses: The Role of Gender in Popular Press Coverage of Women's Health and Biology." In *Man-Made Medicine*, ed. K. L. Moss. Durham, N.C.: Duke University Press.

Bérubé, Michael. 1996. *Life as We Know It: A Father, a Family, and an Exceptional Child*. New York: Pantheon.

Bhabha, Homi. 1983. "The 'Other' Question—the Stereotype and Colonial Discourse." *Screen* 24, no. 6 (November–December): 18–36.

Biggar, Robert J. 1988. "Overview: Africa, AIDS, and Epidemiology." In *AIDS in Africa: The Social and Policy Impact*, ed. Norman Miller and Richard C. Rockwell. Lewiston, N.Y.: Edwin Mellen.

Bird, S. Elizabeth. 1996. "CJ's Revenge: Media, Folklore, and the Cultural Construction of AIDS." *Critical Studies in Mass Communication* 13: 44–58.

Bishop, Katherine. 1987. "Frustrated AIDS Patients Devise Their Own Therapies." *New York Times*, 17 March, 16.

Bishop, Katherine. 1991. "Underground Press Leads the Way on AIDS Advice." *New York Times*, 16 December, 8.

Black, David. 1986. *The Plague Years: A Chronicle of AIDS, the Epidemic of Our Times.* New York: Simon and Schuster. Originally published in *Rolling Stone* in two parts, 1995.

Black, Max. 1962. "Metaphor." In *Models and Metaphors*, ed. M. M. Black. Ithaca, N.Y.: Cornell University Press.

Blasius, Mark, and Shane Phelan, eds. 1997. *We Are Everywhere: A Historical Sourcebook of Gay and Lesbian Politics.* New York: Routledge.

Bleier, Ruth. 1986. *Science and Gender.* London: Pergamon.

Block, Irwin. 1989. "Men Who Don't Use Condoms Called Greatest AIDS Threat." *Montreal Gazette*, 8 June, 10.

Boffey, Philip M. 1988a. "AIDS Panel Wants Wider Drug Tests." *New York Times*, 21 February, 32.

Boffey, Philip M. 1988b. "At Fulcrum of Conflict, Regulator of AIDS Drugs." *New York Times*, 19 August, 12.

Boffey, Philip M. 1988c. "FDA Will Allow AIDS Patients to Import Unapproved Medicines." *New York Times*, 25 July, 1, 10.

Boffey, Philip M. 1988d. "Low AIDS Budget of FDA Said to Slow Drug Approval." *New York Times*, 20 February, 7.

Boffin, Tessa, and Sunil Gupta, eds. 1990. *Ecstatic Antibodies: Revisiting the AIDS Mythology.* London: Rivers Oram.

Bohne, John, Tom Cunningham, Jon Engebretson, Ken Fortunato, and Mark Harrington. 1989. *Treatment and Data Handbook: Treatment Decisions.* New York: ACT UP.

Bolognone, Diane, and Thomas M. Johnson. 1986. "Explanatory Models for AIDS." In *Social Dimension of AIDS: Method and Theory*, ed. Douglas A. Feldman and Thomas M. Johnson. New York: Praeger.

Bolton, Ralph. 1991. "A Selected Bibliography on AIDS and Anthropology." *Journal of Sex Research* 28, no. 2: 307–46.

Bolton, Ralph. 1992. "Mapping Terra Incognita: Sex Research for AIDS Prevention—An Urgent Agenda for the 1990s." *The Time of AIDS: Social Analysis, Theory, and Method.* Newbury Park, California: Sage.

Bond, George C., John Kreniske, Ida Susser, and Joan Vincent, eds. 1997. *AIDS in Africa and the Caribbean.* Boulder, Colo.: Westview.

Bordowitz, Gregg, producer. 1993. *Fast Trip, Long Drop.* New York: Drift Distribution. 16mm film, video.

Bordowitz, Gregg, and Jean Carlomusto, producers. 1988. *Work Your Body.* Living with AIDS Series. New York: Gay Men's Health Crisis. Video.

Bordowitz, Gregg, and Jean Carlomusto, producers. 1989. *Seize Control of the FDA.* Living with AIDS Series. New York: Gay Men's Health Crisis. Video.

Boston Women's Health Book Collective. 1994. *The New Our Bodies, Ourselves.* New York: Simon and Schuster.

Bourdieu, Pierre. [1972] 1977. *Outline of a Theory of Practice.* Translated by Richard Nice. Cambridge: Cambridge University Press.

Bowleg, Lisa. 1992. "Pollutants, Criminals, and Incubators: The Conceptualization of Women under State HIV/AIDS Law 1983 to 1991." *Iris* (Spring/Summer): 11–20.

Boyd, Kenneth M. 1992. "HIV Infection and AIDS: The Ethics of Medical Confidentiality." *Journal of Medical Ethics* 18, no. 4: 173–79.

Braddlee. 1989. "Death in Miami: AIDS, Gender, and Representation." Paper read at the annual meeting of the International Communication Association, 26 May, San Francisco.

Brandt, Allan M. 1987. *No Magic Bullet: A Social History of Venereal Disease in the United States since 1880.* New York: Oxford University Press.

Brandt, Allan M. 1988a. "AIDS and Metaphor: Toward the Social Meaning of Epidemic Disease." *Social Research* 55, no. 3: 413–32.

Bratich, Jack Zeljko. In press. "Injections and Truth Serums: AIDS Conspiracy Accounts and Scientific Authority." In *Conspiracy Nation,* ed. Alisdair Spark and Peter Knight. New York: New York University Press.

Bray, Fiona, and Simon Chapman. 1991. "Community Knowledge, Attitudes, and Media Recall about AIDS, Sydney, 1988 and 1989." *Australian Journal of Public Health* 15, no. 2: 107–13.

Brieger, Gert H. 1980. "History of Medicine." In *A Guide to the Culture of Science, Technology and Medicine,* ed. P. T. Durbin. New York: Free Press.

Bright, Susie. 1995. *Susie Bright's Sexwise.* San Francisco: Cleis.

Bright, Susie. 1997. *Susie Bright's Sexual State of the Union.* New York: Simon and Schuster.

Bristow, Ann, Andrea Devine, and Denise McWilliams. 1987. "AIDS and Women in Prison." Lesbian prisoner supplement, *Gay Community News,* 23 August–5 September, 10–11.

Bronski, Michael. 1987. "Death and the Erotic Imagination." *Radical America* 20, nos. 2–3: 59–65.

Brooke, James. 1988a. "U.S. Culture Plays Well in Africa." *New York Times,* 4 September, A-1.

Brooke, James. 1988b. "Virus Discoveries Help an African Outpost of AIDS Research Gain Notice." *New York Times,* 28 February, A-12.

Brooke, James. 1993. "In Deception and Denial, an Epidemic Looms." *New York Times,* 25 January, 1.

Brooke-Rose, Christine. 1986. "Woman as a Semiotic Object." In *The Female Body in Western Culture: Contemporary Perspectives,* ed. Susan Rubin Suleiman. Cambridge, Mass.: Harvard University Press.

Broullon, Suzanne. 1992. "The Women's Outreach Network of NHF (WONN): A Look at Year Four." *Hemophilia Newsnotes* 11, no. 4 (June): 12–13.

Brown, Raymond Keith. 1986. *AIDS, Cancer, and the Medical Establishment.* New York: Robert Speller.

Browning, Frank. 1988. "AIDS: The Mythology of Plague." Review of *And the Band Played On*, by Randy Shilts. *Tikkun*, March–April, 69–71.

Brunvand, Jan Harold. 1992. *Curses! Broiled Again.* New York: Norton.

Buci-Glucksmann, Christine. 1987. "Catastrophic Utopia: The Feminine as Allegory of the Modern." In *The Making of the Modern Body: Sexuality and Society in the Nineteenth Century*, ed. Catherine Gallagher and Thomas Laqueur. Berkeley and Los Angeles: University of California Press.

Buckley, Stephen. 1997. "Deadly Dowry: Inheriting AIDS in Kenya." *Washington Post*, 8 November, A-1, A-18.

Buckley, William F., Jr. 1986. "Crucial Steps in Combating the AIDS Epidemic: Identify All the Carriers." Opinion, *New York Times*, 18 March, A-27.

Burkett, Elinor. 1995. *The Gravest Show on Earth: America in the Age of AIDS.* Boston: Houghton Mifflin.

Burns, John F. 1989. "Outbreak of AIDS Triples Testing in a Soviet City." *New York Times*, 5 February, 29.

Burr, Chandler. 1997. "The AIDS Exception: Privacy vs. Public Health." *Atlantic Monthly*, June, 57–67.

Burroughs, William S. 1971. *Electronic Revolution.* Cambridge: Blackmoor Head.

Butler, Judith. 1990. *Gender Trouble: Feminism and the Subversion of Identity.* New York: Routledge.

Butler, Judith. 1993. *Bodies That Matter: On the Discursive Limits of "Sex."* New York: Routledge.

Butler, Judith. 1994. "Against Proper Objects." *Differences* 6, nos. 2–3: 1–26.

Buxton, Rodney. 1991. " 'After It Happened . . .': The Battle to Present AIDS in Television Drama." *Velvet Light Trap* 27 (Spring): 37–48.

Buxton, Rodney. 1992. "Broadcast Formats, Fictional Narratives, and Controversy: Network Television's Depiction of AIDS, 1983–1991." Ph.D. diss., University of Texas, Austin.

Bygbjerg, Ib. 1983. Letter to the editor, *Lancet* 2 (23 April): 925.

Byron, Peg. 1985. "Women with AIDS: Untold Stories." *Village Voice*, 24 September, 16–19.

Byron, Peg. 1991. "HIV: The National Scandal." *Ms*, January/February, 24–29.

Cahill, Kevin M., ed. 1983. *The AIDS Epidemic.* New York: St. Martin's.

Calabrese, L. H., and K. V. Gopalakrishna. 1986. "Transmission of HTLV-III Infection from Man to Woman to Man." Letter to the editor, *New England Journal of Medicine* 314: 987.

Califia, Pat. 1988. "A Note on Lesbians, AIDS, and Safer Sex." In *Macho Sluts*. Boston: Alyson.

Califia, Pat. 1997. *Sex Changes: The Politics of Transgenderism.* San Francisco: Cleis.

Callen, Michael, ed. 1987–1988. *Surviving and Thriving with AIDS.* Vols. 1–2. New York: People with AIDS Coalition.

Callen, Michael. 1988. "Media Watch (and It's Still Ticking)." In *AIDS: Cultural Analysis/Cultural Activism*, ed. Douglas Crimp. Cambridge, Mass.: MIT Press.

Callen, Michael. 1989a. "AIDS and Passive Genocide: 30,534 Unnecessary Deaths from PCP due to a Scandalous Failure to Prophylax." *AIDS Forum* 2 (May): 13–16.

Callen, Michael. 1989b. Presentation at the conference "AIDS: The Artists' Response," 10–11 April, Hoyt L. Sherman Gallery, Ohio State University.

Callen, Michael, and Richard Berkowitz, with Joseph Sonnabend and Richard Dworkin. 1983. *How to Have Sex in an Epidemic.* New York: News from the Front.

Callero, Peter L., David V. Baker, Jeannette Carpenter, and Jane Magarigal. 1986. "Fear of AIDS and Its Effects on the Nation's Blood Supply." In *The Social Dimension of AIDS: Method and Theory,* ed. Douglas A. Feldman and Thomas M. Johnson. New York: Praeger.

Campbell, Carole A. 1990a. "Prostitution and AIDS." In *Behavioral Aspects of AIDS,* ed. David Ostrow. New York: Plenum.

Campbell, Carole A. 1990b. "Women and AIDS." *Social Science and Medicine* 30, no. 4: 407–15.

Campbell, Carole A. 1991. "Prostitution, AIDS, and Preventive Health Behavior." *Social Science and Medicine* 32, no. 12: 1367–78.

Campbell, Carole A. 1995. "Male Gender Roles and Sexuality: Implications for Women's AIDS Risk and Prevention." *Social Science and Medicine* 41, no. 2 (July): 197–210.

Camus, Albert. [1947] 1948. *The Plague.* Translated by Stuart Gilbert. New York: Modern Library.

Caplan, Pat. 1987. Introduction to *The Cultural Construction of Sexuality,* ed. Pat Caplan. New York: Tavistock.

Caputo, Robert. 1988. "Uganda: Land beyond Sorrow." *National Geographic,* April, 468–74.

Carey, James W. 1986. "Why and How? The Dark Continent of American Journalism." In *Reading the News,* ed. Robert Karl Manoff and Michael Schudson. New York: Pantheon.

Carlomusto, Jean. 1992. "Focusing on Women: Video as Activism." In *Women, AIDS, and Activism,* ed. ACT UP New York Women and AIDS Book Group. Boston: South End.

Carlomusto, Jean, and Maria Maggenti, producers. 1988. *Doctors, Liars, and Women: AIDS Activists Say No to Cosmo.* New York: Gay Men's Health Crisis. Video.

Carrier, Joseph. 1995. *De Los Otros: Intimacy and Homosexuality among Mexican Men.* New York: Columbia University Press.

Carter, Erica, and Simon Watney, eds. 1989. *Taking Liberties: AIDS and Cultural Politics.* London: Serpent's Tail.

Cartwright, Lisa. 1995. *Screening the Body: Tracing Medicine's Visual Culture.* Minneapolis: University of Minnesota Press.

Caspar, Monica J., and Lisa Jean Moore. 1995. "Inscribing Bodies, Inscribing the Future: Sex, Gender, and Reproduction on the Final Frontier." *Sociological Perspectives* 38 (Summer): 311–33.

Cassileth, Barrie R., and Helene Brown. 1988. "Unorthodox Cancer Medicine." *CA-A Cancer Journal for Clinicians* 38, no. 3: 176–86.

Cathcart, Kevin. 1987. "Soon to Be a Made-for-TV Movie: Randy Shilts, and the Band Played On." Review of *And the Band Played On,* by Randy Shilts. *Radical America* 21, nos. 2–3: 49–57.

Cayleff, Susan. 1989. "The Politics of a Disease: Contemporary Analysis of the AIDS Epidemic." *Radical History Review* 45: 172–80.

Centers for Disease Control (CDC). 1981a. "Pneumocystis Pneumonia—Los Angeles," *Morbidity and Mortality Weekly Report* 30, no. 21 (5 June): 250–52.

Centers for Disease Control (CDC). 1981b. "Kaposi's Sarcoma and *Pneumocystis* Pneumonia among Homosexual Men—New York City and California." *Morbidity and Mortality Weekly Report* 30, no. 25 (3 July): 305–8.

Centers for Disease Control (CDC). 1982a. "Update on Kaposi's Sarcoma and Opportunistic Infections in Previously Healthy Persons—United States." *Morbidity and Mortality Weekly Report* 31 (11 June): 294–301.

Centers for Disease Control (CDC). 1982b. "Opportunistic Infections and Kaposi's Sarcoma among Haitians in the United States." *Morbidity and Mortality Weekly Report* 31 (9 July): 353–61.

Centers for Disease Control (CDC). 1982c. "*Pneumocystis carinii* Pneumonia among Persons with Hemophilia A." *Morbidity and Mortality Weekly Report* 31 (16 July): 365–67.

Centers for Disease Control (CDC). 1982d. "Hepatitis B Virus Vaccine Safety: Report of an Inter-Agency Group." *Morbidity and Mortality Weekly Report* 31 (3 September): 465–67.

Centers for Disease Control (CDC). 1982e. "Update on Acquired Immune Deficiency Syndrome (AIDS) United States." *Morbidity and Mortality Weekly Report* 31 (24 September): 507–14.

Centers for Disease Control (CDC). 1982f. "Unexplained Immunodeficiency and Opportunistic Infections in Infants—New York, New Jersey, California." *Morbidity and Mortality Weekly Report* 31 (17 December): 665–67.

Centers for Disease Control (CDC). 1983a. "Immunodeficiency among Female Sexual Partners of Males with Acquired Immune Deficiency Syndrome." *Morbidity and Mortality Weekly Report* 31 (7 January): 697–98.

Centers for Disease Control (CDC). 1983b. "Prevention of Acquired Immune Deficiency Syndrome (AIDS): Report of Inter-Agency Recommendations." *Morbidity and Mortality Weekly Report* 32 (4 March): 101–4.

Centers for Disease Control (CDC). 1983c. "Acquired Immunodeficiency Syndrome (AIDS) Update—United States." *Morbidity and Mortality Weekly Report* 32 (24 June): 309–11.

Centers for Disease Control (CDC). 1984. "Update: Acquired Immunodeficiency Syndrome (AIDS)—United States." *Morbidity and Mortality Weekly Report* 33 (30 November): 661–64.

Centers for Disease Control (CDC). 1985. *Morbidity and Mortality Weekly Report* 34 (18 January): 21–31.

Centers for Disease Control (CDC). 1986a. "Acquired Immunodeficiency Syndrome—Update." *Morbidity and Mortality Weekly Report* 35 (12 December): 757–60, 765–66.

Centers for Disease Control (CDC). 1986b. "Positive HTLV-III/LAV Antibody Results for Sexually Active Female Members of Social/Sexual Clubs—Minnesota." *Morbidity and Mortality Weekly Report* 35 (14 November): 697–99.

Centers for Disease Control (CDC). 1986c. "Update: Acquired Immunodeficiency Syndrome—United States." Supplement, *Morbidity and Mortality Weekly Report* 35, no. S1 (12 December).

Centers for Disease Control (CDC). 1987a. "Antibody to Human Immunodeficiency Virus in Female Prostitutes." *Morbidity and Mortality Weekly Report* 36 (27 March): 157–61.

Centers for Disease Control (CDC). 1987b. "Human Immunodeficiency Virus Infection in the United States: A Review of Current Knowledge." *Morbidity and Mortality Weekly Report* 36 (18 December): 801–4.

Centers for Disease Control (CDC). 1987c. "Human Immunodeficiency Virus Infection in the United States: A Review of Current Knowledge." Supplement 6, *Morbidity and Mortality Weekly Report*, vol. 36 (18 December).

Centers for Disease Control (CDC). 1989. "CDC Guidelines for Prophylaxis against PCP for Persons Infected with HIV." Supplement 5, *Morbidity and Mortality Weekly Report* 38: 1–9.

Centers for Disease Control (CDC). 1996. "Update: Mortality Attributable to HIV Infection among Persons Aged 25–44 Years—United States, 1994." *Morbidity and Mortality Weekly Report* 45 (16 February): 121–125.

Cerullo, Margaret, and Evelynn Hammonds. 1988. "AIDS in Africa: The Western Imagination and the Dark Continent." *Radical America* 21, nos. 2–3: 17–23.

Charles, Ron. 1989. "HIV Link Over-Emphasized, Say Dissidents." *Montreal Daily News*, 8 June, 5.

Chase, Marilyn. 1986. "Spread of AIDS among Women Poses Widening Challenge to Medical Field." *Wall Street Journal*, 26 June, 1.

Chase, Marilyn. 1988a. "Rich Nations Urged to Help Poor Lands Fight AIDS by Backing WHO Program." *Wall Street Journal*, 17 June, 4.

Chase, Marilyn. 1988b. "U.S.-Sponsored AIDS Drug Trials to Include Private Doctors' Efforts." *Wall Street Journal*, 23 November, B-3.

Check, William A. 1985. "Public Education on AIDS: Not Only the Media's Responsibility." Special supplement, *Hastings Center Report* 15, no. 4 (August): 27–31.

Check, William A. 1990. "U.S. Media Coverage of AIDS in Africa: Presenting the Unthinkable." Paper presented at the conference "The Impact of AIDS on Maternal-Child Health Care Delivery in Africa," 4–6 May, University of Illinois at Urbana-Champaign.

Chick, Jack T. 1991. *Going Home.* Chino, Calif.: Chick Publications. 22 pages.

Chin, James. 1990. "Challenge of the Nineties." *World Health* (November/December): 4–6.

Chirimuuta, Richard C., and Rosalind J. Chirimuuta. [1987] 1989. *AIDS, Africa, and Racism.* London: Free Association.

Chirimuuta, Richard C., Rosalind Harrison, and Davis Gazi. 1987. "AIDS: The Spread of Racism." *West Africa* (9 February): 261–62.

Choi, Keewhan. 1986. "Assembling the AIDS Puzzle: Epidemiology." In *AIDS: Facts and Issues*, ed. Victor Gong and Norman Rudnick. New Brunswick, N.J.: Rutgers University Press.

Chris, Cynthia. 1989. "Policing Desire." Review of *Urinal*, by John Greyson. *Afterimage* 17, no. 5 (December): 19–20.

Chris, Cynthia. 1992. "Transmission Issues for Women." In *Women, AIDS, and Activism*, ed. ACT UP New York Women and AIDS Book Group. Boston: South End.

Christen, Pat. 1989. "The Impact of Television on the Development of AIDS Public Policy and Funding." Paper presented at the conference "AIDS: Communication Challenges," held in conjunction with the annual meeting of the International Communication Association, 27 May, San Francisco.

Christopher, Maurine. 1986. "Nets Stand Fast on Birth Control Ads." *Advertising Age*, 10 November, 36.

Christopher, Maurine. 1987. "AIDS as TV Topic Outstrips Ad Issue." *Advertising Age*, 2 February, 51.

Clark, Matt, with Mariana Gosnell and Mary Hager. 1986. "Women and AIDS." *Newsweek*, 14 July, 60–61.

Clarke, Aileen. 1994. "What Is a Chronic Disease? The Effects of a Re-Definition in HIV and AIDS." *Social Science and Medicine* 39, no. 4: 591–97.

Clifford, James. 1986. "On Ethnographic Allegory." In *Writing Culture*, ed. James Clifford and George E. Marcus. Berkeley and Los Angeles: University of California Press.

Clifford, James, and George E. Marcus, eds. 1986. *Writing Culture*. Berkeley and Los Angeles: University of California Press.

Clines, Francis X. 1987. "Via Addicts' Needles, AIDS Spreads in Edinburgh." *New York Times*, 4 January, 8.

Clumeck, Nathan. 1989. "AIDS in Africa." In *AIDS: Pathogenesis and Treatment*, ed. Jay A. Levy. New York: Marcel Dekker.

Cohen, Cathy Jean. 1993. "Power, Resistance, and the Construction of Crisis: Marginalized Communities Respond to AIDS." Ph.D. diss., University of Michigan.

Cohen, Judith B. 1987. "Three Years Experience Promoting AIDS Prevention among 800 Sexually Active High-Risk Women in San Francisco." Paper presented at the conference "Women and AIDS: Promoting Health Behaviors," an NIMH/NIDA Research Conference, 27–29 September, Bethesda, Md.

Cohen, Judith B., and Constance B. Wofsy. 1989. "Heterosexual Transmission of HIV." In *AIDS Pathogenesis and Treatment*, ed. Jay A. Levy. New York: Marcel Dekker.

Cohen, Jon. 1996. "The Changing of the Guard." *Science* 268, 28 June, 1876–80.

Colby, David C. 1989. "Mass Mediated Epidemic: AIDS and Television News, 1981–87." Paper presented at the conference "AIDS: Communication Challenges," held in conjunction with the annual meeting of the International Communication Association, 27 May, San Francisco.

Colby, David C., and Timothy Cook. 1991. "Epidemics and Agendas: The Politics of Nightly News Coverage of AIDS." *Journal of Health Politics, Policy, and Law* 16, no. 2 (Summer): 215–49.

Colby, David C., and Timothy E. Cook. 1992. "The Mass-Mediated Epidemic: The Politics of AIDS on the Nightly Network News." In *AIDS: The Making of a Chronic Disease*, ed. Elizabeth Fee and Daniel M. Fox. Berkeley and Los Angeles: University of California Press.

Cole, Helen M., and George D. Lundberg, eds. 1987. *AIDS: From the Beginning. See* American Medical Association (1987).

Collins, Monica. 1991. "PBS Flip-Flops on AIDS Shows." *TV Guide*, 31 August–6 September, 27.

Colwell, Stacie A. 1998. "*The End of the Road*: Gender, the Dissemination of Knowledge, and the American Campaign against Venereal Disease during World War I." *The Visible Woman*, ed. Paula A. Treichler, Lisa Cartwright, and Constance Penley. New York: New York University Press.

Concordia University Students' Association (CUSA). 1991. *CUSA Handbook and Agenda, 1991–1992.* Montreal: Concordia University Students' Association.

Condom Advertising and AIDS. See U.S. House (1987).

Cone, Richard A., and Emily Martin. 1998. "The Immune System, Global Economies of Food, and New Implications for Health." *The Visible Woman,* ed. Paula A. Treichler, Lisa Cartwright, and Constance Penley. New York: New York University Press.

Conefrey, Theresa C. 1997. "Discourse in Science Communities: Issues of Language, Authority, and Gender in a Life Sciences Laboratory." Ph.D. diss., University of Illinois at Urbana-Champaign.

Connelly, Mark Thomas. 1984. "Prostitution, Venereal Disease, and American Medicine." In *Women and Health in America,* ed. Judith Leavitt. Madison: University of Wisconsin Press.

Connor, Steve, and Sharon Kingman. 1989. *The Search for the Virus: The Scientific Discovery of AIDS and the Quest for a Cure.* London: Penguin.

Connors, Margaret M., and Janet W. McGrath. 1997. "The Known, Unknown and Unknowable in AIDS Research in Anthropology." *Anthropology Newsletter* 38, no. 3: 1, 4–5.

Consumer Reports. 1986. "AIDS: Deadly but Hard to Catch." *Consumer Reports,* November, 724–28.

Cook, Timothy E. 1989. "Setting the Record Straight: The Construction of Homosexuality on Television News." Paper presented to the Inside/Outside Conference of the Lesbian and Gay Studies Center, October, Yale University, New Haven, Conn.

Cookson, Shari. 1987. *Dying for Love.* Burlington, Vt.: Lifetime Cable Network. Video.

Cooper, Elizabeth, et al. 1992. Letter to the editor, *New England Journal of Medicine* 327 (9 August): 645–46.

Copson, Raymond W. 1987. *AIDS in Africa: Background/Issues for U.S. Policy.* Washington, D.C.: Congressional Research Service, Library of Congress.

Corbin, Alain. 1987. "Commercial Sexuality in Nineteenth-Century France: A System of Images and Regulations." In *The Making of the Modern Body,* ed. Catherine Gallagher and Thomas Laqueur. Berkeley and Los Angeles: University of California Press.

Corea, Gena. 1992. *The Invisible Epidemic: The Story of Women and AIDS.* New York: Harper Collins.

Coucher, Mimi. 1989. "A Girl's Guide to Condoms." *Whole Earth Review,* Spring, 137.

Coughlin, Ellen K. 1992. "Tempers Flare over AIDS Session at Anthropologists' Annual Meeting." *Chronicle of Higher Education,* 16 December: A8.

Council of Europe. Committee of Ministers. 1987. *Concerning a Common European Public Health Policy to Fight the Acquired Immunodeficiency Syndrome (AIDS).* Recommendation R (87) 25. 81st session, 26 November. London.

Cowley, Geoffrey, with Mary Hager. 1991. "Sleeping with the Enemy." *Newsweek,* 9 December, 58–59.

Cowley, Geoffrey, and Mary Hager. 1996. "New AIDS Optimism." *Newsweek,* 22 July, 68.

COYOTE. 1985. Background paper for *1985 COYOTE Convention Summary.* San Francisco, 30 May–2 June.

Crawford, Cookie. 1997. "Building a Better Blow Job." *Sexvibe,* April, 43–46.

Crewdson, John. 1989. "The Great AIDS Quest." *Chicago Tribune,* 19 November, sec. 5, pp. 1–5.

Crimp, Douglas. 1988a. "AIDS: Cultural Analysis/Cultural Activism." In *AIDS: Cul-*

tural Analysis/Cultural Activism, ed. Douglas Crimp. Cambridge, Mass.: MIT Press.

Crimp, Douglas, ed. 1988b. *AIDS: Cultural Analysis/Cultural Activism*. Cambridge, Mass.: MIT Press.

Crimp, Douglas. 1988c. "How to Have Promiscuity in an Epidemic." In *AIDS: Cultural Analysis/Cultural Activism*, ed. Douglas Crimp. Cambridge, Mass.: MIT Press.

Crimp, Douglas. 1989. "Mourning and Militancy." *October* 51 (Winter): 3–18.

Crimp, Douglas. 1992. "Portraits of People with AIDS." In *Cultural Studies*, ed. Lawrence Grossberg, Cary Nelson, and Paula Treichler. New York: Routledge, 1991.

Crimp, Douglas. 1997. "Randy Shilts's Miserable Failure." In *A Queer World: The Center for Lesbian and Gay Studies Reader*, ed. Martin Duberman. New York: New York University Press.

Crimp, Douglas, with Adam Rolston. 1990. *AIDS Demo Graphics*. Seattle: Bay.

Culler, Jonathan. 1982. *On Deconstruction: Theory and Criticism after Structuralism*. Ithaca, N.Y.: Cornell University Press.

Curran, James. 1986. "AIDS Transmission from Infected Mothers." *New York Times*, 13 June, A-1.

Curran, James W. 1988. Interview in *American Medical News*, 15 January, 1, 33–35.

Curran, James, et al. 1985. "The Epidemiology of AIDS: Current Status and Future Prospects." *Science* 229 (September): 1352.

Cussins, Charis. 1997. "Producing Reproduction: Techniques of Normalization and Naturalization in Infertility Clinics." In *Reproducing Reproduction*, ed. Sarah Franklin and H. Ragone. Philadelphia: University of Pennsylvania Press.

Dalton, Harlan L. 1989. "AIDS in Blackface." *Daedalus* (Summer).

Dangerous Bedfellows, eds. 1996. *Policing Public Sex*. Boston: South End.

Daniel, Herbert. 1989. *Life before Death/Vida antes da morte*. Rio de Janeiro: Jaboti.

Daniels, Judith. 1985. "Among Stories of Proms and Birthdays, an Alarming Report." Editor's note, *Life*, July, 6.

Danzig, Alexis. 1992. "Bisexual Women and AIDS." In *Women, AIDS, and Activism*, ed. ACT UP New York Women and AIDS Book Group. Boston: South End.

Danziger, Renee. 1994. "The Social Impact of HIV/AIDS in Developing Countries." *Social Science and Medicine* 39, no. 7: 905–17.

Darril, Rayna E. 1987. *AIDS: The Great Awakening*. Montrose, Colo.: Great Awakening.

Darrow, William W., E. Michael Gorman, and Brad P. Glick. 1986. "The Social Origins of AIDS: Social Change, Sexual Behavior, and Disease Trends." In *The Social Dimension of AIDS: Method and Theory*, ed. Douglas A. Feldman and Thomas M. Johnson. New York: Praeger.

Dawson, Marc H. 1988. "AIDS in Africa: Historical Roots." In *AIDS in Africa: The Social and Policy Impact*, ed. Norman Miller and Richard C. Rockwell. Lewiston, N.Y.: Edwin Mellen.

D'Costa, L. J., F. A. Plummer, I. Bowmer, et al. 1985. "Prostitutes Are a Major Reservoir of Sexually Transmitted Disease in Nairobi." *Sexually Transmitted Disease* 12: 64–67.

Dean, Tim. 1993. "The Psychoanalysis of AIDS." *October* 63 (Winter): 83–116.

Dearing, James W. 1992. "Foreign Blood and Domestic Politics: The Issue of AIDS in Japan." In *AIDS: The Making of a Chronic Disease*, ed. Elizabeth Fee and Daniel M. Fox. Berkeley and Los Angeles: University of California Press.

Dearing, James W., and Everett M. Rogers. 1988. "The Agenda-Setting Process for the Issue of AIDS." Paper presented at the conference of the International Communication Association, 28 May–2 June, New Orleans.

de Beauvoir, Simone. 1953. *The Second Sex.* Translated and edited by H. M. Parshley. New York: Knopf.

Deciding to Enter an AIDS/HIV Drug Trial. 1989. New York: AIDS Treatment Registry.

Defoe, Daniel. [1722] 1960. *A Journal of the Plague Year.* New York: New American Library.

De Kruif, Paul. [1926] 1954. *Microbe Hunters.* Reprint, San Diego: Harcourt Brace Jovanovich.

Delacoste, Fredrique, and Priscilla Alexander, eds. 1987. *Sex Work: Writings by Women in the Sex Industry.* Pittsburgh: Cleis.

De Lauretis, Teresa. 1984. *Alice Doesn't: Feminism, Semiotics, Cinema.* Bloomington: Indiana University Press.

De Lauretis, Teresa, ed. 1991. "Queer Theory: Lesbian and Gay Sexualities." Special issue, *Differences,* vol. 3, no. 2.

D'Emilio, John. 1992. *Making Trouble: Essays on Gay History, Politics, and the University.* New York: Routledge.

Deming, Robert. 1988. "*Kate and Allie:* 'New Women' and the Audience's Television Activity." *Camera Obscura* 16 (January): 155–66.

Demme, Jonathan, director. 1993. *Philadelphia.* Hollywood, Calif.: Tri-Star. Film.

Denenberg, Risa. 1992. "Unique Aspects of HIV Infection in Women." In *Women, AIDS, and Activism,* ed. ACT UP New York Women and AIDS Book Group. Boston: South End.

Des Jarlais, Don C., Samuel R. Friedman, and Jo L. Sotheran. 1992. "The First City: HIV among Intravenous Drug Users in New York City." In *AIDS: The Making of a Chronic Disease,* ed. Elizabeth Fee and Daniel M. Fox. Berkeley and Los Angeles: University of California Press.

Des Jarlais, Don C., Samuel R. Friedman, and David Strug. 1986. "AIDS and Needle Sharing within IV-Drug Use Subculture." In *The Social Dimension of AIDS: Method and Theory,* ed. Douglas A. Feldman and Thomas M. Johnson. New York: Praeger.

Detloff, Madelyn. 1997. "Mean Spirits: The Politics of Contempt between Feminist Generations." *Hypatia* 12, no. 3: 76–99.

De Wolk, Roland. 1990. "Party Opens with a Bleak Prognosis." *Oakland Tribune,* 21 June, A-1.

Dickersin, Kay, and Lauren Schnaper. 1996. "Reinventing Medical Research." In *Man-Made Medicine,* ed. K. L. Moss. Durham, N.C.: Duke University Press.

Dickoff, Micki. 1991. "*Our Sons* Put a Human Face on AIDS Crisis." *Los Angeles Times,* 10 June, F-3.

DiClemente, Ralph J., Jim Zorn, and Lydia Temoshok. 1986. "Adolescents and AIDS: A Survey of Knowledge, Attitudes and Beliefs about AIDS in San Francisco." *American Journal of Public Health* 76, no. 12: 1443–45.

Dieckmann, Katherine. 1987. "Lizzie Borden: Adventures in the Skin Trade." *Village Voice,* 10 March, 33.

Dixon, John. 1990. *Catastrophic Rights: Experimental Drugs and AIDS.* Vancouver: New Star.

Doane, Mary Ann. 1986. "The Clinical Eye: Medical Discourses in the 'Woman's Film' of the 1940s." In *The Female Body in Western Culture: Contemporary Perspectives*, ed. Susan Rubin Suleiman. Cambridge, Mass.: Harvard University Press.

Dobrow, Julie. 1986. "The Symbolism of AIDS: Perspectives on the Use of Language in the Popular Press." Paper presented at the annual meeting of the International Communication Association, May, Chicago.

"Don't Blame Drug Program for AIDS Deaths." 1990. Letter, *New York Times*, 28 March, 18.

Dougherty, Margot. 1988. "AIDS and the Single Woman." *People Weekly*, 14 March, 102–5.

Douglas, Colin. [1975] 1982. *The Intern's Tale*. Reprint, New York: Grove.

Douglas, Paul Harding, ed. 1989. *AIDS: Improving the Odds, 1988*. New York: Columbia Gay Health Advocacy Project.

Douglas, Paul, and Laura Pinsky. 1989. "AIDS and Needless Deaths: How Early Treatment Is Ignored." Paper presented at the seminar "Sex, Gender, and Consumer Culture," 14 April, New York Institute for the Humanities, New York.

Douglas, Paul Harding, and Laura Pinsky. 1996. *The Essential AIDS Fact Book*. New York: Pocket Books.

Douglass, William C. [1987] 1996. "WHO Murdered Africa." In *AIDS Exposed*, ed. Jeffrey Rense. Goleta, Calif.: BioAlert.

Douglass, William C. 1989. *SIDS: The End of Civilization*. Clayton: Valet.

Druck, Michael J. 1992. "Bad Blood." *Village Voice*, 5 December, 10.

Duberman, Martin, ed. 1997. *A Queer World: The Center for Gay and Lesbian Studies Reader*. New York: New York University Press.

Dubos, René [1959] 1987. *Mirage of Health: Utopias, Progress, and Biological Change*. Reprint, New Brunswick, N.J.: Rutgers University Press.

Du Brow, Rick. 1991. "Is TV Too Dirty?" *Montreal Gazette*, 10 November, F-2.

Duesberg, Peter H. 1987. "Retroviruses as Carcinogens and Pathogens: Expectations and Reality." *Cancer Research* 47 (1 March): 1199–1220.

Duggan, Lisa. 1991. "Queer Theory: Deconstructing Identities, Reconstructing Politics." Paper presented to the Colloquium of the Unit for Criticism and Interpretive Theory, University of Illinois at Urbana-Champaign, 29 April.

Duggan, Lisa, and Nan D. Hunter. 1995. *Sex Wars: Sexual Dissent and Political Culture*. New York: Routledge.

Dunlap, David W. 1996. "From AIDS Conference, Talk of Life, Not Death." *New York Times*, 15 July, A-7.

Dunn, Kate. 1989. "Look beyond HIV as the Cause of AIDS, New York Doctor Says." *Montreal Gazette*, 8 June, 10.

Dunning, Jennifer. 1986. "Women and AIDS." *New York Times*, 3 November, 22.

Dunning, Jennifer. 1987. "Suit Filed over Benefit for AIDS." *New York Times*, 27 August, 20.

Durham, Stephen, and Susan Williams. 1986. "AIDS Hysteria: A Marxist Analysis." Seattle: Freedom Socialist Publications. Originally presented at the conference of the Pacific Northwest Marxist Scholars, 11–13 April 1986, University of Washington, Seattle.

Düttman, Alexander García. 1996. *At Odds with AIDS: Thinking and Talking about a Virus*. Translated by Peter Gilgen and Conrad Scott-Curtis. Stanford, Calif.: Stanford University Press.

An Early Frost. 1985. "Monday Night at the Movies." New York: NBC, 11 November.

Echols, Alice. 1985. "The Taming of the Id: Feminist Sexual Politics, 1968–93." In *Pleasure and Danger*, ed. Carol Vance. Boston: Routledge.

Eckholm, Erik. 1985. "Prostitutes' Impact on Spread of AIDS Debated." *New York Times*, 5 November, 15, 18.

Eckholm, Erik. 1986a. "Broad Alert on AIDS: Social Battle Is Shifting." *New York Times*, 17 June, 19–20.

Eckholm, Erik. 1986b. "US Officials Stress AIDS Is Not Spread by Casual Contact." *New York Times*, 27 June, A-17.

Eckholm, Erik. 1987. "AIDS, an Unknown Disease before 1981, Grows into a Worldwide Scourge." *New York Times*, 16 March, 11.

Eckholm, Erik. 1990a. "What Makes the Two Sexes So Vulnerable to the Epidemic." *New York Times*, 16 September, A-11.

Eckholm, Erik. 1990b. "Confronting the Cruel Reality of Africa's AIDS Epidemic." *New York Times*, 19 September, A-1.

Eckholm, Erik, with John Tierney. 1990. "AIDS in Africa: A Killer Rages On." *New York Times*, 16 September, A-1.

Eckman, Anne K. 1996. "From JANE to the Journal of Women's Health: Women's Health as an Emergent Body of Medical Knowledge." Ph.D. diss., University of Illinois at Urbana-Champaign.

Eckman, Anne K. 1998. "Beyond the 'Yentl Syndrome.'" In *The Visible Woman*, ed. Paula A. Treichler, Lisa Cartwright, and Constance Penley. New York: New York University Press, 1998.

Edelman, Lee. 1994. *Homographesis: Essays in Gay Literary and Cultural Theory.* New York: Routledge.

Edgar, Harold, and David J. Rothman. 1990. "New Rules for New Drugs: The Challenge of AIDS to the Regulatory Process." *Milbank Quarterly* 68, suppl. 1: 111–42.

Edgar, Joanne. 1987. "Iceland's Feminists: Power at the Top of the World." *Ms.*, December, 30.

Ehrenreich, Barbara, and Deirdre English. 1973. *Complaints and Disorders: The Sexual Politics of Sickness.* Old Westbury, N.Y.: Feminist.

Eisenberg, David M., et al. 1993. "Unconventional Medicine in the United States: Prevalence, Costs and Patterns of Use." *New England Journal of Medicine* 328 (28 January): 246–83. For responses, see *New England Journal of Medicine*, vol. 329, no. 16.

Eisenstein, Zillah. 1989. *The Female Body and the Law.* Berkeley and Los Angeles: University of California Press.

Elkin, Sandra. 1989. *AIDS Is about Secrets.* New York: HIV Center for Clinical and Behavioral Studies. Videocassette.

Ell, Stephen R. 1986. "The Venetian Plague of 1630–1631: Assessment of a Human Disaster." *Medical Heritage* 2 (March–April): 151–56.

Ellerbrock, T. V., et al. 1991. "Epidemiology of Women with AIDS in the United States, 1981 through 1990: A Comparison with Heterosexual Men with AIDS." *Journal of the American Medical Association* 265: 2971–75.

Ellerbrock, T. V., et al. 1992. "Heterosexually Transmitted Human Immunodeficiency Virus Infection among Pregnant Women in a Rural Florida Community." *New England Journal of Medicine* 327: 1704–9.

Elliot, Beth. 1991. "Does Lesbian Sex Transmit AIDS? GET REAL!" *Off Our Backs*, November, 6.

Elm, Joanna. 1989. "NBC Tones Down *Roe vs. Wade* TV-Movie to Avoid Angering Abortion Pressure Groups." *TV Guide*, 13–20 May, 49–50.

Emerging AIDS Markets: A Worldwide Study of Drugs, Vaccines, and Diagnostics. 1986. New Haven, Conn.: Technology Management Group.

Empson, William. 1967. *The Structure of Complex Words.* Ann Arbor: University of Michigan Press.

"Epidemiologists Were Incensed That the Woman's Doctors Failed to Diagnose AIDS before She Died." 1988. *Edmonton Journal*, 11 October, A-2.

Epstein, Paul, and Randall Packard. 1987. "Ecology and Immunology." *Science for the People* (January–February): 10–17.

Epstein, Robert. 1984. *The Times of Harvey Milk.* San Francisco: Black Sand Productions, 1984.

Epstein, Steven. 1996. *Impure Science: AIDS, Activism, and the Politics of Knowledge.* Berkeley and Los Angeles: University of California Press.

Erni, John Nguyet. 1994. *Unstable Frontiers: Technomedicine and the Cultural Politics of "Curing" AIDS.* Minneapolis: University of Minnesota Press.

Erni, John Nguyet. 1998. "Redressing *Sanuk*: 'Asian AIDS' and the Practices of Women's Resistance." In *Women and AIDS: Negotiating Safer Practices, Care, and Representation*, ed. Nancy L. Roth and Linda K. Fuller. New York: Haworth.

Essoglou, Tracy Ann. 1995. "Louder than Words: A WAC Chronicle." *But Is It Art? The Spirit of Art as Activism*, ed. Nina Felshin. Seattle: Bay Press.

Evans, Alfred S. 1989. "Does HIV Cause AIDS? An Historical Perspective." *Journal of Acquired Immune Deficiency Syndrome* 2 (April): 107–13.

"Exchange." 1997. *Nation*, 29 September, 2, 31–32. Letters responding to Warner (1997).

Fabian's Story. See "AIDS: A National Inquiry."

Fain, Nathan. 1985. "AIDS: An Antidote to Fear." *Village Voice*, 1 October, 35.

Faludi, Susan. 1991. *Backlash: The Undeclared War against American Women.* New York: Crown.

Farber, Celia. 1989. "Sins of Omission: The AZT Scandal." *Spin*, November, 40.

Farber, Stephen. 1991. "A Decade into the AIDS Epidemic, the TV Networks Are Still Nervous." *New York Times*, 30 April, C-13.

Farmer, Paul. 1990. "Sending Sickness: Sorcery, Politics, and Changing Concepts of AIDS in Rural Haiti." *Medical Anthropology Quarterly* 4, no. 1: 6–27.

Farmer, Paul. 1992. *AIDS and Accusation: Haiti and the Geography of Blame.* Berkeley and Los Angeles: University of California Press.

Farmer, Paul, Margaret Connors, and Janie Simmons, eds. 1996. *Women, Poverty, and AIDS: Sex, Drugs, and Structural Violence.* Monroe, Maine: Common Courage.

Farmer, Paul, and Arthur Kleinman. 1989. "AIDS as Human Suffering." *Daedalus* 118, no. 2: 135–60.

Fauci, Anthony S. 1983. "The Acquired Immune Deficiency Syndrome: The Ever-Broadening Clinical Spectrum." Editorial, *Journal of the American Medical Association* 249: 2375–76.

Fausto-Sterling, Anne. 1993. "The Five Sexes." *Sciences* (March/April): 20–25.

Fee, Elizabeth. 1982. "Women and Health Care: A Comparison of Theories." In *Women and Health: The Politics of Sex in Medicine,* ed. Elizabeth Fee. Farmingdale, N.Y.: Baywood.

Fee, Elizabeth. 1988. "Sex Education in Cuba: An Interview with Dr. Celestino Alvarez Lajonchere." *International Journal of Health Services* 18, no. 2: 343–56.

Fee, Elizabeth, and Daniel M. Fox, eds. 1988. *AIDS: The Burdens of History.* Berkeley and Los Angeles: University of California Press.

Fee, Elizabeth, and Daniel M. Fox, eds. 1992a. *AIDS: The Making of a Chronic Disease.* Berkeley and Los Angeles: University of California Press.

Fee, Elizabeth, and Daniel M. Fox, eds. 1992b. "Introduction: The Contemporary Historiography of AIDS." In *AIDS: The Making of a Chronic Disease,* ed. Elizabeth Fee and Daniel M. Fox. Berkeley and Los Angeles: University of California Press.

Feinberg, David. 1989. *Eighty-Sixed.* New York: Penguin.

Feldman, Douglas A. 1986. "AIDS Health Promotion and Clinically Applied Anthropology." In *The Social Dimension of AIDS: Method and Theory,* ed. Douglas A. Feldman and Thomas M. Johnson. New York: Praeger.

Feldman, Douglas A. 1987. "Role of African Mutilations in AIDS Discounted." Letter to the editor, *New York Times,* 7 January, 18.

Feldman, Douglas A. 1991. *Culture and AIDS.* New York: Praeger.

Feldman, Douglas A., and Thomas M. Johnson, eds. 1986. *The Social Dimension of AIDS: Method and Theory.* New York: Praeger.

Feldman, Jamie. 1988. "Social Dialogue, Public Dilemma: French Research Perspectives on AIDS." Paper presented at the seminar "Medical Humanities and Social Sciences," January, University of Illinois at Urbana-Champaign College of Medicine, Urbana.

Feldman, Jamie. 1992. "Gallo, Montagnier, and the Debate over HIV." *Camera Obscura* 28: 101–132.

Feldman, Jamie. 1993. "French and American Medical Perspectives on AIDS: Discourse and Practice." Ph.D. diss., University of Illinois at Urbana-Champaign.

Feldman, Jamie L. 1995. *Plague Doctors: Responding to the AIDS Epidemic in France and America.* Westport, Conn.: Bergin and Garvey.

Feorino, P. M., et al. [1983] 1986. "Lymphadenopathy Associated Virus Infection of a Blood Donor–Recipient Pair with Acquired Immunodeficiency Syndrome." In *AIDS: Papers from Science, 1982–1985,* ed. Ruth Kulstad. Washington, D.C.: American Association for the Advancement of Science.

Fettner, Ann Giudici. 1987. "The AIDS Drug Hustle." *Village Voice,* 2 June, 17–18, 103.

Fettner, Ann Giudici. 1988. "Bad Science Makes Strange Bedfellows." *Village Voice,* 2 February, 25–28.

Fettner, Ann Giudici, and William Check. 1985. *The Truth about AIDS: Evolution of an Epidemic.* New York: Holt, Rinehart and Winston.

Feuer, Jane. 1984. "The MTM Style." In *MTM: "Quality Television,"* ed. Jane Feuer et al. London: BFI.

Fine, Gary Alan. 1987. "Welcome to the World of AIDS: Fantasies of Female Revenge." *Western Folklore* 46: 192–97.

Fischl, Margaret A., et al. 1987a. "The Efficacy of Azidothymidine (AZT) in the Treatment of Patients with AIDS and AIDS-Related Complex." *New England Journal of Medicine* 317, no. 4: 185–97.

Fischl, Margaret A., et al. 1987b. "Evaluation of Heterosexual Partners, Children, and

Household Contact of Adults with AIDS." *Journal of the American Medical Association* 257, no. 5: 640–44.

FitzGerald, Frances. 1986. *Cities on a Hill: A Journey through Contemporary American Cultures.* New York: Simon and Schuster/Touchstone.

Flam, Robin, and Zena Stein. 1986. "Behavior, Infection, and Immune Response: An Epidemiological Approach." In *The Social Dimension of AIDS: Method and Theory,* ed. Douglas A. Feldman and Thomas M. Johnson. New York: Praeger.

Flanders, Laura. 1996. "How Alternative Is It? Feminist Media Activists Take Aim at the Progressive Press." *Extra!* May/June: 14–17.

Fleck, Ludvik. [1935] 1979. *Genesis and Development of a Scientific Fact.* Translated by Fred Bradley and Thaddeus J. Trenn. Edited by Thaddeus J. Trenn and Robert K. Merton. Reprint, Chicago: University of Chicago Press.

Flitterman-Lewis, Sandy. 1988. "All's Well That Doesn't End—Soap Opera and the Marriage Motif." *Camera Obscura* 16 (January): 119–53.

Flood, Ann Barry. 1992. "Empowering Patients: Using Interactive Video Programs to Help Patients Make Difficult Decisions." *Camera Obscura* 29: 225–231.

Flora, June A., et al. 1995. "Communication Campaigns for HIV Prevention: Using Mass Media in the Next Decade." In *Assessing the Social and Behavioral Base for HIV/ AIDS Prevention and Intervention. Workshop Background Papers.* Washington, D.C.: Institute of Medicine.

Foltz, Kim. 1985. "TV, Sex and Prevention." *Newsweek,* 9 September, 72.

Fortin, Alfred J. 1987. "The Politics of AIDS in Kenya." *Third World Quarterly* 9, no. 3 (July): 906–19.

Fortin, Alfred J. 1988. "AIDS and the Third World: The Politics of International Discourse." Paper presented at the Fourteenth World Congress of the International Political Science Association, 28 August–September 1, Washington, D.C.

Foucault, Michel. 1972. *The Archaeology of Knowledge.* Translated by A. M. Sheridan Smith. New York: Pantheon.

Foucault, Michel. 1977. "The Political Function of the Intellectual." *Radical Philosophy* 17: 13–14.

Foucault, Michel. 1979. *The History of Sexuality.* Vol. 1, *An Introduction.* Translated by Robert Hurley. Harmondsworth: Allen Lane/Penguin.

Foucault, Michel. 1985. "Don't Cry for Me, Academia." Interview with Michel Foucault; see Horvitz (1985).

Fox, Daniel M. 1986. "AIDS and American Health Policy: The History and Prospects of a Crisis in Authority." Supplement, *Milbank Quarterly* 64: 7–33.

Francis, Donald P. 1983. "The Search for the Cause." In *The AIDS Epidemic,* ed. Kevin M. Cahill. New York: St. Martin's.

Frank, Francine Wattman, and Paula A. Treichler. 1997. *Language, Gender, and Professional Writing: Theoretical Approaches and Guidelines for Nonsexist Usage.* New York: Modern Language Association.

Franklin, Patricia, et al. 1987. "The AIDS Business." *Business,* April, 42–47.

Frederickson, Donald S. 1983. "Where Do We Go from Here?" In *The AIDS Epidemic,* ed. Kevin M. Cahill. New York: St. Martin's.

Freedman, Benjamin, and McGill Boston Research Group. 1989. "Nonvalidated Therapies and HIV Disease." *Hastings Center Report* 19, no. 3 (May/June): 14–20.

Friedland, Gerald H. 1990. "Early Treatment for HIV: The Time Has Come." *New England Journal of Medicine* 322 (5 April): 1000–1002.

Friedman, Samuel R., Meryl Sufian, Richard Curtis, Alan Neigus, and Don C. Des Jarlais. 1992. "Organizing Drug Users against AIDS." In *The Social Context of AIDS*, ed. Joan Huber and Beth E. Schneider. Newbury Park, Calif.: Sage.

Friedman, Sharon M., Sharon Dunwoody, and Carol L. Rogers. 1986. *Scientists and Journalists: Reporting Science as News*. Washington, D.C.: American Association for the Advancement of Science.

Fujimura, Joan, and Danny Chou. 1994. "Dissent in Science: Styles of Scientific Practice and the Controversy over the Cause of AIDS." *Social Science and Medicine* 38, no. 8: 1017–36.

Fumento, Michael. 1989. *The Myth of Heterosexual AIDS*. New York: Basic.

Fyfe, Gordon, and John Law, eds. 1988. *Picturing Power: Visual Depiction and Social Relations*. New York: Routledge.

Gadsby, Patricia. 1988. "Mapping the Epidemic: Geography as Destiny." *Discover*, April, 28–31.

Gaiman, Neil. 1992. *Death Talks about Life*. Booklet tipped into late run of *Sandman* 46 (February 1993). Illustrator, Dave McKean.

Gaines, Atwood D. 1987. "Cultural Constructivism and Biomedicine: Understanding Ethnomedical Knowledge and Practice." Manuscript in author's collection.

Gaines, Atwood D., and Robert Hahn, eds. 1985. *Physicians of Western Medicine: Anthropological Approaches to Theory and Practice*. Dordrecht: D. Reidel.

Gallagher, Catherine, and Thomas Laqueur, eds. 1987. *The Making of the Modern Body: Sexuality and Society in the Nineteenth Century*. Berkeley and Los Angeles: University of California Press.

Gallo, Robert C. 1987. "The AIDS Virus." *Scientific American*, January, 47–56.

Gallo, Robert C. 1988. "HIV—the Cause of AIDS: An Overview of Its Biology, Mechanisms of Disease Induction, Introduction, and Our Attempts to Control It." *Journal of Acquired Immune Deficiency Syndromes* 1 (December): 521–35.

Gallo, Robert C. 1991. *Virus Hunting: AIDS, Cancer, and the Human Retrovirus*. New York: Basic.

Gallo, Robert C., and Luc Montagnier. 1987. "The Chronology of AIDS Research." *Nature* 362: 435–36.

Gallo, Robert C., and Luc Montagnier. 1988. "AIDS in 1988." *Scientific American* 259, no. 4 (October): 40–48.

Gallo, Robert C., et al. 1983. "Isolation of Human T-Cell Leukemia Virus in Acquired Immune Deficiency Syndrome (AIDS)." *Science* 220: 865–68.

Gallo, Robert C., et al. 1986. "HTLV-III Legend Correction." Letter to the editor, *Science*, 18 April, 307.

Gamson, Joshua. 1989. "Silence, Death, and the Invisible Enemy: AIDS Activism and Social Movement 'Newness.'" *Social Problems* 36 (October): 351–67.

Gamson, Joshua. 1995. "Must Identity Movements Self-Destruct? A Queer Dilemma." *Social Problems* 42 (August): 390–407.

Gamson, Joshua. 1996. "The Organizational Shaping of Collective Identity: The Case of Lesbian and Gay Film Festivals in New York." In *A Queer World: The Center for Lesbian and Gay Studies Reader*, ed. Martin Duberman. New York: New York University Press.

Gander, Cat. 1993. *Double Lives: The Ordinary, Extraordinary Lives of Sex Workers*. Fyshwick, A.C.T.: Workers in Sex Employment.

Garrett, Laurie. 1992. *The Coming Plague*. New York: St. Martin's.

Gathorne-Hardy, Jonathan. 1986. Letter to the editor, *New York Times Book Review,* 29 June, 35.

Geertz, Clifford. 1973. The Interpretation of Cultures. New York: Basic.

Geison, Gerald L. 1995. *The Private Science of Louis Pasteur.* Princeton, N.J.: Princeton University Press.

Geitner, Paul. 1988. "Desperation Draws Victims to Try Unapproved Drugs." *Champaign-Urbana News-Gazette,* 19 June, B-4.

Gendel, Morgan. 1985. "AIDS and *An Early Frost*: The Whisper Becomes a Shout." *Los Angeles Times,* 13 November, sec. 6, p. 1.

Gerard, Jeremy. 1988. "Protestors Disrupt Work on AIDS Episode of a New NBC Series." *New York Times,* 28 October, 9.

Gerbert, Barbara, and Bryan Maguire. 1989. "Public Acceptance of the Surgeon General's Brochure on AIDS." *Public Health Reports* 104, no. 2 (March/April): 130–33.

Gever, Martha. 1988. "Pictures of Sickness: Stuart Marshall's *Bright Eyes.*" In *AIDS: Cultural Analysis/Cultural Activism,* ed. Douglas Crimp. Cambridge, Mass.: MIT Press.

Gieringer, Dale. 1987. "Twice Wrong on AIDS." *New York Times,* 12 January, A-21.

Giese, Jo. 1987. "Of Rubbers and Lovers." *Ms,* September, 100–102.

Gilbert, David. 1996. "AIDS Conspiracy? Tracking the *Real* Genocide." *Covert Action Quarterly* 58 (Fall): 55–64.

Gillespie, Iain, producer/director. 1987. *Suzi's Story.* Sydney: Network Ten and Pro-Image Group.

Gillespie, Marcia Ann. 1991. "Women and AIDS." *Ms,* January/February, 16–22.

Gilman, Sander L. 1985. *Difference and Pathology: Stereotypes of Sexuality, Race, and Madness.* Ithaca, N.Y.: Cornell University Press.

Gilman, Sander L. 1988a. "AIDS and Syphilis: The Iconography of Disease." In *AIDS: Cultural Analysis/Cultural Activism,* ed. Douglas Crimp. Cambridge, Mass.: MIT Press.

Gilman, Sander L. 1988b. *Disease and Representation: Images of Illness from Madness to AIDS.* Ithaca, N.Y.: Cornell University Press.

Gilman, Sander L. 1995. *Picturing Health and Illness: Images of Identity and Difference.* Baltimore: Johns Hopkins University Press.

Gilmore, Norbert. 1992. "An AIDS Chronicle." In *A Leap in the Dark: AIDS, Art and Contemporary Cultures,* ed. Allan Klusaček and Ken Morrison. Montreal: Véhicule Press/Artexte.

Gilmore, Norbert, and Margaret A. Somerville. 1994. "Stigmatization, Scapegoating and Discrimination in Sexually Transmitted Diseases: Overcoming 'Them' and 'Us,'" *Social Science and Medicine* 39, no. 9: 1339–58.

Gitlin, Todd. 1977. "Spotlights and Shadows—TV News." *Cultural Correspondence* 4 (Spring): 3–12.

Gitlin, Todd. 1980. *The Whole World Is Watching: Mass Media in the Making and Unmaking of the New Left.* Berkeley and Los Angeles: University of California Press.

Gitlin, Todd, ed. 1986. *Watching Television.* New York: Pantheon.

Glaser, Vicki. 1988. "AIDS Crisis Spurs Hunt for New Tests." *High Technology Business,* January, 34–39.

Goldberg, Marshall. 1987. "TV Has Done More to Contain AIDS than Any Other Single Factor." *TV Guide,* 28 November, 4–7.

Golden, L. L., and W. T. Anderson. 1992. "AIDS Prevention: Myths, Misinformation, and Health Policy Perceptions." *Journal of Health and Social Policy* 3, no. 3: 37–50.

Goldenberg, Edie N., and Holli A. Semetko. 1989. "Reporters Reporting AIDS: What They Know and What They Think the Public Knows." Paper presented at the conference "AIDS: Communication Challenges," held in conjunction with the annual meeting of the International Communication Association, 27 May, San Francisco.

Goldman, Peter, and Lucille Beachy. 1986. "The AIDS Doctor." *Newsweek*, 21 July, 40–52.

Goldsmith, Barbara. 1993. "Women on the Edge." *New Yorker*, 26 April, 64.

Goldsmith, Marsha F. 1985. "More Heterosexual Spread of HTLV-III Virus Seen." *Journal of the American Medical Association* 253: 3377–79.

Goldsmith, Marsha F. 1988. "Sex Experts and Medical Scientists Join Forces against a Common Foe: AIDS." *Journal of the American Medical Association* 259: 641–43.

Goldsmith, Marsha F. 1989. "Pregnancy Dx? Rx May Now Include Condoms." *Journal of the American Medical Association* 261, no. 5 (February 3): 678–79.

Goldstein, Donna M. 1994. "AIDS and Women in Brazil: The Emerging Problem." *Social Science and Medicine* 39, no. 7: 919–29.

Goldstein, Richard. 1983. "Heartsick: Fear and Loving in the Gay Community." *Village Voice*, 28 June, 13–16.

Goldstein, Richard. 1986. "The New Sobriety." *Village Voice*, 30 December, 23–28.

Goldstein, Richard. 1987a. "AIDS and Race." *Village Voice*, 10 March: 23–30.

Goldstein, Richard. 1987b. "Four Days in the Life." *Village Voice*, 16 June: 21–24.

Goldstein, Richard. 1987c. "Visitation Rites: The Elusive Tradition of Plague Literature." *Voice Literary Supplement* 59 (October): 6–9.

Goldstein, Richard. 1989. "AIDS Arrest: The Cuban Solution." *Village Voice*, 14 February, 18.

Goldstein, Richard, and Robert Massa. 1989. "Compound Q: Hope and Hype; the Making of a New AIDS Drug." *Village Voice*, 30 May, 29–34.

Gong, Victor, and Norman Rudnick, eds. 1986. *AIDS: Facts and Issues.* New Brunswick, N.J.: Rutgers University Press.

Goodfield, June. 1985. *Quest for the Killers.* New York: Hill and Wang.

Goodman, Walter. 1991. "The Story TV Can't Resist." *New York Times*, 17 November, 31.

Gordon, Gill, and Tony Klouda. 1988. *Preventing a Crisis.* London: International Planned Parenthood Federation.

Gordon, Linda. 1976. *Woman's Body, Woman's Right: A Social History of Birth Control in America.* New York: Grossman.

Gorna, Robin. 1996. *Vamps, Virgins and Victims: How Can Women Fight AIDS?* London: Cassell.

Gorna, Robin. 1997. "Feminism and the AIDS Crisis." In *Acting On AIDS*, ed. Joshua Oppenheimer and Helena Reckitt. London: Serpent's Tail.

Gottlieb, Alma. 1990. "Hot Blood, Vengeful Blood: AIDS and Blood Symbolism in Africa." Paper presented at the conference "The Impact of AIDS on Maternal-Child Health Care Delivery in Africa," 4–6 May, University of Illinois at Urbana-Champaign, Urbana.

Gottlieb, M. S., R. Schroff, H. M. Schanker, et al. 1981. "*Pneumocystis carinii* Pneumonia and Mucosal Candidiasis in Previously Healthy Homosexual Men." *New England Journal of Medicine* 305: 1425–31.

Gould, Peter. 1993. *The Slow Plague*. Oxford: Blackwell.

Gould, Robert E. 1988. "Reassuring News about AIDS: A Doctor Tells Why *You* May Not Be at Risk." *Cosmopolitan*, January, 146–47.

Graboys, Angela. 1986. "The Courage of Sunnye Sherman." *Reform Judaism*, Fall, 14–15, 36.

Grady, Christine. 1995. *The Search for an AIDS Vaccine: Ethical Issues in the Development and Testing of a Preventive HIV Vaccine*. Bloomington: Indiana University Press.

Graham, Judith. 1989a. "Ad Industry Rears up at Boycott." *Advertising Age*, 24 July, 16.

Graham, Judith. 1989b. "'New Puritanism' Colors TV Lineup." *Advertising Age*, 29 May, 46.

Gray, Chris Hables, Steven Mentor, and Heidi Figueroa Sarriera, eds. 1994. *The Cyborg Handbook*. New York: Routledge.

Green, Edward C., Bongi Zokwe, and John David Dupree. 1995. "The Experience of an AIDS Prevention Program Focused on South African Traditional Healers." *Social Science and Medicine* 40, no. 4: 503–15.

Green, John, and David Miller. 1986. *AIDS: The Story of a Disease*. London: Grafton.

Greenhouse, Steven. 1988. "Zaire, the Manager's Nightmare: So Much Potential, So Poorly Harnessed." *New York Times*, 23 May, 5.

Greer, William R. 1986. "Violence against Homosexuals Rising, Groups Say in Seeking Protections." *New York Times*, 23 November, 15.

Gregory, Roberta. 1992. "Bialogue." Comic strip, *Out/Look*, Summer, 7.

Greyson, John, director. 1987. *The ADS Epidemic*. Toronto: V Tape. Video.

Greyson, John, director. 1989a. *Angry Initiatives, Defiant Strategies*. Canada: Deep Dish TV. Video.

Greyson, John, director. 1989b. *The Pink Pimpernel*. Tornoto: V Tape. Video.

Greyson, John. 1989c. "Proofing." In *AIDS: The Artists' Response*, ed. Jan Zita Grover. Columbus: Ohio State University.

Greyson, John, director. 1990. *The World Is Sick (Sic)*. Toronto: V Tape. Video.

Greyson, John. 1992. "Still Searching." In *A Leap in the Dark: AIDS, Art, and Contemporary Cultures*, ed. Allan Klusaček and Ken Morrison. Montreal: Véhicule/Artexte.

Greyson, John, director. 1993. *Zero Patience*. Toronto: Zero Patience Productions. Video.

Greyson, John, and Bill Horrigan, compilers. 1990. *Video against AIDS*. Chicago: Video Data Bank; Toronto: V Tape. Video.

GRIA (Haitian Revolutionary Internationalist Group). 1982. "AIDS: Syndrome of an Imperialist Era." Duplicated flyer in the author's collection.

Griffen, Anne. 1994. "Women's Health and the Articulation of Policy Preferences." *Annals of the New York Academy of Sciences* 736 (30 December): 205–216.

Grimes, David A. 1988. "Pregnant Infected Women May Require Additional Medical and Social Support Services." *Journal of the American Medical Association* 259, no. 2 (8 January): 217–18.

Grmek, Mirko D. 1990. *The History of AIDS: Emergence and Origin of a Modern Pandemic*. Translated by Russell C. Maulitz and Jacalyn Duffin. Princeton, N.J.: Princeton University Press.

Gross, Jane. 1987a. "AIDS Victims Grasp at Home Remedies and Rumors of Cures." *New York Times*, 15 May, 13.

Gross, Jane. 1987b. "The Bleak and Lonely Lives of Women Who Carry AIDS." *New York Times*, 27 August, A-1, 14.

Gross, Jane. 1993. "California Inmates Win Better Prison AIDS Care." *New York Times*, 25 January, A12.

Grossberg, Lawrence, Cary Nelson, and Paula A. Treichler, eds. 1992. *Cultural Studies*. New York: Routledge.

Grossman, Arnold H. 1996. "The Virtual and Actual Identities of Older Lesbians and Gay Men." In *A Queer World: The Center for Lesbian and Gay Studies Reader*, ed. Martin Duberman. New York: New York University Press.

Grover, Jan Zita. 1986. "The 'Scientific' Regime of Truth." *In These Times*, 10–16 December, 18–19.

Grover, Jan Zita. 1988a. "AIDS: Keywords." In *AIDS: Cultural Analysis, Cultural Activism*, ed. Douglas Crimp. Cambridge, Mass.: MIT Press.

Grover, Jan Zita. 1988b. "A Matter of Life and Death." *Women's Review of Books*, March, 1, 3.

Grover, Jan Zita. 1988c. Review of *Ground Zero*, by Andrew Holleran. *San Francisco Sentinel*, 7 October, 24, 34.

Grover, Jan Zita. 1989a. *AIDS: The Artists' Response*. Columbus: Ohio State University.

Grover, Jan Zita. 1989b. "Visible Lesions: Images of People with AIDS." *Afterimage* 17, no. 1 (Summer): 10–16.

Grover, Jan Zita. 1992. "AIDS, Keywords, and Cultural Work." In *Cultural Studies*, ed. Lawrence Grossberg, Cary Nelson, and Paula Treichler. New York: Routledge.

Grover, Jan Zita. 1997. *North Enough: AIDS and Other Clear-Cuts*. St. Paul, Minn.: Greywolf.

Guinan, Mary E. 1993. "Black Communities' Belief in 'AIDS as Genocide': A Barrier to Overcome for HIV Prevention." *Annals of Epidemiology* 3, no. 2: 193–95.

Guinan, Mary E., and Ann Hardy. 1987. "Epidemiology of AIDS in Women in the United States: 1981 through 1986." *Journal of the American Medical Association* 257: 2039–42.

Gunn, Albert E., et al. 1988. *AIDS in Africa*. Washington, D.C.: Foundation for America's Future.

Gunn, Thom. 1985. *Lament*. Champaign, Ill.: Doe.

Guthmann, Edward. 1986. "AIDS and the Arts: How the Bay Area Has Been Hit." Datebook special report, *San Francisco Chronicle*, 7 December, 1.

Gutierrez-Gomez, José, and Jose Vergelin, producers. 1987. *Ojos que no ven* (Eyes that fail to see). San Francisco: Adinfinitum Films. Film, 51 minutes, English and Spanish.

Haberman, Clyde. 1987. "Japan Plans to Deny Visas over AIDS." *New York Times*, 1 April, A-18.

Haire, Doris. 1984. *How the F.D.A. Determines the "Safety" of Drugs—Just How Safe Is "Safe"?* Washington, D.C.: National Women's Health Network.

"Haitian AIDS Victim: A Former Playground for Holidayers." 1989. *Macleans*, 24 August, 31.

Hall, Jane. 1985. "A Shattering AIDS TV Movie Mirrors a Family's Pain." *People Weekly*, 18 November, 145.

Hall, Stuart. 1980a. "Cultural Studies: Two Paradigms." *Media, Culture and Society* 2: 57–72.

Hall, Stuart. 1980b. "Encoding and Decoding." In *Culture, Media, Language*, ed. Stuart Hall et al. London: Hutchinson/Center for Contemporary Cultural Studies.

Hall, Stuart. 1992. "Cultural Studies and Its Theoretical Legacies." In *Cultural Studies*, ed. Lawrence Grossberg, Cary Nelson, and Paula A. Treichler. New York: Routledge.

Haller, Scott. 1985. "Fighting for Life." *People Weekly*, 23 September, 28–33.

Hammer, Barbara, 1986. *Snow Job: The Media Hysteria of AIDS*. Chicago: Video Data Bank. Video. 8 min.

Hammonds, Evelynn. 1987. "Race, Sex, AIDS: The Construction of 'Other.'" *Radical America* 20, no. 6: 28–38.

Hammonds, Evelynn. 1992. "Missing Persons: African-American Women, AIDS and the History of Disease." *Radical America* 24, no. 2: 7–23.

Hammonds, Evelynn Maxine. 1993. "The Search for Perfect Control: A Social History of Diphtheria, 1880–1930." Ph.D. diss., Harvard University.

Hammonds, Evelynn. 1994. "Black (W)holes and the Geometry of Black Female Sexuality." *Differences* 6, nos. 2–3: 126–45.

Hammonds, Evelynn. 1997. "Race and Representation: African-Americans and AIDS." Paper given at the symposium "The Culture of AIDS," Humanities Series Colloquium, 5 March, Johns Hopkins University.

Hanawa, Yukiko. 1996. "Inciting Sites of Political Interventions: Queer 'n Asian." In *A Queer World: The Center for Lesbian and Gay Studies Reader*, ed. Martin Duberman. New York: New York University Press.

Handsfield, H. Hunter. 1988. "Heterosexual Transmission of Human Immunodeficiency Virus." *Journal of the American Medical Association* 13, no. 260 (7 October): 1943–44.

Hanna, Leslie. 1997. "Chinese Medicine for HIV Positive Women." *BETA*, September, 39–44.

Hansen, Joseph. 1987. *Early Graves*. New York: Mysterious.

Haq, Cynthia. 1988. "Data on AIDS in Africa: An Assessment." In *AIDS in Africa: The Social and Policy Impact*, ed. Norman Miller and Richard C. Rockwell. Lewiston, N.Y.: Edwin Mellen.

Haraway, Donna J. 1979. "The Biological Enterprise: Sex, Mind, and Profit from Human Engineering to Sociobiology." *Radical History Review* 20 (Spring/Summer): 206–37.

Haraway, Donna J. 1985. "A Manifesto for Cyborgs: Science, Technology, and Socialist Feminism in the 1980s." *Socialist Review* 80 (March/April): 65–108.

Haraway, Donna J. 1989a. "The Biopolitics of Postmodern Bodies: Determinations of Self in Immune System Discourse." *Differences* 1, no. 1: 3–43.

Haraway, Donna J. 1989b. *Primate Visions: Gender, Race, and Nature in the World of Modern Science*. New York: Routledge.

Haraway, Donna J. 1991a. "Overhauling the Meaning Machines: An Interview with Donna Haraway." By Marcy Darnovsky. *Socialist Review* 21, no. 2: 65–84.

Haraway, Donna J. 1991b. *Simians, Cyborgs, and Women*. London: Free Association.

Haraway, Donna J. 1996. *Modest-Witness, Second-Millennium: Femaleman Meets Oncomouse: Feminism and Technoscience*. New York: Routledge.

Harden, Blaine. 1987. "AIDS May Replace Famine as the Continent's Worst Blight." *Washington Post Weekly Review*, 15 June, 16–17.

Harmetz, Aljean. 1987a. "AIDS Is Changing Hollywood Scripts and Lives." *New York Times*, 15 March, 20.

Harmetz, Aljean. 1987b. "Sanitizing a Hot Novel into a Lukewarm Film." *New York Times,* 18 November, 22. Review of the film *Less than Zero.*

Harper, Mary. 1988. "AIDS in Africa—Plague or Propaganda?" *West Africa* (7–13 November): 2072–73.

Harrington, Mark. 1989. "What I Said at the FDA Advisory Committee Meeting on Parallel Track." *ACT UP Reports,* September/October, 5–6.

Harrington, Mark. 1990. *A Critique of the AIDS Clinical Trials Group,* ed. Ken Fortunato. New York: ACT UP Treatment and Data Committee.

Harrington, Mark. 1997. "Some Transitions in the History of AIDS Treatment Activism: From Therapeutic Utopianism to Pragmatic Praxis." In *Acting on AIDS,* ed. Joshua Oppenheimer and Helena Reckitt. London: Serpent's Tail.

Harris, Nigel. 1986. *The End of the Third World: Newly Industrializing Countries and the Decline of an Ideology.* London: Penguin.

Harrison, Barbara Grizzuti. 1986. "It's Okay to Be Angry about AIDS." *Mademoiselle,* February, 96.

Hart, Vada. 1986. "Lesbians and AIDS." *Gossip* 2: 5–10.

Hartouni, Valerie. 1997. *Cultural Conceptions: On Reproductive Technologies and the Remaking of Life.* Minneapolis: University of Minnesota Press.

Havarkos, Harry W. 1993. "Reported Cases of AIDS: An Update." *New England Journal of Medicine* 329, no. 7: 511.

Haver, William. 1996. *The Body of This Death: Historicity and Sociality in the Time of AIDS.* Stanford, Calif.: Stanford University Press.

Hawkins, Christine. 1988. "AIDS Expected to Slow Population Growth." *New African,* August, 25.

Hay, James. 1990. "Advertising as a Cultural Text: Rethinking Message Analysis in a Recombinant Culture." In *Rethinking Communication: Paradigm Exemplar,* vol. 2, ed. Brenda Dervin et al. Newbury Park, Calif.: Sage.

Heise, Lori L., and Christopher Elias. 1995. "Transforming AIDS Prevention to Meet Women's Needs: A Focus on Developing Countries." *Social Science and Medicine* 40, no. 7: 931–43.

Hellinger, Fred J. 1992. "Forecasts of the Costs of Medical Care for Persons with HIV: 1992–1995." *Inquiry* 29 (Fall): 356–65.

Henig, Robin M. 1983. "AIDS: A New Disease's Deadly Odyssey." *New York Times Magazine,* 6 February, 28.

Henig, Robin M. 1994. *A Dancing Matrix: How Science Confronts Emerging Viruses.* New York: Vintage.

Hentoff, Nat. 1987. "The New Priesthood of Death." *Village Voice,* 30 June, 35.

Herdt, Gilbert H. 1981. *Guardians of the Flutes: Idioms of Masculinity.* New York: McGraw-Hill.

Herdt, Gilbert H., and Shirley Lindenbaum, eds. 1992. *The Time of AIDS: Social Analysis, Theory, and Method.* Newbury Park, Calif.: Sage.

Herek, Gregory M., and John P. Capitanio. 1994. "Conspiracies, Contagion, and Compassion: Trust and Public Reactions to AIDS." *AIDS Education and Prevention* 6, no. 4: 365–75.

Herek, Gregory M., and B. Greene, eds. 1995. *AIDS, Identity, and Community: The HIV Epidemic and Lesbians and Gay Men.* Newbury Park, Calif.: Sage.

Herschberger, Ruth. [1948] 1970. *Adam's Rib.* Reprint, New York: Harper and Row.

Herzlich, Claudine, and Janine Pierret. 1989. "The Construction of a Phenomenon: AIDS in the French Press." *Social Science and Medicine* 29: 11.

Hilferty, Robert. 1991. *Stop the Church*. San Francisco: Frameline. Video.

Hill, Jane H. 1988. "Language, Culture, and World Views." In *Linguistics: The Cambridge Survey*, vol. 6, ed. Frederick J. Newmeyer. Cambridge: Cambridge University Press.

Hill, Michael E. 1985. "*An Early Frost* an AIDS Story." *Washington Post TV Week*, 10–16 November, 9–11.

Hill, Ronald Paul, and Andrea L. Beaver. 1991. "Advocacy Groups and Television Advertisers." *Journal of Advertising* 20, no. 1: 18–27.

Hilts, Philip J. 1988. "Out of Africa." *Washington Post's Weekly Journal of Health*, 24 May, 12–17.

Hilts, Philip J. 1989a. "Drug Said to Help AIDS Cases with Virus but No Symptoms." *New York Times*, 18 August, 1.

Hilts, Philip J. 1989b. "Wave of Protests Developing on Profits from AIDS Drugs." *New York Times*, 16 September, 1.

Hilts, Philip J. 1990. "Birth Control Backlash." *New York Times Magazine*, 16 December, 41.

Hoctel, Patrick. 1990. "The Little Movie That Could." *Bay Area Reporter*, 21 June, 49.

Hodgkinson, Neville. 1993. "Why We Won't Be Silenced." *Sunday Times* (London), 12 December, sec. 4, p. 1.

Holland, Dorothy, and Naomi Quinn, eds. 1987. *Cultural Models in Language and Thought*. Cambridge: Cambridge University Press.

Holleran, Andrew. 1988. *Ground Zero*. New York: William Morrow.

Hollibaugh, Amber. [1993] 1997. "Lesbian Leadership and Lesbian Denial in the AIDS Epidemic." In *We Are Everywhere*, ed. Mark Blasius and Shane Phelan. New York: Routledge.

Hollibaugh, Amber, producer. 1987. *The Second Epidemic*. New York: Gay Men's Health Crisis. Video.

Hooper, Ed 1990. *Slim: A Reporter's Own Story of AIDS in East Africa*. London: Bodley Head.

Hopkins, Andrew. 1990. "The Social Recognition of Repetition Strain Injuries: An Australian/American Comparison." *Social Science and Medicine* 30, no. 3: 365–72.

Hornaday, Ann. 1986. "New Theory: AIDS and Women." *Ms*, November, 28.

Horton, Meurig. 1989. "Bugs, Drugs, and Placebos: The Opulence of Truth, or How to Make a Treatment Decision in an Epidemic." In *Taking Liberties: AIDS and Cultural Politics*, ed. Erica Carter and Simon Watney. London: Serpent's Tail.

Horvitz, Philip. 1985. "Don't Cry for Me, Academia." *Jimmy and Lucy's House of K* 2 (August): 78–80. Interview with Michel Foucault.

Hosken, Fran P. 1986. "Why AIDS Pattern Is Different in Africa." Letter, *New York Times*, 15 December, 13.

Hrdy, Daniel B. 1987. "Cultural Practices Contributing to the Transmission of HIV in Africa." *Review of Infectious Diseases* 9, no. 6 (November–December): 1109–19. Reprinted in Koch-Weser and Vanderschmidt (1988).

Huber, Joan, and Beth E. Schneider, eds. 1992. *The Social Context of AIDS*. Newbury Park, Calif.: Sage.

Huestis, Mark, and Wendy Dallas, producers. 1986. *Chuck Solomon: Coming of Age*. San Francisco: Frameline. Video.

Huff, Bob, director. 1987. *The Asshole Is a Tense Hole.* New York: Bob Huff. Video.

Huff, Bob, director. 1989. *Rockville Is Burning.* New York: Bob Huff and Wave 3. Video.

Hughey, Jim D., Robert N. Norton, and Catherine Sullivan. 1986. "Confronting Danger: AIDS in the News." Paper presented at the annual meeting of the Speech Communication Association, November, Chicago.

Hulce, Tom. 1989. "The Subject and the Spectacle." Paper presented at the symposium "SIDART," held in conjunction with the Fifth International Conference on AIDS, 8 June, Montreal.

"The Hunk Who Lived a Lie." 1985. *London Sun,* 3 October.

Hunt, Charles. 1988. "Africa and AIDS." *Monthly Review* 39, no. 9 (February): 10–22.

Hunt, Morton. 1986. "Teaming up against AIDS." *New York Times Magazine,* 2 March, 42–51, 78–83.

Hunter, Nan D. 1992. "Complications of Gender: Women and HIV Disease." In *AIDS Agenda: Emerging Issues in Civil Rights,* ed. Nan D. Hunter and William B. Rubenstein. New York: Free Press.

Ingram, Gordon Brent, Anne-Marie Bouthillette, and Yolanda Retter, eds. 1997. *Queers in Space: Communities/Public Places/Sites of Resistance.* Seattle: Bay.

Ingstad, Benedicte. 1990. "The Cultural Construction of AIDS and Its Consequences for Prevention in Botswana." *Medical Anthropology Quarterly* 4, no. 1: 28–40.

Institute of Medicine. 1997. *The Hidden Epidemic: Confronting Sexually Transmitted Diseases.* Washington, D.C.: National Academy Press.

Institute of Medicine and National Academy of Sciences. 1986. *Confronting AIDS: Directions for Public Health, Health Care, and Research,* ed. David Baltimore and Sheldon M. Wolff. Washington, D.C.: National Academy Press.

Institute of Medicine and National Academy of Sciences. 1988. *Confronting AIDS: Update 1988.* Washington, D.C.: National Academy Press.

International Working Group on Women and AIDS. 1989. Media release. Fifth International AIDS Conference, 8 June, Montreal.

Ireland, Doug. 1989. "Press clips." *Village Voice,* 26 December, 10.

Irigaray, Luce. 1985. *Speculum of the Other Woman.* Translated by Gillian C. Gill. Ithaca, N.Y.: Cornell University Press.

Irvine, Janice M. 1996. "One Generation Post-Stonewall: Political Contests over Lesbian and Gay School Reform." In *A Queer World: The Center for Lesbian and Gay Studies Reader,* ed. Martin Duberman. New York: New York University Press.

Irwin, Susan, and Brigitte Jordan. 1987. "Knowledge, Practice, and Power: Court-Ordered Cesarean Sections." *Medical Anthropology Quarterly* 1, no. 3: 333.

Jacobus, Mary, Evelyn Fox Keller, and Sally Shuttleworth, eds. 1990. *Body/Politics: Women and the Discourses of Science.* New York: Routledge.

James, John S., ed. 1989a. *AIDS Treatment News, Vol. 1.* Berkeley, Calif.: Celestial Arts. Reprints nos. 1–75 (April 1986–March 1989).

James, John S. 1989b. "The Drug-Trials Debacle: 1, What to Do about It." *AIDS Treatment News,* 21 April, 3–6.

James, John S. 1989c. "The Drug-Trials Debacle: 2, What to Do Now." *AIDS Treatment News,* 5 May, 4–8.

James, John S., ed. 1991. *AIDS Treatment News, Vol. 2.* Berkeley, Calif.: Celestial Arts. Reprints nos. 76–125 (April 1989–April 1991).

James, John S., ed. 1994. *AIDS Treatment News, Vol. 3.* Boston: Alyson. Reprints nos. 126–89 (May 1991–December 1993).

James, John S., ed. 1997. *AIDS Treatment News*. Issues 262–85 (January 1997–December 1997).

Jaret, Peter. 1986. "Our Immune System: The Wars Within." *National Geographic*, June, 702–35.

Jaret, Peter. 1994. "Viruses: On the Edge of Life, on the Edge of Death." *National Geographic*, July.

Johnson, Edward S., and Jeffrey Vieira. 1986. "Cause of AIDS: Etiology." In *AIDS: Facts and Issues*, ed. Victor Gong and Norman Rudnick. New Brunswick, N.J.: Rutgers University Press.

Johnson, Hillary. 1996. *Osler's Web: Inside the Labyrinth of the Chronic Fatigue Syndrome Epidemic*. New York: Crown.

Johnson, Paula, Doralba Muñoz, and Jose Pares. 1988. "Multi-Cultural Concerns and AIDS Action: Creating an Alternative." *Radical America* 21, nos. 2–3 (March/April): 18–25.

Johnson, Toby. 1983. "AIDS and Moral Issues." *Advocate*, 27 October, 24–46.

Johnson, Warren D., Jr., and Jean W. Pape. 1989. "AIDS in Haiti." In *AIDS: Pathogenesis and Treatment*, ed. Jay A. Levy. New York: Marcel Dekker.

Jones, Coleman, producer. 1987–89. See "The AIDS Campaigns."

Jones, James H. 1981. *Bad Blood: The Tuskegee Syphilis Experiment: A Tragedy of Race and Medicine*. New York: Free Press.

Jones, Therese. 1997. "As the World Turns on the Sick and the Restless, So Go the Days of Our Lives: Family and Illness in Daytime Drama." *Journal of Medical Humanities* 18, no. 1 (Spring): 5–20.

Jong, Erica. 1986. "Women and AIDS." *New Woman*, April, 42–48.

Jordan, Catherine V., producer. 1987. *All of Us and AIDS*. New York: Peer Education Health Resources. Video.

Jordanova, Ludmilla. 1980. "Natural Facts: A Historical Perspective on Science and Sexuality." In *Nature, Culture and Gender*, ed. Carol P. MacCormack and Marilyn Strathern. Cambridge: Cambridge University Press.

Jordanova, Ludmilla. 1987. "Nature Unveiling before Science: Images of Women and Knowledge." Paper presented at the colloquium "Women, Science, and the Body: Discourses and Representations," May, Cornell University.

Jordanova, Ludmilla. 1989. *Sexual Visions: Images of Gender in Science and Medicine between the Eighteenth and Twentieth Centuries*. Madison: University of Wisconsin Press.

Joseph, Stephen C. 1986. "Intravenous-Drug Abuse Is the Front Line in the War on AIDS." Letter to the editor, *New York Times*, 22 December, 18.

Juengst, Eric, and Barbara Koenig, eds. 1989. *The Meaning of AIDS: Implications for Medical Science, Clinical Practice, and Public Health Policy*. New York: Praeger.

Juhasz, Alexandra, producer. 1988. *A Test of the Nation: Women, Children, Families, and AIDS*. New York: Gay Men's Health Crisis. Video.

Juhasz, Alexandra. 1990a. "The Contained Threat: Women in Mainstream AIDS Documentary." *Journal of Sex Research* 27 (February): 25–46.

Juhasz, Alexandra, producer. 1990b. *We Care: A Video for Care Providers of People Affected with AIDS*. New York: Women's AIDS Video Enterprise. Video.

Juhasz, Alexandra. 1992. "From Within: Alternative AIDS Media by Women." *Praxis* 3: 23–45.

Juhasz, Alexandra. 1995. *AIDS TV: Identity, Community, and Alternative Video.* With videography by Catherine Saalfield. Durham, N.C.: Duke University Press.

Juhasz, Alexandra, and Jean Carlomusto. 1988. *Living with AIDS: Women and AIDS.* New York: Gay Men's Health Crisis.

Julien, Isaac, producer. 1987. *This Is Not an AIDS Advertisement.* New York: Third World Newsreel. Video.

Julien, Isaac, and Pratibha Parmar. 1990. "In Conversation: Isaac Julien and Pratibha Parmar." In *Ecstatic Antibodies: Revisiting the AIDS Mythology,* ed. Tessa Boffin and Sunil Gupta. London: Rivers Oram.

Kaiser, Jon D. 1993. *Immune Power: A Comprehensive Healing Program for HIV.* New York: St. Martin's.

Kaiser Family Foundation. 1996. *AIDS Media Study, 1981–1994.* Menlo Park, Calif.: Kaiser Family Foundation.

Kakoma, Ibulaimu. 1990. "Introductory Overview." Paper presented at the conference "The Impact of AIDS on Maternal-Child Health Care Delivery in Africa," 4–6 May, University of Illinois at Urbana-Champaign, Urbana.

Kalin, Tom. 1988. *They Are Lost to Vision Altogether.* Chicago: Video Data Bank. Video.

Kalisch, Philip A., and Beatrice J. Kalisch. 1985. "When Americans Called for Dr. Kildare: Images of Physicians and Nurses in the Dr. Kildare and Dr. Gillespie Movies, 1937–1947." *Medical Heritage* 1, no. 5: 348–63.

Kalter, Joanmarie. 1987. "Exposing Media Myths: TV Doesn't Affect You as Much as You Think." *TV Guide,* 30 May, 2–5.

Kane, Stephanie. 1990. "AIDS, Addiction and Condom Use: Sources of Sexual Risk for Heterosexual Women." *Journal of Sex Research* 27, no. 3: 427–44.

Kane, Stephanie. 1991. "HIV, Heroin, and Heterosexual Relations." *Social Science and Medicine* 32, no. 9: 1037–50.

Kane, Stephanie. 1993. "Prostitution and the Military: Planning AIDS Intervention in Belize." *Social Science and Medicine* 36: 965–79.

Kane, Stephanie. 1994. "Sacred Deviance and AIDS in a North American Buddhist Community." *Law and Policy* 16, no. 3 (July): 323–39.

Kane, Stephanie C. 1998. *AIDS Alibis: Sex, Drugs, and Crime in the Americas.* Philadelphia: Temple University Press.

Kane, Stephanie, and Theresa Mason. 1992. " 'IV Drug Users' and 'Sex Partners': The Limits of Epidemiological Categories and the Ethnography of Risk." In *The Time of AIDS: Social Analysis, Theory, and Method,* ed. Gilbert Herdt and Shirley Lindenbaum. Newbury Park, Calif.: Sage.

Kant, Harold Sanford. 1985. "The Transmission of HTLV-III." Letter to the editor, *Journal of the American Medical Association* 254: 1901.

Kaplan, E. Ann, ed. 1983. *Regarding Television.* Westport, Conn.: Greenwood.

Kaplan, Helen Singer. 1987. *The Real Truth about Women and AIDS: How to Eliminate the Risks without Giving Up Love and Sex.* New York: Simon and Schuster.

Kaplan, Mark S. 1995. "The Feminization of the AIDS Epidemic." *Journal of Sociology and Social Welfare* 22, no. 2: 5–21.

Karnik, Niranjan S. Forthcoming. "Locating HIV/AIDS and India: Cautionary Notes on the Globalization of Categories." *Science, Technology, and Human Values.*

Karnik, Niranjan S. 1998. "Rwanda and the Media: Imagery, War, and Refuge." *Review of African Political Economy* 78: 611–623.

Karpf, Anne. 1988. *Doctoring the Media: The Reporting of Health and Medicine.* London: Routledge.

Katz, D. H. 1993. "AIDS: Primarily a Viral or an Autoimmune Disease?" *AIDS Research and Human Retroviruses* 9, no. 5: 489–93.

Kayal, Philip M. 1993. *Bearing Witness: Gay Men's Health Crisis and the Politics of AIDS.* Boulder, Colo.: Westview.

Keith, Jim, ed. 1993. *Secret and Suppressed: Banned Ideas and Hidden History.* Portland, Oreg.: Feral.

Kember, Sarah. 1991. "Medical Imaging: The Geometry of Chaos." *New Formations* 15 (Winter): 55–66.

Kendrick, Walter. 1987. "Unsafe Texts." *Voice Literary Supplement* 59, October: 10–13.

Kenny, Lorraine. 1989. "Testing the Limits: An Interview." *Afterimage* 17, no. 3: 4–7.

Kent, Debra. 1995. "Could the Woman Next Door Have AIDS?" *McCall's,* February, 72–73.

Kessler, Suzanne. 1996. "Creating Good-Looking Genitals in the Service of Gender." In *A Queer World: The Center for Lesbian and Gay Studies Reader,* ed. Martin Duberman. New York: New York University Press.

King, Bill. 1985. "*Early Frost* Covers New Ground for Television." *Atlanta Journal/Constitution,* 11 November, TV section, pp. 4–5.

King, Edward. 1993. *Safety in Numbers: Safer Sex and Gay Men.* London: Cassell.

King, Edward. 1997. "HIV Prevention and the New Virology." In *Acting on AIDS,* ed. Joshua Oppenheimer and Helena Reckitt. London: Serpent's Tail.

King, Katie. 1992. "Local and Global: AIDS Activism and Feminist Theory." *Camera Obscura* 28: 79–99.

Kingston, Tim. 1990. "Parallel Track." *San Francisco Bay Times,* May, 4–5.

Kinsella, James. 1989. *Covering the Plague: AIDS and the American Media.* New Brunswick, N.J.: Rutgers University Press.

Kitahata, M. M., T. D. Koepsell, R. A. Deyo, et al. 1996. "Physicians' Experience with the Acquired Immunodeficiency Syndrome as a Factor in Patients' Survival." *New England Journal of Medicine,* 334: 701–6.

Kitzinger, Jenny, and David Miller. 1991. "In Black and White: A Preliminary Report on the Role of the Media in Audience Understandings of 'African AIDS.'" Working paper. Glasgow: AIDS Media Research Project.

Kloser, Patricia, and Jane Maclean Craig. 1994. *The Woman's HIV Sourcebook: A Guide to Better Health and Well-Being.* Dallas: Taylor.

Klusaček, Allan, and Ken Morrison, eds. 1992. *A Leap in the Dark: AIDS, Art, and Contemporary Cultures.* Montreal: Véhicule/Artexte.

Knorr-Cetina, Karin D. 1981. *The Manufacture of Knowledge: An Essay on the Constructivist and Contextual Nature of Science.* Oxford: Pergamon.

Knorr-Cetina, Karin D., and Michael Mulkay, eds. 1983. *Science Observed: Perspectives on the Social Study of Science.* London: Sage.

Koch-Weser, Dieter, and Hannelove Vanderschmidt, eds. 1988. *The Heterosexual Transmission of AIDS in Africa.* Cambridge, Mass.: Abt.

Koehler, Robert. 1990. "Crusade against AIDS by African Pop Singer." *Los Angeles Times,* 3 April, F-9.

Kogan, Rick. 1991. "AIDS Jitters Still Afflict Networks." *Chicago Tribune,* 17 May, sec. 5, p. 1. Review of *Our Sons.*

420   Bibliography

Kohn, Marek, 1987. "Face the Virus: Essential 1980s Biology." *Face*, April, 64–71.

Kolata, Gina. 1988a. "Africa Is Favored for AIDS Testing." *New York Times*, 19 February, 7.

Kolata, Gina. 1988b. "AIDS Patients and Their above-Ground Underground." *New York Times*, 10 July, E-32.

Kolata, Gina. 1988c. "Odd Alliance Would Speed New Drugs." *New York Times*, 26 November, 9.

Kolata, Gina. 1989. "Innovative AIDS Drug Plan May Be Undermining Testing." *New York Times*, 21 November, 1.

Kolata, Gina. 1990. "Odd Surge Found in Deaths of Those Taking AIDS Drug." *New York Times*, 12 March, 1.

Kolata, Gina. 1992. "Who Is Female? Science Can't Say." *New York Times*, 16 February, 6.

Kolata, Gina. 1993. "Targeting Urged in Attack on AIDS." *New York Times*, 7 March, 1, 26.

Kolata, Gina. 1995. "Top Official Says AIDS Fight Is Inefficient." *New York Times*, 3 February, A-9.

Kolata, Gina. 1997. "New View Sees Breast Cancer as 3 Diseases." *New York Times*, 1 April, B-9.

Kolder, Veronika E. B., J. Gallagher, and M. T. Parsons. 1987. "Court-Ordered Obstetrical Interventions." *New England Journal of Medicine* 316: 1192–96.

Konetey-Ahulu, Felix I. D. 1988. "AIDS in Africa: Misinformation and Disinformation." In *The Heterosexual Transmission of AIDS in Africa*, ed. Dieter Koch-Weser and Hannelore Vanderschmidt. Cambridge, Mass.: Abt.

Koop, C. Everett. 1991. *Koop: The Memoirs of America's Family Doctor.* New York: Random House.

Kraft, Scott. 1992. "Africa's Death Sentence." *Los Angeles Times Magazine*, 1 March, 12–16, 32.

Kramer, Larry. 1983. "1,112 and Counting." *New York Native*, March, 14–27.

Kramer, Larry. 1985. *The Normal Heart.* New York: Samuel French.

Kramer, Larry. 1987. "Taking Responsibility for Our Lives: Does the Gay Community Have a Death Wish?" *New York Native*, 29 June, 37–40, 66–67.

Kramer, Larry. 1989a. *Reports from the Holocaust: The Making of an AIDS Activist.* New York: St. Martin's.

Kramer, Larry, 1989b. "Read This and Live: A 14-Point Program to End AIDS." *Village Voice*, 27 June, 24.

Kramer, Larry. 1990. "Second-Rated to Death," *Outweek*, 24 October, 48–50.

Kreiss, Joan K., et al. 1986. "AIDS Virus Infection in Nairobi Prostitutes: Spread of the Epidemic to East Africa." *New England Journal of Medicine* 314, no. 7 (13 February): 414–18.

Krieger, Nancy. 1987. "The Epidemiology of AIDS in Africa." *Science for the People* (January–February): 18–21.

Krieger, Nancy, and Rose Appleman. 1986. *The Politics of AIDS.* Oakland, Calif.: Frontline.

Krieger, Nancy, and Elizabeth Fee. 1992. "Man-Made Medicine and Women's Health: The Biopolitics of Sex/Gender and Race/Ethnicity." In *Man-Made Medicine*, ed. Kary L. Moss. Durham, N.C.: Duke University Press.

Krim, Mathilde. 1985a. "AIDS: The Challenge to Science and Medicine." Special supplement, *Hastings Center Report* 15, no. 4: 2–7.

Krim, Mathilde. 1985b. Interview on "MacNeil/Lehrer News Hour." New York: PBS, 4 September.

Krim, Mathilde. 1986. "A Chance at Life for AIDS Sufferers." *New York Times*, 8 August, A-27.

Krim, Mathilde. 1987. "Making Experimental Drugs Available for AIDS Treatment." *AIDS Public Policy Journal* 2: 1–5.

Kroeber, A. L., and Clyde Kluckhohn, with the assistance of Wayne Untreiner. 1952. *Culture: A Critical Review of Concepts and Definitions.* Papers of the Peabody Museum, Harvard University, vol. 47, no. 1. Cambridge, Mass.: Peabody Museum of American Archaeology and Ethnology.

Kuhn, Thomas S. [1962] 1970. *The Structure of Scientific Revolutions.* Enlarged ed. Chicago: University of Chicago Press.

Kuitenbrouwer, Peter. 1989. "African Girls Need AIDS Facts from Elders: MD." *Montreal Gazette*, 3 June, A-8.

Kulstad, Ruth, ed. 1986. *AIDS: Papers from "Science," 1982–1985.* Washington, D.C.: American Association for the Advancement of Science.

Kulstad, Ruth, ed. 1988. *AIDS 1988: AAAS Symposium Papers.* Washington, D.C.: American Association for the Advancement of Science.

Kwitny, Jonathan. 1992. *Acceptable Risks.* New York: Poseidon.

Kybartas, Stashu. 1987. *Danny.* Chicago: Video Data Bank. Video.

Laclau, Ernesto, and Chantal Mouffe. 1985. *Hegemony and Socialist Strategy: Towards a Radical Democratic Politics.* Translated by Winston Moore and Paul Cammack. London: Verso.

Lakoff, George, and Mark Johnson. 1980. *Metaphors We Live By.* Chicago: University of Chicago Press.

Landers, Timothy. 1988. "Bodies and Anti-Bodies: A Crisis in Representation." *Independent* 11, no. 1: 18–24.

Landesman, Sheldon H., Harold M. Ginzburg, and Stanley H. Weiss. 1985. "The AIDS Epidemic." *New England Journal of Medicine* 312, no. 8: 521–25.

Langone, John. 1985. "AIDS: The Latest Scientific Facts." *Discover*, December, 27–52.

Langone, John. 1988. *AIDS: The Facts.* Boston: Little, Brown.

Laplanche, J., and J. B. Pontalis. 1973. *The Language of Psycho-Analysis.* New York: W. W. Norton.

Laqueur, Thomas. 1987. "Orgasm, Generation, and the Politics of Reproductive Biology." In *The Making of the Modern Body*, ed. Catherine Gallagher and Thomas Laqueur. Berkeley: University of California Press.

Laqueur, Thomas. 1990. *Making Sex: Body and Gender from the Greeks to Freud.* Cambridge, Mass.: Harvard University Press.

LaRouche, Lyndon, Jr. 1987. *My Program against AIDS.* Washington, D.C.: LaRouche Democratic Campaign, 7 February. Pamphlet.

Latour, Bruno. 1987. *Science in Action: How to Follow Scientists and Engineers through Society.* Cambridge, Mass.: Harvard University Press.

Latour, Bruno, and Steve Woolgar [1979] 1986. *Laboratory Life: The Construction of Scientific Facts.* Reprint, Princeton, N.J.: Princeton University Press.

Lauritsen, John. 1987. "Say No to HIV." *New York Native*, July 6, 17–25.

Lauritsen, John, 1989. "The AZT Front." *New York Times,* 2 January, 16–18.

Lauritsen, John. 1997. "The AIDS War." In *We Are Everywhere: A Historical Sourcebook of Gay and Lesbian Politics,* ed. M. Blasius and S. Phelan. New York: Routledge.

Leahy, Michael. 1986. "Why This Young Hunk Risked Playing an AIDS Victim." *TV Guide,* 26 April, 34–38.

Leary, Warren E. 1988. "F.D.A. Pressed to Approve More AIDS Drugs." *New York Times,* 11 October, C-5.

Leary, Warren E. 1993. "Spread of AIDS Is Spurred by Racism, U.S. Panel Says." *New York Times,* 5 January, 1.

Lederer, Robert. 1988. "Origin and Spread of AIDS." *Covert Action Quarterly* 29: 52–67.

Lee, Gary. 1985. "AIDS in Moscow: It Comes from the CIA, or Maybe Africa." *Washington Post National Weekly Edition,* 30 December, 16.

Lehman, Virginia, and Noreen Russell. 1986. "Psychological and Social Issues of AIDS." In *AIDS: Facts and Issues,* ed. Victor Gong and Norman Rudnick. New Brunswick, N.J.: Rutgers University Press.

Lehmann, Daniel J., and Suzy Schultz. 1987. "4 Women among New Cases Here in August." *Chicago Sun-Times,* 3 September, 3.

Leibowitch, Jacques. 1985. *A Strange Virus of Unknown Origin.* Translated by Richard Howard. New York: Ballantine.

Leigh, Carol, producer. 1987. *Safe Sex Slut.* Chicago: Video Data Bank. Video.

Leigh, Carol. 1988. "Speech Presented to the Senate Judiciary Committee." In "AIDS, Cultural Life, and the Arts." Forum on AIDS, *City Lights Review* 2: 21–22.

Leishman, Katie. 1986. "Two Million Americans and Still Counting." *New York Times Book Review,* 27 July, 12. Review of *The Plague Years,* by David Black, and *Mobilizing against AIDS,* by Eve Nichols.

Leishman, Katie. 1987. "Heterosexuals and AIDS: The Second Stage of the Epidemic." *Atlantic,* February 39–58.

Lemp, G. F., et al. 1992. "Survival for Women and Men with AIDS." *Journal of Infectious Diseases* 160 (1 July): 74–79.

Leonard, Terri L. 1990. "Male Clients of Female Street Prostitutes: Unseen Partners in Sexual Disease Transmission." *Medical Anthropology Quarterly* 4, no. 1: 41–55.

Leonard, Zoe. 1992a. "Lesbians in the AIDS Crisis." In *Women, AIDS, and Activism,* ed. ACT UP New York Women and AIDS Book Group. Boston: South End.

Leonard, Zoe. 1992b. "Safe Sex Is Real Sex." In *Women, AIDS, and Activism,* ed. ACT UP New York Women and AIDS Book Group. Boston: South End.

Leonard, Zoe, and Polly Thistlethwaite. 1992. "Prostitution and HIV Infection." In *Women, AIDS, and Activism,* ed. ACT UP New York Women and AIDS Book Group. Boston: South End.

Lerner, Sharon. 1991. "Women . . . AIDS . . . and the Media." *PWA Coalition Newsline* 65 (May): 23–24.

Levine, Carol, N. N. Dubber, and Robert J. Levine. 1991. "Building a New Consensus: Ethical Principles and Policies for Clinical Research on HIV/AIDS." *International Research Bulletin: A Review of Human Subjects Research* 13, nos. 1–2: 1–17.

Levine, Martin P., Peter M. Nardi, and John N. Gagnon, eds. 1997. *In Changing Times: Gay Men and Lesbians Encounter HIV/AIDS.* Chicago: University of Chicago Press.

Levine, Martin P., and Karolynn Siegel. 1992. "Unprotected Sex: Understanding Gay

Men's Participation." In *The Social Context of AIDS*, ed. Joan Huber and Beth E. Schneider. Newbury Park, Calif.: Sage.

Levine, Robert J., and Karen Lebacqz. 1979. "Ethical Considerations in Clinical Trials." *Clinical Pharmacology and Therapeutics* 25 (May): 728–41.

Levy, Dennis. 1997. "Reported Drop in AIDS Death Is Dangerously Misleading." *New York Amsterdam News*, 1 February, 3.

Levy, Jay A. 1993. "Pathogenesis of Human Immunodeficiency Virus Infection." *Microbiological Review* 57 (March): 183–289.

Levy, Jay A., et al. 1984. "Isolation of Lymphocytopathic Retroviruses from San Francisco Patients with AIDS." *Science* 225 (24 August), 840–42.

Levy, Jay A., ed. 1989. *AIDS: Pathogenesis and Treatment.* New York: Marcel Dekker.

Lew, Julie. 1991. "Why the Movies are Ignoring AIDS." *New York Times*, 18 August, Arts and Entertainment section, p. 18.

Lewin, Tamar. 1997. "Fearing Disease, Teens Alter Sexual Practices." *New York Times*, 5 April, 7.

Lewis-Thornton, Rae. 1994. "Facing AIDS." *Essence*, December, 63–64, 124–30.

Lieberson, Jonathan. 1983. "Anatomy of an Epidemic." *New York Review of Books*, 18 August, 17–22.

Lieberson, Jonathan. 1986. "The Reality of AIDS." *New York Review of Books*, 16 January, 43–48.

Limmer, Melissa. 1988. "A World Apart." *Advocate*, 10 October, 26–27.

Lindenbaum, Shirley. 1984. "Variations on a Sociosexual Theme in Melanesia." In *Ritualized Homosexuality in Melanesia*, ed. Gilbert Herdt. Berkeley: University of California Press.

Lindhorst, Taryn. 1988. "Women and AIDS: Scapegoats or a Social Problem?" *Affilia*, Winter, 51–59.

Link, Howard. 1988. *Waves and Plagues: The Art of Masami Teraoka.* Honolulu: Chronicle.

Lippe, Richard. 1987. "Rock Hudson: His Story." *CineAction*, Fall, 47–54.

Lipsitz, George. 1988. "The Meaning of Memory: Family, Class, and Ethnicity in Early Network Television Programs." *Camera Obscura* 16: 79–116.

Little, Matthew A. 1994. "Reporting AIDS: Representation, Rhetoric, and the Construction of Global Geographies of AIDS." M.A. thesis, University of British Columbia.

Litwin, Susan. 1990. "Will America Be Shocked by ABC's *Rock Hudson*?" *TV Guide*, 6 January, 14–17.

Lovejoy, Margot. 1993. *The Book of Plagues.* Philadelphia: Lori Spencer.

Lupton, Deborah. 1994. *Moral Threats and Dangerous Desires: AIDS in the News Media.* London: Taylor and Francis.

Lutaaya, Philly. 1990. *Born in Africa.* Film, biography of Philly Lutaaya, televised on PBS's "Frontline."

Lynch, Michael. 1982. "Living with Kaposi's." *Body Politic* 88 (November): 1–5.

Lynch, Michael, and Steve Woolgar. eds. 1990. *Representation in Scientific Practice.* Cambridge, Mass.: MIT Press.

MacCormack, Carol P., and Marilyn Strathern, eds. 1980. *Nature, Culture and Gender.* Cambridge: Cambridge University Press.

Mack, Arien, ed. 1988. "In Time of Plagues: The History and Social Consequences of Lethal Epidemic Diseases." Special issue. *Social Research* 55, no. 3 (Autumn).

MacNeil, Nancy. 1997. "National Conference on Women and HIV: The Epidemic Is Not Over." *Being Alive Newsletter*, June, 1, 14.

Macro Systems. 1990. *Final Report: Case Study of National AIDS Mailer, Understanding AIDS*. Atlanta, February. Available from Macro Systems, 3 Corporate Square, Atlanta GA 30329.

Mager, Donald. 1986. "The Discourse about Homophobia, Male and Female Contexts." Paper presented at the annual meeting of the Modern Language Association, December, New York.

Maggenti, Maria, ed. 1989. *ACT UP Women's Caucus Women and AIDS Handbook*. New York: ACT UP..

Mahar, Maggie. 1989. "Pitiless Scourge: Separating Out Hype from Hope on AIDS." *Baron's*, 13 March, 6–7, 16, 18, 22–24, 26.

Mains, Geoff. 1985. *Urban Aboriginals: A Celebration of Leathersexuality*. San Francisco: Gay Sunshine.

Malmsheimer, Richard. 1988. *"Doctors Only": The Evolving Image of the American Physician*. New York: Greenwood.

"Managing Our Miracles." 1989. "Frontline." New York: PBS.

Manegold, Catherine S. 1992. "No More Nice Girls: Radical Feminists Just Want to Have Impact." *New York Times*, 12 July, A-20.

Mann, Denise, and Lynn Spigel. 1988. "Television and the Female Viewer." Special issue, *Camera Obscura* 16: 5–7.

Mann, Jonathan M., et al. 1988a. "AIDS Monitor." *New Scientist*, 4 February, 32.

Mann, Jonathan M., et al. 1988b. "The International Epidemiology of AIDS." *Scientific American*, October, 82–89.

Mann, Jonathan, and Daniel J. M. Tarantola, eds. 1996. *AIDS and the World II: Global Dimensions, Social Roots, and Responses*. New York: Oxford University Press.

Mannheim, Karl [1936] 1985. *Ideology and Utopia*. Reprint, New York: Harcourt Brace Jovanovich.

Mannion, Bill. 1997. "Drug Pricing Program Threatened." *Being Alive Newsletter*, June, 13.

Manor, Robert. 1989. "The Language of AIDS." *St. Louis Post-Dispatch*, 1 April, D-1.

Marcus, George E. 1986. "Contemporary Problems of Ethnography in the Modern World System." In *Writing Culture*, ed. James Clifford and George E. Marcus. Berkeley: University of California Press.

Marcus, George E., and Michael M. J. Fischer. 1986. *Anthropology as Cultural Critique: An Experimental Moment in the Human Sciences*. Chicago: University of Chicago Press.

"The Marketplace of HIV/AIDS." 1996. *Science* 272, 28 June, 1880–81

Marmor, Michael, et. al. 1986. "Possible Female-to-Female Transmission of Human Immunodeficiency Virus." Letter to the editor, *Annals of Internal Medicine* 105 (December): 969.

Marshall, Patricia A., and Linda A. Bennett. 1990. "Anthropological Contributions to AIDS Research." *Medical Anthropological Quarterly* 4, no. 1: 3–5.

Marshall, Patricia A., and J. Paul O'Keefe. 1995. "Medical Students' First-Person Narratives of a Patient's Story of AIDS." *Social Science and Medicine* 40, no. 1: 67–76.

Marshall, Stuart. 1989. "Don't Blame Me." *Positively Healthy* 2 (March): 13–14.

Marshall, Stuart, director. 1984. *Bright Eyes*. London: Channel 4.

Martin, Emily. 1987. *The Woman in the Body: A Cultural Analysis of Reproduction.* Boston: Beacon.

Martin, Emily. 1988. "The Cultural Construction of Gendered Bodies: Biology and Metaphors of Production and Destruction." Paper presented at the Vega Day Symposium in Honor of Fredrik Barth, Swedish Society for Anthropology and Geography, 25 April, Stockholm.

Martin, Emily. 1994. *Flexible Bodies: Tracking Immunity in American Culture from the Days of Polio to the Age of AIDS.* Boston: Beacon.

Martin, William G. 1997. *Tuskegee 2? Africa, AIDS, and Us: An ACAS Members' Briefing Packet.* Urbana: University of Illinois, 27 November.

Marx, Jean L. 1984. "Strong New Candidate for AIDS Agent." Research News. *Science* 230 (4 May): 146–51.

Marx, Jean L. 1986a. "AIDS Virus Has New Name—Perhaps." News and Comment, *Science*, 9 May, 699–700.

Marx, Jean L. 1986b. "New Relatives of AIDS Virus Found." Research News, *Science*, 11 April, 540.

Masland, Tom. 1988. "AIDS Threat Turns Shore Leave into Naval Exercise in Caution." *Chicago Tribune*, 17 March, A-13.

Mason, Patrick J., Roberta A. Olson, and Kathy L. Parish. 1988. "AIDS, Hemophilia, and Prevention Efforts within a Comprehensive Care Program." *American Psychologist* 43: 971–76.

Mass, Lawrence D. 1982. "AIDS and What to Do about It." *Gay Community News*, 25 September, 1.

Mass, Lawrence D. 1990. *Homosexuality and Sexuality: Dialogues of the Sexual Revolution.* New York: Harrington Park.

Mass, Lawrence D. [1983] 1997. "Blood and Politics." In *We Are Everywhere: A Historical Sourcebook of Gay and Lesbian Politics*, ed. M. Blasius and S. Phelan. New York: Routledge.

Massa, Robert. 1987. "Why AIDS Activists Target the FDA." *Village Voice*, 18 October, 25.

Masters, William, Virginia Johnson, and Robert C. Kolodny. 1988. *Crisis: Heterosexual Behavior in the Age of AIDS.* New York: Grove.

Mathews, Holly F. 1987. "Doctors and Rootdoctors: Ethnomedicine and the American Medical System." Duplicated paper in the author's files.

Matthews, Gene W., and Verla S. Neslund. 1987. "The Initial Impact of AIDS on Public Health Law in the United States–1986." *Journal of the American Medical Association* 257 (6 January): 344–52.

Maupin, Armistead. 1987. *Significant Others.* New York: Harper and Row.

May, R. M., R. M. Anderson, and A. M. Johnson. 1988. "Patterns of Infectiousness and the Transmission of HIV-1." In *AIDS 1988: AAAS Symposia Papers*, ed. Ruth Kulstad. Washington, D.C.: American Association for the Advancement of Science.

Mayo, Cris. 1997. "Disputing the Subject of Sex: Sexual Identity and School Controversy, New York State, 1986–1993." Ed.D. diss., University of Illinois at Urbana-Champaign.

Mays, Vickie M., and Susan D. Cochran. 1988. "Issues in the Perception of AIDS Risk and Risk Reduction Activities by Black and Hispanic/Latina Women." *American Psychologist* 43: 949–57.

McAllister, Matthew Paul. 1989. "Medicalization in the News Media: A Comparison of AIDS Coverage in Three Newspapers." Ph.D. diss., University of Illinois at Urbana-Champaign.

McAuliffe, Kathleen, et al. 1987. "AIDS: At the Dawn of Fear." *U.S. News and World Report*, 12 January, 60–69.

McCarty, Mary. 1985. "AIDS in Cincinnati: Are We Ready?" *Cincinnati Magazine*, December, 56–60.

McGee, Daniel E. 1996. "Emerging Meanings: Science, the Media, and Infectious Diseases." *Journal of the American Medical Association* 276, no. 13 (2 October): 1095–97.

McGrath, Mark, and Bob Sutcliffe. 1987. "Insuring Profits from AIDS: The Economics of an Epidemic." *Radical America* 20, no. 6: 9–27.

McGrath, Michael S., et al. 1989. "GLQ223: An Inhibitor of Human Immunodeficiency Virus Replication in Acutely and Chronically Infected Cells of Lymphocyte and Mononuclear Phagocyte Lineage." *Proceedings of the National Academy of Sciences* 86 (15 April): 2844–48.

McGrath, Roberta. 1984. "Medical Police." *Ten.8*, no. 14: 13–18.

McGrath, Roberta. 1990. "Dangerous Liaisons: Health, Disease, and Representations." In *Ecstatic Antibodies: Revisiting the AIDS Mythology*, ed. Tessa Boffin and Sunil Gupta. London: Rivers Oram.

McKusick, Leon, ed. 1987. *What to Do about AIDS: Physicians and Mental Health Professionals Discuss the Issues.* Berkeley: University of California Press.

Mendez, Carlos. 1997. "Rebel Yell: Gabriel Rotello's Controversial New Book Calls for an End to Promiscuity as a Way of Stopping AIDS." *Frontiers*, May, 49–86.

Menzies, Christina. 1988. "She Weds AIDS Victim—and Even Has His Baby!" *National Enquirer*, 12 September, 42.

Mercer, Kobena. 1992. "'1968': Periodizing Politics and Identity." In *Cultural Studies*, ed. Lawrence Grossberg, Cary Nelson, and Paula A. Treichler. New York: Routledge.

Meredith, Ann. 1992. "Until the Last Breath." In *AIDS: The Making of a Chronic Disease*, ed. Elizabeth Fee and Daniel M. Fox. Berkeley: University of California Press.

Merritt, Deborah Jones. 1986. "Communicable Diseases and Constitutional Law: Controlling AIDS." *New York University Law Review* 61 (November): 739–99.

Merson, Michael. 1993. "Women and Children with HIV: The Global Experience. Paper presented at the Second International Conference on HIV, 7 September, Edinburgh.

Meyer, Klemens B., and Stephen G. Pauker. 1987. "Screening for HIV: Can We Afford the False Positive Rate?" *New England Journal of Medicine* 317 (23 July): 238–41.

Meyer, Richard. 1989. "Rock Hudson's Body." In *Inside/Out: Lesbian Theories, Gay Theories*, ed. Diana Fuss. New York: Routledge.

Meyer, Richard. 1995. "This Is To Enrage You: Gran Fury and the Graphics of AIDS Activism." *But Is It Art?*, ed. Nina Felshin. Seattle: Bay.

Michaels, Spencer, producer. 1989. *AIDS: Drug Dilemma.* "MacNeil-Lehrer Newshour." New York: PBS, 2 May.

Miller, D. A. 1989. "Sontag's Urbanity." *October* 49: 91–101. Review of *AIDS and Its Metaphors*, by Susan Sontag.

Miller, J. Hillis. 1990. "Narrative." In *Critical Terms for Literary Study*, ed. Frank Lentricchia and Thomas McLaughlin. Chicago: University of Chicago Press.

Miller, James, ed. 1992. *Fluid Exchanges: Artists and Critics in the AIDS Crisis*. Toronto: University of Toronto Press.

Miller, Judith. 1986. "Prostitutes Make Appeal for AIDS Prevention." *New York Times*, 5 October, 6.

Miller, Norman, and Richard C. Rockwell, eds. 1988. *AIDS in Africa: The Social and Policy Impact*. Lewiston, N.Y.: Edwin Mellen.

Millman, Marcia. 1975. "She Did It All for Love: A Feminist View of the Sociology of Deviance." In *Another Voice: Feminist Perspectives on Social Life and Social Deviance*, ed. Marcia Millman and Rosabeth Moss Kanter. Garden City, N.Y.: Anchor, Doubleday.

Millman, Marcia, and Rosabeth Moss Kanter, eds. 1975. *Another Voice: Feminist Perspectives on Social Life and Social Deviance*. Garden City, N.Y.: Anchor, Doubleday.

Minkowitz, Donna. 1989. "Safe and Sappho: An AIDS Primer for Lesbians." *Village Voice*, 21 February, 21.

Minkowitz, Donna. [1990] 1997. "ACT UP at a Crossroads." In *We Are Everywhere*, ed. Mark Blasius and Shane Phelan. New York: Routledge.

Minson, Jeff. 1981. "The Assertion of Homosexuality." *m/f* 5–6: 19–39.

Mitchell, Janet L. 1988. "Women, AIDS and Public Policy." *AIDS and Public Policy Journal* 3, no. 2: 75–86.

Mitchell, Janet L. 1993. "Women and HIV/AIDS." Paper presented to the Second Annual Conference on Women and HIV, 14 November, Los Angeles.

Mohammed, Juanita. 1992. "WAVE in the Media Environment: Camcorder Activism in AIDS Education." *Camera Obscura* 28: 152–55.

Mohanty, Chandra Talpade. 1984. "Under Western Eyes: Feminist Scholarship and Colonial Discourses." *Boundary 2* 12, no. 3/13, no. 1: 333–58.

Mohr, Richard. 1986. "Of Deathbeds and Quarantines: AIDS Funding, Gay Life and State Coercion." *Raritan*, Summer, 38–62.

Moi, Toril. 1985. *Sexual/Textual Politics: Feminist Literary Theory*. New York: Methuen.

Monette, Jean-Françoise, and Peter T. Boullata. 1995. *Anatomy of Desire*. Montreal: National Film Board of Canada and Bare Bones Films. Video.

Montagnier, L., et al. 1984. "A New Human T-Lymphotropic Retrovirus: Characterization and Possible Role in Lymphadenopathy and Acquired Immune Deficiency Syndromes." In *Human T-Cell Leukemia/Lymphoma Virus*, ed. Robert C. Gallo, M. E. Essex, and L. Gross. Cold Spring Harbor, N.Y.: Cold Spring Harbor Laboratory.

Moore, Alexander, and Ronald LeBaron. 1986. "The Case for a Haitian Origin of the AIDS Epidemic." In *The Social Dimension of AIDS*, ed. Douglas A. Feldman and Thomas M. Johnson. New York: Praeger.

Moore, Lisa Jean. 1997. " 'It's Like You Use Pots and Pans to Cook. It's the Tool': The Technologies of Safer Sex." *Science, Technology, and Human Values* 22, no. 4: 434–71.

Moore, Lisa Jean, and Adele E. Clarke. 1995. "Clitoral Conventions and Transgressions: Graphic Representations in Anatomy Texts c. 1900–1991." *Feminist Studies* 21, no. 2 (Summer): 255–301.

Morgan, Tracy. 1993. "Butch-Femme and the Politics of Identity." In *Sisters, Sexperts, Queers*, ed. A. Stein. New York: Plume/Penguin.

Morganthau, Tom, et al. 1986. "Future Shock." *Newsweek*, 24 November, 30–39.

Morse, Stephen S. 1992. "AIDS and Beyond: Defining the Rules for Viral Traffic." In *AIDS: The Making of a Chronic Disease*, ed. Elizabeth Fee and Daniel M. Fox. Berkeley: University of California Press.

Mudimbe, V. Y. 1988. *The Invention of Africa: Gnosis, Philosophy, and the Order of Knowledge*. Bloomington: Indiana University Press.

Murphy, Timothy F., and Suzanne Poirier, eds. 1992. *Writing AIDS: Gay Literature, Language, and Analysis*. New York: Columbia University Press.

Murray, Marea. 1985. "Too Little AIDS Coverage." Letter to the editor, *Sojourner* 10, no. 9 (July): 3.

Musto, Michael. 1987. "Mandatory Macho." *Village Voice*, 30 June, 30.

Nanda, Serena. 1996. "The Hijras of India." In *A Queer World: The Center for Lesbian and Gay Studies Reader*, ed. Martin Duberman. New York: New York University Press.

"National Gay Task Force, Others, Decry Gay Blood Ban by National Hemophilia Foundation." 1983. *Advocate*, 20 January, 8.

National Minority AIDS Council. 1992. *The Impact of HIV on Communities of Color: A Blueprint for the Nineties*. Washington, D.C.: National Minority AIDS Council.

Nelkin, Dorothy. 1984. "Background Paper." In *Science in the Streets: Report of the Twentieth Century Fund Task Force on the Communication of Scientific Risk*. New York: Priority.

Nelkin, Dorothy. 1985. "Managing Biomedical News." *Social Research* 52: 3.

Nelkin, Dorothy. 1987a. "AIDS and the Social Sciences: Review of Useful Knowledge and Research Needs." *Reviews of Infectious Diseases* 9, no. 5: 980–86.

Nelkin, Dorothy. 1987b. *Selling Science: How the Press Covers Science and Technology*. New York: W. H. Freeman.

Nelkin, Dorothy, David P. Willis, and Scott V. Parris, eds. 1991. *A Disease of Society: Cultural and Institutional Responses to AIDS*. Cambridge: Cambridge University Press.

Nelson, Cary. 1985. "Envoys of Otherness: Differences and Continuity in Feminist Criticism." In *For Alma Mater: Theory and Practice in Feminist Scholarship*, ed. Paula A. Treichler, Cheris Kramarae, and Beth Stafford. Urbana: University of Illinois Press.

Netter, Thomas W. 1986. "Cases of AIDS Rise around the World." *New York Times*, 5 October, A-7.

Netter, Thomas W. 1987. "AIDS Spurs Countries to Act as Cases Rise around World." *New York Times*, 22 March 18.

"New Human Retroviruses: One Causes AIDS . . . and the Other Does Not." 1986. *Nature* 320 (3 April): 385.

New York City Task Force on AIDS. 1991. *Policy Document*. New York.

Ng'weno, Hilary. 1987. "The Politics of AIDS in Kenya." *Weekly Review*, 4 September.

Nichols, Eve K. 1986. *Mobilizing against AIDS: The Unfinished Story of a Virus*. Cambridge, Mass.: Harvard University Press.

Nichols, Eve K. 1989. *Mobilizing against AIDS: Newly Revised and Enlarged*. Cambridge, Mass.: Harvard University Press.

Nixon, Nicholas, and Bebe Nixon. 1991. *People with AIDS*. Boston: David R. Godine.

Nordheimer, Jon. 1987. "US Officials Criticized on Efforts to Curb AIDS among Minorities." *New York Times*, 10 August, A-1.

Nordland, Rod, with Ray Wilkinson and Ruth Marshall. 1986. "Africa in the Plague Years." *Newsweek,* 24 November, 44–47.

Norman, Colin. 1986. "A New Twist in AIDS Patent Fight." News and Comment, *Science,* 18 April, 308–9.

Norsigian, Judy. 1996. "The Woman's Health Movement in the United States." *Man-Made Medicine,* ed. Kary L. Moss. Durham, N.C.: Duke University Press.

Norton, Robert, and Jim Hughey, eds. 1990. Special issue, *Communication Research* 17, no. 6: 733–870.

Norton, Robert, Judith Schwartzbaum, and John Whear. 1990. "Language Discrimination of General Physicians: AIDS Metaphors Used in the AIDS Crisis." Special issue, *Communication Research* 17, no. 6: 809–26.

Norwood, Chris. 1985. "AIDS Is Not for Men Only." *Mademoiselle,* September, 198–99, 293–96.

Norwood, Chris. 1986. "Heterosexuals: A New Risk Group." *Village Voice,* 27 May, 19–22.

Norwood, Chris. 1987. *Advice for Life: A Woman's Guide to AIDS Risks and Prevention.* New York: Pantheon.

Norwood, Chris. 1988. "How Real Is *Your* Risk?" *Self,* June, 148–51.

Novick, Alvin. 1987. "Ethical Considerations in Risk Reduction Advising." In *Biobehavioral Control of AIDS,* ed. D. G. Ostrow. New York: Irvington.

Novick, Michael. 1995. *White Lies/White Power.* Monroe, Maine: Common Courage.

Null, Gary, with Trudy Golobic. 1987. "The Secret Battle against AIDS." *Penthouse,* June, 61–68.

Nussbaum, Bruce. 1990. *Good Intentions: How Big Business and the Medical Establishment Have Corrupted the Fight against AIDS.* New York: Atlantic Monthly Press.

O'Connor, John J. 1991a. "Birds Do It, Bees Do It, So Does TV." *New York Times,* 13 October, 29.

O'Connor, John J. 1991b. "Gay Images: TV's Mixed Signals." *New York Times,* 19 May, sec. 2, p. 2.

O'Connor, John J. 1991c. "Three Shows about AIDS (Straight AIDS, That Is)." *New York Times,* 11 April, C-15.

O'Dair, Barbara. 1983. "Anatomy of a Media Epidemic." *Alternative Media* 14, no. 3: 10–13.

Odets, Walt. 1995. *In the Shadow of the Epidemic: Being HIV Negative in the Age of AIDS.* Durham, N.C.: Duke University Press.

Odets, Walt. 1996. "On the Need for a Gay Reconstruction of Public Health." In *A Queer World: The Center for Lesbian and Gay Studies Reader,* ed. Martin Duberman. New York: New York University Press.

Office of Technology Assessment. 1982. *World Population and Fertility Planning Technologies: The Next Twenty Years.* Washington, D.C.: Congress of the United States.

Office of Technology Assessment. 1985. *Review of the Public Health Service's Response to AIDS: A Technical Memorandum.* Washington, D.C.: U.S. Government Printing Office.

"Official Warns of 'Racist, Fascist' Approaches to AIDS." 1987. *American Medical News,* 12 June, 19.

Okware, Samuel I. 1988. "Planning AIDS Education for the Public in Uganda." In *AIDS Prevention and Control: Invited Presentations and Papers from the World Summit of Ministers of Health on Programmes for AIDS Prevention.* Geneva: World Health Organization; Oxford: Pergamon.

Oleske, James, et al. 1983. "Immune Deficiency Syndrome in Children." *Journal of the American Medical Association* 249: 2345–49.

Oppenheimer, Gerald M. 1988. "In the Eye of the Storm." In *AIDS: The Burdens of History*, ed. Elizabeth Fee and Daniel M. Fox. Berkeley: University of California Press.

Oppenheimer, Gerald M. 1992. "Causes, Cases, and Cohorts: The Role of Epidemiology in the Historical Construction of AIDS." In *AIDS: The Making of a Chronic Disease*, ed. Elizabeth Fee and Daniel M. Fox. Berkeley: University of California Press.

Oppenheimer, Joshua, and Helena Reckitt, eds. 1997. *Acting on AIDS: Sex, Drugs, and Politics.* London: Serpent's Tail.

Ortleb, Charles L. 1982. "The Politics of AIDS." *New York Native*, 16 August, 1.

Ortleb, Charles L. 1987. "HBLV in Lake Tahoe: Disease Worse than Originally Thought: Is It AIDS?" *New York Native*, 11 May, 6–8.

Ortleb, Charles. 1997. "Why AIDS Is Really AIDSgate." In *We Are Everywhere: A Historical Sourcebook of Gay and Lesbian Politics*, ed. M. Blasius and S. Phelan. New York: Routledge.

Ortony, Anthony, ed. 1979. *Metaphor and Thought.* Cambridge: Cambridge University Press.

Osborn, June E. 1986. "The AIDS Epidemic: An Overview of the Science." *Issues in Science and Technology* 2, no. 2: 40–55.

Ostrow, David G., ed. 1987a. *Biobehavioral Control of AIDS.* New York: Irvington.

Ostrow, David G. 1987b. "Implications for Prevention of AIDS Transmission among the Heterosexual Population." In *Biobehavioral Control of AIDS*, ed. David G. Ostrow. New York: Irvington.

Ostrow, David G. 1987c. Introduction to *Biobehavioral Control of AIDS*, ed. David G. Ostrow. New York: Irvington.

Ostrow, David G. 1987d. "To Test or Not to Test, That Appears to Be the Question." In *Biobehavioral Control of AIDS*, ed. David G. Ostrow. New York: Irvington.

Ostrow, David G., ed. 1990. *Behavioral Aspects of AIDS.* New York: Plenum.

Ostrow, David G., Steven L. Solomon, Kenneth H. Mayer, and Harry Haverkos. 1987. "Classification of the Clinical Spectrum of HIV Infection in Adults." In *Information on AIDS for the Practicing Physician*, vol. 1. Chicago: American Medical Association.

O'Sullivan, Sue, and Pratibha Parmar. 1992. *Lesbians Talk (Safer Sex).* London: Scarlett.

O'Sullivan, Sue, and Kate Thomson, eds. [1992] 1996. *Positively Women Living with AIDS.* Reprint, London: Pandora.

Oudshoorn, Nelly. 1994. *Beyond the Natural Body: An Archeology of Sex Hormones.* London: Routledge.

Oudshoorn, Nelly. 1996. "A Natural Order of Things? Reproduction, Science and the Politics of Othering." In *Future/Natural: Nature/Science/Culture*, ed. George Robertson et al. London: Routledge.

Our Sons. 1991. "ABC Movie of the Week." New York: ABC, 19 May.

Over, M., et al. 1988. "The Direct and Indirect Costs of HIV Infection in Developing Countries: The Cases of Zaire and Tanzania." Paper presented at the International Conference on the Global Impact of AIDS, 8–10 March, London.

Owens, Craig. 1987. "Outlaws: Gay Men in Feminism." In *Men in Feminism*, ed. Alice Jardine and Paul Smith. New York: Methuen.

Packard, Randall M., and Paul Epstein. 1992. "Medical Research on AIDS in Africa: A Historical Perspective." In *AIDS: The Making of a Chronic Disease*, ed. Elizabeth Fee and Daniel M. Fox. Berkeley: University of California Press.

Packer, Cathy, and Susan Kauffman. 1990. "Reregulation of Commercial Television: Implications for the Coverage of AIDS." *AIDS and Public Policy Journal* 5, no. 2: 82–88.

Padgug, Robert. 1988. "More than the Story of a Virus." *Radical America* 22 nos. 2–3: 35–42.

Padgug, Robert A., and Gerald M. Oppenheimer. 1992. "Riding the Tiger: AIDS and the Gay Community." In *AIDS: The Making of a Chronic Disease*, ed. Elizabeth Fee and Daniel M. Fox. Berkeley: University of California Press.

Pally, Marcia. 1985. "AIDS and the Politics of Despair: Lighting Our Own Funeral Pyre." *Advocate*, 24 December, 8.

Panem, Sandra. 1985. "AIDS: Public Policy and Biomedical Research." Special supplement, *Hastings Central Report* 15, no. 4 (August): 23–26.

Panem, Sandra. 1988. *The AIDS Bureaucracy: Why Society Failed to Meet the AIDS Crisis and How We Might Improve*. Cambridge, Mass.: Harvard University Press.

Pankhurst, Christabel. [1913] 1987. "The Great Scourge and How to End It." In *Suffrage and the Pankhursts*, ed. Jane Marcus. London: Routledge.

Panos Institute. 1986. *AIDS and the Third World*. London: Panos Institute in association with the Norwegian Red Cross; Philadelphia: New Society.

Panos Institute. 1990. *The Third Epidemic: Repercussions of the Fear of AIDS*. London: Panos Institute.

Parker, Richard. 1987. "Acquired Immunodeficiency Syndrome in Brazil." *Medical Anthropology Quarterly* 1, no. 2: 155–75.

Parker, Richard. 1991. *Bodies, Pleasures, and Passions: Sexual Culture in Contemporary Brazil*. Boston: Beacon.

Parker, Richard. 1992. "Sexual Diversity, Cultural Analysis, and AIDS Education in Brazil." In *The Time of AIDS: Social Analysis, Theory and Method*, ed. Gilbert H. Herdt and Shirley Lindenbaum. Newbury Park, Calif.: Sage.

Parmar, Pratibha. 1989. "Other Kinds of Dreams." *Feminist Review* 31 (Spring): 55–65.

Parmar, Pratibha, producer. 1987. *Reframing AIDS*. New York: Video Data Bank. Video.

Pastore, Judith Laurence, ed. 1993. *Confronting AIDS through Literature: The Responsibilities of Representation*. Urbana: University of Illinois Press.

Patton, Cindy. 1983. "National Gay Task Force, Others, Decry Gay Blood Ban by National Hemophilia Foundation." *Advocate*, 20 January, 8.

Patton, Cindy. 1985a. "Feminists Have Avoided the Issue of AIDS." *Sojourner* (October): 19–20.

Patton, Cindy. 1985b. *Sex and Germs: The Politics of AIDS*. Boston: South End.

Patton, Cindy. 1987. "Resistance and the Erotic: Reclaiming History, Setting Strategy as We Face AIDS." *Radical America* 20, no. 6: 68–78.

Patton, Cindy. 1989. "AIDS and Gender Issues." Paper presented at the conference "Opportunities for Solidarity," 2–4 June, Montreal.

Patton, Cindy. 1990. *Inventing AIDS*. New York: Routledge.

Patton, Cindy. 1994. *Last Served: Gendering the HIV Epidemic*. New York: Taylor and Francis.

Patton, Cindy. 1995. "Between Innocence and Safety: Epidemiologic and Popular Constructions of Young People's Need for Safe Sex." *Deviant Bodies: Critical Perspectives on Difference in Science and Popular Culture*, ed. Jennifer Terry and Jacqueline Urla. Bloomington: Indiana University Press.

Patton, Cindy. 1996. *Fatal Advice: How Safe-Sex Education Went Wrong*. Durham, N.C.: Duke University Press.

Patton, Cindy. 1997. "Queer Peregrinations." In *Acting on AIDS*, ed. Joshua Oppenheimer and Helena Reckitt. London: Serpent's Tail.

Patton, Cindy, and Janis Kelly. [1987] 1990. *Making It: A Woman's Guide to Sex in the Age of AIDS*. Rev. ed. Boston: Firebrand.

Payer, Lynn. 1988. *Medicine and Culture: Varieties of Treatment in the United States, England, West Germany, and France*. New York: Henry Holt.

Pear, Robert. 1986. "Ten-Fold Increase in AIDS Death Toll Is Expected by '91." *New York Times*, 13 June, A-1.

Pear, Robert. 1987a. "Three Health Care Workers Found Infected by Blood of Patients with AIDS." *New York Times*, 20 May, A-1.

Pear, Robert. 1987b. "U.S. Seeks to Bar Aliens with AIDS." *New York Times*, 27 March, A-18.

Pearl, Monica. 1991. "Lesbian Sexual Behavior and AIDS." Letter to the editor, *Gay Community News*, 15–21 December, 12.

Pearl, Monica. 1992. "Heterosexual Women and AIDS." In *Women, AIDS, and Activism*, ed. ACT UP New York Women and AIDS Book Group. Boston: South End.

Pearson, Rick. 1997. "Illinois AIDS Cases Edge Upward; African-Americans Hit Hardest." *Chicago Tribune*, 7 February, 1.

Penelhum, Terence. 1967. "Personal Identity." In *Encyclopedia of Philosophy*, vol. 5, ed. Paul Edwards. New York: Macmillan/Free Press.

Penelope, Julia. 1997. "Wimmin- and Lesbian-Only Spaces: Thought into Action." In *We Are Everywhere: A Historical Sourcebook of Gay and Lesbian Politics*, ed. M. Blasius and S. Phelan. New York: Routledge.

Penley, Constance. 1989. *The Future of an Illusion: Film, Feminism, and Psychoanalysis*. Minneapolis: University of Minnesota Press.

Penley, Constance. 1997. *Nasa/Trek: Popular Science and Sex in America*. London: Verso.

People with AIDS Coalition of New York. 1995. *Newsline*. Special section on AIDS/HIV and pregnancy (July–August): 6–32.

Perkins, R., G. Prestage, R. Sharpe, and F. Lovejoy, eds. 1994. *Sex Work and Sex Workers in Australia*. Sydney: University of New South Wales Press.

Perlez, Jane. 1988a. "Africans Weigh Threat of AIDS to Economies." *New York Times*, 22 September, A-16.

Perlez, Jane. 1988b. "Scientists from Western Countries Pressing for AIDS Studies in Africa." *New York Times*, 18 September, B-5.

Perlman, David. 1989. "The Print Media's Response to AIDS." Paper presented at the conference "AIDS: Communication Challenges," held in conjunction with the annual meeting of the International Communication Association, 27 May, San Francisco.

Petchesky, Rosalind Pollack. 1987. "Foetal Images: The Power of Visual Culture in the Politics of Reproduction." In *Reproductive Technologies: Gender, Motherhood, Medicine*, ed. Michelle Stanworth. Minneapolis: University of Minnesota Press.

Peters, Cynthia, and Karen Struening. 1988. "Talking with Women about AIDS." *Zeta,*
   July/August, 133–37.
Petersen, Alan, and Robin Bunton, eds. 1997. *Foucault, Health and Medicine.* New York:
   Routledge.
Picard, Andre. 1989. "Sole Cause of AIDS Queried by Doctor." *Toronto Globe and Mail,*
   8 June, A-12.
Pickering, Andrew. 1995. *The Mangle of Practice: Time, Agency and Science.* Chicago:
   University of Chicago Press.
Pierce, Kenneth M. 1986. "Nowhere to Run, Nowhere to Hide." *Time,* 1 September, 36.
Piot, Peter, et al. 1984. "Acquired Immunodeficiency Syndrome in a Heterosexual Popu-
   lation in Zaire." *Lancet* 2: 65–69.
Piot, Peter, et al. 1988. "AIDS: An International Perspective." *Science* 239: 573–79.
Piot, Peter. 1996. "AIDS: A Global Response." *Science* 272, 28 June, 1855.
Planned Parenthood of America. 1986. "They Did It 9,000 Times on Television Last Year:
   How Come Nobody Got Pregnant?" Advertisement, *Urbana-Champaign News-*
   Gazette, 7 December, A-15.
Plant, Martin, ed. 1990. *AIDS, Drugs, and Prostitution.* London: Routledge.
"Playing It Safe: A Symposium on And the Band Played On." 1994. *Journal of Health*
   Politics, Policy and Law 19, no. 2 (Summer): 449–63.
Pletsch, Carl E. 1981. "The Three Worlds, or the Division of Social Scientific Labor,
   circa 1950–1975." *Comparative Studies in Society and History* 23, no. 4: 565–90.
Poggi, Stephanie. 1987. "*In These Times*: With Friends Like Us, Who Nee [*sic*]." *Gay*
   Community News, 12–13 July, 3.
Poirier, Suzanne, and Louis Borgenicht. 1991. "Physician-Authors—Prophets or Profit-
   eers?" *New England Journal of Medicine* 325, no. 3 (18 July): 212–14.
Pollack, Michael. 1988. *Les homosexuels et le SIDA: Sociologie d'une épidémic.* Paris:
   A. M. Metailie.
Poovey, Mary. 1987. "'Scenes of an Indelicate Character': The Medical 'Treatment' of
   Women." In *The Making of the Modern Body: Sexuality and Society in the Nine-*
   teenth Century, ed. Catherine Gallagher and Thomas Laqueur. Berkeley: University
   of California Press.
Poovey, Mary. 1988. *Uneven Developments: The Ideological Work of Gender in Mid-*
   Victorian England. Chicago: University of Chicago Press.
Poovey, Mary. 1990. "Speaking of the Body: Mid-Victorian Constructions of Female De-
   sire." In *Body/Politics: Women and the Discourses of Science,* ed. Mary Jacobus,
   Evelyn Fox Keller, and Sally Shuttleworth. New York: Routledge.
Poovey, Mary. 1991. Review of *The Body and the Text: Comparative Essays in Literature*
   and Medicine, ed. Bruce Clark and Wendell Aycock. *Bulletin of the History of Medi-*
   cine 65: 291–92.
Potterat, John J., et al. 1987. "Lying to Military Physicians about Risk Factors of HIV
   Infections." Letter to the editor, *Journal of the American Medical Association* 257,
   no. 13 (3 April): 1727.
Pratt, Mary Louise. 1986. "Fieldwork in Common Places." In *Writing Culture,* ed. James
   Clifford and George E. Marcus. Berkeley: University of California Press.
Presidential Commission on the Human Immunodeficiency Virus Epidemic. 1988. *Re-*
   port of the Presidential Commission on the Human Immunodeficiency Virus Epi-
   demic. Washington, D.C.: U.S. Government Printing Office.

President's Commission for the Study of Ethical Problems in Medicine and Biomedical and Behavioral Research. 1983. *Final Report of the President's Commission for the Study of Ethical Problems in Medicine and Biomedical and Behavioral Research.* Washington, D.C.: U.S. Government Printing Office.

Prewitt, Kenneth. 1988. "AIDS in Africa: The Triple Disaster." In *AIDS in Africa: The Social and Policy Impact,* ed. Norman Miller and Richard C. Rockwell. Lewiston, N.Y.: Edwin Mellen.

"Pro and Con: Free Needles to Addicts." 1987. Editorial, *New York Times,* 20 December, 20.

Public Media Center. 1995. *AIDS Stigma and Discrimination: The Attitudes of National Experts and Influentials.* New York: Public Media Center in association with the Ford Foundation and the Joyce Mertz-Gilmore Foundation.

Putnam, Hilary. 1975. *Philosophical Papers.* 2 vols. Cambridge: Cambridge University Press.

PWA Coalition of New York. 1995. "AIDS/HIV and Pregnancy." *PWA Newsline,* July/August, 6–32.

Quick, Linda S. 1986. *AIDS in South Florida and Miami, Florida.* Washington, D.C.: Library of Congress.

Quindlen, Anna. 1987. "For Women, the Condom Campaign Is a Bit Tardy." *New York Times,* 17 June, 19.

Quinn, Thomas C., et al. 1986. "AIDS in Africa: An Epidemiologic Paradigm." *Science,* 21 November, 955–63.

Rabin, Steve. 1991. "Kenya: AIDS as If It Mattered." *Washington Post,* 17 November, C-5.

Raeburn, Paul. 1986. "Doctor Faces Politics of AIDS Research." *Champaign-Urbana News-Gazette,* 25 January, A-8.

Randolph, Laura B. 1988. "The Hidden Fear: Black Women, Bisexuals and the AIDS Risk." *Ebony,* January, 120, 122, 123, 126.

Randolph, Laura B. 1997. "Cookie Johnson on the Magic 'Miracle': The Lord Has Healed Earvin." *Ebony,* April, 72–76.

Rapp, Rayna. 1988. "Chromosomes and Communication: The Discourse of Genetic Counseling." *Medical Anthropology Quarterly* 2: 143–57.

Ratafia, Manny, and Frederick I. Scott Jr. 1987. "AIDS: A Glimpse of Its Impact." *American Clinical Products Review,* May, 26–29.

Raymond, Chris Anne. 1988. "Combating a Deadly Combination: Intravenous Drug Abuse, Acquired Immunodeficiency Syndrome." *Journal of the American Medical Association* 259 (15 January): 329–32.

Reagan, Leslie. 1996. *When Abortion Was a Crime: The Legal and Medical Regulation of Abortion, Chicago, 1880–1973.* Berkeley and Los Angeles: University of California Press.

Rechy, John. 1983. "An Exchange on AIDS." *New York Review of Books,* 15 October, 43–45. Letter to the editor, with reply by Jonathan Lieberson.

Redfield, Robert R., and Donald S. Burke. [1988] 1989. "HIV Infection: The Clinical Picture." In *The Science of AIDS.* New York: W. H. Freeman.

Redfield, Robert R., et al. 1985. "Heterosexually Acquired HTLV-III/LAV Disease (AIDS-Related Complex and AIDS): Epidemiologic Evidence for Female-to-Male Transmission." *Journal of the American Medical Association* 254: 2094–96.

Redfield, Robert R., et al. 1986. "Female-to-Male Transmission of HTLV-III." *Journal of the American Medical Association* 255: 1705–6.

Red, Hot, and Blue. 1990. New York: ABC, 1 December.

Reed, Lori. 1992. "Turned On: A Feminist Critical Analysis of Sexually Explicit Computer Games." M.A. thesis, Ohio State University.

Reed, Paul. 1991. *The Q Journal: A Treatment Diary.* Berkeley, Calif.: Celestial Arts.

Reeves, Jimmy, and Richard Campbell. 1994. *Cracked Coverage: Television News, the Anti-Cocaine Crusade, and the Reagan Legacy.* Durham, N.C.: Duke University Press.

Regush, Nicholas. 1989a. "Focusing on the Cause of AIDS Is a Game of Cat and Mouse." *Montreal Gazette,* 6 June, A-12.

Regush, Nicholas. 1989b. "OK, Bob! Are You Going to Talk Turkey about HIV or Not?" *Montreal Gazette,* 8 June, 11.

Reid, Elizabeth. 1988. "Women and AIDS." *World Health,* March, 20–21.

Reinisch, June Machover, Stephanie A. Sanders, and Mary Ziemba-Davis. 1988. "The Study of Sexual Behavior in Relation to the Transmission of Human Immunodeficiency Virus: Caveats and Recommendations." *American Psychologist* 43: 921–27.

Relman, Arnold. 1985. "Introduction." Special supplement, *Hastings Center Report* 15, no. 4: 1–2.

Renaud, Michelle Lewis. 1996a. Research News. *AIDS and Anthropology Bulletin* 8, no. 4: 7–8.

Renaud, Michelle Lewis. 1996b. *Women at the Crossroads: A Prostitute Community's Response to AIDS in Urban Senegal.* New York: Gordon and Breach.

Rense, Jeffrey, ed. 1996. *AIDS Exposed: Secrets, Lies, and Myths.* Goleta, Calif.: BioAlert.

Restak, Richard. 1985. "AIDS Virus Has No Civil Rights." *Chicago Sun-Times,* 15 September, 1.

Rhodes, Richard. 1997. *Deadly Feasts: Tracking the Secrets of a Terrifying New Plague.* New York: Simon and Schuster.

Ribble, Denise. 1989. "Not Just another Article on Lesbian Safe Sex." *Sappho's Isle,* July, 15.

"Rich Nations Urged to Help Poor Lands Fight AIDS by Backing WHO Program." 1988. *Wall Street Journal,* 17 June, 4.

Richards, I. A. 1936. *The Philosophy of Rhetoric.* London: Oxford University Press.

Richardson, Diane. 1987. *Women and AIDS.* New York: Methuen.

Richardson, Patricia. 1997. "An Old Experiment's Legacy: Distrust of AIDS Treatment." *New York Times,* 21 April, A-1, A-9.

Ricklefs, Roger. 1988. "Gay-Rights Groups and Insurers Battle over Required AIDS Tests." *Wall Street Journal,* 26 April, 41.

Riding, Alan. 1987. "AIDS in Brazil: Taboo of Silence Ends." *New York Times,* 28 October, 8.

Rieder, Ines, and Patricia Ruppelt, eds. 1988. *AIDS: The Women.* Pittsburgh: Cleis.

Roberts, Steven V. 1987. "Politicians Awaken to the Threat of a Global Epidemic." *New York Times,* 7 June, sec. 6, p. 1.

Robertson, Claire, and Iris Berger. 1986. *Women and Class in Africa.* New York: Holmes and Meier.

Rodowick, David N. 1982. "The Difficulty of Difference." *Wide Angle* 5, no. 1: 4–15.

Rodriguez, Ernie. 1997. "Would You Like a Cocktail? (Cocktail of the 90's)." *Sexvibe,* April, 23–24.

Rogers, D. 1988. "AIDS Spreads to the Soaps, Sort Of." *New York Times*, 28 August, sec. 2, p. 29.

Rogers, Everett M. 1989. "The Diffusion of AIDS Information through the Electronic Media, 1981–1988." Paper presented at the conference "AIDS: Communication Challenges," held in conjunction with the annual meeting of the International Communication Association, 27 May, San Francisco.

Roof, Judith. 1996. "The Girl I Never Want to Be: Identity, Identification, and Narrative." In *A Queer World: The Center for Lesbian and Gay Studies Reader*, ed. Martin Duberman. New York: New York University Press.

Root-Bernstein, Robert S. 1993. *Rethinking AIDS: The Tragic Cost of Premature Consensus*. New York: Free Press.

Rosenberg, Howard. 1985. "*An Early Frost*—Brisk Air of Reason in Murky AIDS Arena." *Los Angeles Times*, 11 November, sec. 6, p. 1.

Rosenberg, Howard. 1990a. "ABC Takes Strides with 'Red, Hot'—and Bold—Special." *Los Angeles Times*, 30 November, F-1.

Rosenberg, Howard. 1990b. "*Paul Wynne's Journal*—the Universal Face of AIDS." *Los Angeles Times*, 22 June, F-1.

Rosenberg, Howard. 1991. "ABC's *Our Sons* Handles AIDS with Cliches." *Los Angeles Times*, 17 May, F-26.

Ross, Catherine, and John Mirowsky. 1980. "Theory and Research in Social Epidemiology." Paper presented at the Second Conference on Clinical Applications of the Social Sciences to Health, October, University of Illinois at Urbana-Champaign.

Ross, Judith Wilson. 1988. "Ethics and the Language of AIDS." In *AIDS, Ethics, and Public Policy*, ed. Christine Pierce and Donald VandeVeer. Belmont, Calif.: Wadsworth.

Rotello, Gabriel. 1997. *Sexual Ecology: AIDS and the Destiny of Gay Men*. New York: Dutton.

Roth, Nancy L., and Linda K. Fuller, eds. 1998. *Women and AIDS: Negotiating Safe Sex Practices, Care, and Representation*. New York: Haworth.

Roth, Nancy L., and Katie Hogan, eds. 1998. *The Gendered Epidemic*. New York: Routledge.

Rothman, David J. 1987. "Ethical and Social Issues in the Development of New Drugs and Vaccines." *Bulletin of the New York Academy of Medicine* 63, no. 6: 557–68.

Rothman, David J. 1991. *Strangers at the Bedside*. New York: Basic.

Rothman, David J., and Harold Edgar. 1992. "Scientific Rigor and Medical Realities: Placebo Trials in Cancer and AIDS Research." In *AIDS: The Making of a Chronic Disease*, ed. Elizabeth Fee and Daniel M. Fox. Berkeley: University of California Press.

Rowell, T. E. 1986. "AIDS in Africa." *Weekly Review*, 8 August, 2.

Royce, Rachel A., Arlene Seña, Willard Cates Jr., and Myron S. Cohen. 1997. "Sexual Transmission of HIV." *New England Journal of Medicine* 336, no. 15 (10 April): 1072–78.

Rubin, Gayle S. 1984. "Thinking Sex: Notes for a Radical Theory of the Politics of Sexuality." In *Pleasure and Danger: Exploring Female Sexuality*, ed. Carol S. Vance. New York: Routledge.

Rubin, Gayle S. 1994a. "Sexual Traffic." *Differences* 6, nos. 2/3: 62–99.

Rubin, Gayle S. 1994b. "The Valley of the Kings: Leathermen in San Francisco, 1960–1990." Ph.D. diss., University of Michigan, Ann Arbor.

Rubin, Gayle S. 1997. "Elegy for the Valley of Kings: AIDS and the Leather Community in

San Francisco, 1981–1996." In *In Changing Times: Gay Men and Lesbians Encounter HIV/AIDS*, ed. Martin P. Levine et al. Chicago: University of Chicago Press.

Rudd, Andrea, and Darien Taylor, eds. 1992. *Positive Women: Voices of Women Living with AIDS*. Toronto: Second Story.

Ruiz, Maria V. 1996. "*Alicia*: Hybridity and the Social Construction of SIDA." Paper presented at the Medical Scholars Program conference, September, University of Illinois College of Medicine at Urbana-Champaign.

Russo, Vito. 1987. *The Celluloid Closet: Homosexuality in the Movies*. Revised ed. New York: Harper and Row.

Russo, Vito. 1988. "State of Emergency: A Speech from the AIDS Movement." *Radical America* 21, no. 6: 64–68.

Rutherford, George W., and David Werdegar. 1989. "The Epidemiology of Acquired Immune Deficiency Syndrome." In *AIDS: Pathogenesis and Treatment*, ed. Jay A. Levy. New York: Marcel Dekker.

Ryan, Jane, and Helen Thomas, producers. 1990. "Will Sex Ever Be the Same Again?" Sydney: Australian Broadcasting Co./Radio National. Radio broadcast.

Ryan, Michael, and Avery Gordon, eds. 1994. *Body Politics: Disease, Desire, and the Family*. Boulder, Colo.: Westview.

Ryan White Story, The. 1989. Hollywood: MGM/United Artists.

Saalfield, Catherine. 1992. "AIDS Videos by, for, and about Women." In *Women, AIDS, and Activism*, ed. ACT UP New York Women and AIDS Book Group. Boston: South End.

Saalfield, Catherine. 1993. "Lesbian Marriage . . . (K)not!" In *Sisters, Sexperts, Queers*, ed. A. Stein. New York: Plume/Penguin.

Saalfield, Catherine. 1995. "Videography." In *AIDS TV*, by Alexandra Juhasz. Durham, N.C.: Duke University Press.

Saalfield, Catherine, and Ray Navarro. 1991. "Not Just Black and White: AIDS, Media, and People of Color." *PWA Coalition Newsline* 65 (May): 15–19.

Sabatier, Renée. 1988. *Blaming Others: Prejudice, Race, and Worldwide AIDS*. Washington, D.C.: Panos Institute; Philadelphia: New Society.

Sabatini, Maria T., Kanu Patel, and Richard Hirschman. 1984. "Kaposi's Sarcoma and T-Cell Lymphoma in an Immunodeficient Woman: A Case Report." *AIDS Research* 1, no. 2: 135–37.

Sacks, V. 1996. "Women and AIDS: An Analysis of Media Misrepresentation." *Social Science and Medicine* 42, no. 1, 59–73.

Said, Edward. 1985. "In the Shadow of the West." *Wedge* 7–8 (Winter/Spring): 4–11.

Saiz, Richard, producer. 1990. *AIDS in the 90s*. San Francisco: Group W Television/KPIX, June.

Salter, Stephanie. 1987. "AIDS, Rights." *San Francisco Chronicle*, 16 August, 13.

Sande, Merle A. 1986. "Transmission of AIDS: The Case against Casual Contagion." *New England Journal of Medicine* 314 (6 February): 380–82.

Sanders, Stephanie A., June M. Reinisch, and Mary Ziemba-Davis. 1989. "Self-Labeled Sexual Orientation and Sexual Behavior among Women." Paper presented at the Fifth International Conference on AIDS, 6 June, Montreal.

Sanford Guide to HIV/AIDS Therapy. 1996. 5th ed. (for July 1996–July 1997). Edited by Jay P. Sanford, Merle A. Sande, and David M. Gilbert. Dallas: Roche Laboratories.

San Miguel, Lisa. 1999. "From 'Career Woman's Disease' to 'An Epidemic Ignored': Endometriosis in U.S. Culture since 1948." PhD. diss., University of Illinois at Urbana-Champaign.

Santos, Elizabeth. 1992. "AIDS in Brazil: A Social Epidemiology of Homeless Youth." Ph.D. diss., University of Illinois at Urbana-Champaign.

Saunders, Penelope. 1997. "Successful HIV/AIDS Prevention Strategies in Australia: The Role of Sex Work Organizations." Draft of a paper presented at the White House Conference on Sex Work, 7 November, Washington, D.C.

Saussure, Ferdinand de. (1916) 1988. *Course in General Linguistics.* Trans. Roy Harris. Chicago: Open Court.

Sayers, Dorothy L. [1927] 1987. *Clouds of Witness.* New York: Harper and Row/Perennial.

Scarry, Elaine. 1993. "Watching and Authorizing the Gulf War." *Media Spectacles,* ed. Marjorie Garber, Jann Matlock, and Rebecca L. Walkowitz. New York: Routledge.

Scheper-Hughes, Nancy. 1992. *Death without Weeping: The Violence of Everyday Life in Brazil.* Berkeley and Los Angeles: University of California Press.

Scheper-Hughes, Nancy. 1994. "An Essay: 'AIDS and the Social Body.'" *Social Science and Medicine* 39, no. 7: 991–1003.

Scheper-Hughes, Nancy, and Margaret M. Lock. 1986. "Speaking Truth to Illness: Metaphors, Reification, and a Pedagogy for Patients." *Medical Anthropology Quarterly* 17, no. 5: 137–40.

Schiebinger, Londa. 1993. *Nature's Body: Gender in the Making of the Modern Sciences.* Boston: Beacon.

Schiller, Nina Glick. 1993. "The Invisible Women: Caregiving and the Construction of AIDS Health Services." *Culture, Medicine and Psychiatry* 17, no. 4: 487–512.

Schmemann, Serge. 1988. "Calls of 'Hi Sailor' Get the Heave-Ho." *New York Times,* 14 May, 4.

Schmidt, Nancy. 1990. "African Press Reports on the Social Impact of AIDS on Women and Children in Africa." Paper presented at the conference "Impact of AIDS on Maternal-Child Health Care Delivery in Africa," 4–6 May, University of Illinois at Urbana-Champaign.

Schneider, Beth E. 1988a. "Gender and AIDS." In *AIDS 1988: AAAS Symposia Papers,* ed. Ruth Kulstad. Washington, D.C.: American Association for the Advancement of Science.

Schneider, Beth E. 1988b. "Gender, Sexuality and AIDS: Social Responses and Consequences." In *The Social Impact of AIDS in the U.S.,* ed. Richard A. Berk. Cambridge, Mass.: Abt.

Schneider, Beth E. 1992. "AIDS and Class, Gender and Race Relations." In *The Social Context of AIDS,* ed. Joan Huber and Beth E. Schneider. Newbury Park, Calif.: Sage.

Schneider, Beth E., and Nancy E. Stoller, eds. 1995. *Women Resisting AIDS: Feminist Strategies of Empowerment.* Philadelphia: Temple University Press.

Schneider, David M. 1980. *American Kinship: A Cultural Account.* 2d ed. Chicago: University of Chicago Press.

Schneider, K. 1991. "Women AIDS Victims 'Ignored.'" *Denver Post,* 26 November, 1A, 8A.

Schoepf, Brooke Grundfest. 1991. "Ethical, Methodological, and Political Issues of AIDS Research in Central Africa." *Social Science and Medicine* 33, no. 7: 749–63.

Schoepf, Brooke Grundfest. 1992a. "AIDS, Sex, and Condoms: African Healers and the Reinvention of Tradition in Zaire." *Medical Anthropology* 14, nos. 2–4: 225–42.

Schoepf, Brooke Grundfest. 1992b. "Women at Risk: Case Studies from Zaire." In *The Time of AIDS: Social Analysis, Theory, and Method*, ed. Gilbert H. Herdt and Shirley Lindenbaum. Newbury Park, Calif.: Sage.

Schoepf, Brooke Grundfest, Rukarangira wa Nkara, Claude Schoepf, Walu Engundu, and Payanzo Ntsomo. 1988. "AIDS and Society in Central Africa: A View from Zaire." In *AIDS in Africa: The Social and Policy Impact*, ed. Norman Miller and Richard C. Rockwell. Lewiston, N.Y.: Edwin Mellen.

Schulman, Sarah. 1991. *People in Trouble*. New York: Penguin.

Schulz, L. 1990. "The Made-for-TV Movie: Industrial Practice, Cultural Form, Popular Reception." In *Hollywood in the Age of Television*, ed. T. Balio. Boston: Unwin Hyman.

Schwartz, Harry. 1984. "AIDS in the Media." Appendix to *Science in the Streets: Report to the Twentieth Century Task Force on the Communication of Scientific Risk*. New York: Priority.

Schwartz, John. 1995. "An Outbreak of Medical Myths: News of Ebola Virus Mixes Fact with an Unhealthy Dose of Fiction." *Washington Post National Weekly Edition*, 22–28 May, 38.

Schwartz, Ruth L. 1993. "New Alliances, Strange Bedfellows: Lesbians, Gay Men and AIDS." In *Sisters, Sexperts, Queers*, ed. A. Stein. New York: Plume/Penguin.

"Science and the Citizen." 1987. *Scientific American* 256, no. 1 (January): 58–59.

Scott, Blake. In progress. "Disciplining Diagnosis: Rhetoric, AIDS, and the Technoscience of HIV Testing." Ph.D. diss., Pennsylvania State University.

Scott, Peter. 1997. "White Noise: How Gay Men's Activism Gets Written out of AIDS Prevention." In *Acting on AIDS*, ed. Joshua Oppenheimer and Helena Reckitt. London: Serpent's Tail.

Scott, Sara. 1987. "Sex and Danger: Feminism and AIDS." *Trouble and Strife*, November, 13–18.

Second Laboratory. Shanghai Institute of Experimental Biology. 1976. "Studies on the Mechanisms of Abortion Induced by Tricosanthin." *Sci Sin* 19: 811–27.

Sedgwick, Eve Kosofsky. 1990. *Epistemology of the Closet*. Berkeley and Los Angeles: University of California Press.

Sedgwick, Eve Kosofsky. 1993. *Tendencies*. Durham, N.C.: Duke University Press.

Seftel, David. 1988. "AIDS and Apartheid: Double Trouble." *Africa Report*, November/December, 17–22.

Segal, Lynne. 1987. *Is the Future Female? Troubled Thoughts on Contemporary Feminism*. London: Methuen.

Segal, Lynne. 1989. "Lessons from the Past: Feminism, Sexual Politics, and the Challenge of AIDS." In *Taking Liberties: AIDS and Cultural Politics*, ed. Erica Carter and Simon Watney. London: Serpent's Tail.

Seijo-Maldonado, Haydée, and Christine A. Horak. 1991. "AIDS in Latin American Newsmagazines: A Contest for Meaning." Photocopied research paper in the author's collection.

Selzer, Richard. 1987. "A Mask on the Face of Death: As AIDS Ravages Haiti, a U.S. Doctor Finds a Taboo against Truth." *Life*, August, 58–64.

Setel, Philip. 1990. "AIDS and the Body as Social Space: Epistemologies of Distinction and Difference." Manuscript in the author's collection.

Seven Sisters from Oklahoma [Angie, Ernie, Julie, Lila, Rebecca, Tessa, and Vanessa].

1992. "Pure Lesbian Sex." Letter to the editor, *Gay Community News*, 26 January–1 February, 12.

Sharf, Barbara F., and Vicki S. Freimuth. 1993. "The Construction of Illness on Entertainment Television: Coping with Cancer on 'Thirtysomething.'" *Health Communication* 5, no. 3: 141–60.

Shaw, David. 1987. "Anti-Gay Bias? Coverage of AIDS Story: A Slow Start." *Los Angeles Times*, 20 December, 1.

Shaw, Nancy S. [Nancy E. Stoller]. 1985. "California Models for Women's AIDS Education and Services." San Francisco: San Francisco AIDS Foundation. Report.

Shaw, Nancy S. 1986. "Women and AIDS: Theory and Politics." Paper presented at the annual meeting of the National Women's Studies Association, June, University of Illinois at Urbana-Champaign.

Shaw, Nancy S. 1988. "Preventing AIDS among Women: The Role of Community Organizing." *Socialist Review* 18, no. 4 (October/December): 76–92.

Shaw, Nancy S., and Lyn Paleo. 1987. "Women and AIDS." In *What to Do about AIDS: Physician and Health Professionals Discuss the Issues*, ed. Leon McKusick. Berkeley and Los Angeles: University of California Press.

Shelton, J. D., and J. E. Higgins. 1981. "Contraception and Toxic Shock Syndrome: A Reanalysis." *Contraception* 24: 631–34.

Shenon, Philip. 1993. "Brash and Unabashed, Mr. Condom Takes on Sex and Death in Thailand." *New York Times*, 20 December, 5.

Shenton, Joan, producer and director. 1990. *The AIDS Catch*. London: Meditel. Shown on Channel 4, British television, on 5 March.

Shepherd, Gill. 1987. "Rank, Gender, and Homosexuality: Mombasa as a Key to Understanding Sexual Options." In *The Cultural Construction of Sexuality*, ed. Pat Caplan. New York: Tavistock.

Sher, R., et al. 1987. "Seroepidemiology of Human Immunodeficiency Virus in Africa from 1970 to 1974." *New England Journal of Medicine* 317, no. 7 (13 August): 450–51.

Shilts, Randy. 1987. *And the Band Played On: People, Politics, and the AIDS Epidemic*. New York: St. Martin's.

Shnayerson, Michael. 1987. "One by One." *Vanity Fair*, April, 91–97, 152–53.

Shohat, Ella. 1998. "'Lasers for Ladies': Endo Discourse and the Inscriptions of Science." *The Visible Woman*, ed. Paula A. Treichler, Lisa Cartwright, and Constance Penley. New York: New York University Press.

Shostak, Marjorie. 1983. *Nisa: The Life and Words of a !Kung Woman*. New York: Vintage.

Shoumatoff, Alex. 1988. "In Search of the Source of AIDS." *Vanity Fair*, July, 95.

Showalter, Elaine. 1997. *Hystories: Hysterical Epidemics and Modern Media*. New York: Columbia University Press.

Siebert, Sam., with Alma Guillermo and Ruth Marshall. 1987. "An Epidemic Like AIDS." *Newsweek*, 27 July, 38.

Signorile, Michelangelo. 1997. *Life Outside: The Signorile Report on Gay Men: Sex, Drugs, Muscles, and the Passages of Life*. New York: Harper Collins.

Silverman, Mervyn F. 1989. "The Impact of National Television on AIDS Funding." Paper presented at the conference "AIDS: Communication Challenges," held in conjunction with the annual meeting of the International Communication Association, 27 May, San Francisco.

Silverman, Mervyn F., and Deborah B. Silverman. 1985. "AIDS and the Threat to Public Health." Special supplement, *Hastings Center Report* 15, no. 1: 19–22.

Simon, Roger. 1991. "TV's Failure to Act Seriously Sends Bad Message to Youth." *Champaign-Urbana News-Gazette*, 19 November, p. 4.

Singer, Merrill. 1994. "AIDS and the Health Crisis of the U.S. Urban Poor: The Perspective of Critical Medical Anthropology." *Social Science and Medicine* 39, no. 7: 931–48.

Singer, Merrill, Candida Flores, Lani Davidson, et al. 1990. "SIDA: The Economic, Social, and Cultural Context of AIDS among Latinos." *Medical Anthropology Quarterly* 14, no. 3: 285–306.

Small, Henry, and Edwin Greenlee. 1989. "A Co-Citation Study of AIDS Research." *Communication Research* 16, no. 5: 642–66.

Smith-Rosenberg, Carol. 1985. "The Hysterical Woman: Sex Roles and Role Conflict in Nineteenth-Century America." In *Disorderly Conduct: Visions of Gender in Victorian America.* New York: Knopf.

Sobo, E. J. 1993. "Inner-City Women and AIDS: Psychosocial Benefits of Unsafe Sex." *Culture, Medicine, and Psychiatry* 17, no. 4: 454–85.

"'Social Card' to Reassure Sex Partners." 1985. *San Francisco Chronicle*, 17 October, 30.

Solomon, Nancy. 1991. "Risky Business: Should Lesbians Practice Safe Sex?" *Out/Look*, Spring, 5–8.

Sonnabend, Joseph. 1985. "Looking at AIDS in Totality: A Conversation." *New York Native* 129: 7–13.

Sonnabend, Joseph. 1989. "Review of AZT Multicenter Trial Data Obtained under the Freedom of Information ACT by Project Inform and ACT UP." *AIDS Forum* 1 (January): 9–15.

Sontag, Susan. 1978. *Illness as Metaphor.* New York: Farrar, Straus, Giroux.

Sontag, Susan. 1986. "The Way We Live Now." *New Yorker*, 24 November, 42–51. Reprinted in *The Way We Write Now: Short Stories from the AIDS Crisis*, ed. Sharon Oard Warner (New York: Citadel, 1995).

Sontag, Susan. 1989. *AIDS and Its Metaphors.* New York: Farrar, Straus, Giroux.

Sperber, D. 1985. "Anthropology and Psychology: Towards an Epidemiology of Representations." *Man* 20: 73–89.

Spigel, Lynn. 1988. "Installing the Television Set: Popular Discourses on Television and Domestic Spaces, 1948–1955." *Camera Obscura* 16 (January): 11–45.

Spirit Speaks. 1987. *AIDS: From Fear to Hope: Channeled Teachings Offering Insight and Inspiration.* Miami: New Age.

Spiro, Ellen, director. 1989. *DiAna's Hair ego: AIDS Info Up Front.* Chicago: Video Data Bank. Video.

Spivak, Gayatri Chakravorty. 1988. "Can the Subaltern Speak?" In *Marxism and the Interpretation of Culture*, ed. Cary Nelson and Lawrence Grossberg. Urbana: University of Illinois Press.

Stanley, John. 1988. "Vince Edwards at 59: A Mellowed Rogue." *San Francisco Chronicle*, 14 February, 47.

Stanworth, Michelle, ed. 1987. *Reproductive Technologies: Gender, Motherhood, and Medicine.* Minneapolis: University of Minnesota Press.

Starr, Paul. 1982. *The Social Transformation of American Medicine.* New York: Basic.

Staver, Sari. 1990. "Women Found Contracting HIV via Unprotected Sex." *American Medical News*, 1 June, 4–5.

Stein, Arlene, ed. 1993. *Sisters, Sexperts, Queers: Beyond the Lesbian Nation.* New York: Plume/Penguin.

Stein, Howard F. 1990. "The Story behind the Clinical Story: An Inquiry into Biomedical Narrative." *Family Systems Medicine* 8, no. 2: 213–27.

Steinbrook, Robert. 1985. "Thumbs-Up from Doctors." *Los Angeles Times,* 11 November, sec. 6, p. 9.

Steinbrook, Robert. 1997. "Battling HIV on Many Fronts." *New England Journal of Medicine* 337, no. 11 (11 September): 779–81.

Stephens, P. Clay. 1988. "U.S. Women and HIV Infection." In *The AIDS Epidemic: Private Rights and the Public Interest,* ed. Padraig O'Malley. Boston: Beacon.

Stipp, Horst. 1989. "An Analysis of Trends in NBC's Coverage of AIDS." Paper presented at the conference "AIDS: Communication Challenges," held in conjunction with the annual meeting of the International Communication Association, 27 May, San Francisco.

Stokes, Geoffrey. 1985a. "Press Clips." *Village Voice,* 11 October, 3.

Stokes, Geoffrey. 1985b. "Press Clips." *Village Voice,* 15 October, 4.

Stoller, Nancy E. [see also Nancy S. Shaw] 1995. "Lesbian Involvement in the AIDS Epidemic: Changing Roles and Generational Differences." In *Women Resisting AIDS: Feminist Strategies of Empowerment,* ed. B. E. Schneider and N. E. Stoller. Philadelphia: Temple University Press.

Stone, Laurie. 1987. "The New Femme Fatale." *Ms,* December, 78–79.

Strnad, Patricia. 1990. "Rakolta Seeks Allies in TV Fight." *Advertising Age,* 6 August, 35.

Stroll, Avrum. 1967. "Identity." In *Encyclopedia of Philosophy,* vol. 4, ed. Paul Edwards. New York: Macmillan/Free Press.

Sturken, Marita. 1997. *Tangled Memories: The Vietnam War, the AIDS Epidemic, and the Politics of Remembering.* Berkeley and Los Angeles: University of California Press.

Suleiman, Susan Rubin, ed. 1986. *The Female Body in Western Culture.* Cambridge, Mass.: Harvard University Press.

Sullivan, Ronald. 1987. "Addicts' Deaths from AIDS Are Termed 'Underreported.' " *New York Times,* 26 March, 15.

Susser, Mervyn. 1973. *Causal Thinking in the Health Sciences: Concepts and Strategies of Epidemiology.* New York: Oxford University Press.

Sweet, Ellen. 1988. "Women and AIDS: Who's at Risk?" *Ms,* 26 February, 26.

Switzer, Ellen. 1986. "AIDS: What Women Can Do." *Vogue,* January, 222–23, 264–65.

Switzer, Ellen. 1988. "AIDS: Fear and Loathing." *Vogue,* March, 326.

Symanski, Richard. 1981. *The Immortal Landscape: Female Prostitution in Western Societies.* Toronto: Butterworths.

"Symptoms of Global Malady." 1989. *West Africa,* 19–25 June, 1.

Tagg, John. 1988. *The Burden of Representation: Essays on Photographies and Histories.* Amherst: University of Massachusetts Press.

Tancredi, Laurence R., and Nora D. Volkow. 1986. "AIDS: Its Symbolism and Ethical Implications." *Medical Heritage* 2, no. 1 (January–February): 12–18.

Taussig, Michael T. 1980. "Reification and the Consciousness of the Patient." *Social Science and Medicine* 14B: 3–13.

Teare, Catherine, and Abigail English. 1996. "Women, Girls, and the HIV Epidemic." In *Man-Made Medicine,* ed. K. L. Moss. Durham, N.C.: Duke University Press.

Terry, Jennifer. 1990. "Lesbians under the Medical Gaze: Scientists Search for Remarkable Differences." *Journal of Sex Research* 27, no. 3: 317–39.

Terry, Jennifer, and Jacqueline Urla, eds. 1995. *Deviant Bodies: Cultural Perspectives on Difference in Science and Popular Culture.* Bloomington: Indiana University Press.

Tesh, Sylvia Noble. 1988. *Hidden Arguments: Political Ideology and Disease Prevention Policy.* New Brunswick, N.J.: Rutgers University Press.

Testing the Limits Collective, producers. 1987. *Testing the Limits, Parts 1 and 2.* New York: Gay Men's Health Crisis. Video.

Thomas, Kendall. 1996. "*Corpus Juris (Hetero)Sexualis*: Doctrine, Discourse, and Desire in *Bowers v. Hardwick.*" In *A Queer World: The Center for Lesbian and Gay Studies Reader*, ed. Martin Duberman. New York: New York University Press.

Thompson, Larry. 1989. "Commentary: With No Magic Cure in Sight, Dramatic Epidemic Loses Luster as News Story." *Washington Post*, 13 June, Health Section, p. 7.

Tierney, John. 1990a. "AIDS Tears Lives of the African Family." *New York Times*, 17 September, A-1.

Tierney, John. 1990b. "With 'Social Marketing,' Condoms Combat AIDS." *New York Times*, 18 September, A-1.

Timberlake, Lloyd. 1986. *Africa in Crisis: The Causes, the Cures of Environmental Bankruptcy.* Edited by Jon Tinker. Philadelphia: New Society/Earthscan.

"Toronto Sidewalk Traffic: Growing Fear as AIDS Virus Spreads to General Public." 1987. *Macleans*, 24 August, 31.

Torres, Gabriel. 1989. "New Therapies for PCP." *Treatment Issues* 3 (5 December): 7–10.

Torrey, Barbara Boyle, Peter O. Way, and Patricia Rowe. 1988. "Epidemiology of HIV and AIDS in Africa: Emerging Issues and Social Implications." In *AIDS in Africa: The Social and Policy Impact*, ed. Norman Miller and Richard C. Rockwell. Lewiston, N.Y.: Edwin Mellen.

Toughill, Kelly. 1989. "No Breaks on Price of New AIDS Drug, Firm's Founder Says." *Toronto Star*, 3 April, A-4.

Towle, Lisa H. 1988. "Learn to Read with 'Word Warriors.'" *New York Times*, 31 January, 21.

Treat, John Whittier. 1994. "AIDS Panic in Japan, or How to Have a Sabbatical in an Epidemic." *Positions* 2, no. 2: 629–79.

Trebay, Guy. 1991. "Day of the Dead." *Village Voice*, 10 December, 65.

Treichler, Paula A. 1988a. "AIDS, Gender, and Biomedical Discourse: Current Contests for Meaning." In *AIDS: The Burdens of History*, ed. Elizabeth Fee and Daniel M. Fox. Berkeley and Los Angeles: University of California Press. Reprinted in *American Feminist Thought at Century's End: A Reader*, ed. Linda S. Kaufman (Cambridge: Basil Blackwell, 1993).

Treichler, Paula A. 1988b. "AIDS, Homophobia, and Biomedical Discourse: An Epidemic of Signification." *Cultural Studies* 1, no. 3: 263–305. Reprinted in *AIDS: Cultural Analysis/Cultural Activism*, ed. Douglas Crimp (Cambridge, Mass.: MIT Press, 1988).

Treichler, Paula A. 1989a. "AIDS and HIV Infection in the Third World: A First World Chronicle." In *ReMaking History*, ed. Phil Mariani and Barbara Kruger. New York: Dia Art Foundation. Revised for *AIDS: The Making of a Chronic Disease*, ed. Elizabeth Fee and Daniel M. Fox. (Berkeley: University of California Press, 1992).

Treichler, Paula A. 1989b. "From Discourse to Dictionary: How Sexist Meanings Are Authorized." In *Language, Gender, and Professional Writing: Theoretical Approaches and Guidelines for Nonsexist Usage*, ed. Francine Wattman Frank and Paula A. Treichler. New York: Modern Language Association.

Treichler, Paula A. 1990a. "Feminism, Medicine, and the Meaning of Childbirth." In *Body/Politics: Women and the Discourse of Science*, ed. Mary Jacobus, Evelyn Fox Keller, and Sally Shuttleworth. New York: Routledge.

Treichler, Paula A. 1990b. "Uncertainties and Excesses." *Science*, 6 April, 232–33. Review of *The Myth of Heterosexual AIDS*," by Michael Fumento.

Treichler, Paula A. 1991a. "AIDS, Africa, and Cultural Theory." *Transition* 51: 86–103.

Treichler, Paula A. 1991b. "Beyond *Cosmo*: AIDS, Identity and Feminist Activism." *Camera Obscura* 28: 21–78.

Treichler, Paula A. 1991c. "How to Have Theory in an Epidemic: The Evolution of AIDS Treatment Activism." In *Technoculture*, ed. Constance Penley and Andrew Ross. Minneapolis: University of Minnesota Press.

Treichler, Paula A. 1992a. "AIDS, HIV, and the Cultural Construction of Reality." In *The Time of AIDS: Social Analysis, Theory, and Method*, ed. Gilbert H. Herdt and Shirley Lindenbaum. Newbury Park, Calif.: Sage.

Treichler, Paula A. 1992b. "Seduced and Terrorized: AIDS and Network Television." *Artforum* 28, no. 2: 147–51. Revised for *A Leap in the Dark: AIDS, Art, and Contemporary Culture*, ed. Allan Klusaček and Ken Morrison (Montreal: Véhicule/Artexte, 1992).

Treichler, Paula A. 1993. "AIDS Narratives on Television: Whose Story?" In *Writing AIDS: Gay Literature, Language, and Analysis*, ed. Timothy Murphy and Suzanne Poirier. New York: Columbia University Press.

Treichler, Paula A. 1996. "How to Use a Condom: Bedtime Stories for the Transcendental Signifier." In *Disciplinarity and Dissent in Cultural Studies*, ed. Cary Nelson and Dilip Parameshwar Gaonkar. New York: Routledge.

Treichler, Paula A., and Catherine Warren. 1998. "Maybe Next Year: Feminist Silence and the AIDS Epidemic." In *The Visible Woman*, ed. Paula A. Treichler, Lisa Cartwright, and Constance Penley. New York: New York University Press.

Treichler, Paula A., Lisa Cartwright, and Constance Penley, eds. 1998. *The Visible Woman: Imaging Technology, Science, and Gender*. New York: New York University Press.

"The Trials of AZT." 1989. Editorial, *Positively Healthy* 2 (March): 1.

Tuchman, Barbara. 1978. *A Distant Mirror: The Calamitous 14th Century*. New York: Ballantine.

Tuchman, Gaye. 1978. *Making News*. New York: Free Press.

Tuller, David. 1987. "Trying to Avoid an Insurance Debacle." *New York Times*, 22 February, C-1.

Turner, Bryan A. 1984. *The Body and Society*. New York: Basil Blackwell.

Turner, Charles F., Heather G. Miller, and Lincoln E. Moses, eds. 1989. *AIDS: Sexual Behavior and Intravenous Drug Use*. Washington, D.C.: National Academy Press.

Turow, Joseph. 1990a. *Playing Doctor: Television, Storytelling, and Medical Power*. New York: Oxford University Press.

Turow, Joseph. 1990b. "Television and Institutional Power: The Case of Medicine." In *Rethinking Communication: Paradigm Exemplars*, vol. 2, ed. Brenda Dervin et al. Newbury Park, Calif.: Sage.

Turow, Joseph, and Lisa Coe. 1985. "Curing Television's Ills: The Portrayal of Health Care." *Journal of Communication* 35 (Autumn): 36–51.

Turshen, Meredeth, and Carol Barker. 1986. "Editorial: The Health Issue." *Review of African Political Economy* 36 (September): 1–6.

Udovitch, Mim. 1991. "Full Henhouse: Sitcoms and the Single Girl." *Village Voice*, 22 October, 50–51.

UNAIDS Report on the Global HIV/AIDS Epidemic. 1988. Geneva: UNAIDS and World Health Organization, June.

United Nations Economic and Social Council. 1989. "Effects of the Acquired Immunodeficiency Syndrome (AIDS) on the Advancement of Women." Twenty-third Session of the Commission on the Status of Women, 29 March–7 April, Vienna.

United Nations Educational, Scientific, and Cultural Organization (UNESCO). 1986. "On Prostitution and Strategies against Promiscuity and Sexual Exploitation of Women." *Echo* 1, nos. 2–3: 16–17.

U.S. General Accounting Office. 1989. "AIDS Forecasting: Undercount of Cases and Lack of Key Data Weaken Existing Estimates." GAO/PEMD-89-13. Washington, D.C.: U.S. Government Printing Office.

U.S. House. 1984. *Acquired Immune Deficiency Syndrome: Hearing before the Subcommittee on Health and the Environment of the Committee on Energy and Commerce.* 98th Congress, 2d session, 17 September.

U.S. House. 1987a. *Condom Advertising and AIDS: Hearing before the Subcommittee on Health and the Environment of the Committee on Energy and Commerce.* 100th Congress, 1st session, 10 February.

U.S. House. 1987b. *FDA Proposals to Ease Restrictions on the Use and Sale of Experimental Drugs: Hearing before a Subcommittee of the Committee on Government.* House of Representatives, 100th Congress, 1st session, 29 April.

U.S. House. Select Committee on Hunger. 1988. *AIDS and the Third World: The Impact on Development: Hearing before the Select Committee on Hunger.* 100th Congress, 2d session, 30 June.

U.S. House. Committee on Government Relations. 1989. *Therapeutic Drugs for AIDS: Development, Testing and Availability: A Hearing before the Committee on Government Operations.* 100th Congress, 2d session, 28–29 April.

U.S. Public Health Service, U.S. War Department, and American Social Hygiene Association. 1919. *End of the Road.* Washington, D.C. Film.

U.S. Public Law 100-202. 1987. *Congressional Record* 133, no. 206 (22 December): H12892.

U.S. Surgeon General. 1986. *U.S. Surgeon General's Report on Acquired Immune Deficiency Syndrome.* Washington, D.C.: Public Health Service.

U.S. Surgeon General. 1988. *Understanding AIDS.* Washington, D.C.: Public Health Service.

Valdivia, Angharad N., ed. 1996. *Feminism, Multiculturalism, and the Media.* Thousand Oaks, Calif.: Sage.

Valverde, Mariana. 1987. *Sex, Power and Pleasure.* Philadelphia: New Society.

Van, Jos. 1986. "Cell Researchers Aim to Flush out Body's Terrorists." *Chicago Tribune*, 5 October, 1.

Vance, Carole S. 1984. "Pleasure and Danger." In *Pleasure and Danger*, ed. Carole S. Vance and Paul Kegan. New York: Routledge.

Vance, Carole S. 1987. "A Vagina Surrounded by a Woman: The Meese Commission on Pornography, 1984–1985." Paper presented at the colloquium "Unit for Criticism and Interpretive Theory," April, University of Illinois at Urbana-Champaign.

Vance, Carole S. 1996. "Social Construction Theory: Problems in the History of Sexuality." In *Homosexuality, Which Homosexuality? International Conference on Gay and Lesbian Studies*, ed. Dennis Altman et al. London: GMP.

Van de Perre, P., et al. 1985. "Female Prostitutes: A Risk Group for Infection with Human T-Cell Lymphotropic Virus Type III." *Lancet* 2, no. 5: 24–27.

Van Gelder, Lindsay. 1983. "The Politics of AIDS." *Ms*, May, 103.

Van Gelder, Lindsay. 1987. "AIDS." *Ms*, April, 64–71.

Van Gelder, Lindsay, and Pam Brandt. 1986. "AIDS on Campus." *Rolling Stone* 483: 89–94, 134.

Varmus, Harold. 1989. "Naming the AIDS Virus." In *The Meaning of AIDS*, ed. Eric Juengst and Barbara Koenig. New York: Praeger.

Vaughn, Toni. 1991. "Life Is Day-to-Day War against Despair for HIV-infected Mom." *Champaign-Urbana News-Gazette*, 6 June, A3.

Vedder, Julie. 1996. "Scientific Semen: Cultural Messages and Scientific 'Objectivity' in Pamphlets on Sexually Transmitted Infections." Paper presented at the Science and Literature in Society Conference, 1 October, Atlanta.

Veeder, Mary Harris. 1993. "Authorial Voice, Implied Audiences, and the Drafting of the AIDS National Mailing (1988)." *Risk: Issues in Health and Safety* (Fall): 287–308.

Veeder, Mary Harris. In press. "Authorial Tone and Sexual Relationships in the Drafting of the 1988 AIDS National Mailing." [Journal name, vol., date to come]

Veenstra, Robert J., and Jeannine Cyr Gluck. 1991. "Access to Information about AIDS." *Annals of Internal Medicine* 114, no. 4 (15 February): 320–24.

Veldink, Connie. 1989. "The Honey-Bee Language Controversy." *Interdisciplinary Science Reviews* 14: 166–75.

Venter, A. J. 1988. "AIDS: Its Strategic Consequences in Black Africa." *International Defense Review* 21 (April): 357–59.

Verghese, Abraham. 1994. *My Own Country: A Doctor's Story*. New York: Vintage.

V-Girls. 1995. "Daughters of the ReVolution." *October* 71 (Winter): 121–40.

Voeller, Bruce. 1987. "Nonoxynol-9 and Prevention of Sexual Transmission of HTLV-III/LAV." In *Biobehavioral Control of AIDS*, ed. D. G. Ostrow. New York: Irvington.

Volberding, Paul A. 1996. "Improving the Outcomes of Care for Patients with Human Immunodeficiency Virus Infection." *New England Journal of Medicine* 334: 729–31.

Volberding, Paul A., et al. 1990. "Zidovudine in Asymptomatic Human Immunodeficiency Virus Infection: A Controlled Trial in Persons with Fewer than 500 CD-4-Positive Cells per Cubic Millimeter." *New England Journal of Medicine* 322 (5 April): 941–49.

WAC Stats: The Facts about Women. 1993. New York: Women's Action Coalition.

Wachter, Robert. 1991. *The Fragile Coalition: Scientists, Activists, and AIDS*. New York: St. Martin's.

Wade, Nicholas. 1989. "Cuba's Quarantine for AIDS: A Police State's Health Experiment." Editorial, *New York Times*, 6 February, A-4.

Wain-Hobson, Simon, et al. 1991. "LAV Revisited: Origins of the Early HIV-1 Isolates from the Institut Pasteur." *Science* 252: 961–65.

Waite, Gloria. 1988. "The AIDS Virus and Africa." In *AIDS in Africa: The Social and*

Policy Impact, ed. Norman Miller and Richard C. Rockwell. Lewiston, N.Y.: Edwin Mellen.

Waldby, Catherine. 1996. *AIDS and the Body Politic: Biomedicine and Sexual Difference.* London: Routledge.

Walkowitz, Judith. 1983. *Prostitution and Victorian Society: Women, Class, and the State.* New York: Cambridge University Press.

Wallace, Joyce. 1984. "Acquired Immune Deficiency Syndrome (AIDS) in Prostitutes." In *The Acquired Immune Deficiency Syndrome and Infections of Homosexual Men*, ed. Pearl Ma and Donald Armstrong. New York: Yorke Medical.

Wallace, Rodrick. 1991. "Traveling Waves of HIV Infection on a Low Dimensional 'Socio-Geographic' Network." *Social Science and Medicine* 32, no. 7: 847–52.

Wallace, Rodrick, Mindy Fullilove, Robert Fullilove, Peter Gould, and Deborah Wallace. 1994. "Will AIDS Be Contained within U.S. Minority Urban Populations?" *Social Science and Medicine* 93, no. 8: 1051–62.

Walmsley, Ann. 1986. "Two Women Battle AIDS." *Macleans*, 31 August.

Warren, Catherine A. 1996. "First, Do Not Speak: Errant Doctors, Sexual Abuse, and Institutional Silence." Ph.D. diss., University of Illinois at Urbana-Champaign.

Watney, Simon. 1987a. "A.I.D.S. U.S.A." *Square Peg* (Autumn): 17.

Watney, Simon. 1987b. "People's Perceptions of the Risk of AIDS and the Role of the Mass Media." *Health Education Journal* 46, no. 2: 62–65.

Watney, Simon. 1987c. *Policing Desire: Pornography, AIDS and the Media.* Minneapolis: University of Minnesota Press.

Watney, Simon. 1987d. "Visual AIDS: Advertising Ignorance." *Radical America* 20, no. 6: 79–82.

Watney, Simon. 1988. "The Spectacle of AIDS." In *AIDS: Cultural Analysis/Cultural Activism*, ed. Douglas Crimp. Cambridge, Mass.: MIT Press.

Watney, Simon. 1989. "Missionary Positions: AIDS, 'Africa' and Race." *Differences* 1, no. 1 (Winter): 83–100.

Watney, Simon. 1992. "'The Possibilities of Permutation': Pleasure, Proliferation, and the Politics of Gay Identity in the Age of AIDS." In *Fluid Exchanges*, ed. James Miller. Toronto: University of Toronto Press.

Watney, Simon. 1994. *Practices of Freedom: Selected Writings on HIV/AIDS.* Durham, N.C.: Duke University Press.

Watney, Simon, and Sunil Gupta. 1986. "The Rhetoric of AIDS: A Dossier Compiled by Simon Watney, with Photographer Sunil Gupta." *Screen* 27, no. 1: 72–85.

Watson, Catharine. 1987. "Africa's AIDS Time Bomb: Region Scrambles to Fight Epidemic." *Guardian*, 17 June, 10–11.

Weaver, Frank J., et al. 1988. "Health Care Marketing Minicase: The Impact of AIDS Publicity on Public Perception of a Health Care Organization." *Journal of Health Care Marketing* 8, no. 4 (December): 70–73.

Wechsler, Nancy. 1988. "Diary: FDA Action." *Radical America* 21, no. 6: 71–72.

Weeks, Jeffrey. 1985. *Sexuality and Its Discontents: Meanings, Myths and Modern Sexualities.* London: Routledge and Kegan Paul.

Weeks, Jeffrey. 1987. "Questions of Identity." In *The Cultural Construction of Sexuality*, ed. Pat Caplan. London: Tavistock.

Weinberg, Steven. 1994. *Dreams of a Final Theory.* New York: Vintage.

Weinhouse, Bibi. 1983. "AIDS: The Latest Facts." *Ladies' Home Journal*, November, 100.

Weinstein, Steve. 1990a. "NBC Pulls AIDS-Themed *Lifestories.*" *Los Angeles Times*, 20 November, F-3.

Weinstein, Steve. 1990b. "NBC Puts Message over Money with AIDS Show." *Los Angeles Times*, 18 December, F-1.

Weiss, Ellen, executive producer. 1995. "AIDS in Asia." San Francisco: NPR, 17 February– 6 May. Radio program.

Wendler, I. 1986. "Seroepidemiology of HIV in Africa." *British Journal of Medicine* 293 (27 September): 782–85.

Wenner, Adrian M., and Patrick H. Wells. 1990. *Anatomy of a Controversy: The Question of Language among Bees.* New York: Columbia University Press.

Wermuth, Laurie, Jennifer Ham, and Rebecca L. Robbins. 1992. "Women Don't Wear Condoms: AIDS Risk among Sexual Partners of IV Drug Users." In *The Social Context of AIDS*, ed. Joan Huber and Beth E. Schneider. Newbury Park, Calif.: Sage.

Wheeler, David L. 1986. "More Research Is Urged in Fight against AIDS." *Chronicle of Higher Education*, 5 November, 7.

Whippen, Deb. 1987. "Science Fictions: The Making of a Medical Model for AIDS." *Radical America* 20, no. 6: 39–54.

White, Luise. 1990. *The Comforts of Home: Prostitution in Colonial Nairobi.* Chicago: University of Chicago Press.

White, Luise. 1993. "Cars out of Place: Vampires, Technology, and Labor in East and Central Africa." *Representations* 43 (Summer): 27–50.

Whitehead, Tony L. 1992. "Expressions of Masculinity in a Jamaican Sugartown: Implications for Family Planning Programs." In *Gender Constructs and Social Issues*, ed. Tony L. Whitehead and Barbara V. Reid. Urbana: University of Illinois Press.

Whitmore, George. 1988. "Bearing Witness." *New York Times Magazine*, 31 January, 14.

Wilkinson, Ray, and Ruth Marshall. 1986. "Africa in the Plague Years." *Newsweek*, 24 November, 44–47.

Wilkinson, Stephan. 1985. "Selling Condoms to Women." *Working Woman*, October, 68.

Williams, Bruce A., and Albert R. Mathery. 1995. *Democracy, Dialogue, and Environmental Disputes: The Contested Languages of Social Regulation.* New Haven, Conn.: Yale University Press.

Williams, Raymond. 1973. *The Country and the City.* London: Chatto and Windus.

Williams, Raymond. [1976] 1983. *Keywords: A Vocabulary of Culture and Society.* Revised ed. New York: Oxford University Press.

Williamson, Judith. 1989. "Every Virus Tells a Story: The Meanings of HIV and AIDS." In *Taking Liberties: AIDS and Cultural Politics*, ed. Erica Carter and Simon Watney. London: Serpent's Tail.

Wilson, Carter. 1995. *Hidden in the Blood: A Personal Investigation of AIDS in the Yucatán.* New York: Columbia University Press.

Wilson, Michael B. 1987. "AIDS Prevention Suggestions for 'Safe Sex' Promotional Campaigns." In *Biobehavioral Control of AIDS*, ed. David G. Ostrow. New York: Irvington.

Winik, Marion. 1996. *First Comes Love.* New York: Pantheon.

Winkelstein, Warren, Jr. et al. 1987. "Sexual Practices and Risk of Infection by the Human Immunodeficiency Virus: The San Francisco Men's Health Study." *Journal of the American Medical Association* 257, no. 3 (16 January): 321–25.

Winnow, Jackie. 1989. "Lesbians Working on AIDS: Assessing the Impact of Health Care on Women." *Out/Look*, Summer, 10–18.

Winsten, Jay A. 1985. "Science and the Media: The Boundaries of Truth." *Health Affairs* 4, no. 1 (Spring): 5–23.

Wockner, Rex. 1987. "Back-Door Homophobia." *Chicago Outlines*, Summer, 8.

Woese, Carl R. 1967. *The Genetic Code: The Molecular Basis for Genetic Expression.* New York: Harper and Row.

Wofsy, Constance B. 1987. "Human Immunodeficiency Virus Infection in Women." Editorial, *Journal of the American Medical Association* 257 (17 April): 2074–76.

Wolf, Margery. 1992. *A Thrice-Told Tale: Feminism, Postmodernism, and Ethnographic Responsibility.* Stanford, Calif.: Stanford University Press.

Wolfe, Maxine. 1992. "AIDS and Politics: Transformations of Our Movement." In *Women, AIDS, and Activism*, ed. ACT UP New York Women and AIDS Book Group. Boston: South End. Originally presented at the National Gay and Lesbian Task Force Town Meeting, 6 October 1989, Washington, D.C.

Wolfe, Maxine. 1997. "This Is about People Dying: The Tactics of Early ACT UP and Lesbian Avengers in New York City." In *Queers in Space*, ed. Gordon Brett Ingram, Anne Marie Bouthillette, and Yolanda Retter. Seattle: Bay. Interview by Laraine Sommella.

Wolfe, Maxine, and Iris Long. 1989. "Through the Eye of a Needle: Women's Access to Drug Treatments through Clinical Trials." In *The ACT UP Women's Caucus Women and AIDS Handbook*, ed. Maria Maggenti. New York: ACT UP.

Wolinsky, Howard, and Tom Brune. 1994. *The Serpent and the Staff: The Unhealthy Politics of the American Medical Association.* New York: Putnam's.

"Woman Kills Husband over Condom Packet." 1991. *Kenya Daily Nation*, 9 November, 8.

"Women and AIDS." 1987. London: BBC. Radio program.

"Women and AIDS." 1991. Special section, *Ms*, January/February, 16–33.

Women's AIDS Video Enterprise. 1990a. *A WAVE Taster.* New York: Women's AIDS Video Enterprise. Video.

Women's AIDS Video Enterprise. 1990b. *We Care: A Video for Care Providers of People Affected by AIDS.* New York: Women's AIDS Video Enterprise. Video.

Woodmansee, Martha, and Peter Jaszi, eds. 1994. *The Construction of Authorship: Textual Appropriation in Law and Literature.* Durham, N.C.: Duke University Press.

Woolf, Virginia. 1929. *A Room of One's Own.* New York: Harcourt Brace.

World Health Organization (WHO). 1988a. *AIDS Prevention and Control.* Oxford: Pergamon; Geneva: World Health Organization. Presentations and papers from the World Summit of Ministers of Health on Programmes for AIDS Prevention, jointly organized by the United Kingdom and the World Health Organization, 26–28 January, London.

World Health Organization (WHO). 1988b. *Guidelines for the Development of National AIDS Prevention and Control Programmes.* Geneva: World Health Organization.

World Health Organization (WHO). 1988c. *Guidelines on Sterilization and High-Level Disinfection Methods Effective against Human Immunodeficiency Virus (HIV).* Geneva: World Health Organization.

World Health Organization and Centers for Disease Control (WHO and CDC). 1988. "HIV Not Related to Monkeys." *WHO-CDC AIDS Weekly Report*, 25 July, 8.

World Wide Whore's News. 1985. June. Published by International Prostitutes' Rights Congress.

Worth, Dooley, and Ruth Rodriguez. 1987. "Latina Women and AIDS." *Radical America* 20, no. 6: 63–67.

Wright, Leslie Kirk. 1987. "A Disease of the Other: AIDS Discourse and Homophobia." Paper presented at the conference "Homosexuality, Which Homosexuality? International Scientific Conference on Gay and Lesbian Issues," December, Amsterdam.

Wright, Peter, and Andrew Treacher, eds. 1982. *The Problem of Medical Knowledge: Examining the Social Construction of Medicine.* Edinburgh: University of Edinburgh.

Wuthnow, Robert, James Davison Hunter, Albert Bergensen, and Edith Kurzweil. 1984. *Cultural Analysis: The Work of Peter L. Berger, Mary Douglas, Michel Foucault, and Jürgen Habermas.* London: Routledge and Kegan Paul.

Young, Frank E., et al. 1988. "The FDA's New Procedures for the Use of Investigational New Drugs in Treatment." *Journal of the American Medical Association* 259, no. 15: 2267–70.

Zicklin, Gilbert. 1996. "Media, Science, and Sexual Ideology: The Promotion of Sexual Stability." In *A Queer World: The Center for Lesbian and Gay Studies Reader*, ed. Martin Duberman. New York: New York University Press.

Zinsser, Hans. 1934. *Rats, Lice, and History: The Biography of a Bacillus.* Boston: Little, Brown.

Zones, Jane Sprague. 1986. "AIDS: What Women Need to Know." *National Women's Health Network News* 11, no. 6 (November–December): 1, 3.

Zonona, Victor F. 1988. "Bootstrap AIDS Research Giving Patients Active Role." *Los Angeles Times*, 25 December, I-1.

Zuckerman, Mortimer B. 1987. "AIDS: A Crisis Ignored." Editorial, *U.S. News and World Report*, January 12, 76.

Zuger, Abigail. 1995. *Strong Shadows: Scenes from an Inner City AIDS Clinic.* New York: W. H. Freeman.

Index

Photo captions are indicated by the letter c following the page number.

African Americans, 221; and AIDS, 74; educational materials for, 260c

African media: coverage of AIDS, 121, 209; criticism of "First World" coverage of AIDS in Africa, 209

African Studies Center (University of Illinois at Urbana-Champaign conference), 208

Africa Report, 108, 211; "Dispelling Myths about AIDS in Africa," 108

Aggleton, Peter, et. al. (social scientists), 251

AIDS (Acquired Immune Deficiency Syndrome). *See also* Cultural construction; HIV; individual states, countries, and continents.

"African AIDS," 116; AIDS as real disease, 11; "AIDS belt" (region of Central Africa), 124; "AIDS virus," 30; "celebrity AIDS," 75c, 85; "Central or West African AIDS," 116; "East or West German AIDS," 116; ELISA test for antibodies, 82; epidemiological model to study, 67; "European AIDS," 116; first defined clinically, 46–51, 324, 329, 346 n.9; "foreign or native AIDS," 116; as "gay man's disease," 42–48, 262; "guilty or innocent AIDS," 116; HIV seroprevalence, 54; "infectious-agent hypothesis," 52; "lifestyle hypothesis," 6, 19, 21, 46; "maternal AIDS," 61, 65; panic over "heterosexual AIDS," 57; "pediatric AIDS," 61; persons with AIDS as clinical test subjects, 287–88; politics and problematics of chronologies of, 58; "slim disease" (African term), 124; T-cell ratio testing, 53; "transfusion victims" of, 62; "viral hypothesis," 47

—*other names for:* "epidemic of immunosuppression," 46; "gay cancer," 46; "gay pneumonia," 46; "Gay-Related Immune Deficiency" (GRID), 27, 46–47, 60, 238; "Wrath of God Syndrome" (WOGS), 27, 46

—*transmission of:* anal intercourse, 56; heterosexual contact, 55–56; through "routine household contact," 47, 52, 73;
vaginal intercourse, 56; vertical transmission, 47, 60–61

"AIDS: A Global Crisis" (Wellcome foundation booklet), 150c, 217

AIDS: A Public Inquiry (PBS), 360 n.7

"AIDS: Communication Challenges" (conference), 359 n.2

"AIDS: Drug Dilemma" (TV segment), 130

"AIDS: Science, Ethics, Policy," 350 n.18

"AIDS: What It Does to a Family," 90

"AIDS and the Media" (session at 1990 International AIDS Conference), 213, 216

AIDS and the World, 226

AIDS-associated retrovirus (ARV), 30, 33c

"The AIDS Connection" (call-in TV program), 128

"AIDS Epidemic, Late to Arrive," 308

"AIDS Mary" (urban legend reported by Brunvard), 252

"AIDS Monitor," 356 n.14

"The AIDS Quarterly" (PBS), 129–30, 140–41, 360 n.4

AIDS Targeted Information Newsletter (ATIN), 301

AIDS Treatment News (ATN), 287, 290–92, 306, 379 n.1

Akeroyd, Anne (researcher), 275–76

Albert, Edward (communications scholar), 352 n.23

Alicia (video), 136

All African News Service, 209

Allen, Hilary (scholar), 344 n.4

All the President's Men, 182

Althusser, Louis (philosopher), 155

Altman, Dennis (political scientist, activist), 26, 352 n.27

Altman, Lawrence (print journalist), 64, 121, 124, 308, 336 n.21

Alwood, Edward (communications scholar), 91

America Responds to AIDS (ARTA; education and prevention campaign), 57

America Undercover (TV series), 97

American Anthropological Association (AAA), 218, 374 n.9

American Broadcasting Corporation. *See* ABC

Drug approval by the FDA, 279–90; accelerated approval, 306; clinical trials in approval process, 282–83; "fast-track," 288; history of process for approval, 280–82; time to market, 283. *See also* CRI; IND

Dubos, René (scientist), 109, 116; *Mirage of Health,* 109

Du Brow, Rick (TV critic), 370 n.14

Duesberg, Peter (virologist), 115, 163, 166, 306–7, 338 n.25, 347 n.9, 364 n.11, 384 n.11

Duggan, Lisa (historian), 86, 95, 215, 376 n.7

Durham, Stephen, and Susan Williams, 332 n.4

An Early Frost (NBC made-for-TV movie), 8, 134, 145, 176–204, 360 n.6, 365 n.1, 366 n.3, 367 n.6, 370 n.14, 371 n.18; Aidan Quinn in, 134, 184, 189, 193, 360 n.6, 372 n.24; D. W. Moffett in, 371 n.18; *characters in:* Michael Pierson (Chicago attorney), 176–79, 184–95, 199, 201; Peter (Michael's lover), 179c, 184–94, 201; Nick and Kay (Michael's parents), 176–77, 189, 193–97; Bea (Michael's grandmother), 176–77, 193; Susan (Michael's sister), 177, 199; Victor (AIDS patient), 186, 190; Redding (Michael's doctor), 188–92

Ebony: CJ story (urban legend), 252–53

Eckholm, Eric (print journalist), 205, 207, 254; "What Makes the Two Sexes So Vulnerable to the Epidemic," 207

Eckman, Anne (communications scholar), 342 n.1, 380 n.3

Eisenberg, David (physician, scientist), 383 n.10

ELISA test for antibodies, 82. *See also* AIDS

Ell, Stephen (medical historian), 349 n.14

Elliot, Beth (print journalist): "Does Lesbian Sex Transmit AIDS? Get Real!," 259–62

Emerging AIDS Markets, 120

Emerging Infectious Diseases (journal), 321

Empson, William (literary critic), 369 n.13

End of the Road (World War I anti-VD film), 44

England (U.K.), 116, 322; English society, 110

English language, 123, 153

Epidemic: awareness of AIDS beyond the gay community, 202; biological, measured by statistics, 110–13; as cultural crisis, 45; discursive representation of, 45; global, interpretations of, 110–15, 120–22, 226; semantic/signification, 171, 315; social parameters of, 99, 149, 223, 233; transformation of AIDS from acute to chronic epidemic, 325; types of AIDS epidemic (patterns I, II, and III), 111; written record of AIDS epidemic, 324

"Epidemic of signification," 1, 11, 19, 172, 315; epidemiology of signification, 39

"Epidemiology of AIDS in Women," 68

Epstein, Steven (sociologist), 71, 73, 279, 347 n.9, 380 n.1, 385 nn.13 and 15

"ER" (TV series), 144; Jeanie Boulet (character), 144

Essence, 253; story of Rae Lewis-Thornton, 253

Essex, Myron (Max) (scientist), 29–30, 160

Ethan Hoffman Archive, 80c

Ethiopia, 113

Ethnography, 103–5, 152–54, 218–22, 245; dialogue as metaphor for, 159; experimental, 218; as mediated production of knowledge, 119, 153; medical, 191, 275; as source of information, 104

Europe, 320; Eastern Europe, 141, 215; European medicine, 121; *MMWR* report on, 53; Western Europe, 111

Experimental subject, 284–85

Fabian's Story. See AIDS: A Public Inquiry

Fain, Nathan (print journalist), 335 n.15

Farber, Celia (print journalist), 384 n.11; "AIDS: Words from the Front" column, 384 n.11

Farber, Stephen (TV critic), 198

Far East, 112

Farmer, Paul (physician, anthropologist), 65, 151, 234, 254–55, 308

Fatal Attraction (film), 253

Fauci, Anthony (scientist, director of NIAID), 60–61, 290, 294–95

Fayetteville, Arkansas, 195–96

Federal Bureau of Investigation (FBI), 322

Federal guidelines for AIDS treatment, 306

Fee, Elizabeth (historian of medicine and public health), 59, 324, 357 n.18; *AIDS: The Burdens of History*, 324–25, 341; *AIDS: The Making of a Chronic Disease*, 325; and Daniel Fox, 324

Feldman, Douglas (anthropologist), 67

Feldman, Jamie (physician, anthropologist), 115, 338 n.26, 348 n.12, 359 n.25

Feminism, 236, 258–62, 266, 276–77, 341 n.1; AIDS epidemic as feminist issue, 271; failure of U.S. feminists to challenge AIDS biomedical discourses, 46, 86–98; feminist sex wars, 268–69; and identity politics, 215–216. *See also* Gender; Women

Fettner, Ann Giudici (print journalist), 20

"First World," 99–103, 106c, 109, 112, 116, 119–20, 125–26, 205–11, 219, 222, 272, 303, 353 n.1; representation of AIDS epidemic in Africa, 104–9, 205; as source of narratives about AIDS, 99, 102, 109, 120, 222; stereotypes about the "Third World," 206, 209–10. *See also* "The West"; Western medical science

Fit to Fight (World War I anti-VD film), 44

FitzGerald, Frances (print journalist), 39, 291, 334 n.11, 336 n.19

Flam, Robin (epidemiologist), 67–68

Fleck, Ludvik (historian of science), 157, 170, 343 n.2

Flora, June A., et. al. (communications scholars): "Communication Campaigns for HIV Prevention," 144

Food and Drug Administration. *See* U.S. Food and Drug Administration

Fortin, Alfred J. (political scientist), 122–24; "Politics of AIDS in Kenya," 123

Foucault, Michel (philosopher, historian of ideas), 39, 139, 157, 170, 279–80, 285, 341 n.34, 345 n.6

"4 Sisters Only" (booklet), 261c

"Fragile urethra," 17

France, 115, 214, 247, 293, 348 n.12; the French, 163; French AIDS, 115

Frank, Francine, and Paula Treichler (linguists), 347 n.9

Franklin, Patricia, et. al., 380 n.4

Freedom of Information Act (U.S.), 161, 287, 302

Freimuth, Vicki S. (communications scholar), 76

Friedland, Gerald R. (physician), 14c, 307; editorial in *New England Journal*, 305

"Frontline" (PBS program): *AIDS: A Public Inquiry*, 134; *Fabian's Story*, 134

Fumento, Michael (science writer, social critic), 248, 253, 273, 377 n.16; *Myth of Heterosexual AIDS*, 248

Fung, Richard (filmmaker), 215–16

Fury, Gran (art collective), 381 n.4

Gagnon, John (sociologist), 323

Gaiman, Neil (writer): *Sandman*, 261c

Gaines, Atwood (anthropologist), 363 n.6; and Robert Hahn, 159; *Physicians of Western Medicine*, 159, 363 n.6

Gallo, Robert (scientist), 28–30, 32c, 130, 133, 160–63, 165–67, 170, 333 n.7, 337 n.24, 338 n.26, 364 n.11, 365 n.14

Garland, Judy (cultural icon), 180

Garrett, Colin (former Peace Corps volunteer), 227–30, 375 n.11

Garrett, Laurie (science writer), 213, 308

"Gatekeeping": as control of scientific information, 158, 161

Gay: community, 291–93; disease, 247; men, 134, 192, 291; plague, 238. *See also* Activism; Homosexual; Queer

Gay and Lesbian Town Meeting (Boston), 293

Gay Community News (Boston), 86, 88

Gay Men's Health Crisis, 89, 251, 335 n.12, 341 n.35, 379 n.26

Haiti (*cont.*)

114; claims about voodoo in, 114; Haitians, 26, 51, 59, 102, 106; Haitians living in United States as risk group, 47–50 (*see also* Risk groups); heterosexual transmission of AIDS in, 64; Ministry of Tourism, 102; patients who are Haitian, 49, 109

Haitian Women's Program, 135

Hall, Jane (TV producer), 184, 192

Hall, Stuart (cultural critic), 3, 158

Hammer, Barbara (video artist): *Snow Job*, 131

Hammonds, Evelynn (historian of medicine), 86–88

Hankins, Catherine (physician), 255

Hannan, Tom (AIDS activist), 297

Haraway, Donna (historian of science), 31, 32c, 159, 170, 311, 324, 374 n.9; "Manifesto for Cyborgs," 266

Hardy, Ann (epidemiologist), 68–69, 71

Harlow, Harry (primate researcher), 159

Harmison, Lowell (PHS official), 294–95

Harrington, Mark (AIDS activist), 280, 285, 290, 309, 385 n.15; "Some Transitions in the History of AIDS Treatment Activism," 280

Harrison, Barbara Grizutti (writer): "It's Okay to Be Angry about AIDS," 91–92

Haseltine, William (virologist), 62

Health care model (tripod model), 304

"The Health Quarterly" (PBS, formerly "AIDS Quarterly"), 360 n.4

Heape, Walter (nineteenth-century zoologist), 342 n.2

Heckler, Margaret (former Secretary of HHS), 334 n.12

Hefner, Maria (partner of man with AIDS): David (man with AIDS), 78c; marriage at St. Patrick's Cathedral, 78c

Helms, Jesse (U.S. Senator), 83c; Helms amendment, 57, 83c, 96, 231

Hemophilia, people with, 38, 47, 50, 53; "persons with hemophilia A" risk group, 50, 59

Henig, Robin Marantz (science writer), 73

Hepatitis B virus vaccine (as possible source of HIV infection), 50, 291

Herdt, Gilbert (anthropologist), 218

Heroin addicts. *See* IV drug users

Herschberger, Ruth (science writer): *Adam's Rib*, 344 n.4

Heterosexuality, 143, 236, 241; AIDS in Africa as heterosexual, 16; as classification, 118; fantasies of homosexuality, 23; heterosexuals as IV drug users, 50; heterosexuals as risk group, 18; and identity, 247–48; perceived social threat of heterosexual transmission, 46, 57, 82; and promiscuity, 56; and prostitution, 54; transmission of AIDS through heterosexual contact, 45–55, 143, 243–44

Hilferty, Robert (video producer): *Stop the Church* (AIDS documentary, PBS's failure to air), 180. See also *Stop the Church*

Hill, Ronald Paul, and Andrea L. Beaver (communications scholars), 368 n.8, 370 n.15

Hilts, Philip J. (science writer), 108, 357 n.20; "Out of Africa," 108

Hippocrates, 42

Hirohito, 43

Hitler, Adolf, 43

HIV (human immunodeficiency virus), 30, 33c, 40, 61, 167–70. *See also* Cultural construction; International Committee on the Taxonomy of Viruses

Hoffman Laroche (pharmaceutical firm), 381 n.4

Holland, Dorothy, and Naomi Quinn (anthropologists), 363 n.6

Holleran, Andrew (writer): *Ground Zero*, 371–72 n.19

Hollibaugh, Amber (media activist, writer, producer), 89, 135; *The Second Epidemic* (video), 89, 135

Hollywood, 179c, 181–82, 360 n.6

Home Box Office (HBO), 368 n.9

Homosexuality, 5; as an activity, 38; in Africa, 217; AIDS as gay disease, gay plague, 6, 12, 15, 20, 22–23, 26; AIDS as "toxic cock syndrome," 21; anal intercourse, as associated with, 18, 22, 25;

and bisexuality, 45; as classification, 118; construction of, 256; gay baths, 16; "gay lifestyle" as related to AIDS, 6, 19, 21, 46; heterosexual, as opposite of, 6; homophobia, 6, 21, 36–37; homosexual men, 16, 18; lack of public health information directed toward, 83c (see also Helms amendment); media representations of, 134–38; as "mental disorder," 291; and mothers, 199; television and, 176–81, 184; transmission of HIV, 244; as "unnatural activity" leading to HIV infection, 239, 240–41

Hooper, Ed (photographer), 106, 107c, 108; *Slim: A Reporter's Own Story of AIDS in Africa*, 107c, 108, 354 n.7

Hopkins, Andrew (policy analyst), 364–65 n.12

Horton, Meurig (author, health researcher), 280, 310, 380 n.2; "Bugs, Drugs, and Placebos," 280, 310

Horvitz, Philip (interview with Foucault), 341 n.34

The Hot Zone, 321

House of Lords (U.K.), 97

"How to Have Sex in an Epidemic" (booklet), 24, 292

Hrdy, Daniel (anthropologist), 357 n.17, 373 n.4

Hudson, Rock (actor), 13, 14, 19, 46, 61, 72–77, 80, 139, 177, 189, 202, 334 n.11, 373 n.27; as canonical person with AIDS, 74

Huestis, Mark, and Wendy Dallas (video artists), 131; "Chuck Solomon: Coming of Age," 131, 360 n.7

Huff, Bob (video artist), 141c; "The Asshole Is a Tense Hole," 360–61 n.9; "Rockville Is Burning," 141, 142, 284, 290, 298, 311, 380 n.4

Hulce, Tom (actor), 360 n.6, 371 n.18

Human Immunodeficiency Virus. *See* HIV

Human Retrovirus Subcommittee of the International Committee on the Taxonomy of Viruses, 30, 167, 346–47 n.9. *See also* Varmus, Harold

"Human Sexuality and Issues of Sex Workers" (session at 1990 International AIDS Conference), 214–15

Human T-cell leukemia viruses (HTLV), 28–30, 337 n.24, 365 n.14

Human T-cell lymphotropic virus type III (HTLV-III), 28–31, 33c, 61, 167; HTLV-III/LAV (compound name), 30, 167. *See also* Cultural Construction; HIV

Hunter, Nan (legal scholar), 97, 263

Hussein, Saddam, 140

Identification, 8; with characters on television, 200–202

Identity, 8, 135, 235, 237–38; biological, 241–47; clinical, 249; feminist, 258–62; heterosexual, 247–48; media portrayal of gay identity, 134–36, 191–92, 195; multiple identities, 216; personal identity, 238; psychological identity, 238; statistical identity, 242–43; types of identity and identification, 236–38

Identity politics, 215–16, 266

Ideology, as used by Mannheim, 154, 172, 308

Immigration policy, U.S., 212

Immunodeficiency-associated virus (IDAV), 30

Immunology, 2, 140

IND (investigational new drug), 283; compassionate use IND, 283; treatment IND, 284, 288. *See also* Drug approval by the FDA

Influenza, 31

Ingstad, Benedicte (anthropologist): "Cultural Construction of AIDS," 151–52

Inside/Out Lesbian and Gay Studies Conference at Yale, 375

Institute of Medicine/National Academy of Science, 25, 333 n.10, 339 n.30

Intelligence, urgent need for, 2

Intercourse, sexual, 219; anal, 138, 240–41; "normal," 236

International AIDS Center (Harvard AIDS Institute), 226

International Committee on the Taxonomy of Viruses. *See* Human Retrovirus Subcommittee

Rubin, Gayle (anthropologist), 268–69, 276, 345 n.6, 350 n.16; and Judith Butler (political theorist), 268–69

"Rugged vagina," 6, 17, 37, 69, 82, 92, 227, 231, 239–41

Ruiz, Maria V. (communications scholar), 136

"Rules of Attraction" (conference), 215

Russo, Vito (film scholar), 181, 192, 295, 371 n.18; *The Celluloid Closet* (video), 181; *Consenting Adults*, 181

Rwanda, 29, 113, 122; Butare, 113; Rwandan Red Cross, 224c

Ryan, Jane, and Helen Thomas (radio producers), 133

Sabatier, René, 119, 354 n.8, 356 n.13

Sagan, Carl (scientist), 129

Said, Edward (cultural critic), 109

"Sally Jessie Rafael" (TV talk show), 379 n.27

San Diego, 293

Sanford Guide to HIV/AIDS Therapy, 300, 384 n.11

San Francisco, 12, 26, 38, 55, 63, 116, 211–12, 320, 345 n.6; AIDS Foundation, 70, 379 n.26; *A.I.D.S. Show*, 26, 39, 336 n.19; Castro district, 76, 291; Golden Gate Bridge, 296; International AIDS Conference, 211–15; KQED, 130; Moscone Center (location of International AIDS Conference), 211, 214; network affiliates, 140; Project AWARE, 69 (*see also* Project AWARE)

San Francisco Chronicle, 128

San Francisco Gay and Lesbian Film Festival, 215–16

Sango language (of Central African Republic), 151, 227–28

"Saturday Night Live" (TV series), 145–46, 360 n.6; Ellen Cleghorn (as former U.S. Surgeon General Jocelyn Elders), 146

Saussure, Ferdinand de (linguist), 174

Scarlet Alliance (Australian national sex worker organization), 274

The Scarlet Pimpernel, 290

Scarry, Elaine (literary and cultural critic), 361 n.12

Schable, Charles (CDC), 377 n.13

Scheper-Hughes, Nancy (anthropologist), 357 n.18; and Margaret Lock (anthropologist), 171

Schmidt, Nancy: "African Press Reports," 209

Schoepf, Brooke Grundfest (anthropologist), 117–18, 276, 358 n.21, 361 n.10

Schulman, Sarah (writer): *People in Trouble*, 176, 370 n.16

Science, 19, 22, 31, 51, 56, 150, 160–61, 167, 333 n.7

Science: idealized in the media, 129–30; as social construction, 155–58, 165, 309, 321. *See also* Western medical science

Science fiction, 13

Scientific American, 32c, 33, 34, 38, 84, 161, 249, 251

Scriptographic booklets, 24

The Second Epidemic (video), 89

"Second World," 99, 353 n.1

Segal, Lynne (cultural critic), 268

Selzer, Richard (physician, writer), 101–6, 109, 114, 353 n.5 n.9

Se met ko (video), 135–6, 137c

Seroconversion, 197

Setel, Philip (author), 161

Seventeen (magazine), 93

Sexuality: medical model of, 255–56, 260; as socially constructed, 118, 219. *See also* Heterosexuality; Homosexuality; Lesbians; Media: representations of hetero/homosexuality

Sexually transmitted diseases (STDs), 46, 88, 164, 220

Shalala, Donna (U.S. secretary of HHS under Clinton), 143

Shandera, Wayne (researcher), 48

Shanti Project, 251

Sharf, Barbara (communications scholar), 76

Shaw, Nancy (sociologist, now Nancy Stoller), 54, 70, 266, 335 n.12; and Lyn Paleo, 246, 275

Shea Stadium, 272, 296

Shepherd, Gill (anthropologist), 256, 363 n.7

Sherwood, Bill (filmmaker): *Parting Glances*, 181

Shilts, Randy (print journalist, writer), 48, 52, 60, 63, 68, 72–73, 145, 182, 186; *And the Band Played On*, 182, 292, 312–13, 346 n.9, 350 nn.15 and 16, 351 n.22, 368 n.9; lack of women in *And the Band Played On*, 63

Shostak, Marjorie (anthropologist): *Nisa*, 100, 104

Shoumatoff, Alex (print journalist), 207

SIDART (conference), 360 n.6

Silverman, Mervyn (scientist, public health official), 133, 338 n.27

Slim: A Reporter's Own Story of AIDS in Africa, 107c, 108

Snead, Eva Lee ("Dr."), 359 n.3

Sociology of knowledge, 154–57, 211

Sociology of science, 321

Sojourner, 92

Solomon, Nancy, 377 n.13

Sonnabend, Joseph (physician, scientist), 25, 46, 68, 163–66, 169, 302–5, 337 n.23, 339 n.29, 364 n.12

Sontag, Susan (cultural critic), 15, 332 n.4

South Africa: apartheid, 116; Johannesburg, 116

Southern Christian Leadership Conference, 87

Soviet Union, 12, 29, 112, 140, 215, 355 n.13

Spigel, Lynn (communications scholar), 202

Staley, Peter (AIDS activist), 214

Starr, Paul (sociologist), 45

Statistics: as potentially misleading, 112–15, 206, 209–10, 219; as source of information and knowledge, 110, 112–14, 206; women and AIDS, 242–43

St. Cyr, Marie (director, Women and AIDS Resource Network, NY), 71

Stein, Howard (ethnographer), 191

Stein, Zena (epidemiologist), 67–8, 378 n.25

Stephens, Clay (social scientist), 246, 271

Stereotypes: cultural, 327–28; of "Third World peoples," 206, 210, 236; of women with AIDS, 269

Stokes, Geoffrey (print journalist): "Press Clips" (column), 352 n.23

Stoller, Nancy (AIDS activist and writer, formerly Nancy Shaw), 266, 350 n.17

Stop the Church (documentary), 180, 368 n.7

St. Patrick's Cathedral, 78c

Stroll, Avrum (philosopher), 235–37

Sullivan, Louis (former secretary of HHS under Bush), 384 n.11

Sunday Times (London), 115

Susser, Mervyn (epidemiologist), 248

Sutton, Terry (AIDS activist), 291–92

Suzi's Story (Australian documentary), 97, 253

Swahili, 124

Switzer, Ellen (print journalist), 90

Sydney, Australia, 97

Syphilis, 44, 164, 281, 343 n.2, 345 n.6

Tagg, John (art historian, cultural critic): *The Burden of Representation*, 110

Tanzania, 29, 105, 113, 224c, 231, 358 n.24; CHAWAHATA (Tanzanian Media Women's Association), 231–32; Ministry of Health, 224c, 225c

Taussig, Michael (physician, anthropologist), 160, 307; "Reification and the Consciousness of the Patient," 160

Teare, Catherine, and Abigail English (authors), 270

Television: as educational about AIDS, 178, 189–90; failure to examine role in cultural construction, 131–34; made-for-television movies about AIDS, 145, 176–204; medical dramas, 182–83, 191; narratives about AIDS, 182–83, 204; network coverage influenced by the market, 139, 179–80; omission of social and political concerns, 181–82, 204; public service announcements, 136; reports of AIDS, 128–36; representation of AIDS and construction of reality,

Weekly Review (journal), 108, 122–24, 354 n.8

Weekly World News, 12, 78c; "AIDS Victim to Wed in St. Patrick's Cathedral," 78; "Wife Murders Hubby with AIDS Cocktail," 78

Weeks, Ned (as Larry Kramer's alter ego), 74

Weicker, Lowell (former U.S. senator), 83c

Weinhouse, Bibi (print journalist), 90

Weiss, Theodore (U.S. congressperson), 26

"Welcome to the World of AIDS" (urban legend reported by Fine), 252

Wellcome Foundation (philanthropic arm of Burroughs-Wellcome), 150c, 217–18, 223, 229. *See also* Burroughs-Wellcome

Wenner, Adrian (scientist), 362 n.4

Wenner-Gren Symposium (1990), 218, 374 n.9; "AIDS Research: Issues for Anthropological Theory, Method, Practice" in Estes Park, CO, 218–9

"The West," 121–23, 171, 209, 213

West Africa, 113, 364 n.9

Western liberal humanism, 190, 317–18

Western medical science, 103, 105; as cultural construct, 153, 155, 157–74, 309; as discoverer of "truth," 149–52; as ideology, 160; and power, 307; as privileged narrative, 151, 160–62, 191; racism and, 215, 221; subordination of social science to biomedicine, 150, 159, 161–63; as transcultural model, 119. *See also* Science

WHAM (activist health group), 273

White(s), 248. *See also* Risk groups

White, Allan (print journalist), 213

White, Luise (anthropologist), 222

White, Ryan, 14, 75c; as "celebrity PWA," 81

White, Steve (TV executive), 184

Whitmore, George (journalist with AIDS), 80–81

Williams, Bruce A., and Albert R. Mathery (communications and policy analysts): *Democracy, Dialogues, and Environmental Disputes*, 142

Williams, Raymond (cultural studies scholar), 110, 115, 120, 153–54; *The Country and the City*, 110, 355 n.10; *Keywords*, 355 n.10

Windom, Robert (HHS official), 294–95

Wofsy, Constance (physician), 61, 69

WOGS (Wrath of God Syndrome), 27

Wolf, Margery (anthropologist), 95

Wolfe, Maxine, and Iris Long (AIDS activists and authors), 250, 266

Women: and activism, 237, 263–65, 271; African women, 254–55; and AIDS, 42–98, 235–77; as category, 9; denial of AIDS in, 235, 249, 270; dichotomies about, 235, 272–74; exclusion from clinical trials of drugs, 67–68, 250–51, 285; factors related to HIV vulnerability, 240–41; as "inefficient" transmitters of HIV, 239; IV drug users, 63–64; lesbians, 245; maternal transmission of HIV, 52, 60–61, 65, 245, 274; media representation of, 252–53, 269; as "other" in AIDS discourse, 243, 273; and "pediatric AIDS," 61; in prison, 71; and race, 86–98; reproductive legislation, 263, 267; as reservoirs of HIV, 186, 239, 263; as "risk group," 57–98; sexism, 44; statistics about AIDS in women, 242–43; women's bodies as pathological, 42; women's health movement, 7; women's magazines, 7, 86–98; women's organizing efforts around AIDS, 67. *See also* Feminism; Gender

Women, AIDS, and Activism, 97, 264, 379 n.26

Women and AIDS Resource Network (WARN, in New York), 71

Women in Love. See Kramer, Larry.

Women's Action Coalition: *Stats*, 86

Women's Outreach Network of the National Hemophilia Foundation (WONN), 245

World Health Organization (WHO), 7, 53, 57, 64, 100, 111–13, 166, 208, 322, 333 n.10; categorization of "Pattern I, II, and III" countries, 62, 111, 239, 355–56 n.13; Declaration of Helsinki, 281;

Paula A. Treichler is Professor in the College of Medicine, the Institute of Communications Research, and
the Women's Studies Program at the University of Illinois, Urbana-Champaign. She is the author and editor
of a number of books, including *A Feminist Dictionary*
(with Cheris Kramarae), *The Visible Woman: Imaging
Technologies, Gender, and Science* (with Lisa Cartwright and Constance Penley), and *Cultural Studies*
(with Lawrence Grossberg and Cary Nelson).

Library of Congress Cataloging-in-Publication Data

Treichler, Paula A.
How to have theory in an epidemic : cultural
chronicles of AIDS / Paula A. Treichler.
Includes bibliographical references and index.
ISBN 0-8223-2286-2 (cloth : alk. paper). —
ISBN 0-8223-2318-4 (pbk. : alk. paper)
1. AIDS (Disease)—Social aspects.   2. Culture—
Philosophy.   3. AIDS (Disease) in mass media.
I. Title.
RA644.A25T78   1999
362.1'969792—dc21   98-50855 CIP